D1219470

# PRACTICAL ESSENTIALS OF INTENSITY MODULATED RADIATION THERAPY

## SECOND EDITION

# PRACTICAL ESSENTIALS OF INTENSITY MODULATED RADIATION THERAPY

## SECOND EDITION

*Editor*

## K. S. CLIFFORD CHAO, MD

*Associate Professor of Radiation Oncology*
*University of Texas*
*MD Anderson Cancer Center*
*Houston, Texas*

*Assistant Editors*

## SMITH APISARNTHANARAX, MD

*Postdoctoral Fellow*
*University of Texas*
*MD Anderson Cancer Center*
*Houston, Texas*

## GOKHAN OZYIGIT, MD

*Instructor of Radiation Oncology*
*Hacettepe University, Faculty of Medicine*
*Ankara, Turkey*

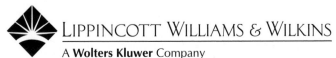

LIPPINCOTT WILLIAMS & WILKINS
A **Wolters Kluwer** Company
Philadelphia · Baltimore · New York · London
Buenos Aires · Hong Kong · Sydney · Tokyo

Property of Library
Cape Fear Community College
Wilmington, NC

*Acquisitions Editor:* Jonathan Pine
*Developmental Editor:* Joanne Bersin
*Marketing Manager:* Adam Glazer
*Production Editor:* David Murphy
*Compositor:* Maryland Composition, Inc.
*Printer:* Quebecor/Kingsport

© 2005 by LIPPINCOTT WILLIAMS & WILKINS
530 Walnut St.
Philadelphia, PA 19106 USA
www.LWW.com

First edition 2003, Lippincott Williams & Wilkins

All rights reserved. This book is protected by copyright. No part of this book may be reproduced in any form or by any means, including photocopying, or utilized by any information storage and retrieval system without written permission from the copyright owner, except for brief quotations embodied in critical articles and reviews. Materials appearing in this book prepared by individuals as part of their official duties as U.S. government employees are not covered by the above-mentioned copyright.

Printed in the USA

**Library of Congress Cataloging-in-Publication Data**

Practical essentials of intensity modulated radiation therapy / editor, K. S.
    Clifford Chao, assistant editors, Smith Apisarnthanarax, Gokhan Ozyigit.
    —2nd ed.
       p.; cm.
    Rev. ed. of: Intensity modulated radiation therapy for head and neck
cancer, ©2003.
    Includes bibliographical references and index.
    ISBN 0-7817-5279-5
    1. Cancer—Radiotherapy.   2. Radiation—Dosage.   I. Chao, K. S.
Clifford.   II. Apisarnthanarax, Smith.   III. Ozyigit, Gokhan.   IV. Intensity
modulated radiation therapy for head and neck cancer.
    [DNLM:   1. Head and Neck Neoplasms—radiotherapy.   WE 707
P8946 2005]
    RC271.R3P715   2005
    616.99′40642—dc22                                    2004018388

Care has been taken to confirm the accuracy of the information presented and to describe generally accepted practices. However, the authors, editors, and publisher are not responsible for errors or omissions or for any consequences from application of the information in this book and make no warranty, expressed or implied, with respect to the currency, completeness, or accuracy of the contents of the publication. Application of this information in a particular situation remains the professional responsibility of the practitioner.

The authors, editors, and publisher have exerted every effort to ensure that drug selection and dosage set forth in this text are in accordance with current recommendations and practice at the time of publication. However, in view of ongoing research, changes in government regulations, and the constant flow of information relating to drug therapy and drug reactions, the reader is urged to check the package insert for each drug for any change in indications and dosage and for added warnings and precautions. This is particularly important when the recommended agent is a new or infrequently employed drug.

Some drugs and medical devices presented in this publication have Food and Drug Administration (FDA) clearance or limited use in restricted research settings. It is the responsibility of the health care provider to ascertain the FDA status of each drug or device planned for use in their clinical practice.

10 9 8 7 6 5 4 3 2 1

*To our patients from whom we have learned to excel.*

*To our patients from whom we have learned to excel.*

*To Helen, David, and Nick whose support have made this book possible.*

# CONTENTS

# CONTRIBUTING AUTHORS

**Anesa Ahamad, M.D.** Assistant Professor of Radiation Oncology, University of Texas, MD Anderson Cancer Center, Department of Radiation Oncology, Houston, Texas

**Kie-Kian Ang, M.D.** Professor of Radiation Oncology, University of Texas, MD Anderson Cancer Center, Department of Radiation Oncology, Houston Texas

**Smith Apisarnthanarax, M.D.** Postdoctoral Fellow, University of Texas, MD Anderson Cancer Center, Department of Experimental Radiation Oncology, Houston, Texas

**Angel Blanco, M.D.** Assistant Professor of Radiation Oncology, University of Texas, MD Anderson Cancer Center, Department of Radiaton Oncology, Houston, Texas

**Thomas A. Buchholz, M.D.** Associate Professor of Radiation Oncology, University of Texas, MD Anderson Cancer Center, Department of Radiation Oncology, Houston, Texas

**Eric L. Chang, M.D.** Assistant Professor of Radiation Oncology, University of Texas, MD Anderson Cancer Center, Department of Radiation Oncology, Houston, Texas

**K. S. Clifford Chao, M.D.** Associate Professor of Radiation Oncology, University of Texas, MD Anderson Cancer Center, Department of Radiation Oncology, Houston, Texas

**James D. Cox, M.D.** Professor and Chairman of Radiation Oncology, University of Texas, MD Anderson Cancer Center, Department of Radiation Oncology, Houston, Texas

**Lei Dong, Ph.D.** Assistant Professor of Radiation Physics, University of Texas, MD Anderson Cancer Center, Department of Radiation Physics, Houston, Texas

**Steven J. Feigenberg, M.D.** Assistant Professor of Radiation Oncology, Fox Chase Cancer Center, Department of Radiation Oncology, Philadelphia, Pennsylvania

**Kenneth M. Forster, Ph.D.** Assistant Professor of Radiation Physics, University of Texas, MD Anderson Cancer Center, Department of Radiation Physics, Houston, Texas

**Adam S. Garden, M.D.** Professor of Radiation Oncology, University of Texas, MD Anderson Cancer Center, Department of Radiation Oncology, Houston, Texas

**Eric M. Horwitz, M.D.** Associate Professor of Radiation Oncology, Fox Chase Cancer Center, Department of Radiation Oncology, Philadelphia, Pennsylvania

**Anuja Jhingran, M.D.** Associate Professor of Radiation Oncology, University of Texas, MD Anderson Cancer Center, Department of Radiation Oncology, Houston, Texas

**Michael V. Knopp, M.D.** Division of Imaging Research, Department of Radiology, Ohio State University, University Hospitals, Columbus, Ohio

**Ritsuko Komaki, M.D.** Professor of Radiation Oncology, University of Texas, MD Anderson Cancer Center, Department of Radiation Oncology, Houston, Texas

**Nancy Y. Lee, M.D.** Associate Professor of Radiation Oncology, Memorial Sloan Kettering Cancer Center, Department of Radiation Oncology, New York, New York

**Zhongxing Liao, M.D.** Assistant Professor of Radiation Oncology, University of Texas, MD Anderson Cancer Center, Department of Radiation Oncology, Houston, Texas

**Homer A. Macapinlac, M.D.** Associate Professor of Nuclear Medicine, University of Texas, MD Anderson Cancer Center, Department of Nuclear Medicine, Houston, Texas

**Nina A. Mayr, M.D.** Professor and Director of Radiation Oncology, Vice Chair of Radiological Sciences, University of Oklahoma Health Sciences Center, Department of Radiological Sciences, Oklahoma City, Oklahoma

**Shawn W. McNeeley, M.S.** Medical Physicist, Fox Chase Cancer Center, Department of Radiation Oncology, Philadelphia, Pennsylvania

**Cynthia Ménard, M.D.** Radiation Oncology Branch, NCI, NIH, DHHS, Bldg 10, Rm B3B69, 9000 Rockville Pike, Bethesda, Maryland

**Radhe Mohan, Ph.D.**   Professor and Chair of Radiation Physics, University of Texas, MD Anderson Cancer Center, Department of Radiation Physics, Houston, Texas

**Allen R. Molloy, M.D.**   Resident in Diagnostic Radiology, University of Oklahoma Health Sciences Center, Department of Radiological Sciences, Oklahoma City, Oklahoma

**Gokhan Ozyigit, M.D.**   Instructor of Radiation Oncology, Hacettepe University, Faculty of Medicine, Department of Radiation Oncology, Ankara, Turkey

**Alan Pollack, M.D., Ph.D.**   Professor and Chair of Radiation Oncology, Fox Chase Cancer Center, Department of Radiation Oncology, Philadelphia, Pennsylvania

**Robert A. Price, Ph.D., D.A.B.R.**   Assistant Professor, Chief Clinical Physicist, Fox Chase Cancer Center, Department of Radiation Oncology, Philadelphia, Pennsylvania

**Ugur Selek, M.D., Ph.D.**   Fellow of Radiation Oncology, University of Texas, MD Anderson Cancer Center, Department of Radiation Oncology, Houston, Texas

**W. Roy Smythe, MD**   Department of Thoracic and Cardiovascular Surgery, The University of Texas, MD Anderson Cancer Center, Houston, Texas

**Craig Stevens, M.D., Ph.D.**   Associate Professor of Radiation Oncology, University of Texas, MD Anderson Cancer Center, Department of Radiation Oncology, Houston, Texas

**Wade L. Thorstad, MD**   Department of Radiation Oncology, Washington University School of Medicine, St. Louis, Missouri

**Franz Wippold II, M.D.**   Associate Professor of Radiology, Chief of Neuroradiology, Mallinckrodt Institute of Radiology, Washington University Medical Center, St. Louis, Missouri

**Ping Xia, Ph.D.**   Assistant Professor of Radiation Physics, University of California, San Francisco, Department of Radiation Oncology, San Francisco, California

**William T.C. Yuh, M.D., M.S.E.E.**   Professor and Bob Eaton Chair of Radiology, University of Oklahoma Health Sciences Center, Department of Radiological Sciences, Oklahoma City, OK 73190, Oklahoma City, Oklahoma,

# FOREWORD

## PRACTICAL ESSENTIALS OF INTENSITY MODULATED RADIATION THERAPY

A revolution has been taking place in radiation oncology over the last 15 years. Although it began many years before, the evolution of conformal radiation therapy (CRT) escalated dramatically between 1993 and 1996. Treatment planning for CRT migrated from very progressive individual institutions to commercial availability and widespread use in the radiation oncology community. Treatment planning systems have continued to evolve over the past decade and treatment delivery capability has largely caught up with the planning capability. It has also become possible to archive three-dimensional images including dose distributions. This permits research relating normal tissue volumes to toxicity and holds the promise of better defining normal tissue complication probabilities based on volumes irradiated.

Whereas three-dimensional CRT has become standard, intensity modulated radiation therapy (IMRT) is still evolving. The broad field of image guided radiation therapy of which IMRT is an important part, is constantly developing as a function of improved imaging of tumors and surrounding normal tissues. The ability to fuse images, especially anatomic and metabolic images, is only beginning to be appreciated with reference to specific clinical problems. Although there is broad availability of IMRT planning and delivery capability, there is still much uncertainty about proper use of IMRT. In addition, limited numbers of medical physicists limit implementation of IMRT.

The second edition of *Practical Essentials of Intensity Modulated Radiation Therapy* is very ambitious. It sets the stage for a contemporary exposé of IMRT physics, treatment planning, and quality assurance. It explores the imaging techniques available for image-guided radiation therapy in multiple anatomic locations. Great emphasis is placed on malignant tumors arising in the head and neck. The anatomic constraints and issues related to target delineation in these locations help define the problems and possibilities clearly when there is no motion related to the tumor location day to day. However, in the thorax, and even in the pelvis, tumor motion is a matter of concern. The anatomic location of the tumor must be established daily or the tumor must be immobilized with a great degree of certainty. These efforts are progressing at a very rapid rate, to assure optimal utilization of IMRT and even set the seen for proton beam therapy in the few institutions where such capability is or will be available.

As was the case for the first edition of this important textbook, the reader will find a clear articulation of current state of the art in advanced treatment planning, target determination, target delineation, and dose delivery with the heaviest emphasis on IMRT. It provides a strong foundation upon which the medical community is continuing to build. Practical issues and constraints related to target delineation are elaborated extensively in this text. What also becomes clear is the continued evolution in this exciting and demanding domain in radiation oncology. Although it is critical to have such capability articulated carefully and fully in the second edition of this important work, the need for additional editions is apparent from the rate of change, indicated by the progress that has been made between the first and second editions of this work.

James Cox, M.D.

# PREFACE

Intensity modulated radiation therapy (IMRT) offers an excellent opportunity to optimize the therapeutic ratio in radiation oncology through maximizing tumor coverage and sparing normal tissue by appropriate clinical input and precise computer algorithms. This cutting edge technology is being used not only in academic institutions, but also in community clinics. The increasing need for essential practical guidelines to address clinical indication, imaging interpretation, target delineation, and plan optimization has inspired the genesis of the 2nd edition of *Practical Essentials of Intensity Modulated Radiation Therapy*.

In this book, a practical overview of IMRT physics, quality assurance, and treatment planning and optimization are first given in Chapters 1 and 2. Because successful implementation of IMRT depends on proficient understanding in anatomical imaging (computed tomography and magnetic resonance imaging), pertinent information to update readers on this topic is provided in Chapters 3 and 4 for brain, head and neck, urological, and gynecological cancers. Further, integrating functional imaging to assist in more accurate target delineation or for dose escalation may soon be a clinical reality, we elicit the process and caution of incorporating functional images for IMRT planning in Chapter 5.

In the first edition, we provided practical guidance for IMRT in the management of head and neck cancer patients.

Because IMRT utilization has become more widespread, the 2nd edition expands the breadth of coverage to include concise, relevant overviews of the natural course, diagnostic criteria, therapeutic options, as well as up-to-date IMRT treatment guidelines for other various tumor sites. Chapters 6 through 14 provide updated information and results on head and neck cancers with a new Chapter 13 on thyroid carcinoma. New chapters encompassing breast, thoracic, esophageal, prostate, and gynecological cancers are included with high quality of illustration to assist reader in target determination and delineation (Chapters 15 to 18 and 20 to 21).

We emphasize the importance of understanding basic anatomy and the corresponding imaging sections that are being used for target and normal tissue determination and delineation. Accordingly, more than 350 full-color, detailed illustrations are provided to clarify each step in the clinical implementation of IMRT. We believe this new edition will assist residents, fellows, and clinicians of radiation oncology in learning the practical essentials for the clinical evaluation, decision-making, and technical proficiency of IMRT for multiple disease sites. The information presented in this book will continue to be refined, as rapid accumulation of clinical experience and evolution of imaging and targeting techniques have become so evident.

# ACKNOWLEDGMENTS

Special thanks to colleagues and friends at M.D. Anderson Cancer Center, Memorial Sloan-Kettering Cancer Center, and Washington University. Through countless critics and debates, we have refined the target determination and delineation for the benefit that best serves our patients.

# 1

# INTENSITY-MODULATED RADIATION THERAPY PHYSICS AND QUALITY ASSURANCE

## LEI DONG
## RADHE MOHAN

## 1. INTRODUCTION

- Intensity-modulated radiation therapy (IMRT) represents one of the major technical innovations in modern radiation therapy (RT). IMRT is an advanced three-dimensional (3D) conformal treatment that uses nonuniform beam intensity patterns with computer-aided optimization to achieve superior dose distribution.[1,2]
- Because of this new capability in manipulating the intensities of individual rays within each beam, IMRT allows greater control of dose distributions that, when combined with various image-guided techniques to precisely delineate target volumes and deliver the planned treatments, may improve tumor control and reduce normal tissue toxicity.

## 1.1. Features and Benefits of Intensity-Modulated Radiation Therapy

### 1.1.1. Dose Conformality

- The biggest advantage of IMRT is the ability to produce much higher conformality of dose distributions than those achievable with conventional 3D conformal radiation therapy (3DCRT) by using uniform beam intensities. In particular, IMRT can produce concave-shaped isodose distributions that may more closely follow the shapes or boundaries of the target and critical structures in three dimensions.
- In contrast, the isodose distributions designed for 3DCRT plans are convex, which may be suboptimal in treating certain disease sites. Examples of prostate cancer isodose distributions using a four-field 3DCRT plan (4F-CRT), a seven-field 3DCRT plan (7F-CRT), a dynamic IMRT plan using the NOMOS Peacock system (MIMiC, NOMOS Corp., Sewickley, PA), and a step-and-shoot ten-field IMRT plan (10F-segmental multileaf collimator [SMLC]) are shown in Figure 1-1. The prescribed dose was 75.6 Gy to the 95% volume of the

planning target volume (PTV). Figure 1-1 clearly demonstrates the more conformal dose distributions provided by the two IMRT plans.

### 1.1.2. Normal Organ Sparing

- The ability to shape dose distributions can be exploited to create sharp dose fall-off near the boundaries of the target and critical structures. This means that the volumes of the critical structures receiving a high dose could be greatly reduced. This may allow escalation of tumor dose, reduction of normal tissue doses, or both, potentially leading to improved outcome. This is analogous to inventing a more effective drug (using dose escalation) that causes fewer side effects (reducing radiation toxicities to normal organs).
- To illustrate the dosimetric advantage of IMRT over conventional 3DCRT techniques, the dosimetries of twenty consecutive prostate cancer cases were compared (Fig. 1-2). Similar to Figure 1-1, all twenty patients had 4F-CRT, 7F-CRT, MIMiC, and 10F-SMLC plans and were normalized to the prescription dose of 75.6 Gy at 95% PTV coverage.
- The statistics for the mean dose and minimum doses are shown in Figure 1-2, which indicates that limited dose escalation can be reached when keeping the same target coverage (minimum dose and the percent of volume at the prescription dose level).
- Figure 1-3 demonstrates the statistical significance of IMRT over 3DCRT techniques in sparing critical structures (rectum and bladder) at dose levels greater than 70 Gy. It was reported that patients with more than 25% of the rectum receiving 70 Gy or greater had a 5-year risk of grade 2 or higher complications of 37% compared with 13% for patients with 25% or less ($P = .05$).[3] Figure 1-3 shows that a significant portion of the 3DCRT plans (for both 4F-CRT or the 7F-CRT plans) failed to meet this 25% volume criterion for the rectum receiving greater

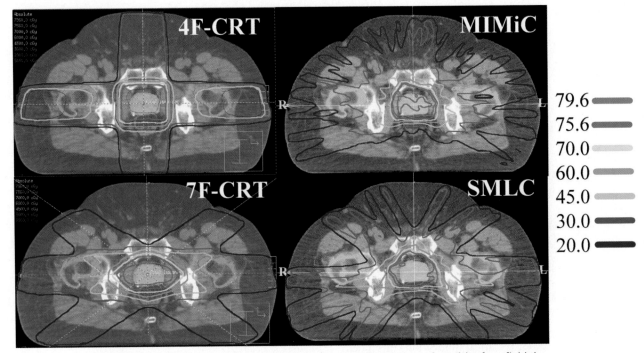

**FIGURE 1-1.** Typical isodose distributions for treating prostate cancer from (1) a four-field three-dimensional conformal radiation therapy (3DCRT) plan (4F-CRT), (2) a seven-field 3DCRT plan (7F-CRT), (3) an intensity-modulated radiation therapy (IMRT) plan delivered by serial tomotherapy using MIMiC (NOMOS Corp., Sewickley, PA), and (4) a ten-field step-and-shoot segmental multi-leaf collimator (SMLC) plan.

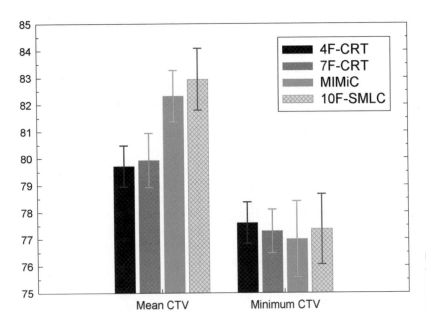

**FIGURE 1-2.** Comparison of mean and minimum doses to clinical target volume (CTV) in 3DCRT and IMRT techniques for prostate cancer. Twenty sequential patients with prostate cancer were selected for this planning study.

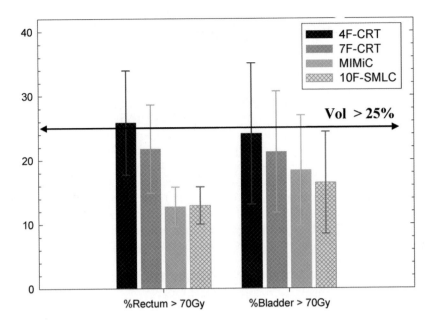

**FIGURE 1-3.** Comparison of dose to critical organs (rectum and bladder) among two 3DCRT plans and two IMRT plans. The risk for rectal bleeding is substantially higher when the volume of rectum receiving more than 70 Gy is more than 25%. A significant portion of 3DCRT plans (especially the 4F-CRT plans) failed to meet this planning constraint, but all IMRT plans satisfied the same constraint.

than 70 Gy, whereas all of the IMRT plans satisfied the same criterion, thus demonstrating the superior dosimetric advantage of IMRT.

### 1.1.3. Multiple Simultaneous Treatments

- Traditionally, multiple targets and boost fields of different dose prescriptions are treated sequentially and require separate dose plans, which may be inefficient for in-treatment management (e.g., matching junctions of multiple plans and coordinating the start of boost treatments).
- With IMRT, multiple targets (gross disease, subclinical extensions, and electively treated nodes) and boost fields can be integrated into a single treatment plan during the entire course of treatment.[4–9] This strategy not only is more efficient but also optimizes the overall doses by considering the interactions of different dose prescriptions.
- An integrated boost treatment may offer an additional radiobiologic advantage in terms of lower dose per fraction to normal tissues while delivering higher dose per fraction to the target volume. Higher dose per fraction also reduces the number of fractions and thus lowers the cost of a treatment course.

## 1.2. Medical Necessity of Intensity-Modulated Radiation Therapy

- The American College of Radiology (ACR) and the American Society for Therapeutic Radiology and Oncology (ASTRO) Joint Economic Committee recommend the determination of certain medical requirements when choosing IMRT for treatments.

- Examples of these requirements are the following: the target is irregularly shaped and in close proximity to critical structures; IMRT is the only option to cover the volume with narrow margins to protect adjacent structures; there is a nearby previously irradiated area; and a conformal dose distribution is required for concave treatment target(s).

## 1.3. Limitations and Risks of Intensity-Modulated Radiation Therapy

- When a major innovation is introduced, there are many new issues that may challenge existing technology or clinical knowledge. In this book, we describe many examples of using IMRT for certain clinical problems in radiation oncology.
- We recognize that there are many unresolved technical difficulties and lack of clinical knowledge that may limit our capability to extend the use of IMRT. Although some of the limitations may be overcome, the risks of misusing IMRT can still be significant. Some of the risks and limitations of IMRT are described next.

### 1.3.1. Defining Clinical Target Volume

- To take advantage of numeric optimization, IMRT requires a clear and quantitative definition of the target volume and critical organs. Uncertainties in defining tumor extension and clinically important target volumes can have a direct impact on treatment outcome.
- Because the final dose plan is highly conformal to the target(s), IMRT is less forgiving of uncertainties in defining clinical target volumes (CTVs) and critical structures. For this reason, great emphasis is placed in this book on

how to define CTVs on the basis of clinical experience and with the aid of advanced imaging techniques.

### 1.3.2. Uncertainties in Dose-Response Data

- In contrast with typical IMRT treatments, large and uniform treatment fields are commonly used in conventional external beam radiotherapy.
- Our previous clinical experience with dose tolerances is based largely on uniformly irradiated organs. IMRT dose distributions can have sharp dose gradients, a factor that challenges our clinical knowledge about the dose-volume relationship, especially for critical organs in which the dose gradients usually occur.
- The risk of a small volume receiving a high dose versus a large volume receiving a low dose is still unknown in many cases. In addition, the effect of fraction sizes used in integral boost IMRT for tissues embedded within the CTV is uncertain and may present an increased risk of injury or failure to achieve local control if used inadequately.[5]
- Adequate understanding of radiobiologic characteristics, dose, dose-volume, and functional characteristics of normal tissues is critical in prescribing IMRT treatments.

### 1.3.3. Defining Adequate Planning Target Volume

- Uncertainties of various types such as those related to daily (interfraction) positioning, displacement and distortions of internal anatomy, and intra-fraction motion may limit the applicability and efficacy of IMRT.[10–15]
- There may be an increased risk that the high degree of conformality associated with IMRT may lead to missing a portion of the target and to subsequent recurrences, especially for disease sites where positioning and motion uncertainties play large roles.
- A large margin could be added to the CTV (to form a larger PTV); however, a large PTV may create more overlaps with nearby critical structures, increasing the risk of radiation-induced morbidity.
- To take full advantage of sharp gradients and tight dose conformations, IMRT treatments should be accompanied by better immobilization and target localization techniques.[16]

### 1.3.4. Uncertainties in Plan Optimization, Dose Calculation, Plan Evaluation, and Treatment Delivery

- IMRT typically uses many small "pencil" beams to achieve beam intensity modulation and optimization. This presents a significant technical challenge in dose measurement, dose calculation, and treatment delivery.
- Current IMRT planning and delivery systems can be classified as first-generation systems, which, in general,

lack the ability to account for the limitations of the delivery system in the plan optimization process.[17]
- Certain dose distributions designed by the IMRT planning system may not be physically achievable or may not be delivered with good fidelity. In addition, limitations of the mathematic formalism of clinical problems may prevent the best solutions. Imperfect mathematic formalism can also create unexpected dose distributions, such as the "dose dumping" effect in unspecified tissues.
- IMRT dose distributions can also be difficult to interpret, which may increase the risk of unforeseen complications. Although some of these difficulties may be resolved in the future, there is conceivable risk in using current IMRT systems in the short-term.

## 2. INTENSITY-MODULATED RADIATION THERAPY TERMINOLOGY

- Because IMRT is an emerging technology, it is essential to know the definitions of some of the important nomenclature used in IMRT planning and delivery.[1]
- *Beamlet (bixels or rays):* The beamlet is a small photon intensity element used to subdivide an intensity-modulated beam for the purposes of intensity distribution optimization or dose calculation. Sometimes, the beamlets are also called "bixels," "rays," or "pencil beams." The intensity of the beamlet can either be in the unit of particle fluence or the energy fluence, depending on the particular dose calculation algorithm.
- *Dynamic multileaf collimator (DMLC):* The DMLC is an IMRT delivery mode in which the leaves continuously move and shape the beam intensity while the radiation is turned on. This mode has the advantage of higher spatial resolution and quick treatment delivery; however, it requires more accurate synchronization of leaf positions with beam-on time. Typical examples of this mode are the sliding window technique using conventional multileaf collimators (MLCs) or the NOMOS MIMiC system using binary collimators in arc treatment mode.[18–20]
- *SMLC:* The SMLC is an IMRT delivery mode in which the leaves only move when the radiation beam is turned off and remain in their predefined positions while the required radiation doses are being delivered. This is usually called the "step-and-shoot" delivery technique.[1,21]
- *Segment:* This is the shaped aperture (usually formed by MLCs) with uniform beam intensity. A segment is the basic unit in an SMLC treatment delivery. Sometimes a segment is also called a "control point."
- *Objective function:* This function is a mathematic formalism of clinical requirements. These clinical requirements can be (1) dose based, such as the minimum or maximum doses for a target or critical structure; (2) dose-volume based, which specifies a fractional volume that can receive certain doses; and (3) dose-response based,

which usually uses limited clinical data to translate the dose requirements into certain clinical outcomes. These clinical indicators (outcomes) may include, but are not limited to, tumor control probability, normal tissue complication probability, and equivalent uniform doses.

- *Score (cost):* The score is a numeric value of the objective function that represents a figure of merit indicating the quality of a treatment plan. The numeric score is a key parameter for IMRT optimization.
- *Inverse planning:* This is the term used to describe an optimization process that translates the mathematic formalism of clinical requirements into deliverable intensity patterns. Although the word "optimization" is used, it does not always guarantee that a global optimal solution is found for the clinical problem. The numeric solution can be trapped into a local minimum during the optimization process. The solution is also subject to the mathematic description of the clinical problem. A flawed objective function can lead to erroneous or clinically inferior solutions.
- *Forward planning:* Forward planning is a trial-and-error process in which the treatment fields or beam weights are modified iteratively (usually manually) to achieve acceptable clinical solutions. The process is commonly used in designing 3DCRT plans, although the same process can be used to create simple "field-in-field" intensity-modulated treatments. Sometimes a simple beam-weight optimization may be used in the forward planning process, but a forward planning process, in general, does not take full advantage of mathematic optimization using beamlets. Because of the limitations in current IMRT planning systems, the forward planning process can be effective in solving certain clinical problems. For example, the "field-in-field" planning technique has been used successfully in designing breast cancer radiation treatments in which the goal was to improve the dose uniformity in a parallel-opposed beam arrangement.[22,23] There is also reported success in head and neck and prostate treatments, but, in general, the solutions are inferior compared with the inverse planning approach.[24,25]
- *Leaf sequencing and deliverable optimization:* The leaf sequence is a set of leaf positions and the corresponding monitor units (MUs) (beam-on time) to be delivered by the treatment machine. In some of the IMRT planning systems, the optimization process is separated into two consecutive steps. The first step is to generate the ideal fluence patterns that satisfy the optimum solution for the objective function. Then the ideal fluence patterns are converted into deliverable leaf sequences in the second step. If the optimization process does not take into account some of the limitations of the deliverable system (e.g., leakage and head scatters), there will be a degradation in the final deliverable treatment plan. Sometimes the optimization process can create leaf sequences that are not physically deliverable. A deliverable optimization

process takes into account the constraints and characteristics of the leaves and reoptimizes leaf sequences on the basis of deliverable fluence distributions and the original objective function.[26,27] The deliverable optimization will improve the quality or the deliverability of an IMRT plan.

- *Aperture-based IMRT:* To improve deliverability and reduce beam-on time, a subset of IMRT solutions is sought by dividing the treatment portal into predefined segments or apertures. The rule of aperture segmentation varies depending on different implementations.[28–30] When the beam apertures are defined, the optimization process becomes a standard beam-weight optimization, which can be solved quickly. Because aperture-based IMRT does not take full advantage of beamlet optimization, the solution is usually inferior to a pencil-beam–based inverse planning algorithm.
- *Class solution:* This involves the use of historical experience based on solving similar cases with the same treatment technique or the same approach. Typical IMRT class solutions include a set of fixed gantry angles or a set of partial volume dose prescriptions for a particular treatment site. A clinical protocol, such as the Radiation Therapy Oncology Group (RTOG) phase I and II study of conformal and IMRT treatments for oropharyngeal cancer (RTOG H-0022, http://www.rtog.org), contains many important clinical guidelines, but it may not include sufficient treatment directives for actual IMRT planning. An example of class solution for ethmoid sinus cancer was described by Claus et al.[31]
- *Multimodality image fusion:* As target delineation becomes an important step in IMRT planning, the use of two or more imaging techniques to provide additional spatial or functional information about the treatment target(s) has become common. Image fusion refers to a process that combines two or more signals from different images of the same subject into one single dataset. In most situations, the additional information from the fused image is transcribed to the computed tomography image dataset as contoured structures, which will be used for IMRT planning.
- *Image registration:* This is a process to find the geometric transformation that brings one image in precise spatial correspondence with another image. Image registration is frequently used in both single modality and multimodality image fusion.
- *Digital imaging and communications in medicine (DICOM):* This is a standard protocol for medical image transmission and management (http://medical. nema.org/). Most diagnostic images are transferred from one system to another by using the latest DICOM 3.0 protocol, maintained by the combined effort of the ACR and the National Electrical Manufacturers Association.
- *DICOM RT:* This is the RT extension of the DICOM protocol. The current RT objects include, but are not

limited to, the RT structure set (contours are delineated from the images for each named structure), RT image (e.g., digitally reconstructed radiographs and portal images), RT plan (e.g., treatment parameters, including gantry angles, collimator settings, MUs, and MLC leaf positions), and RT dose (calculated dose matrix).

# 3. INTENSITY-MODULATED RADIATION THERAPY PROCESS

- A general IMRT process is shown in Figure 1-4. The details of the implementation may be vendor- or delivery system-dependent, but the general flow is similar. The IMRT process can also be grouped into four sequential phases: target delineation, treatment planning and optimization, quality assurance (QA), and treatment delivery. Each will be explained in more detail next.

## 3.1. Delineation of Target Volume and Critical Structures

- Similar to conventional 3DCRT, the treatment planning process begins with the delineation of the gross target volume, the CTV, and the critical normal structures considered to be at risk.[32]

- One important difference between conventional 3DCRT and IMRT is the quantitative definition of the target volume and critical organs. To take advantage of computer optimization, both the target(s) and the critical organ(s) should be identified and quantified (outlined) accurately by using one or more imaging techniques.
- IMRT is also called "image-guided" radiotherapy because the use of volumetric image information is almost compulsory. The success of IMRT depends on how accurately the target volume or critical organs are determined.
- Multimodality imaging can enhance our knowledge about the extent that diseases should be treated and will therefore play an important role in the IMRT process. Many of the subsequent chapters will focus on the site-specific target delineation and dose prescription.

## 3.2. Treatment Planning and Optimization

- The core of IMRT is in the treatment planning and optimization processes, which are enclosed by the dashed box in Figure 1-4. These processes translate clinical requirements for a specific clinical problem into machine-deliverable commands. They can be further divided into several components to be described next.

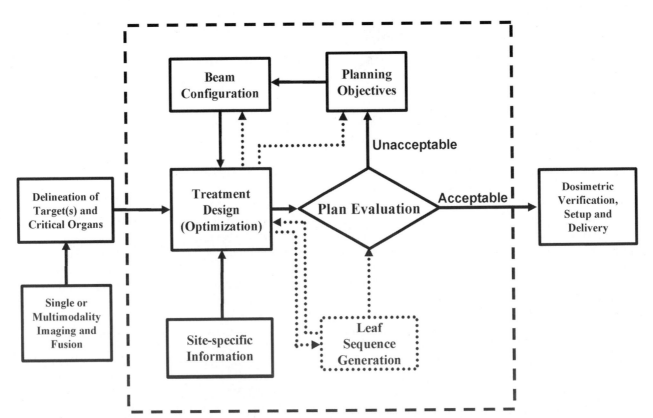

**FIGURE 1-4.** IMRT planning and delivery process. Core of the IMRT optimization process (*large dashed box*). Optimization loops that may be optional or still in development (*dotted arrows and boxes*).

### 3.2.1. Site-Specific Information and Class Solutions

- *PTV determination:* After the radiation oncologists determine the treatment targets (CTVs), a supplemental margin should be added to allow for uncertainties related to the movement of the tumor volume from treatment to treatment and for potential intra-fraction organ motion. This will establish the PTVs.[32] The size of the margin depends on the particular treatment site and the specific treatment technique used, especially the immobilization and localization techniques. Each institution should evaluate what the proper margin for IMRT treatments should be.[10,13,16] It is conceivable that IMRT planning would be much easier when a smaller margin is used. However, it is essential to make sure that the margins assigned are such that tumor coverage is ensured during the actual treatment delivery. Determination of site-specific margins is one of the important tasks that should not be overlooked.

- Similarly, the International Commission on Radiation Units and Measurements Report 62 proposed a concept of planning organ-at-risk volume, which is a margin around the organ at risk to account for uncertainties in determining the position of the organ during actual treatments. The effect of using planning organ-at-risk volume for IMRT planning was studied by Manning et al.[33]

- The site-specific information also includes the previous clinical experience in treating similar cases. It usually includes the range of dose prescription for each target, tolerance doses for critical structures, fractionation scheme, and strategies for treating subclinical disease. A subset of such information is usually used as the basis for plan evaluation. The site-specific information is different from the class solution, which contains more specific planning instructions and site-specific clinical guidelines.

- The fractionation scheme is somewhat unique to IMRT treatments. As indicated earlier, IMRT is capable of performing multiple simultaneous treatments. Such a treatment strategy has been called the simultaneous integrated boost (SIB).[5] The SIB-IMRT strategy not only can produce superior dose distributions but also is an easier, more efficient, and perhaps a less error prone method of planning and delivering IMRT because it involves the use of the same plan for the entire course of treatment. It also avoids the problem of field matching and junctioning encountered in many multifield boost treatment strategies.

- One of the issues involved in the use of the SIB technique is that each of the target regions receives different doses per fraction, which may create disproportionate corresponding biologic effects. However, the fraction sizes may be estimated by using an iso-effect relationship based on the linear-quadratic model and the values of its parameters (e.g., alpha-beta ratios and tumor doubling time).[5] Continued investigations and clinical trials are required to develop more reliable time-dose fractionation models to produce better estimates of their parameters and to evaluate alternate SIB-IMRT fractionation strategies for all sites.

- For example, in the head and neck RTOG H-0022 protocol (http://www.rtog.org), thirty daily fractions are used to simultaneously deliver 66 Gy (2.2 Gy/fraction) to the PTV, 60 Gy (2 Gy/fraction) to high-risk subclinical disease ("first echelon nodes or dissected neck area containing lymph node metastases"), and 54 Gy (1.8 Gy per fraction) to subclinical disease. These are biologically equivalent to 70, 50, and 50 Gy, respectively, if given in 2 Gy per fraction. The maximum dose to the brainstem, spinal cord, and mandible is to be maintained below 54, 45, and 70 Gy, respectively. The mean dose to the parotids is to be maintained below 26 Gy, or 50% of one of the parotids is to be maintained below 30 Gy, or at least 20 cc of the combined volume of both parotids is constrained to receive no more than 20 Gy.

### 3.2.2. Beam Configuration

- Beam configuration (selection of gantry angle or couch angle combinations) is usually required before performing the "in-field" beam intensity optimization in linac-based fixed-beam delivery systems. Beam angle selection may have a considerable impact on the quality of the final optimized IMRT plans.

- However, beam angle optimization is not a trivial problem to solve. For example, selecting 7 of 36 uniformly spaced coplanar beams would require the intercomparison of 8,347,680 IMRT plans.

- Currently, beam configuration optimization is usually not a part of the IMRT optimization (as indicated by the dotted line in the IMRT flow diagram, Fig. 1-4); however, there were some attempts to incorporate this optimization with the general IMRT optimization process.[28,34,35]

- The general observations regarding beam orientation selection for IMRT can be summarized as follows:

  □ Because IMRT has the ability to modulate beam intensities and usually uses multiple beams, the effectiveness of parallel-opposed beam arrangement seems to be lessened; therefore, directly parallel-opposed beams should be avoided.

  □ Beam angle optimization might not be very important when a large number of beams (e.g., eight or more) are used. Figure 1-5 shows the comparison of prostate IMRT plans for a number of optimally placed beams from a pool of eighteen equally spaced angles. A lower score indicates a better treatment plan. It can be seen that the percentage of better plans increases when more beam angles are used (the peak moves toward a low score end).

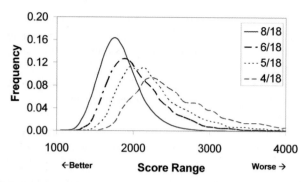

**FIGURE 1-5.** Effect of beam angle optimization for IMRT planning of prostate cancer treatment. The normalized score distribution is plotted for using four, five, six, and eight beam angles from a pool of eighteen equispaced coplanar beams. A lower score indicates a better treatment plan. When more beams are used, the solution is usually better. However, fewer beam angles can attain good solutions if the angles are optimally placed.

◻ Figure 1-5 also demonstrates that the plans with fewer but optimally placed beams could be as good as or better than plans using a larger number of suboptimally or uniformly placed beams. This demonstrates the importance of beam orientation optimization, which could lead to more efficient IMRT treatments.

### 3.2.3. Planning Objectives

- As discussed earlier, a cost function has to be defined to perform optimization in IMRT. The planning objectives are the mathematic translation of clinical objectives. As a figure of merit, a planning objective tries to quantify the underlining clinical goal.
- For example, the response of the tumor and normal tissues is a function not only of radiation doses but also of the volumes subjected to each level of dose (to varying degrees depending on the tissue type). In this case, a dose-volume–based objective function can be used.[36,37] Dose-volume–based objective functions are expressed in terms of the limits on the volumes of each structure that may be allowed to receive a certain dose or higher.
- Figure 1-6 shows a simple schematic example of one organ at risk. The dose-volume constraint is specified as $V$ $(>D_1) < V_1$ (point A in Fig. 1-6). In other words, the volume receiving doses greater than $D_1$ should be less than $V_1$. To implement such a constraint into the objective function, we seek another dose value $D_2$ so that the current dose-volume histogram (DVH) $V(D_2)$ equals $V_1$. The objective function component for this organ at risk may then be written mathematically as:

$$p_n \cdot \sum_j H(D_2 - D_j) \cdot H(D_j - D_1) \cdot (D_j - D_1)^2$$

in which "H" is a step function and $p_n$ is an organ-specific weighting factor. This objective function implies that only the points with dose values between $D_1$ and $D_2$

contribute to the score. Therefore, they are the only ones penalized.

- Because of imperfect mathematic formalism, planning objectives can also be considered as planning tools to achieve the real clinical goals. Frequently, the planning objectives have to be modified to drive the plan to a better clinical solution.
- The IMRT planners have to intervene and interactively set new planning objectives to get a better dose distribution for the particular case. This is usually the most time-consuming part of the IMRT planning process.
- Currently, the planning objectives themselves are not considered a part of IMRT optimization, but it is possible that the planning objectives can be a part of the IMRT optimization loop in the future, as indicated by the dotted line in Figure 1-4. If this is true, the time spent in fine-tuning planning objectives could be greatly reduced.
- Examples of deficiencies in the formalism of objective functions are shown in Figure 1-7, in which a constraint has been specified so that no more than 25% of the volume receives 50 Gy. All three DVHs shown meet this criteria. However, the DVH represented by the solid curve clearly causes the least damage.

### 3.2.4. Plan Evaluation

- Plan evaluation plays a central role in both defining the original objectives and evaluating the final optimization results. There are numerous dose, dose-volume, or dose-response models to quantitatively evaluate the merits of different IMRT plans.

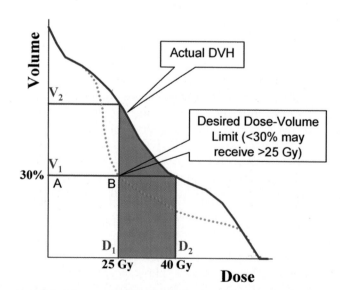

**FIGURE 1-6.** A method of incorporating dose-volume constraints in IMRT optimization. Adapted from: Wu Q, Mohan R. Algorithms and functionality of an intensity modulated radiotherapy optimization system. *Med Phys* 2000;27:701–711, with permission.

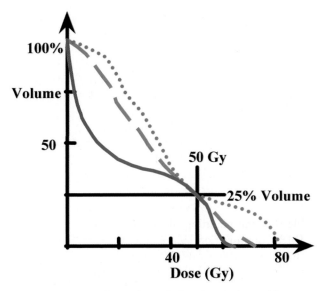

**FIGURE 1-7.** One limitation of the dose-volume histogram (DVH) prescription: one DVH control point (at 50 Gy and 25% of the volume) can have multiple DVH lines of inequitable clinical implications.

- Practically, however, slice-by-slice review of individual isodose distributions is almost always used. In fact, it is important to review every slice in the CT-based IMRT plan because a single anomalous target voxel may be accidentally drawn too near or distal to the anatomy of interest, causing potential radiation injury.
- Prescription isodose lines should be reviewed with special attention to the target coverage and PTV margin. Margin propinquity may cause underdosing of the target during actual treatment delivery.
- Special attention should also be paid to the hot and cold spots; both can cause damage in target or normal tissues. It is useful to add extra isodose lines when reviewing an IMRT plan. These may reveal some unexpected dose distributions.
- Sometimes it is necessary to review the absolute volume instead of the normalized volume, as commonly used in DVH comparisons.

### 3.2.5. Leaf Sequencing Generation

- We used the term "leaf sequencing" to describe the general process to convert an IMRT optimized dose distribution into machine-deliverable parameters. In the case of delivery treatments using a linac-based MLC, this means the creation of the leaf position sequences as a function of MUs.
- *Why is a separate leaf sequence generator required?* Unfortunately, modeling the dosimetry of MLC can be a complex and computational-intensive task.[26,38,39] To reduce computation time, most IMRT optimization algorithms use variable degrees of dose approximations. The result of

this dose approximation can result in inaccurate or unrealistic, undeliverable leaf sequences. This also means that the final deliverable plan may no longer be an optimal plan. Many investigators have been attempting to improve the accuracy and efficiency of the leaf sequencer,[17,26,40–49] whereas others are trying to incorporate leaf sequencing into the IMRT optimization loop or develop direct aperture-based or leaf position-based optimization methods that do not require a separate leaf sequencer.[17,27,29,30]

- It is recommended that the dose distribution using the final deliverable leaf sequences should be calculated and reviewed. This will ensure, to the limit of the dose calculation algorithm, that the final IMRT plan represents the actual treatment.

### 3.2.6. Connectivity Issues

- Parallel to the IMRT process are flows of information and data from and to the IMRT treatment planning system (Fig. 1-4).
- Examples of input data are the anatomic images, structural contours (if they are delineated outside the treatment planning system), and landmarks for treatment setup.
- Examples of output data include treatment parameters (gantry, collimator and couch angles, MLC leaf positions and MUs for each beam, isocenter positions, and reference digitally reconstructed radiographs for patient setup verifications).
- The connectivity (the ability to perform data transfer) among equipment of multiple vendors becomes an important issue when starting and maintaining the IMRT process.
- Physicists should review the capabilities of equipment for the whole IMRT process, including the hospital information system, scheduling, imaging studies, contouring, planning, QA, record and verification system, and patient treatments.
- Excessive manual entry or data transfer will reduce staff productivity and increase the risk for error. In most situations, the data transfer protocol will transfer only a subset of data. Nevertheless, it is important to keep a centralized database, which can simplify the pathway for further data-transfer requirements.
- There are several treatment planning-related data-transfer protocols, including the RTPconnect, initially developed by IMPAC (IMPAC Medical Systems, Mountain View, CA), and the DICOM-RT protocol, which will become an industrial standard in the near future. When selecting equipment in a multivendor environment, one should consider the matching of different data transfer protocols to ensure connectivity. Several vendors, including IMPAC and Varian (Varian Oncology Systems, Palo Alto, CA), provide system integration solutions,

which can be an efficient way to establish the necessary infrastructure for future growth.

## 4. QUALITY ASSURANCE FOR INTENSITY-MODULATED RADIATION THERAPY

### 4.1. The Importance of Intensity-Modulated Radiation Therapy Quality Assurance

- Because of the use of mathematic optimization and beam intensity modulation, IMRT treatment planning and delivery are more complex than the conventional 3DCRT technique. IMRT plans are difficult to interpret and less intuitive.
- When a linac-based MLC is used for IMRT delivery, the leaf movement is much more complex and requires precise synchronization to the cumulative delivered dose index. Many small and irregular fields present a challenge in data collection, beam modeling, and dose verification.
- QA in each of these steps in a complete IMRT treatment process is required, especially for these first-generation IMRT systems.
- Dose accuracy is important for RT. It has been reported that a 7% to 10% difference in dose delivery could produce significant change in tumor control probability (International Commission on Radiation Units and Measurements 1976). It is conceivable that the potential for dose error can be greater for IMRT treatments because a much steeper dose gradient is usually used and is near the boundaries of tumor and critical structures.
- The general QA requirements for conventional 3DCRT has been discussed by Fraass et al.[50] However, IMRT uses more computer-aided processes and has a greater mechanical demand for the delivery system; therefore, additional QA procedures are required to ensure that "what you plan is what you get."

### 4.2. Intensity-Modulated Radiation Therapy Dosimetry and Measurement Equipment

- IMRT treatments can be made entirely of small fields, such as in the serial tomotherapy treatments using MIMiC or a combination of small and large subfields in SMLC or DMLC.
- In all situations, the composition of small fields is essential in IMRT treatment, which may present a challenge because many of the conventional radiation detectors may be too large to be covered entirely by these small fields.
- The effect of detector size and lack of lateral electronic equilibrium in the small fields and steep dose gradient regions may present a challenge for the dosimetry of IMRT. In addition, IMRT treatments are usually deliv-

ered from many beam orientations, which require the accurate accumulation of weak signals from scattered radiation and leakage.
- Ionization chambers are most often used in RT for point dose measurement because of their excellent stability, linear response to radiation, low directional dependence, and low energy response. For IMRT field measurements, spatial resolution can be important.[51–57]
- A partial list of common small volume ion chambers and diodes is shown in Table 1-1. The dimensions, radiation responses, and leakage characteristics are based on the manufacturer's specifications.
- For very small microchambers, the central electrode is usually made of high-Z materials because of constructional considerations. For example, the central collecting electrode is made of steel in both the PinPoint™ PTW Freiburg, Germany and the Wellhöfer/Scanditronix, Scanditronix Wellhöfer AB, Sweden CC01 chambers. This will cause overresponse to low-energy scattered photons, which are abundant in large treatment fields or under heavily blocked areas.
- The p-type semiconductor detectors have some useful characteristics for small-field measurements. Diode detectors usually have very small active volume and high sensitivity to radiation. Comparison of the diode detectors in Table 1-1 reveals that the sensitivity of these diodes is 20 to 100 times higher than ion chambers. The high signal-to-noise ratio can be very useful in measuring weak signals from leakage or scattered radiation. However, the relative high atomic number of silicon in the diode detector can lead to a higher sensitivity to low-energy photons. Therefore, a diode detector is generally applied in small-field measurements in which the relative composition of low-energy photons is usually low.[58]
- Another disadvantage of a single diode detector is the relatively large directional dependence in detector sensitivity. In general, the magnitude of this directional dependence is less than or equal to 3%. However, under extreme conditions when comparing a vertex beam angle and a coplanar beam angle, the difference in sensitivity can be as high as 15% (technical data sheet, Scanditronix). In addition to directional dependence, some reports also indicate long-term irreversible radiation damage that changes the sensitivity of diodes over time. Therefore, it is recommended to use diodes for relative dose measurements only.
- The diamond detector also shows a high sensitivity to radiation, which is an alternative to small ionization chambers or silicon diodes. Bucciolini et al.[53] demonstrated that the diamond detector can produce clinically identical results to a p-type silicon diode for small treatment fields ($2.6 \times 2.6$–$10 \times 10$ cm). However, there are some drawbacks in the use of a diamond detector: (1) Its signal shows a dose rate dependence that must be accounted for, (2) it has a relatively slow response in time to obtain signal stability, and (3) it is relatively more expensive

**TABLE 1-1. COMMERCIALLY AVAILABLE SMALL-VOLUME IONIZATION CHAMBERS AND DIODES**

| Vendors | Description | Model | Appr. Vol. (cc) | Eff. Length (mm) | Eff. Dia. (mm) | Response (nC/Gy) | Leakage $10^{(-15)}$A | Central Electrode | Wall Material |
|---|---|---|---|---|---|---|---|---|---|
| Capintec | Cylinderical | PR-05PW | 0.07 | 5 | 4 | 2.1 | 10 | Air-eq plastic | Air-eq plastic |
| PTW | Cylinderical (Pinpoit™) | T31006 | 0.015 | 5 | 2 | 0.4 | 4 | Steel | acrylic+graphite |
| PTW | Cylinderical (Semiflex) | T31002 | 0.125 | 6.5 | 5.5 | 4 | 4 | Aluminum/ graphite | acrylic+graphite |
| Scanditronix | Cylinderical | CC01 | 0.01 | 3.6 | 2 | 0.33 | 0.75 | Steel | Shonka C552 |
| | Cylinderical | CC04 | 0.04 | 3.6 | 4 | 1 | 0.5 | Shonka C552 | Shonka C552 |
| | Cylinderical | CC08 | 0.08 | 4 | 6 | 2.7 | 4 | Shonka C552 | Shonka C552 |
| | Cylinderical | CC13 | 0.13 | 5.8 | 6 | 4 | 4 | Shonka C552 | Shonka C552 |
| Standard Imaging | Cylinderical | A1/A1SL/ M1/T1 | 0.05 | 4.35 | 4 | 1.7 | 1 | See model letter | See model letter |
| | Hemi-spherical | A14/A14SL/ T14 | 0.009 | 2 | 4 | 0.3 | 1 | See model letter | See model letter |
| | Planar | A14P/T14P | 0.002 | 1.5 | 2.5 | 0.08 | 1 | See model letter | See model letter |
| | Cylinderical | A16 | 0.007 | 1.8 | 2.4 | 0.3 | 1 | Shonka C552 | Shonka C552 |
| Scanditronix | Photon filed diode | PFD_DEB010 | ~0 | 0.5 | 2 | 35 | | | p-type Silicon |
| | Stereotactic field diode | SFD_DEB050 | ~0 | 0.5 | 0.6 | 6 | | | p-type Silicon |

For Standard Imaging/Exradin ionization chambers, the chamber materials are designated as Model A, Shonka C552; Model M, pure magnesium; and Model T, Shonka A150. Capintee, Inc., Ramsey, NJ, Standard Imaging, Middleton, WI.

than other detectors. Because of these reasons, diamond detectors are rarely used in IMRT field measurements.

- The basic requirements for electrometers are (1) accuracy, (2) linearity, (3) stability, (4) minimum charge collection, (5) minimum current collection, (6) high impedance, and (7) low leakage. It is important to point out that the leakage of electrometers is usually comparable to that of ionization chambers. Leakage should be carefully evaluated as a part of the dosimetry chain in performing dose measurements. The newer electrometers usually have much lower leakage than most older models.

- The correct selection of radiation detectors depends on the type of IMRT measurements and the IMRT delivery characteristics. For example, when the IMRT treatment is delivered with many small beamlets as in the MIMiC tomotherapy delivery, a microchamber (with <0.02 cc) can be a good choice because the relative percentage of low-energy photons in the beam can be lower, which reduces the effect of high-Z electrodes used in the microchamber.

- Similarly, diodes may be used in these applications, although the directional dependence is still a concern. For most step-and-shoot or dynamic MLC treatments, the field size can be a mixture of large fields and small fields. The particular mix of large and small fields depends on the type of IMRT delivery system, the IMRT treatment planning system, and the specific patient case. To minimize the detector overresponse to variable low-energy

photons, an ion chamber with tissue- or air-equivalent materials is recommended. In addition, low leakage dosimetry system (detector, cable, and electrometer) and the small directional dependence of the detector are important factors in choosing the proper equipment.

- Because of the rapid dose gradient and the composition of small fields seen in IMRT plans, it is essential to have adequate spatial resolution when performing these measurements. Although it is possible to use large volume ionization chambers in IMRT dose measurement, it is important to include the volume of the detector in the calculation instead of using "point" dose calculation. Even with the smallest ionization chamber, the effective volume is not zero. Therefore, when comparing IMRT dose calculations, it is unwise to compare calculated point dose with the dose measured using a detector of finite size.

- Physicists should try to outline the active volume of the detector and compare the mean calculated value to the measurement. This is particularly important when a large ionization chamber, such as the Farmer-type chamber (0.6 cc), is used. It is also recommended to expand the outlined volume slightly to include the uncertainty in positioning the detector during measurement. Most IMRT treatment planning systems allow you to obtain dosimetric statistics over an outlined or expanded volume.

- The selection of a good measurement point should be based on (1) the clinical importance (this is typically inside a treatment target or a critical structure), (2) the least sensitivity to setup uncertainties in the measurement, and (3) a useful reference point for dose normalization, which is usually in conjunction with composite or planar 2D measurements such as films.

- Selection of the cable that connects the ionization chamber with the electrometer can be important. Leakage of the dosimetry system (ionization chamber, cable, and electrometer) can affect the accurate measurement of weak signals from scatters and leakage in an IMRT delivery. Sometimes a straight (through-the-door) cable connection between the ionization chamber and the electrometer can greatly reduce the leakage compared with a patch panel connection. Although convenient for setup (unwinding the through-the-door cables is not necessary), a patch panel increases the number of connections and therefore increases the probability of high leakage in the dosimetry chain. The ionization chamber should also be pre-irradiated, and the dosimetry system should be tested to ensure good signal stability.

- Electrometers may exhibit a slow warm-up period, which causes the measured leakage for the dosimetry chain to vary during the initial 25 minutes. Some manufacturers recommend a 15-minute warm-up before using the electrometer. Therefore, it is also prudent to routinely warm up the electrometer while the phantom is being set up for measurement.

- The sensitivity of a small-volume ionization chamber can be unstable, and the output of a linac can also vary. It is recommended to use relative measurements for IMRT point dose measurement in patient-specific QA. This implies that a calibration procedure for the detector should be established before IMRT measurements. For example, Dong et al.[54] described a calibration procedure that used bilateral parallel-opposed large fields (10 × 10 cm) to obtain the "dose calibration factor" of the day for the ionization chamber, assuming a perfectly calibrated linac (1 MU is calibrated to 1 cGy under standard conditions). The procedure focuses on the comparison of an IMRT plan, which assumes a perfectly calibrated linac. If the absolute dose measurements were used, it would not be possible to distinguish whether the difference in the measurement was caused by the errors in the IMRT plan or by the daily output fluctuation of the linac. Although the absolute dose matters for the patient, this method assumes that other standard QA procedures will ensure that the output of a linac is calibrated properly.

- Sometimes it is necessary to provide output factor measurements for IMRT commissioning. When performing these measurements, we have to be aware of the limitations of the detectors used for these measurements. For example, diode detectors and microchambers with a volume less than 0.02 cc can be a good choice for small-field output measurements, but they are usually overresponding to low-energy photons, which are more apparent in large fields. Whereas a large volume ion chamber can be excel-

lent in large-field measurements, their large dimensions may discourage their use in small-field measurements.

- During output factor measurement, the response of the chambers or diodes should be frequently measured and compared with a reference field. This will minimize any potential drifting or changing in detector sensitivity during measurements. The drifts in ionization chamber or diode can be attributable to a number of reasons, for example, the temporal change in machine output, the temperature change of the measurement medium, or the stability of small volume ion chambers themselves. Special corrections for volume averaging, such as the deconvolution method, can be used to improve data accuracy.[55,59-61] The literature for small-field measurements in stereotactic radiosurgery could also be useful, although most of the small-field IMRT treatments are off-axis, which may be different from typical stereotactic treatments.

- Occasionally, it is necessary to provide profile and percent depth dose measurements for IMRT commissioning. Before performing the measurement, it is important to read the instructions. For example: (1) How far along the tail of a profile should measurements be performed? (2) What is used to define the profile, MLC, or secondary photon jaws? If the profile is defined by an MLC, what are the positions of the secondary photon jaws? (3) Which profiles should be measured at what depths and along which direction (in-plane or cross-plane)? (4) What is the spatial resolution required for the measurements? Because various detectors may have different dimensions along the length and the diameter directions (Table 1-1), optimizing the detector orientation is important for profile and depth dose measurements. It is recommended to use the smallest dimension in the scanning direction to give the best spatial resolution. The diode detector may be an exception because of the directional dependence.

## 4.3. Overview of Quality Assurance Process

- To implement a new treatment technology into routine clinical use, there are usually three distinct but closely related phases:

  □ *Acceptance tests:* This is the initial set of tests that ensures the hardware and software meet the factory or customer-provided specifications. Usually, but not always, the written specifications contain the necessary instructions or guidelines for these tests (to avoid legal ambiguity in the measurements). It is also a good opportunity for the users to establish some performance baselines, especially for the hardware purchased.

  □ *Commissioning tests:* The IMRT commissioning is a process used to implement IMRT treatments by using the customer's hardware and beam data. Various groups have studied the general guidelines for commissioning a treatment planning system.[50,62] The process usually starts with collection of essential beam data for beam modeling. The parameters of the dose calculation algorithm are then tuned to provide the best performance for the user's beam. Additional tests should be performed to evaluate the limitations of the treatment planning system, and a solution or a workaround should be found if the problem is clearly identified. Then IMRT phantom measurements should be performed to test the accuracy of the delivery system and data connectivity. If the accuracy is judged to be acceptable, the system can be released to the clinic after the necessary user training and procedural implementations. It is recommended that a small (interdisciplinary) focus group be assigned to lead the IMRT implementation in the clinic. The "train-the-trainer" approach has proven to be effective in translating new technology into routine clinical practice.

☐ *Ongoing QA*: After the system is released to the clinic, it is important to establish a routine QA program. The performance of various steps involved in performing IMRT treatments should be tracked so that the quality of the treatments can be maintained. The ongoing QA program can be separated into patient-specific QA and equipment QA, which will be described in more detail next.

## 4.4. Patient-Specific Quality Assurance

- Because of the complexity of irregular field shapes, small-field dosimetry, and time-dependent deliverable leaf sequences, it is recommended by the American Association of Physicists in Medicine (AAPM) and ASTRO that patient-specific QA should be performed as a part of the IMRT management process and a requirement for billing for IMRT services. Figure 1-8 shows the general categories of patient-specific QA.

- Patient setup, although not specific to IMRT dosimetry, is considered a key step in ensuring accurate IMRT treatments. A variety of image-guided localization techniques has been proposed for use with IMRT treatments, from simple orthogonal portal films to the beam's eye view portal film with IMRT intensity pattern overlays,[63] daily electronic portal imaging of implanted fiducial markers,[64–66] daily ultrasound-guided localization,[67–69] and most integrated tomotherapy solutions.[16] A detailed discussion of these specific image-guided procedures is beyond the scope of this book, but QA in patient positioning remains an important issue for IMRT.

- The implementation of patient-specific QA depends highly on each institution. For example, dosimetric measurements of MU settings can be verified for each beam individually (usually in a flat [slab] phantom geometry) or for the composite treatment plan (usually in a specially

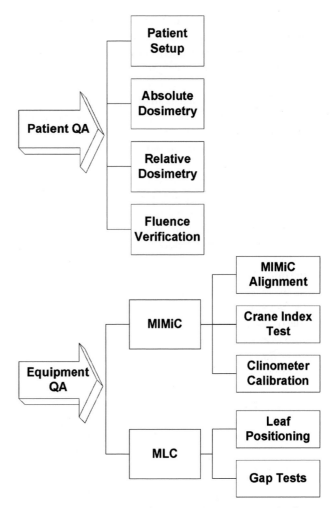

**FIGURE 1-8.** Separation of IMRT quality assurance (QA) into patient-specific and equipment-specific QA.

designed phantom, but it is also possible to use the simple slab phantom setup).

- Unlike single beam verification in which the single beam dose distribution can be significantly different from the original patient plan, the advantage of measuring the composite treatment plan in a phantom (regardless of the shape of the phantom) is that the composite dose distribution or the dose "pattern" generated in a phantom is usually similar to that in the original patient plan. This can be useful in selecting the measurement points or visualizing potential dose errors.

- Absolute dosimetry is usually referred to as "MU verification" for IMRT. The traditional manual process for MU verification is virtually impossible to perform because of the large number of fields involved and the irregular shape and size of the treatment segments.

- Attempts have been made to verify MU settings in an IMRT plan using alternative calculation methods.[70–72] However, these alternative calculation methods cannot predict the uncertainties during the actual delivery at the treatment machines and are also subject to limitations and approximations in their dose calculation models. Currently, the most reliable and practical technique for IMRT MU verification is still the ion chamber-based point dose measurement in a phantom.

- Absolute dose measurement in a phantom is usually performed through a process called the "hybrid phantom plan." In this plan, all beam angles and deliverable intensity patterns for a patient plan are transferred to the phantom, and doses in the phantom are computed for QA. The basic assumption in this process is that if the dose calculated in the phantom agrees with the measurement in the phantom, then the dose delivered to the patient agrees with the dose calculated in the patient.

- Relative dosimetry is usually performed with radiographic films or 2D array detectors. The process is similar to absolute dose measurement by using the hybrid phantom plan technique. For film dosimetry, it is important to convert film density into relative dose using a film calibration process.[73] Because of the additional dimensionality, it becomes difficult to define good numeric criteria for evaluating relative 2D and 3D measurements. Various numeric indicators (e.g., the distance to agreement, gamma,[74–76] or normalized agreement test[77]) were proposed. In particular, the concept of gamma, combining the dose difference and distance to agreement, is appealing in evaluating 2D or 3D dose distributions.[74]

- For clinical applications, the most reliable and practical way to evaluate 2D distribution is to overlay the measurement isodose lines with the calculated ones. Special attention should be paid to the low-dose regions near critical structures in the original patient plan. Attention should also be paid to the systematic shifts of isodose lines, which may reveal whether the isocenter or any reference setup point may be off. The relative dosimetry verification for IMRT should be performed in conjunction with the absolute dose verification for IMRT. It would be useful if the relative dose distribution can be normalized to the absolute dose measurement point, which converts the relative dose measurement into absolute dose distributions.

- 2D fluence verification of intensity patterns gained popularity with the invention of 2D array detectors and the necessary software.[78,79] Fluence verification usually is performed for each IMRT beam at a fixed gantry angle with or without a flat phantom geometry. The purpose of fluence verification is to make sure the intensity patterns created in each IMRT plan can be faithfully delivered under ideal conditions (2D and beam's eye view). Fluence verification should be combined with other patient-specific and equipment QAs to make sure that IMRT treatments are executed accurately.

## 4.5. Equipment Quality Assurance

- IMRT delivery system is equipment-specific, which usually requires special design of QA procedures. In general, IMRT QA is a subset of general equipment QA processes. Many of the sources of uncertainties in RT and IMRT applications have been discussed in the AAPM report (TG-40),[80] the IMRT working group report,[1] and many individual investigations.[18,49,81–84]

- In 2003, the AAPM organized an IMRT summer school that covered many of the relevant topics (proceedings to be published soon). Examples include IMRT delivery using serial tomotherapy, static MLC IMRT, dynamic IMRT delivery, and computer-controlled linacs. The technology of IMRT and techniques for QA are also evolving. It is strongly suggested that users of IMRT should attempt to attend national meetings and technology conferences or training courses so that their knowledge about the use of IMRT can be updated regularly.

- To illustrate the separation of equipment QA into several elements, Figure 1-8 shows the three major steps in performing serial tomotherapy QA (the NOMOS MIMiC): the MIMiC alignment test (which aligns the leaves relative to the beam isocenter), the crane index test (which calibrates the advancement of the couch to achieve the best match between slices of the treated volume), and the clinometer test (which calibrates the gantry angles for the MIMiC treatment head).

- Similarly, for IMRT using a linac-based MLC, the leaf-positioning test is necessary as well as the leaf light-field and radiation-field offset test (gap test). The gap test usually uses a 2-cm matching strip with variable leaf offsets (in steps of 0.2 mm). The best leaf offset is obtained by finding the best inter-strip dosimetric overlap. Figure 1-9 shows an example of the MIMiC alignment, and Figure 1-10 shows the MLC leaf offset measurement and the leaf positioning test.

## 4.6. Tolerances and Action Levels

- As mentioned previously, IMRT treatments may be more sensitive to geometric accuracy in positioning treatment beams. Difficulties in small-field dosimetry and the risk of mathematic optimization, which may generate undeliverable leaf sequences, could also reduce the accuracy of IMRT treatments. Although there is little clinical evidence on how accurate IMRT treatments should be, it is generally accepted that dose delivery accuracy should be maintained within 5%.[85]

- The tolerances for IMRT treatments should also be site-specific. Each treatment site, such as the prostate, head and neck, and lung, presents a different problem in patient setup (related to the PTV margin determination) and IMRT planning. The overall uncertainty is a combination of uncertainties in target delineation, patient-

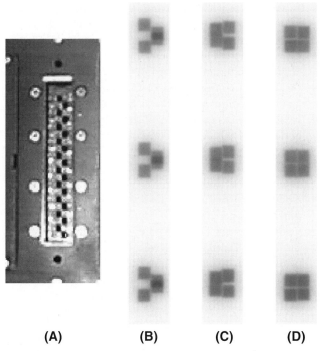

**(A)      (B)      (C)      (D)**

**FIGURE 1-9.** Equipment QA for NOMOS MIMiC shows verification of the alignment of leaf positions relative to the collimator axis of rotation. **A:** MIMiC. **B** and **C:** Unacceptable alignments. **D:** Good alignment.

specific dose prescriptions, treatment planning, and treatment delivery. Developing site-specific tolerance and guidelines for IMRT treatments is important and essential for the quality of patient care.

■ The action level is closely related to the site-specific treatment and the delivery system. For example, a 2-mm leaf positioning accuracy may be sufficient for conventional 3DCRT treatments but is not sufficient for SMLC or DMLC treatments. The machine's output changes rapidly with the decrease in field sizes, which makes leaf-

positioning accuracy important for IMRT. It is conceivable that DMLC using dynamic treatment delivery would also have a tighter action level than SMLC treatments using the step-and-shoot technique.

■ The specific guidelines and action levels for various treatment devices have not been determined because of the constantly changing technology and exploratory use of IMRT at the present time. More controlled clinical studies should be conducted to investigate the real clinical benefits and risks of IMRT. At this time, it is suggested to maintain a good consistency and follow general good practice and common sense in RT.

## 5. GUIDELINES FOR STARTING AN INTENSITY-MODULATED RADIATION THERAPY PROGRAM

### 5.1. Intensity-Modulated Radiation Therapy Benefits

■ The technical benefits of IMRT are of interest to hospital administrators. If the clinical benefits of IMRT can be realized, that is, if improved local control and low incidence of morbidity can be demonstrated with the use of IMRT, it will be an effective and economic alternative treatment for patients with cancer. The benefits for hospital administrators can be summarized as follows:

  □ Cost-effective therapy
  □ Development of a service niche in providing cutting-edge cancer treatment
  □ New markets and referrals
  □ Revenue enhancement

■ Hospital administrators may be pressed to offer IMRT services to compete with other health care providers. In addition, the current reimbursement policy favors IMRT treatments, although significant investment has to be made in equipment, staff, and staff training.

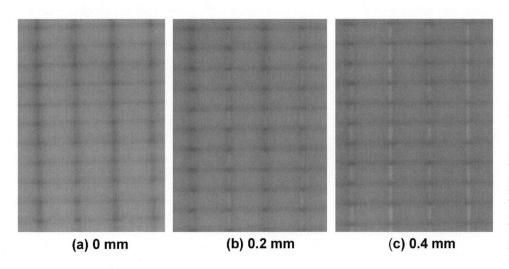

**(a) 0 mm          (b) 0.2 mm          (c) 0.4 mm**

**FIGURE 1-10.** MLC QA. The light-field and radiation-field offset is measured by sequentially exposing a 2-cm strip with different leaf offsets. The best leaf offset is obtained by judging the dosimetric overlap in the junction line. In this case, the 0.2-mm leaf offset gives the best match between two adjacent strips. The position of the junction line also indicates the absolute leaf positions across the field.

## 5.2. Intensity-Modulated Radiation Therapy Program Preparation

- The first step in starting an IMRT program is to organize an interdisciplinary team or task force and perform a self-assessment. The assessment should consider past referring patterns in the primary and secondary service areas, market competence, patient population and disease sites, current equipment, upgradeability, staffing levels, local expertise, and so forth. Although IMRT can be and has been applied to different treatment sites, patients with prostate and head and neck cancers are considered the primary candidates for IMRT applications.
- Ideal tumor sites for IMRT should have the following characteristics:
  - A positive response to radiation dose (potential for dose escalation to improve local control).
  - Proximity to critical normal structures or near a previously treated area (to take advantage of the sharp gradient in IMRT).
  - Setup or organ motion uncertainty is small (increased treatment margin will minimize the effectiveness of IMRT).

## 5.3. Equipment Selection

- *Linear accelerators with IMRT capability*: Vendors may provide marketing materials for their equipment, but it is important to perform a site visit and see the performance of different linear accelerators in delivering IMRT treatments. If head and neck cancers will be one of the major treatment sites for IMRT, a smaller MLC leaf width will be helpful because it provides better spatial resolution. The machine uptime and the quality of local service providers should be considered in addition to the package and financial considerations for a specific vendor. Different options to update existing treatment units should be considered. Sometimes, it is useful to have matched (or backup) machines to provide redundancy and efficiency in patient scheduling. Additional considerations should be the routine maintenance of the equipment, replacement parts, installation time, and system integration issues.
- The choice of photon beam energy is less sensitive when using IMRT.[16,86] If IMRT is the primary modality for treating patients, a linac with single photon energy can be configured, which reduces the capital expenses. However, IMRT usually requires 2 to 10 times more MUs for treatment delivery; therefore, the room shielding should be carefully revisited. The additional MUs are usually spent in beam intensity modulation, which increases the total leakage exposure, but the target dose per fraction usually remains unchanged. Therefore, the secondary barriers should be thickened according to the IMRT treatment techniques and the estimated workload, but

the primary barrier is similar to the conventional designs. If a high-energy photon beam is used for IMRT, the whole-body neutron dose can become significant.[87]

- Careful selection of dosimetry equipment for performing commissioning and routine IMRT QA is important. The quality and configuration of the dosimetry equipment can make a difference in the staff's productivity.
- IMRT increases the activity of contouring target volumes and critical structures; therefore, having a good CT-simulation system is important. The RT facility should determine whether a dedicated CT-simulation workstation should be added.
- *Connectivity*: Because of the large amount of treatment parameters generated by an IMRT planning system (more treatment fields and leaf set files should be transferred from the planning system to the treatment unit), it is mandatory to have an integrated or an effective record and verification system to assist with data transfer and treatment verification for IMRT. A good record and verification system can significantly increase treatment efficiency and reduce treatment operation errors.

## 5.4. Implementation Steps

- Start with a proven IMRT treatment site, for example, the prostate. A team approach is essential because the staff (physicians, dosimetrists, physicists, and therapists) should know what their roles will be and how long each step of implementation will take.
- A "dry run" is a good idea for the entire team before treating the first patient.
- Site visits and peer review are good ideas to maintain safety and quality.
- Communication among different groups is important, and it is prudent to keep everyone involved; oftentimes, the imaging study is performed outside of the RT department.
- To use the new technology appropriately, careful patient selection is important. Because IMRT is more sensitive to treatment margin and setup uncertainties, improper selection of patient cases or immobilization techniques may even deteriorate the treatment quality.
- Although there are billing codes for IMRT service, the local billing policy should be reviewed so that the revenue from IMRT is appropriately ensured. The selection for IMRT treatments should follow ACR's and ASTRO's recommendation for the medical necessity of using IMRT and AAPM's recommendation for patient-specific QA.
- Finally, staff training is essential for the success of an IMRT program. Staff at all levels should be educated about the benefits, risks, and pitfalls of IMRT for patient management. Staff members should be encouraged to attend and learn various IMRT techniques at local or national meetings organized by various professional soci-

eties. The real risk of IMRT is to apply it routinely without fully understanding the rationale for its use and its clinical aspects and physics.

## REFERENCES

1. Group ICW. Intensity-modulated radiotherapy: current status and issues of interest. *Int J Radiat Oncol Biol Phys* 2001;51:880–914.
2. Ezzell GA, Galvin JM, Low D, et al. Guidance document on delivery, treatment planning, and clinical implementation of IMRT: report of the IMRT subcommittee of the AAPM radiation therapy committee. *Med Phys* 2003;30:2089–2115.
3. Storey MR, Pollack A, Zagars G, et al. Complications from radiotherapy dose escalation in prostate cancer: preliminary results of a randomized trial. [Comment.] *Int J Radiat Oncol Biol Phys* 2000;48:635–642.
4. Butler EB, Teh BS, Grant WH 3rd, et al. Smart (simultaneous modulated accelerated radiation therapy) boost: a new accelerated fractionation schedule for the treatment of head and neck cancer with intensity modulated radiotherapy. *Int J Radiat Oncol Biol Phys* 1999;45:21–32.
5. Mohan R, Wu Q, Manning M, et al. Radiobiological considerations in the design of fractionation strategies for intensity-modulated radiation therapy of head and neck cancers. *Int J Radiat Oncol Biol Phys* 2000;46:619–630.
6. Wu Q, Manning M, Schmidt-Ullrich R, et al. The potential for sparing of parotids and escalation of biologically effective dose with intensity-modulated radiation treatments of head and neck cancers: a treatment design study. *Int J Radiat Oncol Biol Phys* 2000;46:195–205.
7. Amosson CM, Teh BS, Van TJ, et al. Dosimetric predictors of xerostomia for head-and-neck cancer patients treated with the smart (simultaneous modulated accelerated radiation therapy) boost technique. *Int J Radiat Oncol Biol Phys* 2003;56:136–144.
8. Suzuki M, Nakamatsu K, Kanamori S, et al. Feasibility study of the simultaneous integrated boost (SIB) method for malignant gliomas using intensity-modulated radiotherapy (IMRT). *Jpn J Clin Oncol* 2003;33:271–277.
9. Wu Q, Mohan R, Morris M, et al. Simultaneous integrated boost intensity-modulated radiotherapy for locally advanced head-and-neck squamous cell carcinomas. I: dosimetric results. *Int J Radiat Oncol Biol Phys* 2003;56:573–585.
10. Langen KM, Jones DT. Organ motion and its management. *Int J Radiat Oncol Biol Phys* 2001;50:265–278.
11. McKenzie A, van Herk M, Mijnheer B. Margins for geometric uncertainty around organs at risk in radiotherapy. *Radiother Oncol* 2002;62:299–307.
12. Antolak JA, Rosen II. Planning target volumes for radiotherapy: how much margin is needed? *Int J Radiat Oncol Biol Phys* 1999;44:1165–1170.
13. Jaffray DA, Yan D, Wong JW. Managing geometric uncertainty in conformal intensity-modulated radiation therapy. *Semin Radiat Oncol* 1999;9:4–19.
14. van Herk M, Remeijer P, Lebesque JV. Inclusion of geometric uncertainties in treatment plan evaluation. *Int J Radiat Oncol Biol Phys* 2002;52:1407–1422.
15. van Herk M, Remeijer P, Rasch C, et al. The probability of correct target dosage: dose-population histograms for deriving treatment margins in radiotherapy. *Int J Radiat Oncol Biol Phys* 2000;47:1121–1135.
16. Mackie TR, Kapatoes J, Ruchala K, et al. Image guidance for precise conformal radiotherapy. *Int J Radiat Oncol Biol Phys* 2003;56:89–105.
17. Litzenberg DW, Moran JM, Fraass BA. Incorporation of realistic delivery limitations into dynamic MLC treatment delivery. *Med Phys* 2002;29:810–820.
18. Chui CS, Spirou S, LoSasso T. Testing of dynamic multileaf collimation. *Med Phys* 1996;23:635–641.
19. Curran B. Where goest the peacock? *Med Dosim* 2001;26:3–9.
20. Chao KS, Low DA, Perez CA, et al. Intensity-modulated radiation therapy in head and neck cancers: the Mallinckrodt experience. *Int J Cancer* 2000;90:92–103.
21. Sharpe MB, Miller BM, Yan D, et al. Monitor unit settings for intensity modulated beams delivered using a step-and-shoot approach. *Med Phys* 2000;27:2719–2725.
22. Kestin LL, Sharpe MB, Frazier RC, et al. Intensity modulation to improve dose uniformity with tangential breast radiotherapy: initial clinical experience. *Int J Radiat Oncol Biol Phys* 2000;48:1559–1568.
23. Thilmann C, Zabel A, Nill S, et al. Intensity-modulated radiotherapy of the female breast. *Med Dosim* 2002;27:79–90.
24. Vineberg KA, Eisbruch A, Coselmon MM, et al. Is uniform target dose possible in IMRT plans in the head and neck? *Int J Radiat Oncol Biol Phys* 2002;52:1159–1172.
25. Xia P, Pickett B, Vigneault E, et al. Forward or inversely planned segmental multileaf collimator IMRT and sequential tomotherapy to treat multiple dominant intraprostatic lesions of prostate cancer to 90 Gy. *Int J Radiat Oncol Biol Phys* 2001;51:244–254.
26. Mohan R, Arnfield M, Tong S, et al. The impact of fluctuations in intensity patterns on the number of monitor units and the quality and accuracy of intensity modulated radiotherapy. *Med Phys* 2000;27:1226–1237.
27. Siebers JV, Lauterbach M, Keall PJ, et al. Incorporating multileaf collimator leaf sequencing into iterative IMRT optimization. *Med Phys* 2002;29:952–959.
28. Das S, Cullip T, Tracton G, et al. Beam orientation selection for intensity-modulated radiation therapy based on target equivalent uniform dose maximization. *Int J Radiat Oncol Biol Phys* 2003;55:215–224.
29. De Gersem W, Claus F, De Wagter C, et al. An anatomy-based beam segmentation tool for intensity-modulated radiation therapy and its application to head-and-neck cancer. *Int J Radiat Oncol Biol Phys* 2001;51:849–859.
30. Shepard DM, Earl MA, Li XA, et al. Direct aperture optimization: a turnkey solution for step-and-shoot IMRT. *Med Phys* 2002;29:1007–1018.
31. Claus F, De Gersem W, De Wagter C, et al. An implementation strategy for IMRT of ethmoid sinus cancer with bilateral sparing of the optic pathways. *Int J Radiat Oncol Biol Phys* 2001;51:318–331.
32. Purdy JA. Dose-volume specification: new challenges with intensity-modulated radiation therapy. *Semin Radiat Oncol* 2002;12:199–209.
33. Manning MA, Wu Q, Cardinale RM, et al. The effect of setup uncertainty on normal tissue sparing with IMRT for head-and-neck cancer. *Int J Radiat Oncol Biol Phys* 2001;51:1400–1409.
34. Pugachev A, Xing L. Incorporating prior knowledge into beam orientation optimization in IMRT. *Int J Radiat Oncol Biol Phys* 2002;54:1565–1574.
35. Bedford JL, Webb S. Elimination of importance factors for clinically accurate selection of beam orientations, beam weights and wedge angles in conformal radiation therapy. *Med Phys* 2003;30:1788–1804.
36. Bortfeld T. Optimized planning using physical objectives and constraints. *Semin Radiat Oncol* 1999;9:20–34.
37. Wu Q, Mohan R. Algorithms and functionality of an intensity modulated radiotherapy optimization system. *Med Phys* 2000;27:701–711.

38. Arnfield MR, Siebers JV, Kim JO, et al. A method for determining multileaf collimator transmission and scatter for dynamic intensity modulated radiotherapy. *Med Phys* 2000;27:2231–2241.

39. Siebers JV, Keall PJ, Kim JO, et al. A method for photon beam Monte Carlo multileaf collimator particle transport. *Phys Med Biol* 2002;47:3225–3249.

40. Xia P, Verhey LJ. Multileaf collimator leaf sequencing algorithm for intensity modulated beams with multiple static segments. *Med Phys* 1998;25:1424–1434.

41. Boyer AL, Yu CX. Intensity-modulated radiation therapy with dynamic multileaf collimators. *Semin Radiat Oncol* 1999;9:48–59.

42. Kuterdem HG, Cho PS. Leaf sequencing with secondary beam blocking under leaf positioning constraints for continuously modulated radiotherapy beams. *Med Phys* 2001;28:894–902.

43. Langer M, Thai V, Papiez L. Improved leaf sequencing reduces segments or monitor units needed to deliver IMRT using multileaf collimators. *Med Phys* 2001;28:2450–2458.

44. Crooks SM, McAven LF, Robinson DF, et al. Minimizing delivery time and monitor units in static IMRT by leaf-sequencing. *Phys Med Biol* 2002;47:3105–3116.

45. Xia P, Hwang AB, Verhey LJ. A leaf sequencing algorithm to enlarge treatment field length in IMRT. *Med Phys* 2002;29:991–998.

46. Meyer RR, Gunawardena A, D'Souza W, et al. Leaf sequencing via difference matrices reduces aperture number and beam-on time in IMRT. *Int J Radiat Oncol Biol Phys* 2003;57:S267–S268.

47. Kamath S, Sahni S, Li J, et al. Leaf sequencing algorithms for segmented multileaf collimation. *Phys Med Biol* 2003;48:307–324.

48. Spirou SV, Fournier-Bidoz N, Yang J, et al. Smoothing intensity-modulated beam profiles to improve the efficiency of delivery. *Med Phys* 2001;28:2105–2112.

49. Chui CS, Chan MF, Yorke E, et al. Delivery of intensity-modulated radiation therapy with a conventional multileaf collimator: comparison of dynamic and segmental methods. *Med Phys* 2001;28:2441–2449.

50. Fraass BA, Lash KL, Matrone GM, et al. The impact of treatment complexity and computer-control delivery technology on treatment delivery errors. *Int J Radiat Oncol Biol Phys* 1998;42:651–659.

51. Low DA, Mutic S, Dempsey JF, et al. Quantitative dosimetric verification of an IMRT planning and delivery system. *Radiother Oncol* 1998;49:305–316.

52. Martens C, De Wagter C, De Neve W. The value of the PinPoint ion chamber for characterization of small field segments used in intensity-modulated radiotherapy. *Phys Med Biol* 2000;45:2519–2530.

53. Bucciolini M, Buonamici FB, Mazzocchi S, et al. Diamond detector versus silicon diode and ion chamber in photon beams of different energy and field size. *Med Phys* 2003;30:2149–2154.

54. Dong L, Antolak J, Salehpour M, et al. Patient-specific point dose measurement for IMRT monitor unit verification. *Int J Radiat Oncol Biol Phys* 2003;56:867–877.

55. Laub WU, Wong T. The volume effect of detectors in the dosimetry of small fields used in IMRT. *Med Phys* 2003;30:341–347.

56. Leybovich LB, Sethi A, Dogan N. Comparison of ionization chambers of various volumes for IMRT absolute dose verification. *Med Phys* 2003;30:119–123.

57. Low D, Parikh P, Dempsey J, Wahab S, et al. Ionization chamber volume averaging effects in dynamic intensity modulated radiation therapy beams. *Med Phys* 2003;30:1706–1711.

58. Westermark M, Arndt J, Nilsson B, et al. Comparative dosimetry in narrow high-energy photon beams. *Phys Med Biol* 2000;45:685–702.

59. Garcia-Vicente F, Delgado JM, Peraza C. Experimental determination of the convolution kernel for the study of the spatial response of a detector. *Med Phys* 1998;25:202–207.

60. Bednarz G, Saiful Huq M, Rosenow UF. Deconvolution of detector size effect for output factor measurement for narrow Gamma Knife radiosurgery beams. *Phys Med Biol* 2002;47:3643–3649.

61. Low DA, Dempsey JF, Markman J, et al. Toward automated quality assurance for intensity-modulated radiation therapy. *Int J Radiat Oncol Biol Phys* 2002;53:443–452.

62. Van Dyk J, Barnett RB, Cygler JE, et al. Commissioning and quality assurance of treatment planning computers.[comment]. *Int J Radiat Oncol Biol Phys* 1993;26:261–273.

63. Xing L, Curran B, Hill R, et al. Dosimetric verification of a commercial inverse treatment planning system. *Phys Med Biol* 1999;44:463–478.

64. Kitamura K, Shirato H, Shimizu S, et al. Registration accuracy and possible migration of internal fiducial gold marker implanted in prostate and liver treated with real-time tumor-tracking radiation therapy (RTRT). *Radiother Oncol* 2002;62:275–281.

65. Verellen D, Soete G, Linthout N, et al. Quality assurance of a system for improved target localization and patient set-up that combines real-time infrared tracking and stereoscopic X-ray imaging. *Radiother Oncol* 2003;67:129–141.

66. Murphy MJ. Fiducial-based targeting accuracy for external-beam radiotherapy. *Med Phys* 2002;29:334–344.

67. Lattanzi J, McNeeley S, Hanlon A, et al. Ultrasound-based stereotactic guidance of precision conformal external beam radiation therapy in clinically localized prostate cancer. *Urology* 2000;55:73–78.

68. Serago CF, Chungbin SJ, Buskirk SJ, et al. Initial experience with ultrasound localization for positioning prostate cancer patients for external beam radiotherapy. *Int J Radiat Oncol Biol Phys* 2002;53:1130–1138.

69. Chandra A, Dong L, Huang E, et al. Experience of ultrasound-based daily prostate localization. *Int J Radiat Oncol Biol Phys* 2003;56:436–447.

70. Kung JH, Chen GT, Kuchnir FK. A monitor unit verification calculation in intensity modulated radiotherapy as a dosimetry quality assurance. *Med Phys* 2000;27:2226–2230.

71. Xing L, Chen Y, Luxton G, et al. Monitor unit calculation for an intensity modulated photon field by a simple scatter-summation algorithm. *Phys Med Biol* 2000;45:N1–7.

72. Chen Z, Xing L, Nath R. Independent monitor unit calculation for intensity modulated radiotherapy using the MIMiC multileaf collimator. *Med Phys* 2002;29:2041–2051.

73. Childress NL, Dong L, Rosen II. Rapid radiographic film calibration for IMRT verification using automated MLC fields. *Med Phys* 2002;29:2384–2390.

74. Low DA, Harms WB, Mutic S, et al. A technique for the quantitative evaluation of dose distributions. *Med Phys* 1998;25:656–661.

75. Depuydt T, Van Esch A, Huyskens DP. A quantitative evaluation of IMRT dose distributions: refinement and clinical assessment of the gamma evaluation. *Radiother Oncol* 2002;62:309–319.

76. Kapulsky A, Mullokandov E, Gejerman G. An automated phantom-film QA procedure for intensity-modulated radiation therapy. *Med Dosim* 2002;27:201–207.

77. Childress NL, Rosen II. The design and testing of novel clinical parameters for dose comparison. *Int J Radiat Oncol Biol Phys* 2003;56:1464–1479.

78. Jursinic PA, Nelms BE. A 2-D diode array and analysis software for verification of intensity modulated radiation therapy delivery. *Med Phys* 2003;30:870–879.

79. Li JG, Dempsey JF, Ding L, et al. Validation of dynamic MLC-controller log files using a two-dimensional diode array. *Med Phys* 2003;30:799–805.

80. Kutcher GJ, Coia L, Gillin M, et al. Comprehensive QA for radiation oncology: report of AAPM Radiation Therapy Committee Task Group 40. *Med Phys* 1994;21:581–618.

81. Burman C, Chui CS, Kutcher G, et al. Planning, delivery, and quality assurance of intensity-modulated radiotherapy using dynamic multileaf collimator: a strategy for large-scale implementation for the treatment of carcinoma of the prostate. *Int J Radiat Oncol Biol Phys* 1997;39:863–873.

82. Low DA, Mutic S, Dempsey JF, et al. Quantitative dosimetric verification of an IMRT planning and delivery system. *Radiother Oncol* 1998;49:305–316.

83. Saw CB, Ayyangar KM, Zhen W, et al. Quality assurance procedures for the Peacock system. *Med Dosim* 2001;26:83–90.

84. Ma LJ, Phaisangittisakul N, Yu CX, et al. A quality assurance method for analyzing and verifying intensity modulated fields. *Med Phys* 2003;30:2082–2088.

85. Dische S, Saunders MI, Williams C, et al. Precision in reporting the dose given in a course of radiotherapy. [Comment.] *Radiother Oncol* 1993;29:287–293.

86. Pirzkall A, Carol MP, Pickett B, et al. The effect of beam energy and number of fields on photon-based IMRT for deep-seated targets. *Int J Radiat Oncol Biol Phys* 2002;53:434–442.

87. Followill D, Geis P, Boyer A. Estimates of whole-body dose equivalent produced by beam intensity modulated conformal therapy. *Int J Radiat Oncol Biol Phys* 1997;38:667–672.

# 2

# OPTIMIZATION OF INTENSITY-MODULATED RADIATION THERAPY TREATMENT PLANNING

## PING XIA

## 1. FORWARD TREATMENT PLANNING

- Intensity-modulated radiation therapy treatment (IMRT) plans can be created by using either the "forward planning" or the "inverse planning" method.[1] Figure 2-1 shows a flow chart depicting both forward and inverse planning processes.
- The forward planning method is similar to the method normally used in conventional three-dimensional conformal radiation therapy (3DCRT). In this method, planners first specify beam directions, shapes, and intensities (or weightings), and the computer calculates the resulting dose distributions. The planners then manually adjust beam directions, bean shapes, and beam intensities on the basis of their planning experience and intuition.
- The forward planning method works well for tumors with simple shapes (e.g., brain tumors) that are not surrounded by numerous critical structures. For complex tumor geometries (e.g., concave tumors and tumors surrounded by sensitive structures), the forward planning method may be limited by the experience of the individual planner and the restricted beam intensity variation inside each beam.
- One step beyond forward planning is the so-called aperture-based optimization, in which the planner designs one or several beam shapes for each beam angle, and computer optimization determines the intensities (or weightings) of these beam shapes in all beam angles.[2] Another variation of the aperture-based optimization is for the planner to select the number of segments (subfields) allowed for each beam and for computer optimization to determine the shape of each segment and its associated intensity (or weighting).[3]
- The advantage of the aperture-based optimization method is that the planner can control the complexity of a treatment, yet the plan quality is less dependent on the expertise of the individual planner as in forward planning. For tumor sites that are not involved with many sensitive structures, such as the breast or brain, this approach may have advantages with comparable plan quality when compared with plans produced by inverse planning, but with much simpler treatment delivery.[4]

## 2. INVERSE TREATMENT PLANNING

- The inverse planning method starts with a desired dose distribution and finishes with fluence distributions that, when taken together, approximate the desired dose distribution.[5] The main differences between forward planning and inverse planning are that the plan quality is evaluated by a score rather than by the planner's intuition and that the number of parameters adjusted by the computer is extremely large in inverse planning.
- Inverse planning includes three key components: formulation of the score function, input of dose constraints to the tumor targets and normal organs of interests, and methods of computer optimization that search for optimal plans.
- The computer optimizer first divides each broad beam into many pixels ("beamlets" or "pencil beams") and then iteratively adjusts the relative weight of each pixel. Figure 2-2 illustrates how a $2 \times 2$ cm$^2$ broad beam is divided into four $1 \times 1$ cm$^2$ beamlets.
- A score, defined by a cost function, evaluates the quality of a plan. The cost function is usually defined as the square of the difference between the current dose distributions and the desired dose distributions, summed over all points of interest.[6]
- Specification of dose constraints for each clinical case is to specify the parameters in the cost function, although the formulation of the cost function in most inverse planning systems is predetermined. Specification of dose constraints, therefore, is the only direct input from users to the inverse planning system. Table 2-1 shows a set of dose constraints for a patient with head and neck cancer.

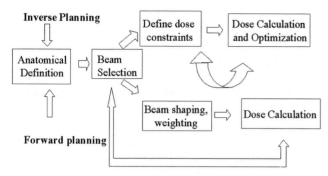

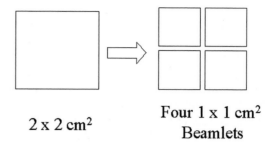

**FIGURE 2-2.** A 2 × 2 cm² broad beam is divided into four 1 × 1 cm² beamlets.

**FIGURE 2-1.** Flow chart for both forward and inverse planning processes.

As shown in Table 2-1, inverse planning requires planners to specify a 3D dose distribution with numeric values of dose constraints. The spatial description is missing in these numeric values.

- The methods used for computer optimization can be either deterministic or stochastic.[7,8] The deterministic optimization only accepts a change in plan with a decreased value of the cost function. With a probability, the stochastic optimization may accept a change in plan with an increase of the cost function.

- The deterministic algorithms often lead to a rapid descent toward a minimum cost that is interpreted as the optimum plan. However, if there are multiple minima in the cost function distribution, the deterministic optimization method may interpret a local minimum cost as the optimum plan. In this situation, only stochastic optimization methods can find the global minimum of the cost function.[6,9]

## 3. TUMOR TARGET AND SENSITIVE STRUCTURE DELINEATIONS

- IMRT plans generated through inverse planning critically depend on the delineation of tumor target volumes and sensitive structures of interest. The target delineation in IMRT, therefore, becomes very important. Radiation oncologists and planners (physicists or dosimetrists) work closely as a team to determine what to treat, what to spare, and how to compromise if conflicts arise.[10]

- It is often necessary to use multiple-image modalities to delineate target volume, such as magnetic resonance imaging spectroscopy (MRIS), and positron emission tomography scans. If necessary, an imaging fusion tool can be used to translate tumor volumes from other image modalities to the planning computed tomography (CT) images. It must be kept in mind, however, that the image

**TABLE 2-1. PLANNING DOSE CONSTRAINTS USED FOR AN ADVANCED CASE OF NASOPHARYNGEAL CANCER**

| Targets | Goal | Volume Below | Minimum Dose | Maximum Dose | Structure Type |
|---|---|---|---|---|---|
| PTV-GTV | 70.0 Gy | 5% | 59.4 Gy | 75.0 Gy | Basic |
| PTV-CTV | 59.4 Gy | 5% | 58.0 Gy | 70.0 Gy | Basic |

| Structures | Limits | Volume Above | Minimum Dose | Maximum Dose | Type |
|---|---|---|---|---|---|
| Spinal cord | 40.0 Gy | 5% | 10.0 Gy | 45.0 Gy | Basic |
| Brainstem | 43.0 Gy | 5% | 25.0 Gy | 54.0 Gy | Basic |
| Parotid glands | 22.0 Gy | 30% | 15.0 Gy | 60.0 Gy | Parallel |
| Chiasm | 48.0 Gy | 2% | 25.0 Gy | 52.0 Gy | Basic |
| Optic nerve | 34.4 Gy | 5% | 25.0 Gy | 42.0 Gy | Basic |
| Eye | 22.0 Gy | 5% | 15.0 Gy | 35.0 Gy | Basic |
| Lens | 4.0 Gy | 2% | 2.0 Gy | 8.0 Gy | Expendable |
| Ear | 49.6 Gy | 50% | 25.0 Gy | 60.0 Gy | Expendable |
| Tongue | 50.0 Gy | 10% | 30.0 Gy | 60.0 Gy | Expendable |
| Temporal lobe | 50.0 Gy | 5% | 25.0 Gy | 60.0 Gy | Basic |
| Mandible | 50.0 Gy | 33% | 30.0 Gy | 55.0 Gy | Expendable |
| Larynx | 45.0 Gy | 10% | 25.0 Gy | 55.0 Gy | Expendable |
| TMJs | 38.0 Gy | 50% | 30.0 Gy | 60.0 Gy | Expendable |
| Neck skin | 55.0 Gy | 10% | 30.0 Gy | 60.0 Gy | Expendable |

PTV, planning target volume; GTV, gross tumor volume; TMJ, temporomandibular joint.

fusion tool from commercial treatment planning systems may not register two image sets precisely, particularly when the patients are in different positions during the image acquisitions.

■ Precisely delineating sensitive structures becomes a new and important task in inverse planning. To advise the optimization algorithm how to form desired 3D dose distributions, many normal tissues in the vicinity of the tumor target volume should be explicitly contoured.

■ Both radiation oncologists and planners should possess an adequate knowledge of cross-sectional image anatomy.

■ Sensitive structures can be divided into parallel organs and serial organs. A parallel organ will lose its functionality only if all the subvolumes of the organ are damaged. A serial organ will be damaged even if only one of its subvolumes is damaged.

■ Because of the different characteristics between parallel organ and serial organs, it is important to contour the entire parallel organ even if a portion of the organ is not proximal to the target volume. Table 2-2 lists example parallel and serial organs contoured for a typical nasopharyngeal case.

## 4. MARGINS

■ Delineation of beam and tumor volume margins is another challenge in inverse-planned IMRT because the block shapes cannot be directly adjusted to tighten or loosen margins. Margins to account for tumor localization and patient positioning uncertainties (referred to as

**TABLE 2-2. EXAMPLES OF PARALLEL AND SERIAL ORGANS INVOLVED IN A TYPICAL CASE OF NASOPHARYNGEAL CANCER**

| Structures | Organs |
| --- | --- |
| Serial | Spinal cord |
| | Brainstem |
| | Optic chiasm |
| | Optic nerves (Rt, Lt) |
| | Optic lens (Rt, Lt) |
| | Brain |
| | Eyes (Rt, Lt) |
| | Mandible |
| | Temporal lobes |
| Parallel | Parotid glands (Rt, Lt) |
| | Ears (Rt, Lt) |
| | TMJs (Rt, Lt) |
| Others | Tongue |
| | Oral cavity |
| | Larynx |
| | Neck skin |
| | Posterior neck |
| | Airway |

TMJ, temporomandibular joint; Rt, right; Lt, left.

tumor margins) must be explicitly specified during planning. In addition, margins to account for beam penumbra (referred to as beam margins) are often included during optimization.

■ In conventional radiotherapy, margins include both the tumor margins and the beam margins. Depending on the specific beam energy and linear accelerator, the beam penumbra for a single beam is approximately 6 to 8 mm.[11] If a margin of 1.5 cm is used in conventional planning, a margin of 0.8 cm should be specified in the inverse planning to account for tumor localization and patient positioning uncertainties.

■ Similar to the tumor margins, one can also create individual margins for each sensitive structure to achieve better sensitive sparing. For example, the Radiation Therapy Oncology Group protocols for oropharyngeal and nasopharyngeal cancers suggest using 0.5-cm margins for the spinal cord.

■ 2D or 3D tumor margins can be created. 2D tumor margins are created by expanding the tumor contours in every image slice and manually extrapolating the tumor volume in the superior and inferior directions. A computer program (as a tool in planning systems) can create 3D tumor margins by expanding the entire tumor volume in three dimensions. The computer program interpolates tumor volumes from multiple image slices. Figure 2-3 demonstrates the differences between 2D and 3D tumor margins for two involved lymph nodes in a patient with head and neck cancer. In Figure 2-3B, the planning system interpolated the tumor volume from its neighboring images to create 3-mm 3D margins.

■ In principle, 3D tumor margins are more accurate than 2D tumor margins when taking into account patient positioning and tumor target localization uncertainties. The clinical tumor volume plus the 3D margins are considered the planning target volume (PTV).

■ Some planning systems (i.e., Pinnical ADAC System, Phillips Medical Systems, Bothell, WA) can create such PTVs explicitly, allowing planners to directly give dose constraints to the PTV. Other inverse planning systems (i.e., Corvus 5.0, NOMOS Corp., Sewickley, PA) are not able to create PTVs explicitly before computer optimization. To control the dose constraints to the PTV in the latter planning systems, planners may create a PTV explicitly by expanding the clinical target volume (CTV) in every image slice.

## 5. DOSE CONSTRAINTS

■ Specification of dose constraints is the only direct input from users to steer the inverse planning system toward the desired plan in their minds. Unrealistic constraints may lead the computer optimization to produce an inferior plan.

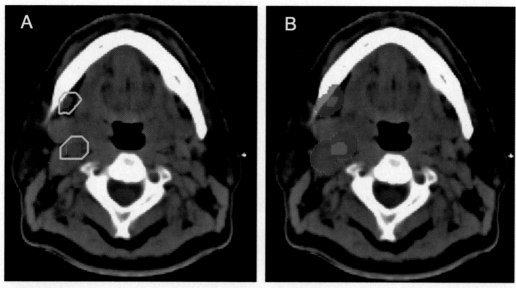

**FIGURE 2-3. A:** Two lymph nodes in red with 3-mm two-dimensional margins (*light blue*). **B:** Two lymph nodes in red with 3-mm three-dimensional margins (*red*).

- To specify appropriate dose constraints, planners should learn the relationship between the dose constraints and resulting dose distributions for the specific inverse planning system they are using. This learning process involves a systematic trial and error approach, which is often less intuitive than the trial and error planning process involved in 3DCRT planning.

- For a typical case of head and neck cancer with a centrally located tumor volume, one can start a plan with nine equally spaced axial beam angles and five non-zero intensity levels for each beam. These geometric parameters are often sufficient to produce a high-quality plan, although a careful beam angle selection can reduce the number of beams or complexity of intensity modulation of each beam while keeping the same quality of the plan (to be discussed later).[12]

- In these geometric parameter settings, a case with advanced stage nasopharyngeal cancer is presented as an example. Figure 2-4 displays the tumor volumes in selected axial, coronal, and sagittal images. In this particular case, the PTV-gross tumor volume (GTV) and the PTV-CTV were delineated in each axial image by an attending radiation oncologist. Table 2-1 lists planning dose constraints, developed on the basis of our previous planning experience for nasopharyngeal cancer with a commercial treatment planning system (Corvus, NOMOS Corp., Sewickley, PA).[13] In this planning system, the relative weighting factors were associated with the type of structure (last column of Table 2-1). In order of importance, the two basic types of a tumor are homogenous and basic; the three basic types of sensitive structures are critical, basic, parallel, and expendable.

- The treatment goal for this example case is to deliver a dose of 70 Gy to more than 95% of the PTV-70 and a

dose of 59.4 Gy to more than 95% of the PTV-59.4 simultaneously. The evaluation endpoint for serial sensitive structures is the maximum dose, and the evaluation endpoint for parallel sensitive structures is the mean dose. Table 2-3 lists the expected tolerance endpoint doses for selected sensitive structures.

- The most time-consuming part of IMRT planning is to find a compromise between the dose coverage of the tumor volumes and the sparing of the sensitive structures. A systematic trial and error approach is the only way to accomplish this.

- In Trial 1 for the example case, the top priority is given to the tumor target coverage, which associates heavier weighting factors for all tumor volumes (choose "homogeneity" for the tumor volumes). The weighting factor for all sensitive structures is relatively lower (choose "expendable" for all sensitive structures) in comparison with the tumor volumes. The resultant endpoint doses for the tumor coverage and selective important sensitive structures are shown in Table 2-4. The prescription isodose line is chosen in such a way that at least 95% of the GTV and CTV are adequately covered by the prescribed doses. The maximum dose is normalized as 100%.

- In Trial 1, the focus was on finding the best dose uniformity for the tumor targets without emphasis on sensitive structures. Not surprisingly, the resultant endpoint doses of the sensitive structures, especially the serial structures, exceeded their tolerance. This plan is not clinically acceptable, but does display the best achievable dose uniformity for the tumor targets.

- In Trial 2 the critical sensitive structures, such as the spinal cord, brainstem, optic chiasm, and optic nerves, were given heavier weights (choose "critical" for the

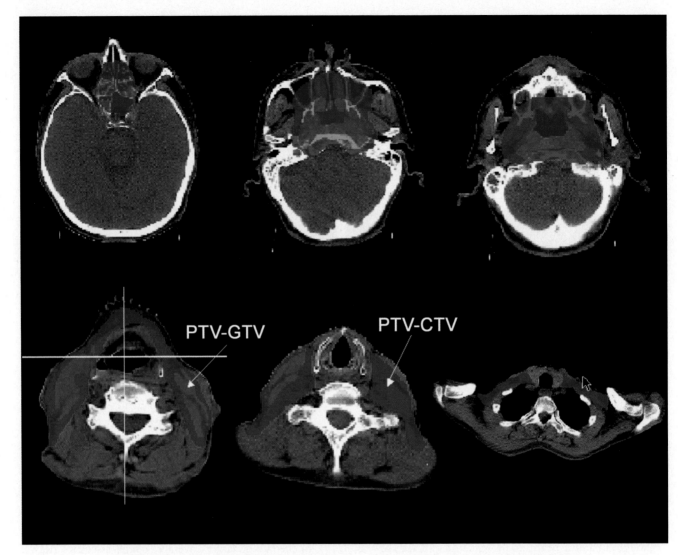

**FIGURE 2-4.** Isodose distributions for the example case of nasopharyngeal cancer in multiple images. *Aqua-blue:* 79.2 Gy, *dark-blue:* 70.0 Gy, *yellow:* 59.4 Gy, *red:* 54.0 Gy, *green:* 45.0 Gy.

## TABLE 2-3.  BASIC PLAN ACCEPTANCE CRITERIA FOR CASES OF HEAD AND NECK CANCER

|  |  | Priority* |
| --- | --- | --- |
| PTV-GTV | >95% volume received Rx dose<br>>99% volume received 93% of Rx dose | 2 |
| PTV-CTV | >95% volume received Rx dose<br>>99% of volume received 93% of Rx dose | 2 |
| Spinal cord | Maximum <45 Gy, or no more than 1 cc of volume >45 Gy | 1 |
| Brainstem | Maximum <54 Gy, or no more than 1% of volume >54 Gy | 1 |
| Optic structures | Maximum <54 Gy | 2 |
| Eye/retina | Maximum <50 Gy | 3 |
| Parotid glands | Mean <26 Gy, or 50% of volume <30 Gy | 3 |
| Mandible | Maximum <70 Gy, or no more than 1 cc of volume >70 Gy | 3 |

PTV, planning target volume; GTV, gross tumor volume; CTV, clinical target volume; Rx, treatment.
* 1 is the highest priority.

**TABLE 2-4. SELECTED ENDPOINT DOSES (GY) FOR A CASE OF NASOPHARYNGEAL CANCER IN FOUR EXAMPLE TRIALS**

|  | Trial 1 | Trial 2 | Trial 3 | Trial 4 |
|---|---|---|---|---|
| Rx-IDL | 88% | 85% | 81% | 84% |
| Spinal cord | 68.0 | 41.2 | 45.4 | 42.1 |
| Brainstem | 68.4 | 53.1 | 57.5 | 53.7 |
| Left OPN | 58.5 | 43.7 | 47.5 | 45.4 |
| Right OPN | 56.9 | 43.2 | 48.8 | 45.9 |
| Mandible | 73.2 | 70.4 | 66.1 | 67.1 |
| Right eye | 53.7 | 44.9 | 39.3 | 38.3 |
| Left eye | 48.9 | 42.2 | 38.9 | 35.0 |
| Optic chiasm | 60.5 | 52.3 | 55.3 | 52.5 |
| Left parotid | 41.9 | 32.4 | 28.6 | 26.3 |
| Right parotid | 42.1 | 33.9 | 29.1 | 27.5 |

Rx-IDL, percentage isodose line prescribed to gross tumor volume; OPN, optic nerve.

structure type); the other sensitive structures were assigned lower weighting factors (choose "expendable" for the structure type); and the tumor volumes were designated with the "basic" type. The resultant endpoints are also shown in Table 2-4.

- Trial 2 focuses on the lowest possible doses for the critical structures at a cost of reduced dose uniformity inside the tumor targets and at a cost of sparing of other sensitive structures. The resultant endpoint doses are listed in Table 2-4. In this trial, the endpoint doses for the spinal cord, brainstem, and optic structures are significantly reduced compared with the corresponding endpoint doses in Trial 1. The dose uniformity inside targets is decreased from 88% to 85%. The drawback of this plan is that the mean dose to the parotid glands exceeds the desired dose limit of 26 Gy. This trial shows the lowest possible dose for the critical structures.

- In Trial 3, all sensitive structures and tumor volumes are assigned with the basic type of structure. The resultant endpoint doses are also listed in Table 2-4. In this plan, the dose uniformity is reduced to 81%, and the maximum dose to the brainstem is increased to 57.5 Gy. This plan demonstrates that to obtain a reasonable plan, one has to give priority to protecting some critical structures.

- In Trial 4, some structures are assigned with less weighting factors, such as the expendable structures. The resultant endpoint doses are listed in Table 2-4. Figure 2-5 shows isodose distributions in several axial, coronal, and sagittal images. Figure 2-6 displays the dose-volume histograms (DVHs).

- These trial-and-error processes can be initially time-consuming. After learning the relationship between the dose constraints and the resulting dose distributions for the specific inverse planning system, one can develop a disease-specific dose constraint template. Table 2-1 is a dose constraint template developed in our institution for advanced stage nasopharyngeal cancer. Because of the patient-to-patient anatomic variations, however, the dose constraint templates can only be used as good starting points. With a good starting point, one can reduce the number of trials from an average of five to ten per patient plan to an average of two to five per patient plan.

## 6. PLAN EVALUATION

- The tools required to evaluate an IMRT plan are similar to those required for a 3DCRT plan, including dose distributions displayed on each CT image and a DVH of each structure with defined endpoints, such as the maximum, minimum, and mean doses. Some treatment planning systems will automatically generate a statistics report of the maximum, minimum, and mean doses, and percentage of the volume exceeding planning dose limits. Figure 2-7 is a statistics report for some structures in the Trial 4 plan for the example case discussed in the previous section. This report can be a useful tool for a quick plan evaluation, provided the planner knows the plan acceptance criteria (to be discussed in the next section).

- For an inverse IMRT plan, planners often examine the statistics spreadsheet first to assess whether the plan acceptance criteria are met. DVH information is also used for evaluating the fraction of the defined volumes receiving high and low doses.

- If the criteria are met, planners further examine the dose distribution displayed in each CT image and pay special attention to the dose conformity and locations of hot and cold spots.

- If the criteria are not met, one should find out what the key limiting factors are. The first step is to examine whether there are dose constraints that are physically impossible to achieve. It is useful to remember that the most achievable dose gradient for a single beam is approximately 10% per millimeter. Scatter doses from other beams in a treatment plan that uses multiple beams and the leakage dose from the multileaf collimator make the dose gradient shallower than 10% per millimeter. For example, if the spinal cord is adjacent to the CTV, it would be impractical to require the maximum dose of the cord to be less than 50% of the prescribed CTV dose without underdosing the CTV.

- To control the spatial dose distribution, contouring additional structures is helpful. For example, to deposit a

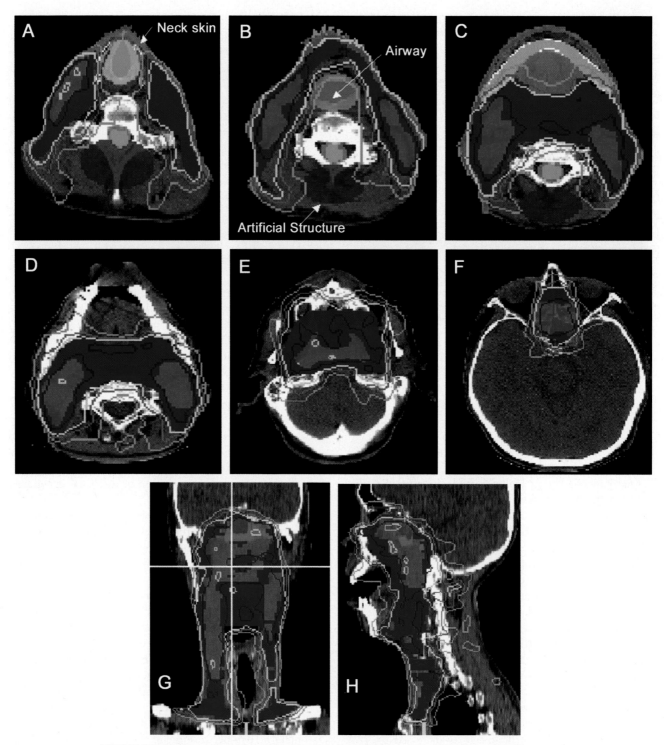

**FIGURE 2-5.** Tumor volumes for a case of nasopharyngeal cancer in selected axial **(A–F)**, coronal **(G)**, and sagittal images **(H)**. PTV-GTV, planning target volume of the gross tumor volume (*red*); PTV-CTV, planning target volume of the clinical target volume (*purple*).

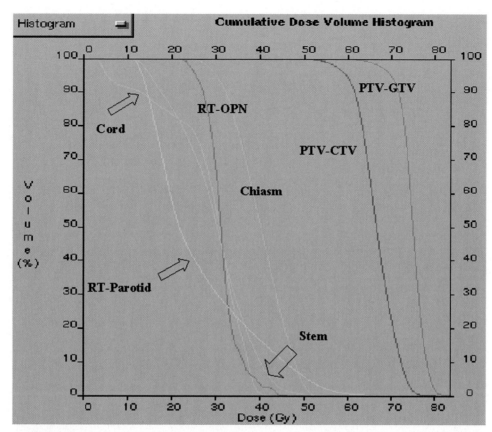

**FIGURE 2-6.** Dose-volume histograms (DVHs) for the PTV-GTV, PTV-CTV, brainstem, spinal cord, optic chiasm, right optic nerve, and right parotid gland. The DVHs for the left optic nerve and parotid gland are omitted because of the similarity to the right side of the organs. PTV-GTV, planning target volume of the gross tumor volume; PTV-CTV, planning target volume of the clinical target volume.

hot spot into a specific region inside the target, one can contour that part of the target separately and allow a relatively large dose inhomogeneity in it. Likewise, defining subsections of a sensitive structure, especially a large volume structure, can also improve spatial dose distributions. In Figure 2-5, to control the dose distribution in the posterior neck, an artificial structure was contoured in that area. Defining these subsections is a useful strategy to control the special dose distributions because most cost functions used in inverse planning lack spatial information.

## 7. PLAN ACCEPTANCE CRITERIA

- Plan acceptance criteria for each specific site should be developed among attending physicians, planners, and therapists according to clinical requirements, physics limitations, and practical limitations.
- The basic plan acceptance criteria for cases of head and neck cancer that were developed in our institution are listed in Table 2-3. In addition to these criteria, the min-

imum prescription isodose line to the PTV-GTV (which often receives a higher dose than the PTV-CTV) should be greater than 80% and the maximum dose should be normalized to 100%, reflecting allowable dose uniformity inside the target.

- Plan acceptance criteria developed on the basis of the Radiation Therapy Oncology Group protocol of H0225 for nasopharyngeal cancer can be found at their website (www.rtog.org).

## 8. BEAM ANGLE SELECTIONS

- As mentioned in the previous section, for a centrally located tumor such as nasopharyngeal cancer, one can often start a plan with nine equally spaced axial beam angles and five non-zero intensity levels for each beam, because these geometric parameters are often sufficient to produce a high-quality plan.[12] A careful beam angle selection can reduce the number of beams or complexity of intensity modulation of each beam while maintaining the same quality of the plan.

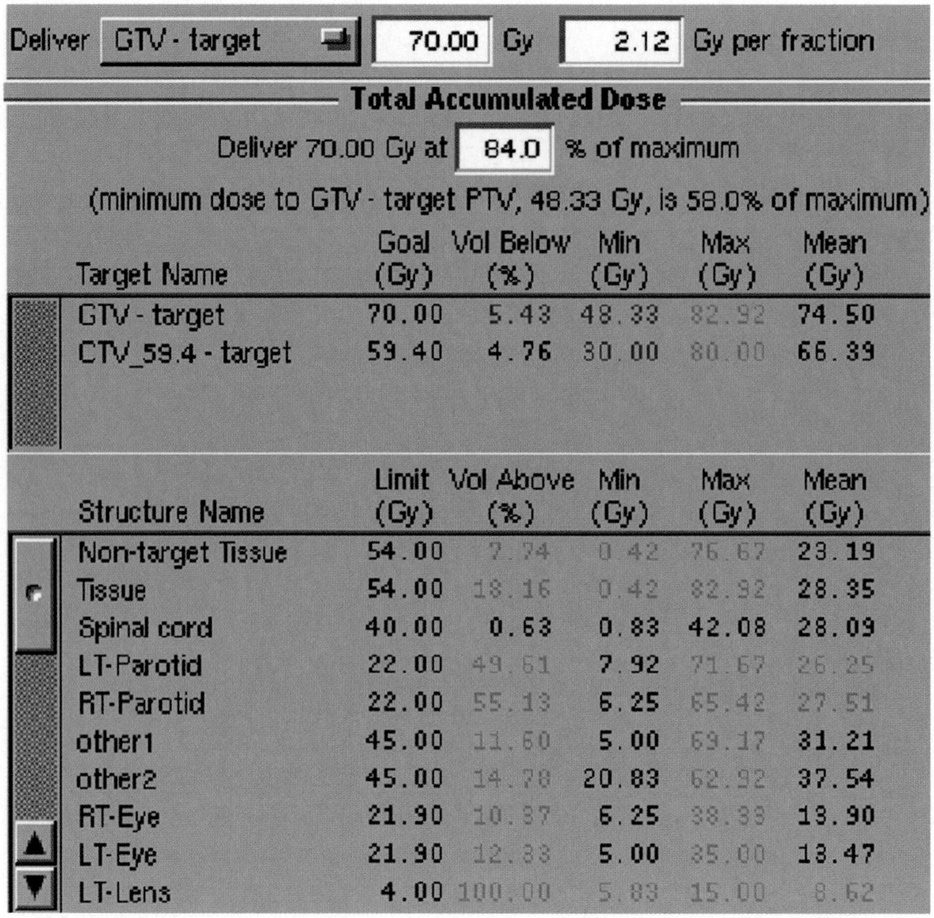

Deliver GTV - target 70.00 Gy 2.12 Gy per fraction

Total Accumulated Dose

Deliver 70.00 Gy at 84.0 % of maximum

(minimum dose to GTV - target PTV, 48.33 Gy, is 58.0% of maximum)

| Target Name | Goal (Gy) | Vol Below (%) | Min (Gy) | Max (Gy) | Mean (Gy) |
|---|---|---|---|---|---|
| GTV - target | 70.00 | 5.43 | 48.33 | 82.92 | 74.50 |
| CTV_59.4 - target | 59.40 | 4.76 | 30.00 | 80.00 | 66.39 |

| Structure Name | Limit (Gy) | Vol Above (%) | Min (Gy) | Max (Gy) | Mean (Gy) |
|---|---|---|---|---|---|
| Non-target Tissue | 54.00 | 7.74 | 0.42 | 76.67 | 23.19 |
| Tissue | 54.00 | 18.16 | 0.42 | 82.92 | 28.35 |
| Spinal cord | 40.00 | 0.63 | 0.83 | 42.08 | 28.09 |
| LT-Parotid | 22.00 | 49.61 | 7.92 | 71.67 | 26.25 |
| RT-Parotid | 22.00 | 55.13 | 6.25 | 65.42 | 27.51 |
| other1 | 45.00 | 11.60 | 5.00 | 69.17 | 31.21 |
| other2 | 45.00 | 14.78 | 20.83 | 62.92 | 37.54 |
| RT-Eye | 21.90 | 10.37 | 6.25 | 38.33 | 13.90 |
| LT-Eye | 21.90 | 12.33 | 5.00 | 35.00 | 13.47 |
| LT-Lens | 4.00 | 100.00 | 5.83 | 15.00 | 8.62 |

**FIGURE 2-7.** Statistics report excerpt for the example case of nasopharyngeal cancer.

- With the dose constraints listed in Table 2-1, the example nasopharyngeal case was planned with fifteen, eleven, nine, and eight beam angles. However, the eight beam angles were not arranged with an equally spaced separation, whereas the other beam angles were arranged in an equally spaced separation. The eight beam angles were 0, 50, 90, 140, 220, 260, 290, and 330 degrees (with 0 degrees for anterior-posterior direction).
- Table 2-5 lists the resultant endpoint doses for the selected structures and shows that increasing the number of beams from nine to fifteen did not significantly improve the plan quality, whereas the quality of the plan with eight beam angles was comparable to the other plans.
- The basic principles in beam angle selection that are used in 3DCRT forward planning are still valid in inverse planning, including choosing the shortest pathway to irradiate the tumor, avoiding direct irradiation to the critical structures, and keeping a large beam separation if possible. Because of the power of intensity modulation, the third principle in inverse planning is more important than the other two principles.

**TABLE 2-5. SELECTED ENDPOINT DOSES (GY) FOR A NASOPHARYNGEAL CASE PLANNED WITH FOUR DIFFERENT NUMBERS OF BEAM ANGLES**

| No. of Beams | Cord | Brainstem | Left OPN | Right OPN | Mandible | Right Eye | Left Eye | Chiasm | Left Parotid | Right Parotid |
|---|---|---|---|---|---|---|---|---|---|---|
| 15 | 42.6 | 54.4 | 44.3 | 46.8 | 68.7 | 39.2 | 36.3 | 52.7 | 26.6 | 28.4 |
| 11 | 41.9 | 52.5 | 45.2 | 46.0 | 68.0 | 38.7 | 38.7 | 53.7 | 25.2 | 26.3 |
| 9 | 42.1 | 53.7 | 45.4 | 45.9 | 67.1 | 38.3 | 35.0 | 52.5 | 26.3 | 27.5 |
| 8 | 43.3 | 54.7 | 46.4 | 46.8 | 71.3 | 39.8 | 35.9 | 56.0 | 28.0 | 28.1 |

OPN, optic nerve.

**TABLE 2-6. ESTIMATED TREATMENT TIME, TOTAL MONITOR UNITS, AND TOTAL NUMBER OF SEGMENTS FOR FOUR PLANS WITH DIFFERENT NUMBERS OF BEAM ANGLES**

| No. of Beams | Rx-IDL | No. of Segments | No. of MUs | Treatment Time (min) |
|---|---|---|---|---|
| 15 | 83% | 284 | 1,868 | 37.6 |
| 11 | 86% | 203 | 1,680 | 28.1 |
| 9 | 84% | 155 | 1,467 | 22.1 |
| 8 | 80% | 140 | 1,529 | 20.7 |

Rx-IDL, percentage isodose line prescribed to gross tumor volume; MU, monitor unit.

- It is also true that inverse planning requires more beam angles than conventional planning in obtaining a similar quality plan. For example, two tangential beams are good choices for the treatment of breast cancer. By using the same two tangential beams, however, the inverse planning system cannot create a plan comparable to the conventional plans because of the lack of variables in optimization.
- To make use of more beam variables, directly opposing beams are less useful in inverse planning.

## 9. TREATMENT TIME CONSIDERATIONS

- Although pressured to produce good-quality plans, planners can easily create a complex treatment plan by using more than ten beams in inverse planning. Both clinicians and planners should carefully assess the balance between the plan quality and efficiency and accuracy of treatment delivery.
- For the plans that use eight, nine, eleven, and fifteen beam angles, Table 2-6 lists the estimated treatment time, total number of segments, and total monitor units (MUs). The treatment time was estimated on the basis of Siemens linear accelerators by using a step-and-shoot delivery technique, including the pausing time between segments (6 seconds), 300 MU per minute dose rate, and pausing time between gantry angles (12 seconds).
- As seen in Table 2-6, the plan with fifteen beam angles requires the longest treatment time and the largest total MUs, yet the quality of the plan did not significantly improve when compared with the plans with less beam angles (Table 2-5).
- Complex plans that use many beams and great levels of intensity modulations increase "indirect radiation" to the patient because of scatter and leakage doses. These indirect radiation doses cannot be predicted accurately in the currently dose calculation algorithms.[14]

- Therefore, complex IMRT plans may introduce larger dosimetric uncertainties than the simple plans and decrease radiation efficiency. The decrease in radiation efficiency results in prolonged treatment time and increased total body dose to the patient.
- Radiation oncologists should attempt to keep the plan as simple as possible by using less beam angles whenever possible and should always challenge the planner to try another plan by using less beams while keeping the same quality of plans.
- Radiation oncologists should also bear in mind to accept a plan with a reasonable delivery time. Estimated treatment time depends on the specific treatment machines and IMRT delivery techniques. In our institution, we prefer to keep a maximum treatment time less than 30 minutes, not including patient setup time.

## REFERENCES

1. Intensity Modulated Radiation Therapy Collaborative Working Group. Intensity-modulated radiotherapy: current status and issues of interest. *Int J Radiat Oncol Biol Phys* 2001;51:880–914.
2. Xiao Y, Galvin J, Hossain M, et al. An optimized forward-planning technique for intensity modulated radiation therapy. *Med Phys* 2000;27:2093–2099.
3. Shepard DM, Earl MA, Li XA, et al. Direct aperture optimization: a turnkey solution for step-and-shoot IMRT. *Med Phys* 2002;29:1007–1018.
4. Vicini FA, Sharpe M, Kestin L, et al. Optimizing breast cancer treatment efficacy with intensity-modulated radiotherapy. *Int J Radiat Oncol Biol Phys* 2002;54:1336–1344.
5. Brahme A. Optimization of stationary and moving beam radiation therapy techniques. *Radiother Oncol* 1988;12:129–140.
6. Bortfeld T. Optimized planning using physical objectives and constraints. *Semin Radiat Oncol* 1999;9:20–34.
7. Spirou SV, Chui CS. A gradient inverse planning algorithm with dose-volume constraints. *Med Phys* 1998;25:321–333.
8. Webb S. Optimizing the planning of intensity-modulated radiotherapy. *Phys Med Biol* 1994;39:2229–2246.
9. Wu Q, Mohan R. Multiple local minima in IMRT optimization based on dose-volume criteria. *Med Phys* 2002;29:1514–1527.
10. Eisbruch A, Marsh LH, Martel MK, et al. Comprehensive irradiation of head and neck cancer using conformal multisegmental fields: assessment of target coverage and noninvolved tissue sparing. *Int J Radiat Oncol Biol Phys* 1998;41:559–568.
11. Huq MS, Das IJ, Steinberg T, et al. A dosimetric comparison of various multileaf collimators. *Phys Med Biol* 2002;47:N159–170.
12. Stein J, Mohan R, Wang XH, et al. Number and orientations of beams in intensity-modulated radiation treatments. *Med Phys* 1997;24:149–160.
13. Lee N, Xia P, Quivey JM, et al. Intensity-modulated radiotherapy in the treatment of nasopharyngeal carcinoma: an update of the UCSF experience. *Int J Radiat Oncol Biol Phys* 2002;53:12–22.
14. Mohan R, Arnfield M, Tong S, et al. The impact of fluctuations in intensity patterns on the number of monitor units and the quality and accuracy of intensity modulated radiotherapy. *Med Phys* 2000;27:1226–1237.

# 3

# COMPUTED TOMOGRAPHY AND MAGNETIC RESONANCE IMAGING OF BRAIN, SKULL BASE, AND NECK CANCERS

## FRANZ J. WIPPOLD II

## 1. BASICS OF CROSS-SECTIONAL IMAGING

- Cross-sectional imaging has become an indispensable tool in the characterization and staging of brain, skull base, and neck pathology. Noninvasive imaging of these regions is currently performed with high-resolution rapid computed tomography (CT) and magnetic resonance imaging (MRI).
- In regard to the brain, MRI has emerged as the primary method for detailed evaluation of intraaxial and extraaxial lesions. CT is usually reserved for analyzing bony involvement and monitoring post-therapy complications such as hemorrhage and hydrocephalus.[1]
- In regard to the skull base and neck, both CT and MRI provide essential information about the deep extension of clinically detected masses, delineate additional clinically unsuspected lesions, assist in definitive therapy planning, and provide a method of surveillance after therapy.[2,3]

### 1.1. Computed Tomography Imaging

- CT uses x-rays and digital computer analysis of x-ray data to create cross-sectional images of the brain, skull base, and neck.

#### 1.1.1. Brain Imaging

- CT scanning of the brain should begin with an unenhanced survey of axial slices extending from the skull vertex to the skull base (Fig. 3-1).
- After intravenous contrast administration, the scan is repeated, covering skull vertex to skull base.
- Detailed scans including the use of thin slices, zoomed fields of view, and bone detail algorithms can be applied in special circumstances.

#### 1.1.2. Head and Neck Imaging

- CT scanning of the neck should begin with a general neck survey examination before more detailed and focused protocols.
- Scanning should cover the region from the base of the skull to the clavicles. A digital lateral scout radiograph may assist in planning.
- Spiral (helical) CT scanning, especially with multi-row detector scanners, permits rapid scanning of large volumes of tissues during quiet respiration.[4] Helical data permit optimal multiplanar and three-dimensional (3D) reconstructions.[5,6]
- Intravenous contrast administered with a power injector through a venous catheter is essential.
- Advanced CT techniques, such as 3DCT, may be useful for radiotherapy planning. With the use of special computer software, traces of selected anatomic structures are reformatted into a 3D-wire diagram that can then be manipulated to reveal the most optimum radiation port. This technique limits extraneous collateral radiation to other organs such as the salivary glands.[7]

### 1.2. Magnetic Resonance Imaging

- MRI uses magnetic fields and radio frequency to create cross-sectional images of the brain, skull base, and neck.

#### 1.2.1. Brain Imaging

- Imaging is best performed with a head coil.
- T1-weighted images display anatomic relationships (Fig. 3-2A). T1-weighted sagittal images are especially useful for evaluating the corpus callosum, sella, and foramen magnum. The T1-weighted sequence is also helpful for analyzing blood products.

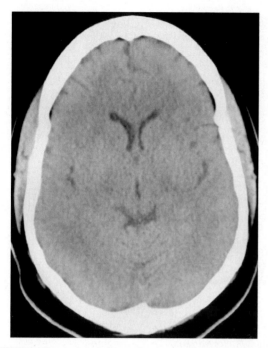

**FIGURE 3-1.** Normal unenhanced computed tomography (CT) of the brain. On axial imaging, the brain anatomy is symmetric in structure and density. Hypodense cerebrospinal fluid is contained within the ventricles and cisterns. Cerebral hemispheres and scalp soft tissues are intermediate density, and the skull is hyperdense.

- Fluid-attenuated inversion recovery (FLAIR) (Fig. 3-2B) and T2-weighted images (Fig. 3-2C) portray edema especially well.[8]
- Gadolinium-enhancing T1-weighted images (Fig. 3-2D and E) improve delineation of tumor margins. Enhancement also assists in post-therapy detection of tumor recurrence and radiation necrosis identification.[9]
- MR spectroscopy uses MRI data to quantify tissue metabolites. Diffusion-weighted images, perfusion images, T2-weighted gradient images, and functional images all have special roles in specific problem solving, such as the detection of infarcted tissue or the presence of blood.

### 1.2.2. Head and Neck Imaging

- MRI limited to the suprahyoid neck region and base of the skull can be performed with a head coil. Examinations that include the infrahyoid region require a neck coil.
- T1-weighted images display anatomic relationships and detect lesions such as lymph nodes embedded within fat. T1-weighted coronal images define the false cords, true cords, laryngeal ventricle, and floor of the mouth.[10] T1-weighted sagittal images are useful for evaluating the preepiglottic space, paraglottic spaces, and nasopharynx.
- T2-weighted images characterize tissue, detect tumor within muscle, demonstrate cysts, and assist differentiation of post-therapy fibrosis from recurrent tumor.[11]
- Gadolinium-enhanced T1-weighted images improve delineation of margins in many tumors,[12] although lesions

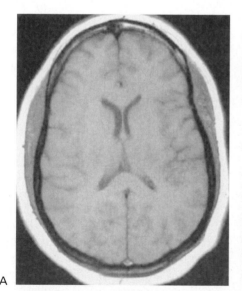
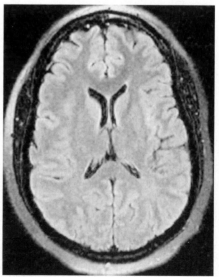

A                                                                          B

**FIGURE 3-2.** Normal magnetic resonance imaging (MRI) of the brain. **A:** T1-weighted axial image. Cerebrospinal fluid is hypointense compared with the cerebral hemispheres. Cortical bone, such as the inner and outer table of the calvarium, is markedly hypointense without evidence of signal. Fat within the scalp and diploic space of the calvarium is hyperintense on this sequence. **B:** Fluid-attenuated inversion recovery (FLAIR) image. This T2-weighted sequence displays cerebrospinal fluid as hypointense rather than hyperintense. The advantage of this sequence is the conspicuity of periventricular lesions. FLAIR imaging is excellent for tracking edema and gliosis.

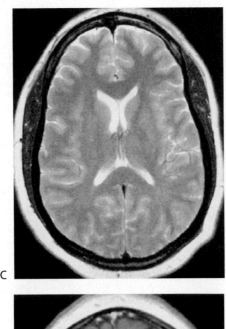

C

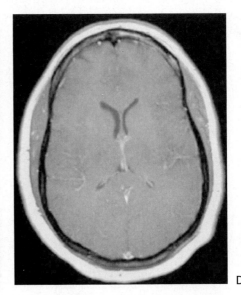

D

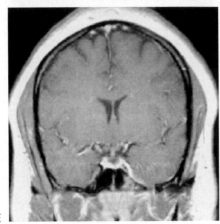

E

**FIGURE 3-2.** *(continued)* **C:** T2-weighted image. The conventional fast spin echo T2-weighted sequence displays fluid as hyperintense. Gray matter is slightly hyperintense compared with the white matter. **D:** Enhanced T1-weighted image. After administration of intravenous gadolinium, vascular structures typically enhance. This sequence is excellent for identifying blood–brain barrier breakdown, such as seen in tumors and other pathologies. **E:** Coronal-enhanced T1-weighted image. This image demonstrates the multiplanar capability of MRI. Display of pathology in three planes is possible with MRI.

embedded in fat may be obscured unless fat-saturation techniques are used (Fig. 3-3).[13] Enhanced normal aerodigestive mucosa may also obscure small mucosal tumors. Gadolinium-enhanced, fat-suppressed T1-weighted images are especially useful in staging nodal disease.

- The magnetization transfer technique uses the transfer of magnetization between restricted protons that are associated with macromolecules and free water protons to improve the contrast between lesions and background tissue.[14] Magnetization transfer may be useful in differentiating enhancing lesions from background tissue and in defining unenhanced lesions.

- New open-bore MRI units are being used for MRI guidance of biopsies.[15]

## 1.3. Comparison of Computed Tomography and Magnetic Resonance Imaging

- CT and MRI have different and often complementary roles. MRI is the preferred modality in brain imaging.[1]

Although both CT and MRI provide comparable anatomic information on the neck in most cases, CT is preferred as a screening modality.

- An advantage of CT includes the fast scanning speed, especially with the spiral technique, which enables rapid assessment of the patient who may be dyspneic from a comorbidity such as chronic airway obstruction. Spatial resolution of anatomy is superb with modern scanners. Calcifications are also well depicted (Fig. 3-4).

- Disadvantages of CT include limitation of scanning to the transverse plane, although the spiral-imaging technique has markedly improved coronal and sagittal reformation capabilities. Dental amalgam, metal instrumentation, and large shoulders may create annoying scan artifacts. Intravenous iodinated contrast agents used in CT carry a definite risk of anaphylaxis and further compromise of impaired renal function in select patients. The newer nonionic contrast agents may be safer than the older agents for use in patients with previous contrast reactions or compromised renal function.[16]

- The advantages of MRI include its superb soft tissue contrast, multiplanar display (Fig. 3-2), and minimal arti-

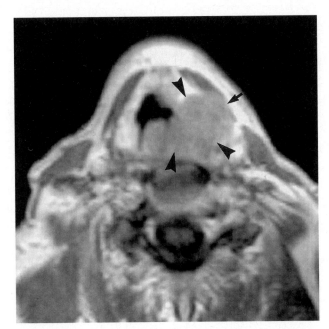

**FIGURE 3-3.** Transglottic carcinoma. Enhanced axial T1-weighted MRI demonstrating a supraglottic soft tissue mass (*arrowheads*) invading the left paraglottic space, left thyroid cartilage, and paraglottic muscles (*arrow*). Hyperintense fat on T1-weighted images provides excellent natural soft tissue contrast for detecting the less hyperintense tumor. (From: Wippold FJ II. Neck. In: Lee JKT, Sagel SS, Stanley RJ, et al., eds. *Computed Body Tomography with MRI Correlation, 3rd ed.* Philadelphia: Lippincott-Raven, 1998:107–182, with permission.)

facts from shoulders, dental amalgam, and densely calcified or ossified cartilages. Noniodinated gadolinium MRI enhancement compounds are generally well tolerated by individuals with impaired kidneys.[17] MRI is ideally suited for evaluation of the masticator, parapharyngeal, and parotid spaces, skull base, and floor of the mouth.[18]

- The disadvantages of MRI include degradation of images because of motion artifacts from breathing, carotid artery pulsations, swallowing, and often lengthy examinations.
- Contraindications for MRI include patients with cerebral aneurysm clips, cardiac pacemakers, or a history of intraorbital ferromagnetic foreign bodies.

## 1.4. Fundamentals of Interpretation

- Interpretation of cross-sectional imaging requires a thorough knowledge of normal brain, skull base, and neck anatomy and an appreciation of the changes that occur with surgery and radiation.
- The brain and neck tissues are symmetric in anatomy, image density, and signal intensity on axial images.
- Asymmetric soft tissue masses, CT densities, or MRI signal intensities should always be viewed with suspicion for tumor unless an alternative explanation such as atrophy, prior trauma, or an anatomic normal variant applies (Figs. 3-5 and 3-6).
- On CT images, brain tumors usually appear hypodense or isodense on unenhanced images and are frequently surrounded by hypodense edema. Occasionally, tumors may be hyperdense, especially if densely cellular or hemorrhagic. Tumors typically enhance with administration of intravenous iodine. Necrosis may be evident as a hypodense core.
- On CT images, neck tumors usually appear as dense, enhancing soft tissue abnormalities.

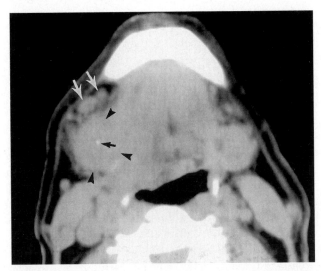

**FIGURE 3-4.** Submandibular nodes in a patient with sialadenitis. CT images showing multiple submandibular lymph nodes (*white arrows*) adjacent to an inflamed submandibular salivary gland (*arrowheads*). Note the calculus within the gland (*black arrow*).

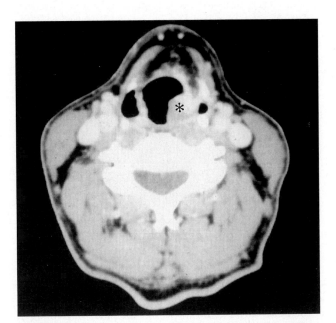

**FIGURE 3-5.** Carcinoma of the aryepiglottic fold. CT scan revealing asymmetric thickening of the left aryepiglottic fold (*asterisk*) caused by a supraglottic carcinoma of the larynx. Soft tissue asymmetry provides a helpful clue for identifying pathology. On CT images, tumors typically appear as dense soft tissue masses.

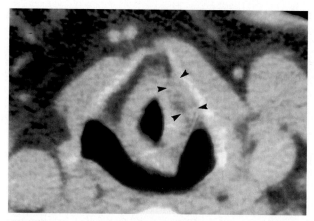

**FIGURE 3-6.** Supraglottic carcinoma. Axial CT scan reveals soft tissue density (*arrowheads*) within the fat of the paraglottic space. High-resolution CT imaging often reveals subtleties of pathologic anatomy not readily appreciated with conventional CT imaging. Soft tissue asymmetry is a helpful clue for detecting pathology. (From: Wippold FJ II. Neck. In: Lee JKT, Sagel SS, Stanley RJ, et al., eds. *Computed Body Tomography with MRI Correlation, 3rd ed.* Philadelphia: Lippincott-Raven, 1998:107–182, with permission.)

- On MRI, brain and neck tumors usually appear hypointense to isointense on T1-weighted images, hyperintense on T2-weighted images, and hyperintense on gadolinium-enhanced T1-weighted images (Fig. 3-3).
- Subtle soft tissue changes, hemorrhagic components, and anatomic variants may be misinterpreted by the untrained eye (Fig. 3-7). This issue is especially important in the patient with neck cancer in whom multiple sites of disease may coexist or in whom successful therapy has virtually eliminated the original pathology. In addition, many exceptions to the basic previously stated imaging appearances exist. For difficult cases, reliance on a trained neuroradiologist is crucial.

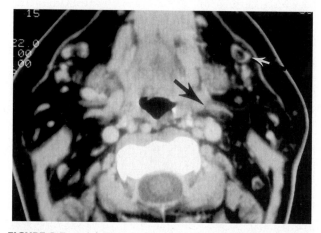

**FIGURE 3-7.** Axial CT scan demonstrating normal lymph nodes (*arrows*) with hypodense fat within the hila. These findings should not be confused with necrosis. (From: Wippold FJ II. Neck. In: Lee JKT, Sagel SS, Stanley RJ, et al., eds. *Computed Body Tomography with MRI Correlation, 3rd ed.* Philadelphia: Lippincott-Raven, 1998:107–182, with permission.)

## 2. IMAGING APPROACH TO BRAIN ANATOMY AND PATHOLOGY

### 2.1. Anatomy

- Brain anatomy can be conveniently divided into a supratentorial compartment containing the cerebral hemispheres and an infratentorial compartment containing the cerebellum and brainstem.[19,20]
- The cerebral hemispheres contain white matter surrounded by the gray matter cortex. Deep gray matter nuclei include the basal ganglia and thalami.
- The cerebellum includes the laterally positioned cerebellar hemispheres and the midline vermis.
- The brainstem can be further divided into the midbrain, pons, and medulla.
- Cerebrospinal fluid envelops the brain within the subarachnoid cisterns. Cerebrospinal fluid also flows within the two lateral ventricles, third ventricle, and fourth ventricle located deep within the brain.

### 2.2. Pathology

- For imaging purposes, tumors can be divided into extraaxial lesions that arise from the skull or meninges and intraaxial lesions that arise from the brain itself. Common extraaxial lesions include the benign meningioma (Fig. 3-8) and dural metastases. Primary intraaxial tumors include gliomas (Fig. 3-9).[1,21]
- Tumors typically distort the normal anatomic symmetry of the brain. The usual normal symmetry of CT density or MRI intensity is usually violated as well (Figs. 3-8 and 3-9).
- Conventionally, the margins of enhancement have been used to mark the boundaries of tumors. Most gliomas, however, infiltrate beyond the enhancing margins. Tumors are often surrounded by nonenhancing vasogenic edema (Fig. 3-9).
- Complications of tumors that are readily imaged include hemorrhage, hydrocephalus, and herniation.

### 2.3. Post-Therapy Brain

- Imaging evaluation of the patient post-therapy requires knowledge of the procedures and the timing of the therapy. Comparison with pretreatment films is essential.
- Residual or recurrent tumors are usually enhanced after administration of intravenous contrast and enlarge over time. Vasogenic edema may also increase over sequential studies.
- Radiation necrosis may also be enhanced and have associated edema (Fig. 3-10). Differentiation from recurrent tumor with CT or MRI may be impossible. Positron emission tomography may be useful to distinguish metabolically active tumors from metabolically inactive necrosis.[22]

*Text continues on page 37.*

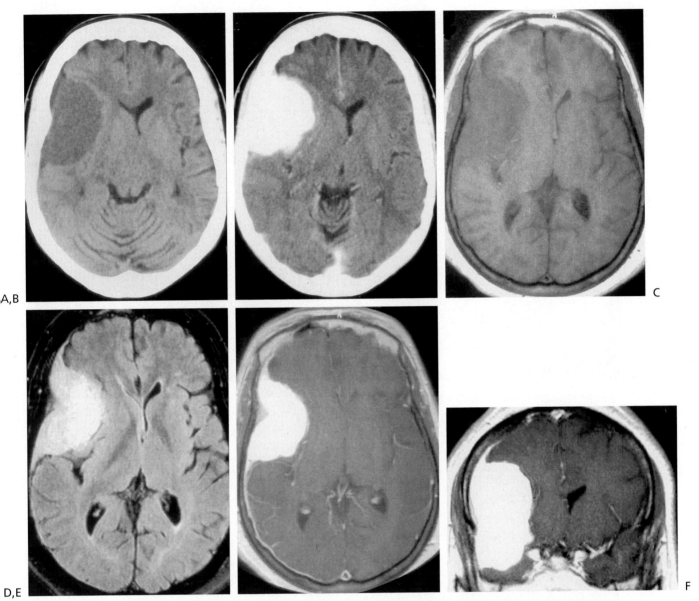

**FIGURE 3-8.** Meningioma. **A:** Unenhanced CT scan shows a large right frontal dural-based extraaxial hypodense mass with little mass effect given its size. **B:** Enhanced axial CT image shows dense enhancement. **C:** T1-weighted MRI in same patient demonstrates that the mass is hypointense. **D:** FLAIR MRI reveals little edema surrounding the hyperintense lesion. **E:** The mass intensely and homogeneously enhances on the enhanced T1-weighted image. The thickened adjacent enhancing trailing edges of the meninges have been termed the "dural tail sign." **F:** Coronal-enhanced T1-weighted images demonstrate the utility of multiplanar imaging.

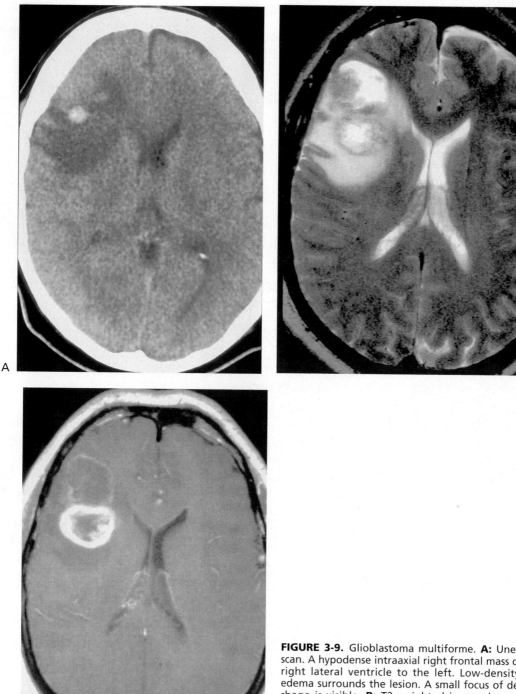

**FIGURE 3-9.** Glioblastoma multiforme. **A:** Unenhanced CT scan. A hypodense intraaxial right frontal mass displaces the right lateral ventricle to the left. Low-density vasogenic edema surrounds the lesion. A small focus of dense hemorrhage is visible. **B:** T2-weighted image demonstrates the moderately hyperintense complex mass with hyperintense vasogenic edema. The ventricles are hyperintense on this sequence. **C:** Enhanced T1-weighted image reveals the irregularly ring-enhancing margins of the tumor embedded within the edema.

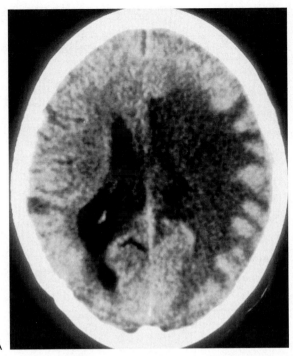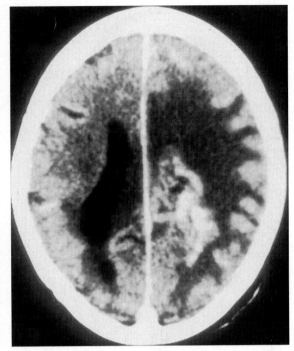

A                                                                                              B

**FIGURE 3-10.** Radiation necrosis. **A:** Unenhanced CT image shows an irregular region of vaso-genic edema in the left cerebral hemisphere of a previously radiated patient. **B:** After intravenous administration of contrast an irregularly enhancing lesion, ultimately shown to be necrosis, appears within the edema. Appearance of radiation necrosis may be indistinguishable from recurrent tumor on cross-sectional imaging.

## 3. IMAGING APPROACH TO NECK ANATOMY AND PATHOLOGY

### 3.1. Spaces of the Neck

- The deep cervical fascia of the neck consists of three layers: a superficial investing layer, middle visceral layer, and deep prevertebral layer.[23,24] The neck can be divided into spaces or compartments based on the deep cervical fascial planes.[24–28] This method of compartmentalization is ideal for analysis of cross-sectional images (Figs. 3-11 and 3-12).

#### 3.1.1. Normal Anatomy

- The cervical spaces of the suprahyoid and infrahyoid neck include the sublingual space, submandibular space, buccal space, parotid space, parapharyngeal space, carotid space, masticator space, pharyngeal mucosal space, visceral space, retropharyngeal space, posterior cervical space, and prevertebral space (Table 3-1) (Figs. 3-11 and 3-12).

#### 3.1.2. Pathology

- Of the spaces of the neck, the epithelial-lined suprahyoid pharyngeal mucosal space and the infrahyoid visceral space are especially important sites of primary carcinoma.

- The surrounding spaces, such as the parapharyngeal space, masticator space, and retropharyngeal space, are important sites of secondary tumor invasion.
- The pharyngeal mucosal space includes the mucosal surfaces and immediate submucosa of the nasopharynx and oropharynx. The oral cavity and the suprahyoid portion of the hypopharynx can also be conveniently included in this discussion.
- Imaging signs of nasopharyngeal cancer, a common pharyngeal mucosal space lesion, include blunting of the fossa of Rosenmüller, displacement of the parapharyngeal fat, and thickening of the retropharyngeal and prevertebral spaces.[29] The sphenoid and ethmoid sinuses, eustachian tube, pterygoid canal, skull base, and intracranial cavity may be invaded. MRI is especially useful in establishing soft tissue and dural invasion, although CT is useful in depicting bony invasion at the base of the skull. Oral cavity and oropharyngeal cancers may spread to involve the mandible.
- The midline visceral space extends from the hyoid bone to the mediastinum. This space is important because it contains the larynx and hypopharynx, thyroid and parathyroid glands, trachea and esophagus, paratracheal lymph nodes, and recurrent laryngeal nerves, and is the site for many primary carcinomas.[27,30]

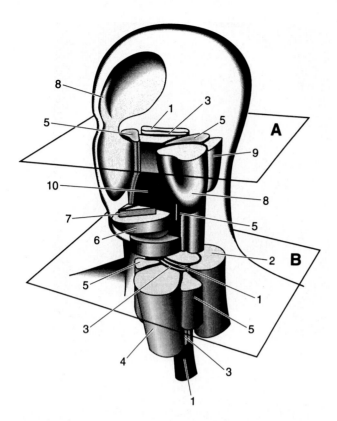

**FIGURE 3-11.** Diagram of the spaces of the neck defined by the deep cervical fascia. Axial slices through the suprahyoid **(A)** and infrahyoid **(B)** levels illustrating cross-sectional relationships of the spaces. Perivertebral space, anterior compartment (1), perivertebral space, posterior compartment (2), retropharyngeal space (3), visceral space (4), prestyloid parapharyngeal space and poststyloid parapharyngeal space (carotid space) (5), submandibular space (6), sublingual space (7), masticator space (8), parotid space (9), and pharyngeal mucosal space (10). (From: Smoker WRK. Normal Anatomy of the Neck. In: Som PM, Curtin HD, eds. *Head and Neck Imaging, 3rd ed.* St. Louis: Mosby-Yearbook, 1996:711–771, with permission. Wippold FJ II. Neck. In: Lee JKT, Sagel SS, Stanley RJ, et al., eds. *Computed Body Tomography with MRI Correlation, 3rd ed.* Philadelphia: Lippincott-Raven, 1998:107–182, with permission.)

- Axial and sagittal T1-weighted MRI best demonstrate preepiglottic space and paraglottic space tumor infiltration (Fig. 3-3). In large tumors, MRI is superior in demonstrating cartilage involvement and bone marrow infiltration. Circumferential attachment of a tumor 270° or greater of the carotid diameter implies carotid involvement with a sensitivity approaching 100%.[27]

## 3.2. Lymph Nodes of the Neck

### 3.2.1. Normal Anatomy

- Ten major groups of cervical lymph nodes are recognized: occipital, mastoid, parotid, submandibular, facial, submental, sublingual, retropharyngeal, and paired anterior and lateral cervical chains (Figs. 3-4, 3-13–3-18).[24,27,31] Of these groups, the submental, sub-

## TABLE 3-1. LOCATION OF ANATOMIC SPACES OF THE NECK

| Space | Suprahyoid | Infrahyoid |
|---|---|---|
| Buccal | X | |
| Sublingual | X | |
| Submandibular | X | |
| Parotid | X | |
| Parapharyngeal | | |
|   Prestyloid (parapharyngeal) | X | |
|   Poststyloid (carotid) | X | X |
| Masticator | X | |
| Retropharyngeal | X | X |
| Perivertebral | X | X |
| Posterior cervical | X | X |
| Pharyngeal mucosal | X | |
| Visceral | | X |

mandibular, retropharyngeal, and lateral cervical chains play especially important roles in the spread of head and neck disease.

- The American Joint Committee on Cancer and the American Academy of Otolaryngology—Head and Neck Surgery have established guidelines using a terminology that divides the lymph node groups into a series of levels that have prognostic importance (Fig. 3-19).[32,33]
- Level I consists of the sublingual, submental, and submandibular nodes (Figs. 3-4, 3-15, 3-16). These nodes lie above the hyoid bone, below the mylohyoid muscle, and anterior to the posterior margin of the submandibular gland. Level IA contains the sublingual and submental nodes, and level IB includes the submandibular nodes.
- Level II includes the internal jugular chain nodes extending from the base of the skull to the carotid bifurcation at the level of the hyoid bone (Fig. 3-18). They lie posterior to the submandibular gland and anterior to the posterior margin of the sternocleidomastoid muscle. Level IIA nodes are anterior, medial, or lateral to the internal jugular vein. If posterior to the vein, the nodes are inseparable from the vein. Level IIB nodes are posterior to the internal jugular vein with a fat plane separating the vein from the nodes.
- Level III corresponds to the internal jugular nodes from the carotid bifurcation to the omohyoid muscle at the level of the cricoid cartilage. They lie anterior to the posterior margin of the sternocleidomastoid muscle.
- Level IV refers to all nodes in the internal jugular group from the omohyoid muscle to the clavicle. They lie anterior to the posterior margin of the sternocleidomastoid muscle and lateral to the carotid arteries.

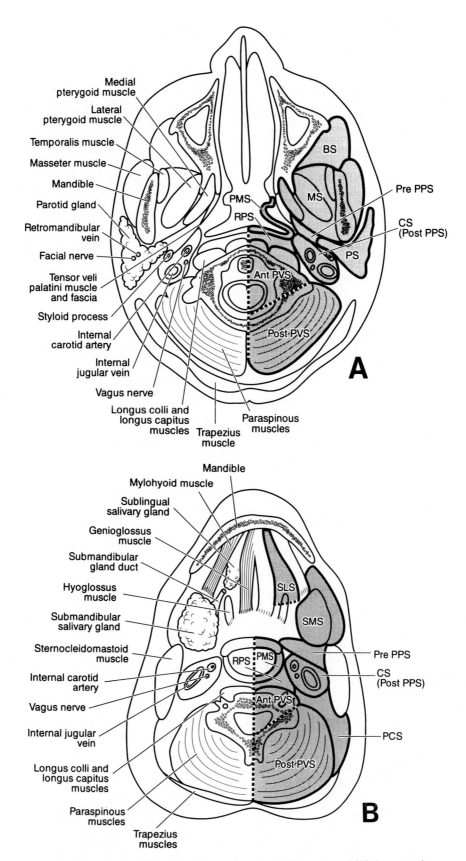

**FIGURE 3-12.** Axial diagrams of the neck to the high suprahyoid **(A)**, low suprahyoid **(B)**, and infrahyoid

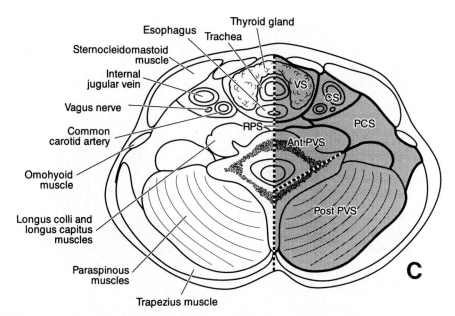

**FIGURE 3-12.** *(continued)* **(C)** levels showing the relationships of the sublingual space (SLS); submandibular space (SMS); buccal space (BS); parotid space (PS); prestyloid parapharyngeal space (PrePPS); carotid space (CS) (also known as the poststyloid parapharyngeal space [PostPPS] in the suprahyoid neck); masticator space (MS); pharyngeal mucosal space (PMS); visceral space (VS); retropharyngeal space (RPS); posterior cervical space (PCS); anterior compartment of the prevertebral space (AntPVS); and posterior compartment of the perivertebral space (PostPVS). (From: Harnsberger HR. The Perivertebral Space. In: Harnsberger HR, ed. *Head and Neck Imaging, 2nd ed.* St. Louis: Mosby-Yearbook, 1995:105–119, with permission. Smoker WRK. Normal Anatomy of the Neck. In: Som PM, Curtin HD, eds. *Head and Neck Imaging, 3rd ed.* St. Louis: Mosby-Yearbook, 1996:711–771, with permission. Wippold FJ II. Neck. In: Lee JKT, Sagel SS, Stanley RJ, et al., eds. *Computed Body Tomography with MRI Correlation, 3rd ed.* Philadelphia: Lippincott-Raven, 1998:107–182, with permission.)

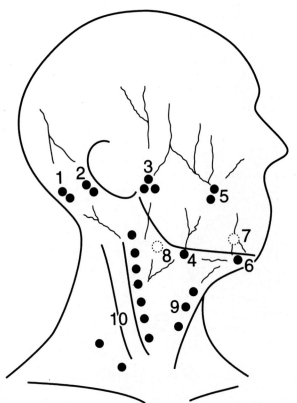

**FIGURE 3-13.** Diagram of the cervical lymph nodes. Major groups of the cervical lymph nodes include: occipital (1), mastoid (2), parotid (3), submandibular (4), facial (5), submental (6), sublingual (concealed by the deep structures of the neck) (7), retropharyngeal (concealed in the deep structures of the neck) (8), anterior cervical (9), and lateral cervical (10). (From: Wippold FJ II. Neck. In: Lee JKT, Sagel SS, Stanley RJ, et al., eds. *Computed Body Tomography with MRI Correlation, 3rd ed.* Philadelphia: Lippincott-Raven, 1998:107–182, with permission.)

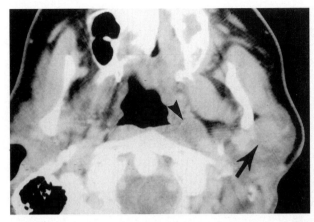

**FIGURE 3-14.** Parotid node. Prominent parotid lymph node (*arrow*) in CT scan of a patient with lymphoma. Retropharyngeal lymph node (*arrowhead*). (From: Wippold FJ II. Neck. In: Lee JKT, Sagel SS, Stanley RJ, Heiken JP, eds. *Computed Body Tomography with MRI Correlation, 3rd ed.* Philadelphia: Lippincott-Raven, 1998:107–182, with permission.)

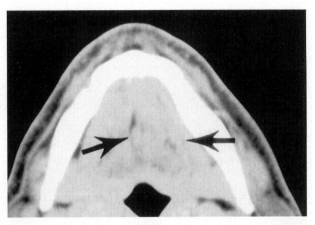

**FIGURE 3-16.** Sublingual lymph nodes. CT scan showing several small lymph nodes (*arrows*) within the sublingual space adjacent to the sublingual salivary glands and mylohyoid muscle. Nodes are also seen in the midline, between the genioglossus muscles. (From: Wippold FJ II. Neck. In: Lee JKT, Sagel SS, Stanley RJ, et al., eds. *Computed Body Tomography with MRI Correlation, 3rd ed.* Philadelphia: Lippincott-Raven, 1998:107–182, with permission.)

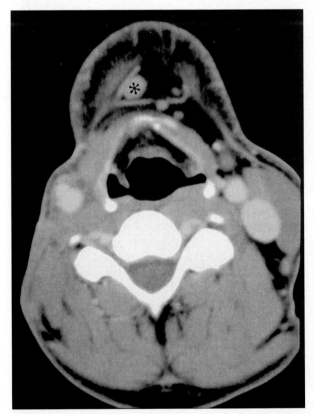

**FIGURE 3-15.** Submental lymph node. CT scan in a patient with cancer after right radical neck dissection demonstrating a prominent submental lymph node (*asterisk*). The right sternocleidomastoid muscle, right internal jugular vein, and right cervical lymph nodes have been removed. (From: Wippold FJ II. Neck. In: Lee JKT, Sagel SS, Stanley RJ, et al., eds. *Computed Body Tomography with MRI Correlation, 3rd ed.* Philadelphia: Lippincott-Raven, 1998:107–182, with permission.)

- Level V consists of spinal accessory and transverse cervical nodes that occupy the posterior cervical triangle. They lie posterior to the posterior margin of the sternocleidomastoid muscle. Level VA extends from the skull base to the inferior margin of the cricoid arch, and level VB extends from the cricoid arch to the clavicle.

- Level VI contains the pretracheal, prelaryngeal, and paratracheal nodes. These nodes lie between the carotid arteries from the hyoid bone to the manubrium.

- Level VII includes the nodes in the tracheoesophageal groove and upper mediastinum. They lie between the carotid arteries below the manubrium and above the innominate vein.[33]

### 3.2.2. Pathology

- Imaging criteria for lymphadenopathy are based on nodal size, internal heterogeneity, presence of clusters, shape, and associated findings.[32,34,35]

- The maximum transaxial diameter of a node in levels I or II should not exceed 1.5 cm, and the minimum transaxial diameter should not exceed 1.1 cm (Figs. 3-18 and 3-20). For levels III to VII, maximum and minimum transaxial diameter should be no greater than 1.0 cm.

- Internal lymph node heterogeneity is one of the most reliable criteria for recognizing abnormal lymphadenopathy. Central regions within nodes displaying hypodensity on CT, hypointensity on T1-weighted MRI, and hyperintensity on T2-weighted MRI should be regarded as abnormal and usually signify necrosis (Fig. 3-20). Necrosis generally is proportional to nodal size; however, this finding should be considered abnormal regardless of

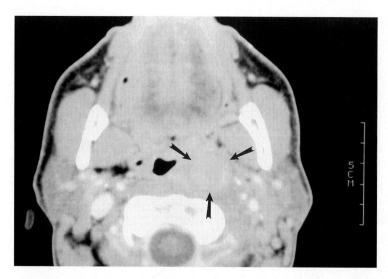

**FIGURE 3-17.** Retropharyngeal node. CT scan showing an enlarged left retropharyngeal lymph node (*arrows*) in a patient with nasopharyngeal carcinoma.

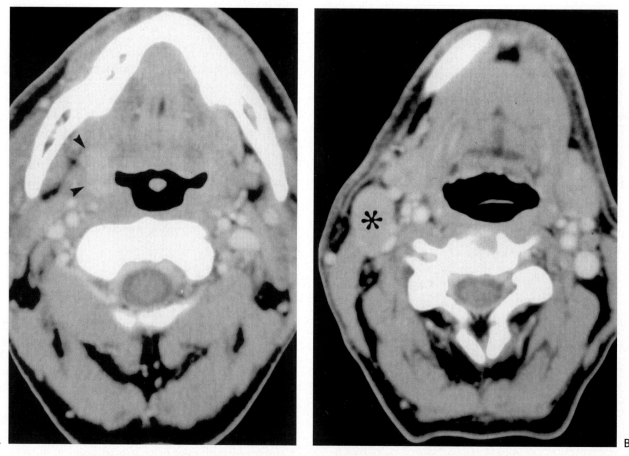

A                                                                                          B

**FIGURE 3-18.** Tonsillar carcinoma with internal jugular lymphadenopathy. **A:** Axial CT scan revealing dense right tonsillar mass (*arrowheads*). **B:** Enlarged right internal jugular lymph node (*asterisk*) superior to the hyoid bone (level II lymphadenopathy).

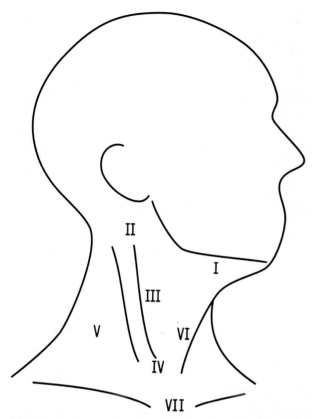

**FIGURE 3-19.** Cervical lymph node levels defined by the American Joint Committee on Cancer (AJCC). Level I consists of the submental and submandibular lymph nodes. Levels II, III, and IV consist of the high, middle, and lower internal jugular chain nodes. Level V corresponds to the spinal accessory and transverse cervical lymph node chains. Level VI consists of pretracheal and paratracheal lymph nodes. Level VII corresponds to the nodes in the tracheoesophageal groove and upper mediastinum. (From: Wippold FJ II. Neck. In: Lee JKT, Sagel SS, Stanley RJ, et al, eds. *Computed Body Tomography with MRI Correlation, 3rd ed.* Philadelphia: Lippincott-Raven, 1998:107–182, with permission.)

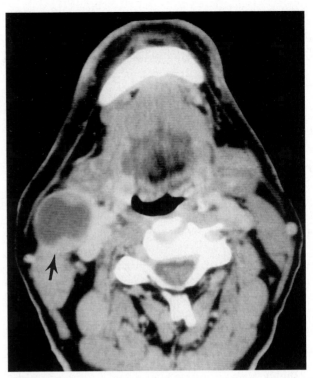

**FIGURE 3-20.** Metastatic internal jugular lymph node. CT scan of an enlarged right internal jugular lymph node (level II) (*arrow*) demonstrating internal inhomogeneity consistent with necrosis.

- Additional imaging signs of lymphadenopathy are the presence of enhancement and calcification within nodes. Calcification of a node may be seen in granulomatous disease, such as tuberculosis, previously radiated neoplastic nodes, and metastatic thyroid carcinoma.

nodal size. The hilum of a normal node may contain hypodense fat on CT imaging and should not be mistaken for necrosis (Fig. 3-7).

- Clusters are defined as three or more contiguous ill-defined nodes within the same level ranging from 8 to 15 mm in size. Clusters may be seen in inflammation, cancer, or lymphoma (Fig. 3-21). Small cancerous nodes, seemingly normal by size criteria, may be clustered with larger obviously malignant nodes.
- Shape is no longer thought to be reliable in differentiating normal from pathologic nodes. Round nodes tend to be neoplastic, whereas elliptical or bean-shaped nodes are generally normal or hyperplastic; however, many exceptions may be encountered.
- Tumor spread beyond the capsule of a node is manifested by capsular enhancement, ill-defined nodal margins, obliterated fat planes surrounding the node, and edema or thickening in the adjacent soft tissues.

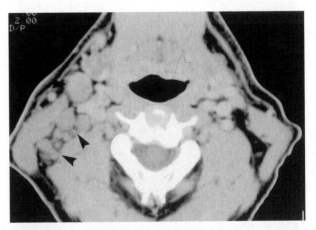

**FIGURE 3-21.** Lymphoma with abnormal lymph node clusters. Axial CT scan in a patient with squamous cell cancer demonstrating multiple small lymph nodes (*arrowheads*) within the lateral cervical chain. Although several of the nodes are normal by size criteria, the multiplicity indicates lymphadenopathy. Clusters are also present in the left side of the neck. (From: Wippold FJ II. Neck. In: Lee JKT, Sagel SS, Stanley RJ, et al., eds. *Computed Body Tomography with MRI Correlation, 3rd ed.* Philadelphia: Lippincott-Raven, 1998:107–182, with permission.)

### 3.3. Post-Therapy Neck

- Therapy for head and neck cancer may involve surgery, radiation, chemotherapy, immunotherapy, or combined modalities. Surgical treatment can be divided into surgery for the primary lesion (e.g., laryngectomy for laryngeal cancer), adjunctive surgery for spread of disease (e.g., neck dissection for cervical lymphadenopathy), and reconstructive surgery (e.g., construction of myocutaneous flaps).[27,36]

- The imaging evaluation of the patient post-therapy begins with a thorough understanding of the procedures that are performed coupled with pretreatment images that identify the original lesion.

- Primary and adjunctive surgery usually entail partial or complete removal of the lesion. Discussion with the surgeon about the extent of the procedure assists in the appreciation of anatomic alterations typically seen on imaging. In these instances, key anatomic structures will be absent on post-therapy scans (Figs. 3-22 and 3-23). Reconstructive surgery usually entails augmentation of residual tissues or transplanting distant tissues for cosmetic and functional effect. Again, the surgeon can supply essential information about the procedure that facilitates understanding of the anatomic alterations seen on imaging. In these instances, anatomic structures not present on the pretherapy scans will be visible (Fig. 3-24).[27,36–38]

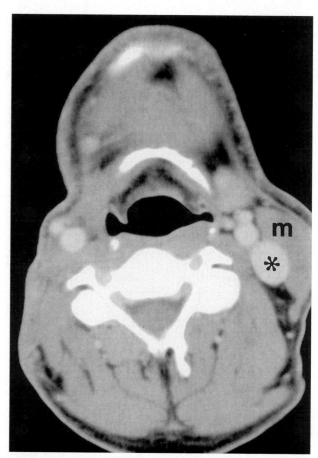

**FIGURE 3-23.** Axial CT scan after a right radical neck dissection. The asymmetry of the neck is striking. Note the absent right jugular vein and sternocleidomastoid muscle compared with the normal left sternocleidomastoid muscle (*m*) and left internal jugular vein (*asterisk*).

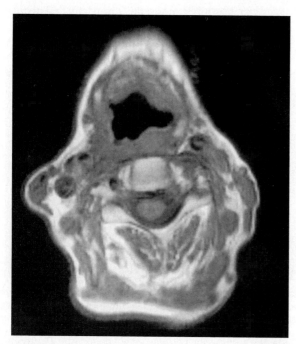

**FIGURE 3-22.** Supraglottic laryngectomy. T1-weighted MRI of a patient with a supraglottic laryngectomy. Neopharyngeal tissues are thickened. Recognition of the surgery depends on the appreciation of absent anatomy (e.g., the epiglottis).

- Patients receiving radiation therapy develop soft tissue and bony changes on imaging with doses of 6,500 to 7,000 cGy. Depending on the ports and doses of radiation, these changes may include thickening of the skin and platysma; stranding of the subcutaneous fat; fibrosis of the muscles of mastication; enhancement and eventual atrophy of the major and minor salivary glands; stranding of the fat containing preepiglottic and paraglottic spaces; thickening of the epiglottis, aryepiglottic folds, false vocal cords, and true cords; enhancement of mucosal surfaces; contraction of the thyrohyoid membrane; chondronecrosis and cartilage collapse; fatty infiltration of the radiated bone marrow; osteoradionecrosis of the mandible; atrophy because of cranial neuropathies; and diminished vascular flow because of accelerated atherosclerotic disease, and, rarely, sarcomas (Figs. 3-25–3-27).[27,37,39] 3D radiation port planning may ameliorate post-therapy xerostomia by shielding of the parotid glands.[7]

- For patients with successful surgical therapy, scans should remain stable over time, with the exceptions that

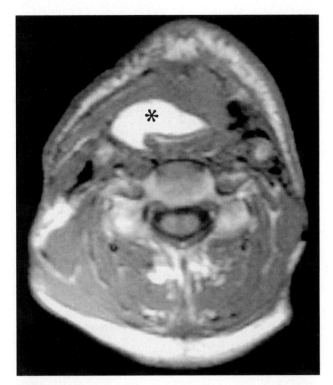

**FIGURE 3-24.** Myocutaneous graft in a patient with hypopharyngeal carcinoma treated with radical neck dissection. T1-weighted MRI revealing the hyperintense fat-containing graft (*asterisk*) and surrounding soft tissue thickening after a total laryngectomy.

bulky, fatty reconstruction flaps usually atrophy and fibrotic scar develops. Tissue planes become more defined as postsurgical edema subsides, but they may remain somewhat obscured compared with the preoperative images. The complete or nearly complete resolution of the

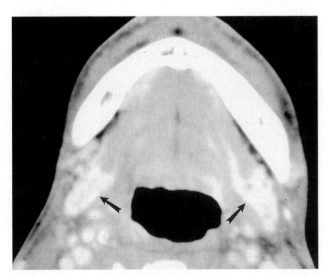

**FIGURE 3-25.** Radiation sialadenitis. Axial CT scan revealing densely enhancing submandibular salivary glands (*arrows*) after radiation for neck carcinoma.

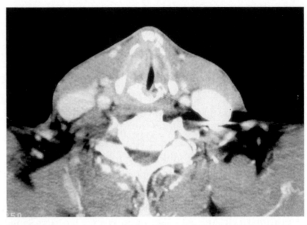

**FIGURE 3-26.** Mucosal edema after radiation therapy. Enhanced CT demonstrates asymmetric thickening of the true vocal cords with irregular enhancement and airway narrowing after radiation therapy for a glottic carcinoma.

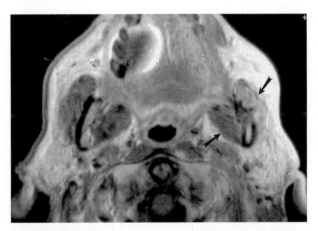

**FIGURE 3-27.** Masticator space changes after radiation therapy. Atrophied and hyperintense, contrast-enhancing changes in the left masseter and medial pterygoid muscles (*arrows*) on enhanced T1-weighted images after radiation therapy.

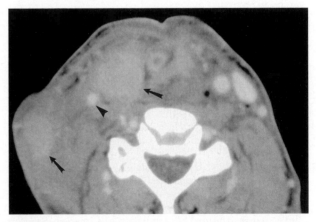

**FIGURE 3-28.** Recurrent carcinoma in a patient with a total laryngectomy. Axial CT scan reveals dense masses (*arrows*) representing recurrent carcinoma within the neck. Note the absent right internal jugular vein after the patient's radical neck dissection. Normal laryngeal structures are absent. Note the small right carotid artery (*arrowhead*). Skin is thickened, and subcutaneous fat is edematous after radiation therapy.

primary lesion on imaging is one of the best criterion for a successful radiation response.

- The development of a focal, dense, and necrotic mass within the original surgical bed or the reconstructed tissue or the appearance of enlarging lymph nodes draining the surgical site usually indicate recurrent tumor (Fig. 3-28). Residual mass of greater than 50% of the original tumor volume indicates a radiation therapy failure.[40]

- A baseline imaging study in patients who are especially at risk for recurrence should not be performed for a least 1 month because of the persistence of potentially confusing postsurgical hemorrhage and edema. Scanning at intervals of 4 to 6 months for the first 1 to 3 years is then appropriate.[38] Annual examinations are then performed unless a change in clinical status prompts a more timely scan.[38]

## REFERENCES

1. Ricci PE. Imaging of adult brain tumors. *Neuroimaging Clin N Am* 1999;9:651–669.
2. Russell EJ. The radiologic approach to malignant tumors of the head and neck, with emphasis on computed tomography. *Clin Plast Surg* 1985;12:343–374.
3. Wortham DG, Hoover LA, Lufkin RB, et al. Magnetic resonance imaging of the larynx: a correlation with histologic sections. *Otolaryngol Head Neck Surg* 1986;94:123–133.
4. Suojanen JN, Mukherji SK, Dupuy DE, et al. Spiral CT in evaluation of head and neck lesions: work in progress. *Radiology* 1992;183:281–283.
5. Suojanen JN, Mukherji SK, Wippold FJ. Spiral CT of the larynx. *AJNR Am J Neuroradiol* 1994;15:1579–1582.
6. Zeiberg AS, Silverman PM, Sessions RB, et al. Helical (spiral) CT of the upper airway with three-dimensional imaging: technique and clinical assessment. *AJR Am J Roentgenol* 1996;166:293–299.
7. Emami B, Purdy JA, Simpson JR, et al. 3-D conformal radiotherapy in head and neck cancer. *Front Radiat Ther Oncol* 1996;29:207–220.
8. Tsuchiya K, Mieutani Y, Hachiya J. Preliminary evaluation of fluid-attenuated inversion-recovery MR in the diagnosis of intracranial tumors. *AJNR Am J Neuroradiol* 1996;17:1081–1086.
9. Muroff LR, Runge VM. The use of MR contrast in neoplastic disease of the brain. *Top Magn Reson Imaging* 1995;7:137–157.
10. Hudgins PA, Gussack GS. MR imaging in the management of extracranial malignant tumors of the head and neck. *AJR Am J Roentgenol* 1992;159:161–169.
11. Glazer HS, Niemeyer JH, Balfe DM, et al. Neck neoplasms: MR imaging. Part II. Posttreatment evaluation. *Radiology* 1986;160:349–354.
12. Hasso AN, Brown KD. Use of gadolinium chelates in MR imaging of lesions of the extracranial head and neck. *J Magn Reson Imaging* 1993;3:247–263.
13. Barakos JA, Dillon WP, Chew WM. Orbit, skull base, and pharynx: contrast-enhanced fat suppression MR imaging. *Radiology* 1991;179:191–198.
14. Balaban RS, Ceckler TL. Magnetization transfer contrast in magnetic resonance imaging. *Magn Reson Q* 1992;8:116–137.
15. Lambre H, Anzai Y, Farahani K, et al. Interventional magnetic resonance imaging of the head and neck and new imaging techniques. *Neuroimaging Clin N Am* 1996;6:461–472.
16. Harris KG, Smith TP, Cragg AH, et al. Nephrotoxicity from contrast material in renal insufficiency: ionic versus nonionic agents. *Radiology* 1991;179:849–852.
17. Haustein J, Niendorf HP, Krestin G, et al. Renal tolerance of gadolinium-DTPA/dimeglumine in patients with chronic renal failure. *Invest Radiol* 1992;27:153–156.
18. Som PM. The present controversy over imaging method of choice for evaluating the soft tissues of the neck. *AJNR Am J Neuroradiol* 1997;18:1869–1872.
19. Gado M, Hanaway J, Frank R. Functional anatomy of the cerebral cortex by computed tomography. *J Comput Assist Tomogr* 1979;3:1–19.
20. Chong BW, Levine JD. The Normal Brain. In: Orrison WW, ed. *Neuroimaging*. Philadelphia: W.B. Saunders, 2000:517–547.
21. Smirniotopoulos JG. The new WHO classification of brain tumors. *Neuroimaging Clin N Am* 1999;9:595–613.
22. Nelson SJ. Imaging of brain tumors after therapy. *Neuroimaging Clin N Am* 1999;9:801–817.
23. Grodinsky M, Holyoke EA. The fasciae and fascial spaces of the head, neck and adjacent regions. *Am J Anat* 1938;63:367–407.
24. Williams DW III. An imager's guide to normal neck anatomy. *Semin Ultrasound CT MR* 1997;18:157–181.
25. Harnsberger HR. The Perivertebral Space. In: Harnsberger HR, ed. *Head and Neck Imaging*, 2nd ed. St. Louis: Mosby-Yearbook, 1995:105–119.
26. Smoker WRK. Normal Anatomy of the Neck. In: Som PM, Curtin HD, eds. *Head and Neck Imaging*, 3rd ed. St. Louis: Mosby-Yearbook, 1996:711–771.
27. Wippold FJ II. Neck. In: Lee JKT, Sagel SS, Stanley RJ, et al., eds. *Computed Body Tomography with MRI Correlation*, 3rd ed. Philadelphia: Lippincott-Raven, 1998:107–182.
28. Mukherji SK, Castillo M. A simplified approach to the spaces of the suprahyoid neck. *Radiol Clin North Am* 1998;36:761–780.
29. Chong VFH, Fan Y-F, Mukherji SK. Carcinoma of the nasopharynx. *Semin Ultrasound CT MR* 1998;19:449–462.
30. Wippold FJ II. Diagnostic Imaging of the Larynx. In: Cummings CW, Fredrickson JM, Harker LA, et al., eds. *Otolaryngology—Head and Neck Surgery*, 3rd ed. St. Louis: C.V. Mosby, 1998:1895–1919.
31. Rouvier H. *Anatomy of the Human Lymphatic System*. Ann Arbor, MI: Edwards Brothers, 1938:1–82.
32. Kaji AV, Mohuchy T, Swartz JD. Imaging of cervical lymphadenopathy. *Semin Ultrasound CT MR* 1997;18:220–249.
33. Som PM, Curtin HD, Mancuso AA. An imaging-based classification for the cervical nodes designed as an adjunct to recent clinically based nodal classifications. *Arch Otolaryngol Head Neck Surg* 1999;125:388–396.
34. Som PM. Lymph nodes of the neck. *Radiology* 1987;165:593–600.
35. van den Brekel MWM, Stel HV, Castelijns JA, et al. Cervical lymph node metastasis: assessment of radiologic criteria. *Radiology* 1990;177:379–384.
36. Wippold FJ II. Postoperative Pharynx. In: Gore RM, Levine MS, eds. *Textbook of Gastrointestinal Radiology*, 2nd ed. Philadelphia: W.B. Saunders, 2000:257–270.
37. Wippold FJ II. Imaging the treated oral cavity and oropharynx. *Europ J Radiol* 2002;44:96–107.
38. Som PM, Urken ML, Biller H, et al. Imaging the postoperative neck. *Radiology* 1993;187:593–603.
39. Tartaglino LM, Rao VM, Markiewicz DA. Imaging of radiation changes in the head and neck. *Semin Roentgen* 1994;29:81–91.
40. Mukherji SK, Mancuso AA, Kotzur IM, et al. Radiologic appearance of the irradiated larynx. Part II. Primary site response. *Radiology* 1994;193:149–154.

# 4

# COMPUTED TOMOGRAPHY AND MAGNETIC RESONANCE IMAGING OF THE PROSTATE, UTERUS, AND CERVIX

NINA A. MAYR
CYNTHIA MÉNARD
ALLEN R. MOLLOY
MICHAEL V. KNOPP

## 1. PROSTATE IMAGING

### 1.1. Magnetic Resonance Imaging Technique and Protocol

- Magnetic resonance imaging (MRI) techniques and interpretation are traditionally not as familiar to radiation oncologists as computed tomography (CT) imaging techniques and interpretation. It is therefore important to understand the basics of MRI technology to fully comprehend MRI-based treatment planning, particularly in regard to the prostate, uterus, and cervix. A brief introduction to MRI techniques will be presented.

### 1.1. Axial T2-Weighted Fast Spin Echo

- These images provide optimal definition of the prostatic subzonal anatomy and can depict malignant tumors in the peripheral zone of the prostate gland.
- The prescription recommendation is as follows: 3- to 4-mm slice thickness, no spacing or gap, from apex to seminal vesicles, repetition time 3500 to 6000 ms, echo time 90 to 120 ms, and phase encode right to left (to minimize propagation of motion or endorectal coil artifact over the prostate).
- Contraindications to MRI include ferromagnetic devices such as aneurysm clips, cochlear implants, implanted electrodes, and drug infusion pumps. Pacemakers may be deactivated in the magnetic field. Orthopedic hardware such as hip prosthesis, although generally safely imaged, may produce significant artifacts. If there is any question of safety, consultation with the radiologist is recommended.

### 1.1.1. Coronal or Sagittal T2-Weighted Fast Spin Echo

- These images are useful for defining the location of the base and apex of the gland and to characterize pathologic processes at those sites.
- The prescription recommendation is the same as stated previously.

### 1.1.2. Axial T1-Weighted Fast Spin Echo

- These images are useful to detect the presence of intraglandular hemorrhage after prostate biopsy, which is of high signal intensity secondary to the T1-shortening effects of methemoglobin. It is also useful to identify the neurovascular bundle.
- The prescription recommendation is as follows: 4- to 6-mm slice thickness, no spacing or gap, repetition time 600 to 700 ms, echo time 12 ms, and phase encode anterior to posterior (to prevent obscuration of pelvic nodes by endorectal coil motion artifact), including the pelvis from the aortic bifurcation to the pubic symphysis.
- The field of view (FOV) acquired should balance those requirements for image coregistration to the treatment planning CT scans and anatomic resolution. To maximize anatomic resolution, a small FOV (usually 14 cm) should be used.
- The endorectal coil can significantly improve the signal-to-noise ratio of the image but will distort the shape of the prostate gland (Fig. 4-1). For diagnostic images, the endorectal coil must be positioned such that there is no rotation of the coil on axial images to avoid asymmetry in the signal acquired from the peripheral zone. It must also overlap both the base and apex of the prostate gland on

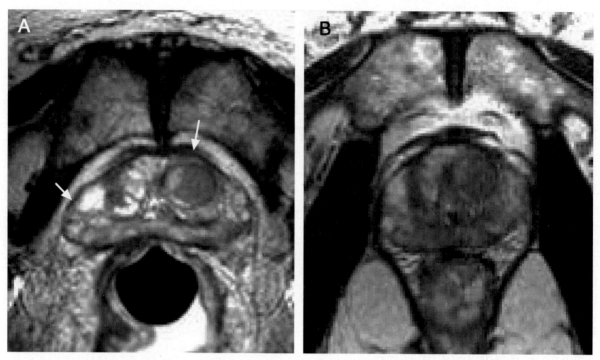

**FIGURE 4-1.** Axial T2-weighted images of the prostate gland acquired with **(A)** and without **(B)** an endorectal coil in the same patient. The endorectal coil deforms the prostate gland but improves the quality of the image and definition of the zonal anatomy. The peripheral zone is bounded by the dark band of the prostate capsule *(arrows)*.

sagittal images (Fig. 4-2). Corrections for inhomogeneous signal intensity from the endorectal coil can be applied to improve visualization of posterior anatomic structures (Fig. 4-3).[1,2]

## 1.2. Magnetic Resonance Imaging Anatomy

- There are two important subdivisions of the prostate gland on MRI: the *peripheral zone* (Fig. 4-1) and the *central gland.* The peripheral zone consists of normal glandular tissue and is normally hyperintense on T2-weighted images. The central gland is composed of the periurethral, transitional, and central zones, and thus contains both glandular and stromal tissue. It is usually heterogeneously hypointense in signal intensity. Benign prostatic hyperplasia predominantly involves the transition zone, whereas prostate cancer predominantly involves the peripheral zone (Figs. 4-4 and 4-5).
- A thin rim of low T2 signal intensity, which represents the anatomic or true *capsule* (Fig. 4-1), surrounds the prostate gland.[3]
- The hypointense central *base* of the prostate is difficult to distinguish from the muscle wall of the bladder on axial images. Delineation of the prostatic margin at the base is best depicted on sagittal or coronal images. Similarly, the

location of the prostatic *apex* is best depicted on sagittal images (Figs. 4-3 and 4-6), which can then be translated to the corresponding axial image.

- The proximal *urethra* is rarely identifiable, unless a Foley catheter is present or a transurethral resection has been performed. The distal prostatic urethra can be seen as a low T2 signal intensity ring in the lower prostate (Fig. 4-7) because it is enclosed by an additional layer of muscle.[3]
- The *neurovascular bundles,* which contain nerves and vessels responsible for erectile function, lie immediately adjacent to the mid-prostatic capsule in the rectoprostatic angle at approximately 4 and 8 o'clock (Fig. 4-8). At the apex, the neurovascular bundles lie immediately adjacent to the membranous urethra in the same orientation. The nerve then passes through the genitourinary membrane as several fine branches diverging 4 to 12 mm lateral to the urethra to innervate the corpus spongiosum and corpus cavernosa.[3] At the level of the mid-gland, the neurovascular bundles can be identified as areas of low signal intensity within the high-intensity triangle of periprostatic fat. They are best visualized on T1-weighted images.
- The *penile root* contains structures involved in erection, including the corpora cavernosa and corpus spongiosum (Fig. 4-7). The posterior part of the corpus spongiosum is expanded, forming the bulb of the penis. These structures are readily delineated on MRI. Cavernosal dysfunction may contribute to erectile dysfunction after radiotherapy.

*Text continues on page 52.*

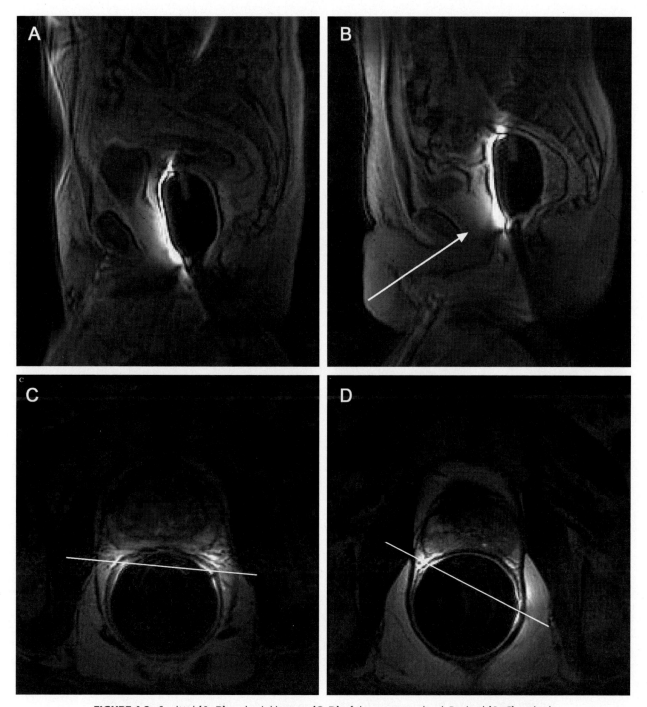

**FIGURE 4-2.** Sagittal **(A, B)** and axial images **(C, D)** of the prostate gland. Desired **(A, C)** and suboptimal **(B,D)** positions of the inserted endorectal coil are demonstrated. The coil in sagittal image **(B)** is inserted too far and does not adequately cover the apex of the gland *(arrow)*. The coil in axial image **(D)** is rotated and creates higher signal intensity on the right compared with the left peripheral zone.

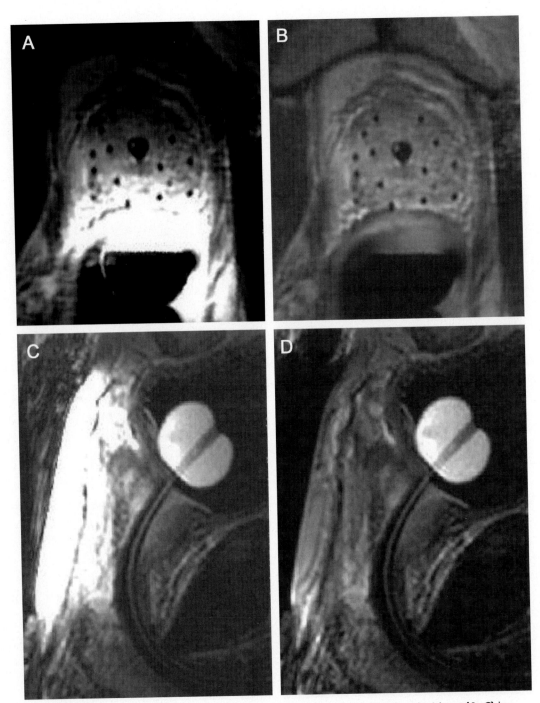

**FIGURE 4-3.** Axial **(A, B)** and sagittal **(C, D)** prostate images with **(B, D)** and without **(A, C)** intensity correction for the endorectal coil. The posterior demarcation of the prostate gland and the rectal mucosa are more clearly identified on corrected images. The images were acquired at the end of a prostate brachytherapy procedure, whereas the brachytherapy catheters are seen as sites of signal void on the axial images.

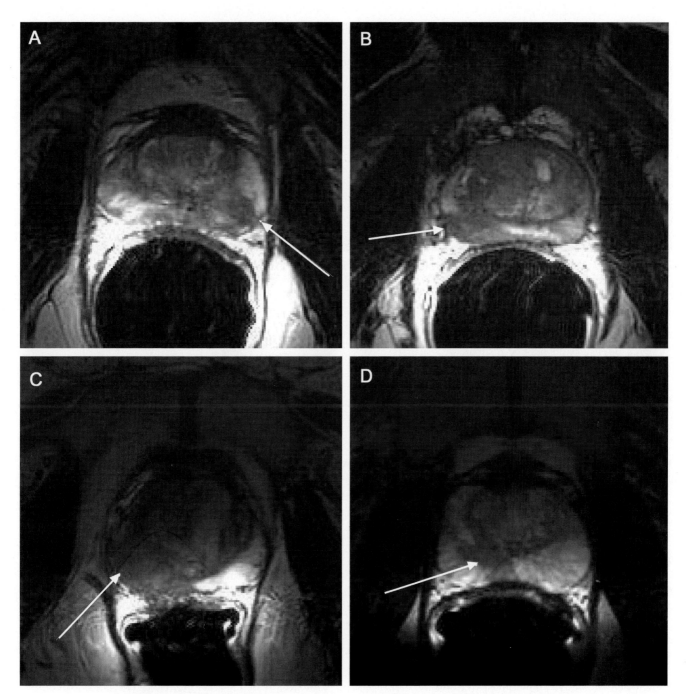

**FIGURE 4-4.** Axial T2-weighted images of four patients **(A–D)** with prostate cancer. Areas of low-signal intensity on T2-weighted images are highly suspicious for malignant disease in the peripheral zones of these patients *(arrows)*.

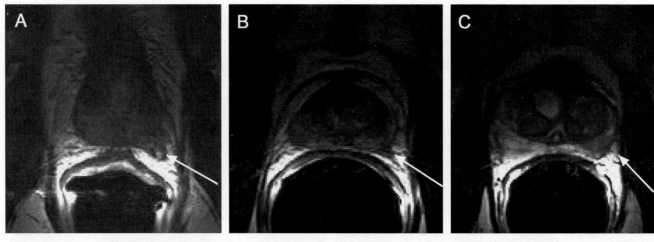

**FIGURE 4-5.** Axial images showing evidence of extracapsular extension *(arrows)* in three patients with prostate cancer. Obliteration of the rectoprostatic angle **(A, B)** and hypointense stranding **(C)** of the periprostatic fat are demonstrated.

- The *rectal mucosa* is depicted by a thin rim of low T2 signal intensity and may be difficult to visualize when no intensity correction is applied to the endorectal coil (Fig. 4-7).
- Superiorly, the *muscles* (Fig. 4-7) lateral to the prostate are the obturators interni, and more inferiorly the prostate is flanked by the levator ani. Radiation injury to the levator ani may contribute to gastrointestinal symptoms.[3]
- The *seminal vesicles* are bilateral structures superior to the prostate (Fig. 4-7). Laterally, the vesicles are high in signal on T2-weighted images lined by a thin, low signal rim. Medially, the paired vas deferens are lower in signal and lined by a thick rim of low signal.

## 1.3. Prostate Cancer

- Prostate cancer usually manifests as abnormal areas of low signal intensity within the homogeneous high signal intensity background of the normal peripheral zone (Figs. 4-4 and 4-5). Postbiopsy hemorrhage, prostatitis, and prior therapy may also appear as low T2 signals in the peripheral zone.
- Evidence of extraprostatic spread of tumor includes hypointense stranding in the periprostatic fat, obliteration of the rectoprostatic angle, or clear-cut extracapsular extension (Figs. 4-4B,C and 4-5 ).[3] Staging accuracies for high (1.5T) field strength MR images are 82% to 88% in single institutional series.[3–6]
- Findings indicative of seminal vesicle invasion include asymmetry of the seminal vesicle caused by abnormal low signal intensity on T2-weighted images, loss of the normal fat plane between the base of the prostate and the inferior aspect of the seminal vesicle (best seen on the coronal images), focal or diffuse wall thickening, low signal intensity mass, and nonvisualization of the ejaculatory ducts or seminal vesicle walls.[3]

## 1.4. Image-Based Treatment Planning

### 1.4.1. Computed Tomography-Based Treatment Planning

- Standard of care for radiotherapy of the prostate involves treatment planning based on CT images of the pelvis acquired with the patient in the treatment position. This approach permits accurate three-dimensional spatial representation of the anatomy.
- Unfortunately, the boundaries of the prostate gland and adjacent normal structures at risk of injury are poorly discriminated because of limited soft tissue contrast on CT. The MR images can be registered or "fused" to the CT images to aid in target delineation.
- MR images of the prostate destined for registration with treatment-planning CT scans should be acquired with the patient in the same position as the CT scan, and image spatial distortion must be corrected for gradient nonlinearity.
- The imaging coils should not physically distort the anatomy. For this reason, an endorectal coil is not recommended, because it compresses and changes the shape of the prostate gland (Fig. 4-1). The posterior component of the pelvic phased-array coil should be placed beneath a flat table overlay onto which the patient is positioned. The anterior component of the pelvic phased-array coil should be loosely placed on the skin and not compress the pelvis.

### 1.4.2. Magnetic Resonance Imaging Registration with Bony Landmarks

- MR images can be registered to the CT images on the basis of common bony landmarks. For this, MR images with a large FOV encompassing the pelvic bone structures are required.

*Text continues on page 56.*

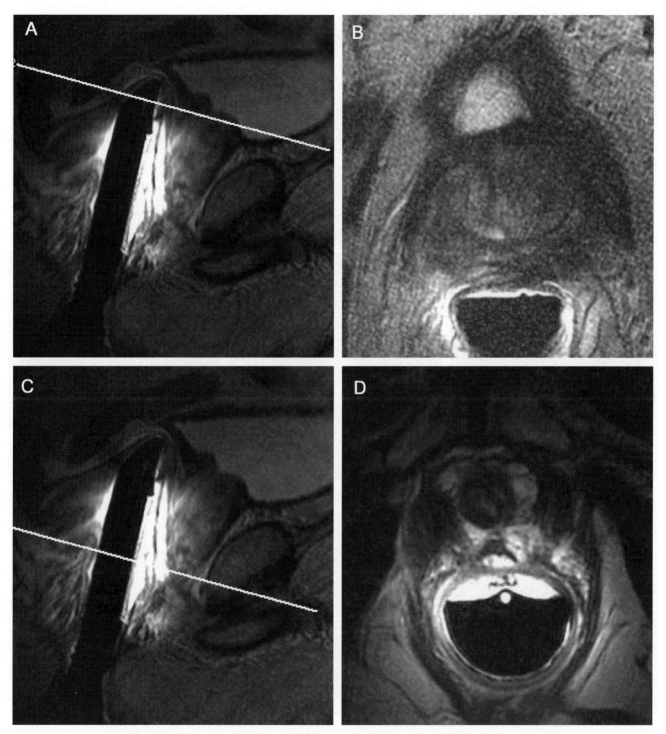

**FIGURE 4-6.** The location of the base **(A, B)** and apex **(C, D)** of the prostate gland is clearly delineated on sagittal images **(A, C)**, and the corresponding axial image **(B, D)** can be determined.

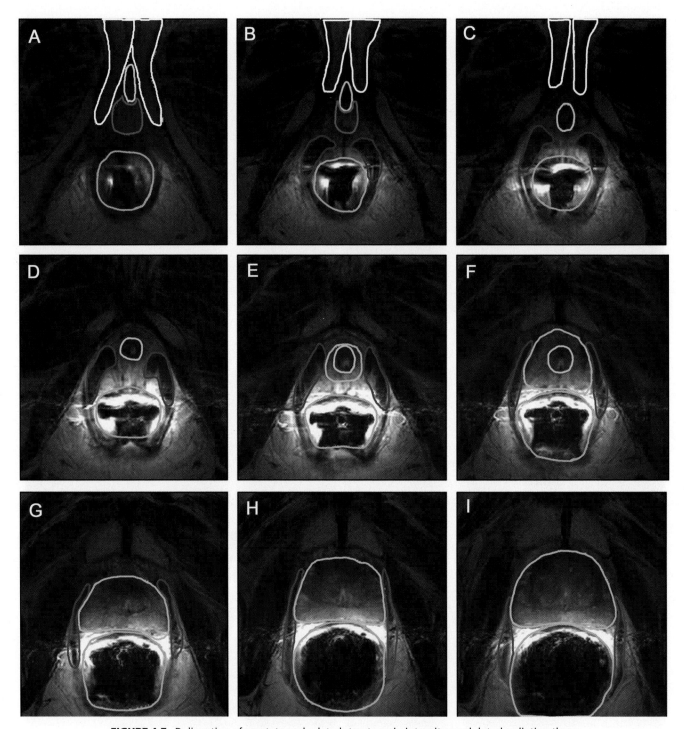

**FIGURE 4-7.** Delineation of prostate and related structures in intensity-modulated radiation therapy (IMRT) planning. The prostate gland *(pale blue)*, rectum *(pink)*, distal urethra *(yellow)*, levator ani *(purple)*, corpus spongiosum *(red)*, and corpora cavernosa *(white)* are visible on axial magnetic resonance imaging (MRI) superior sections (**A–I**) and can be delineated for IMRT planning.

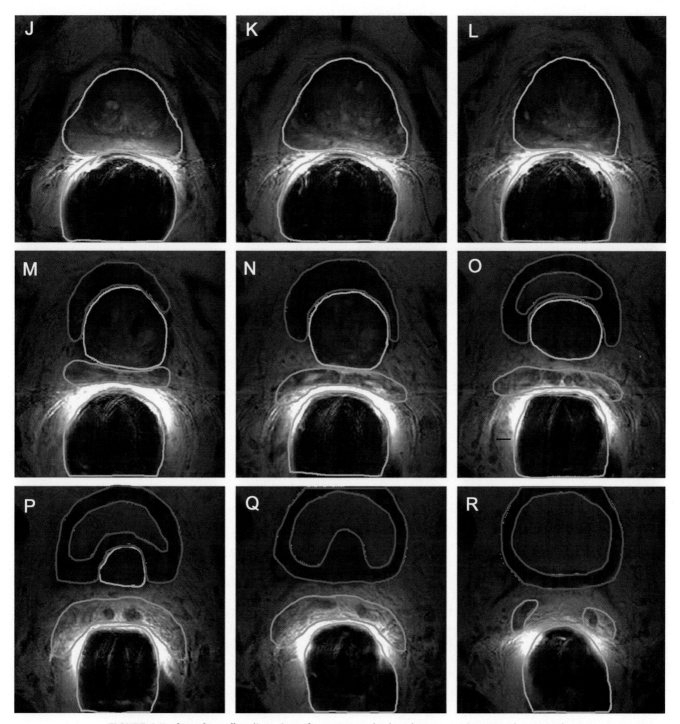

**FIGURE 4-7.** *(continued)* Delineation of prostate and related structures in IMRT planning. The prostate gland *(pale blue)*, rectum *(pink)*, seminal vesicles *(orange)*, and bladder wall *(green)* are visible on axial MRI inferior sections **(J–R)** and can be delineated for IMRT planning.

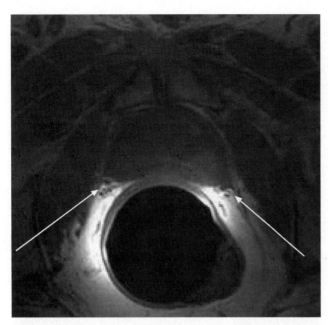

**FIGURE 4-8.** The neurovascular bundles *(arrows)* are visualized at the rectoprostatic angle on an axial T1-weighted image.

- Discordance between the apparent location of the prostate gland on the registered CT and MR images may be caused by (1) registration error or (2) motion of the prostate gland relative to bony landmarks.

### 1.4.3. Magnetic Resonance Imaging Registration with Fiducial Markers

- MR images can be registered to the CT images on the basis of fiducial markers previously implanted into the prostate gland. For this, MR images with a small FOV encompassing the prostate gland and seminal vesicles are sufficient.
- Fiducial markers commonly consist of pure gold or gold alloy seeds measuring 0.8 to 1.3 mm in diameter and 3 to 5 mm in length, which can be placed through a needle.[7] The optimal MRI technique is dependent on the metal alloy introduced into the prostate gland. Small pure gold fiducial markers are not clearly visualized on T2-weighted fast spin echo images and are best visualized on gradient echo techniques.

### 1.4.4. Magnetic Resonance Imaging-Based Treatment Planning

- Treatment planning directly based on MR images is actively being investigated.[8] This approach strives to reduce the error introduced with coregistration of images.
- Limitations to address include (1) the generation of digitally reconstructed radiographs for treatment verification, (2) the correction of spatial distortions caused by nonuniform magnetic field gradients with accurate ren-

dering of surface contours, and (3) an adaptation of the planning software for tissue inhomogeneity correction.

### 1.5. Biologic Magnetic Resonance Imaging Techniques

- A number of emerging MRI techniques promise to improve the accuracy of staging and "tumor mapping" within the prostate gland. These techniques may also shed light on the physiology, biochemistry, or radiobiology of a given tumor.

#### 1.5.1. Magnetic Resonance Spectroscopy Imaging

- MR spectroscopy imaging (MRSI) of the prostate depicts the altered metabolism associated with prostate cancer and is performed in conjunction with standard endorectal MRI.
- MRSI findings in prostate cancer are characterized by elevated levels of choline or reduced levels of citrate, or both. Voxels in which there is good signal-to-noise ratio, no partial volume effects, and a ratio of choline and creatine to citrate of greater than 0.61 are considered most likely to be malignant.[9]
- Preliminary studies suggest that MRSI may provide information that could be used to increase staging accuracy for less experienced readers and thereby reduce interobserver variability.[10]

#### 1.5.2. Dynamic Contrast-Enhanced Magnetic Resonance Imaging

- Dynamic contrast-enhanced MRI consists of a sequential acquisition of gradient echo images of the prostate gland during the passage of a contrast agent (gadolinium-diethylenetriamine pentaacetic acid). MRI signal intensity can be plotted over time for various regions of interest within the prostate and reflects physiologic parameters such as tissue perfusion, blood flow, vascular density, and vascular permeability.
- Preliminary studies suggest that malignant tumors demonstrate a more rapid and intense uptake of contrast, as well as a more rapid washout, compared with the normal peripheral zone.[11] This may be consistent with angiogenesis in malignant sites within the prostate gland.

## 2. UTERUS AND CERVIX IMAGING

### 2.1. Magnetic Resonance Imaging Technique and Protocol

- Patient preparation: Glucagon 1 mg is given intramuscularly 10 minutes before the imaging to reduce the artifact caused by intestinal movement. If sedation is required, the patient should receive nothing by mouth according to the center's protocol. A tampon may be used in some instances to improve visualization of the lumen of the vagina.

- Contraindications to MRI include ferromagnetic devices such as aneurysm clips, cochlear implants, implanted electrodes, and drug infusion pumps. Pacemakers may be deactivated in the magnetic field. Intrauterine devices are safely imaged.[12] Orthopedic hardware such as hip prosthesis, although generally safely imaged, may produce significant artifacts. If there is any question of safety, consultation with the radiologist is recommended.

### 2.1.1. Axial and Sagittal T2-Weighted Fast Spin Echo

- T2-weighted axial images allow for excellent depiction of the zonal anatomy of the uterus and cervix. Sagittal images depict the uterus and cervix longitudinally and show relationships with adjacent structures and the fat planes that separate them. These planes are important components of tumor staging by MRI (Fig. 4-9).[13–18]

### 2.1.2. Axial and Sagittal T1-Weighted Images

- T1-weighted images emphasize the differences between fat and muscle and are useful for evaluating pelvic lymphadenopathy (Fig. 4-9).[13–18]

## 2.2. Magnetic Resonance Imaging Anatomic Delineation

- The fundus, corpus, and cervix comprise the three major segments of the uterus (Fig. 4-9). The uterus is supported by the broad ligaments, round ligaments, uretrosacral ligaments, and ligaments formed by condensations of the subperitoneal pelvic connective tissues. The uterus is further divided into the endometrium with its columnar epithelium; the myometrium with its mixed collection of smooth muscle, fibrous, and elastic elements; and the surrounding visceral fascia of the parametrium and paracervix. These zones and the uterus itself vary in size depending on the age of the patient and the presence or lack of hormonal influence.[19–22]

- Three distinct uterine zones can be recognized by T2-weighted images (Fig. 4-9A).[13] From internally to externally:

  □ The high signal endometrium and secretions.
  □ The junctional zone that comprises the innermost myometrium with its low signal.
  □ The intermediate signal of the outer myometrium.

- The cervix is defined from the external os to the internal os. T2-weighted images demonstrate three zones and the

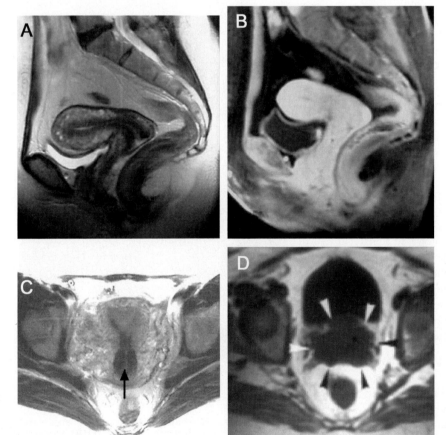

**FIGURE 4-9.** Sagittal **(A, B)** and axial **(C, D)** MRI of the uterus. Sagittal T2-weighted **(A)** and post-contrast T1-weighted **(B)** MRI shows an anteverted uterus. The uterus shows a high signal intensity endometrial canal **(A)**, surrounded by a relatively low signal intensity junctional zone. The myometrium shows intermediate signal intensity, whereas the bladder shows high signal intensity on the T2-weighted sagittal images **(A)**. The relatively high signal intensity endometrial canal *(arrow)* on the axial T2-weighted image **(C)** again is noted, surrounded by the relatively lower signal intensity of the myometrium. The parametrial involvement *(arrowheads)* and vascular structures are better appreciated on the axial T1-weighted image **(D)**.

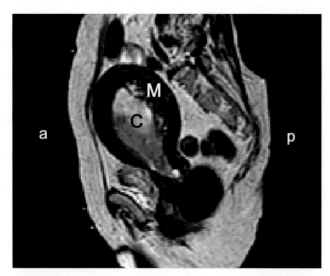

**FIGURE 4-10.** Sagittal T2-weighted image shows an endometrial cancer as an enlarged uterus with a distended endometrial cavity filled with a hyperintense mass (*C*). Myometrial invasion (*M*) is evident as an irregular interphase between the tumor and the myometrium at the posterior fundus. Anterior (*a*), posterior (*p*).

mucus within the canal (Fig. 4-9A).[13] From internally to externally:

- □ The high signal endocervix.
- □ The low signal surrounding stroma.
- □ The intermediate signal of the peripheral smooth muscle, which is continuous with the outermost myometrium of the uterus.

## 2.3. Dynamic Contrast Magnetic Resonance Imaging

- ▪ The addition of MRI contrast agents with sequential acquisition of gradient echo images, which can be displayed mathematically, allows for a physiologic view of the tumor. With this technique, parameters such as tissue perfusion, blood flow, vascular density, and vascular permeability can be studied.[23]

## 2.4. Endometrial Cancer

- ▪ Endometrial cancer usually manifests as increased signal on T2-weighted images (Fig. 4-10). The tumor usually demonstrates less enhancement than the surrounding uterine tissue after contrast administration.[13,18,24–27]
- ▪ MR appearance by the International Federation of Gynecology and Obstetrics staging on the basis of T2-weighted images and post-contrast T1-weighted images is as follows:

  - □ *Stages 0 and I:* Carcinoma in situ or confined to the corpus may appear normal or have a thickened endometrial stripe. The inner myometrium may be involved, but the outer myometrium is preserved.
  - □ *Stage II:* Tumor extension to the cervix is demonstrated by widening of the internal cervical os and abnormal high signal in the cervical stroma.

- □ *Stage III:* Tumor extension is beyond the uterus but within the true pelvis demonstrated by increased signal in the outer myometrium and architectural distortion of the outer myometrium. An increased signal in the vaginal wall and pelvic lymph nodes greater than 1 cm may be seen.
- □ *Stage IV:* Tumor outside of the true pelvis or invasion of the bladder or rectal mucosa is demonstrated by loss of the normal fat planes with increased signal in the involved organs and distant metastasis.

## 2.5. Cervical Cancer

- ▪ Cervical cancer, like uterine cancer, demonstrates increased T2 signal compared with the normal stroma (Fig. 4-11). Although postcontrast MR images are of limited

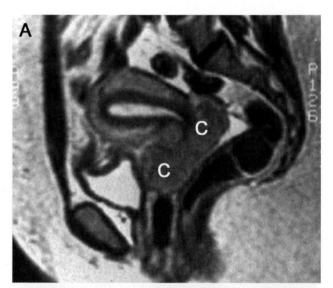

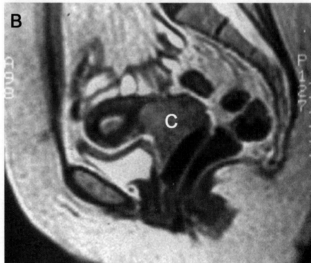

**FIGURE 4-11.** Sagittal T2-weighted images demonstrate two cervical cancers (*C*) in two different patients (**A** and **B**). Moderate obstruction is evident by increase of the diameter of the endometrial canal.

value (Fig. 4-9B), dynamic contrast images may have the potential to provide the physiologic information that may improve treatment outcome.

- MR appearance of cervical cancer based on the International Federation of Gynecology and Obstetrics staging and T2-weighted images[13–18]:

  □ *Stages 0 and I:* Carcinoma in situ or confined to the cervix may appear normal or demonstrate increased signal, which does not extend beyond the cervical stroma.

  □ *Stage II:* Tumor beyond the cervix, but not involving the pelvic sidewall or lower third of the vagina, is demonstrated by increased signal extending beyond the fibrous stroma (IIB) or into the upper two-thirds of the vagina (IIA).

  □ *Stage III:* Tumor extending to the lower third of the vagina, pelvic sidewall, or uretral obstruction is demonstrated by increased signal outside the uterine stroma or into the lower third of the vagina. Increased signal in the levator ani, pyriformis, or obturator internus as well as a dilated ureter signify stage III.

  □ *Stage IV:* Tumor outside of the true pelvis or invasion of the bladder or rectal mucosa is demonstrated by loss of the normal fat planes with increased signal in the involved organs and distant metastasis.

## 2.6. Magnetic Resonance Spectroscopy Imaging

- Although few studies have been reported and no clinical use has been established, MRSI may be used to evaluate tissue biochemistry in the future. This holds promise in evaluating the changes in the metabolic activity in the tissues affected by malignancy.[28–30]

## 2.7. Magnetic Resonance Imaging and Computed Tomography for Treatment Planning

- Radiation therapy for gynecologic cancer frequently includes a significant portion of sensitive normal tissues because of the close vicinity of the target regions (tumor

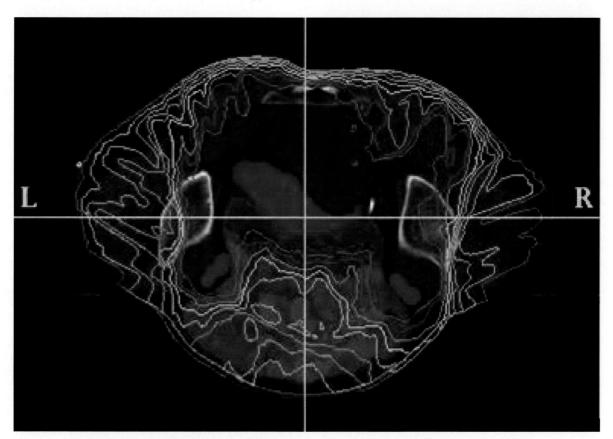

**FIGURE 4-12.** Sample IMRT dose distribution in a patient with cervical cancer who is in a prone position. The dose distribution highly conforms to the target structures including the uterus *(red)* and parametrial and pelvic lymph nodes *(orange)*, whereas the dose to the small bowel *(aqua)* is minimized. In the prone position, the small bowel *(light blue)* is displaced anteriorly and away from the target creating a gap between target and a large portion of the small bowel. Color coding for the isodose lines ranges from the 100% isodose line *(pink)* to the 10% isodose line *(dark blue)*.

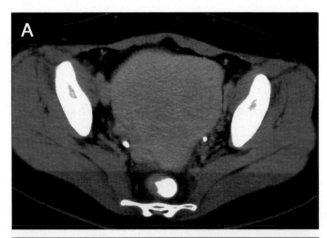

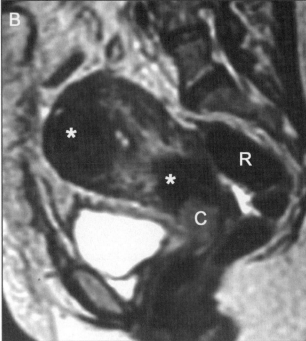

**FIGURE 4-13.** Axial computed tomography (CT) image **(A)** demonstrates enlargement of the cervix and uterus in a patient with cervical cancer. The cervical cancer cannot be readily differentiated from the remainder of the uterus. Sagittal T2-weighted MRI **(B)** clearly demonstrates the enlarged uterus with fibroids (*asterisk*) from the small cervical cancer *(C)*. The close proximity of the rectum *(R)* can be clearly seen.

and lymph nodes) to the bowel and bladder. In pelvic and para-aortic radiation, bowel complications have remained among the most common short- and long-term toxicities of pelvic radiation therapy in patients with gynecologic cancer.[31–34] Traditionally, it has been difficult to reduce the radiation dose to bowel and other normal tissues to decrease the chance of complications.

- With the increasing use of imaging-based therapy planning, radiation delivery techniques have advanced rapidly, and the recent availability of intensity-modu-

lated radiation therapy (IMRT) has greatly improved highly conformal radiation therapy delivery to target tissues while reducing the dose to critical surrounding normal structures (Fig. 4-12). The effectiveness of IMRT in reducing small bowel dose in gynecologic pelvic radiation therapy has been demonstrated in recent studies.[34–37]

- These studies[34–37] have been largely based on CT imaging (Fig. 4-12). However, compared with CT, MRI has been shown to have higher accuracy and better delineation of tumor and normal tissue in patients with gynecologic cancer (Fig. 4-13).[38–44] The incorporation of MRI data into the planning process has the potential to further improve target definition for IMRT in gynecologic cancer. In particular, the extent of extrauterine parametrial tumor extension can be more successfully integrated into the therapeutic algorithm. This may allow for further dose intensification to target structures while reducing radiation dose to sensitive normal tissues.

## REFERENCES

1. Susil RC, Camphausen K, Choyke P, et al. MRI-guided prostate interventions in a standard 1.5T magnet. Submitted 2003.
2. Liney GP, Turnbull LW, Knowles AJ. A simple method for the correction of endorectal surface coil inhomogeneity in prostate imaging. *J Magn Reson Imaging* 1998;8:994–997.
3. Coakley FV, Hricak H. Radiologic anatomy of the prostate gland: a clinical approach. *Radiol Clin North Am* 2000;38:15–30.
4. Tempany CM, Zhou X, Zerhouni EA, et al. Staging of prostate cancer: results of Radiology Diagnostic Oncology Group project comparison of three MR imaging techniques. *Radiology* 1994; 192:47–54.
5. Hricak H, White S, Vigneron D, et al. Carcinoma of the prostate gland: MR imaging with pelvic phased-array coils versus integrated endorectal-pelvic phased-array coils. *Radiology* 1994;193: 703–709.
6. D'Amico AV, Whittington R, Malkowicz SB, et al. Critical analysis of the ability of the endorectal coil magnetic resonance imaging scan to predict pathologic stage, margin status, and postoperative prostate-specific antigen failure in patients with clinically organ-confined prostate cancer. *J Clin Oncol* 1996;14: 1770–1777.
7. Parker CC, Damyanovich A, Haycocks T, et al. Magnetic resonance imaging in the radiation treatment planning of localized prostate cancer using intra-prostatic fiducial markers for computed tomography co-registration. *Radiother Oncol* 2003;66: 217–224.
8. Ramsey CR, Oliver AL. Magnetic resonance imaging based digitally reconstructed radiographs, virtual simulation, and three-dimensional treatment planning for brain neoplasms. *Med Phys* 1998;25:1928–1934.
9. Kurhanewicz J, Vigneron DB, Hricak H, et al. Three-dimensional H-1 MR spectroscopic imaging of the in situ human prostate with high (0.24–0.7-cm3) spatial resolution. *Radiology* 1996;198:795–805.
10. Yu KK, Scheidler J, Hricak H, et al. Prostate cancer: prediction of extracapsular extension with endorectal MR imaging and three-dimensional proton MR spectroscopic imaging. *Radiology* 1999;213:481–488.

11. Padhani AR, Gapinski CJ, Macvicar DA, et al. Dynamic contrast enhanced MRI of prostate cancer: correlation with morphology and tumour stage, histological grade and PSA. *Clin Radiol* 2000;55:99–109.
12. Pasquale SA, Russer TJ, Foldesy R, et al. Lack of interaction between magnetic resonance imaging and the copper-T380A IUD. *Contraception* 1997;55:169–173.
13. Kubik-Huch RA, Reinhold C, Semelka RC, et al. Uterus and cervix. In: Semelka RC. *Abdominal-pelvic MRI.* New York: Wiley-Liss, 2002:1049–1122.
14. Sironi S, De Cobelli F, Scarfone G, et al. Carcinoma of the cervix: value of plain and gadolinium-enhanced MR imaging in assessing the degree of invasiveness. *Radiology* 1993;188:797–801.
15. Hawighorst H, Knapstein PG, Weikel W, et al. Cervical carcinoma: comparison of standard and pharmacokinetic MR imaging. *Radiology* 1996;201:531–539.
16. Semelka RC, Hricak H, Kim B, et al. Pelvic fistulas: appearances on MR images. *Abdom Imaging* 1997;22:91–95.
17. Scheidler J, Heuck AF, Steinborn M, et al. Parametrial invasion in cervical carcinoma: evaluation of detection at MR imaging with fat suppression. *Radiology* 1998;206:125–129.
18. Hamm B, Kubich-Huch RA, Fleige B, et al. MR imaging and CT of the female pelvis: radiologic-pathologic correlation. *Eur Radiol* 1999;9:3–15.
19. McCarthy S, Tauber C, Gore J, et al. Female pelvic anatomy: MR assessment of variations during the menstrual cycle and with use of oral contraceptives. *Radiology* 1986;160:119–123.
20. Demas BE, Hricak H, Jaffe RB. Uterine MR imaging: effects of hormonal stimulation. *Radiology* 1986;159:123–136.
21. Wiczyk HP, Janus CL, Richards CJ, et al. Comparison of magnetic resonance imaging and ultrasound in evaluating follicular and endometrial development throughout the normal cycle. *Fertil Steril* 1988;49:969–972.
22. Janus CL, Bateman B, Wiczyk H, et al. Evaluation of the stimulated menstrual cycle by magnetic resonance imaging. *Fertil Steril* 1990;54:1017–1020.
23. Mayr NA, Tali ET, Yuh WTC, et al. Cervical cancer: application of MR imaging in radiation therapy. *Radiology* 1993;189:601–608.
24. Yamashita Y, Mizutani H, Torashima M, et al. Assessment of myometrial invasion by endometrial carcinoma: transvaginal sonography vs. contrast-enhanced MR imaging. *AJR Am J Roentgenol* 1993;161:595–599.
25. Hricak H, Rubinstein LV, Gherman GM, et al. MR imaging evaluation of endometrial carcinoma: results of an NCI cooperative study. *Radiology* 1991;179:829–832.
26. Sironi S, Colombo E, Villa G, et al. Myometrial invasion by endometrial carcinoma: assessment with plain and gadolinium-enhanced MR imaging. *Radiology* 1992;185:207–212.
27. Hricak H, Stern JL, Fisher MR, et al. Endometrial carcinoma staging by MR imaging. *Radiology* 1987;162:297–305.
28. Allen JR, Prost RW, Griffith OW, et al. In vivo proton (H1) magnetic resonance spectroscopy for cervical carcinoma. *Am J Clin Oncol* 2001;24(5):522–529.
29. Lee JH, Cho KS, Kim YM, et al. Localized in vivo 1H nuclear MR spectroscopy for evaluation of human uterine cervical carcinoma. *AJR Am J Roentgenol* 1998;170(5):1279–1282.
30. Kunnecke B, Delikatny EJ, Russell P, et al. Proton magnetic resonance and human cervical neoplasia. II. Ex vivo chemical-shift microimaging. *J Magn Reson B* 1994;104(2):135–142.
31. Perez CA, Breaux S, Bedwinek JM, et al. Radiation therapy alone in the treatment of carcinoma of the uterine cervix. II. Analysis of complications. *Cancer* 1984;54:235–246.
32. Corn BW, Lanciano RM, Greven KM, et al. Impact of improved irradiation technique, age, and lymph node sampling on the severe complication rate of surgically staged endometrial cancer patients: a multivariate analysis. *J Clin Oncol* 1994;12:510–515.
33. Snijders-Keiholz A, Griffioen G, Davelaar J, et al. Vitamin B12 malabsorption after irradiation for gynaecological tumors. *Anticancer Res* 1993;13:1877–1881.
34. Roeske JC, Lujan A, Rotmensch J, et al. Intensity-modulated whole pelvic radiation therapy in patients with gynecologic malignancies. *Int J Radiat Oncol Biol Phys* 2000;48:1613–1621.
35. Mundt AJ, Roeske JC, Lujan AE, et al. Initial clinical experience with intensity modulated whole-pelvis radiation therapy in women with gynecologic malignancies. *Gynecol Oncol* 2001;82:456–463.
36. Mundt AJ, Lujan AE, Rotmensch J, et al. Intensity-modulated whole pelvic radiotherapy in women with gynecologic malignancies. *Int J Radiat Oncol Biol Phys* 2002;52:1330–1337.
37. Portelance L, Chao KSC, Grigsby PW, et al. Intensity-modulated radiation therapy (IMRT) reduces small bowel, rectum, and bladder doses in patients with cervical cancer receiving pelvic and para-aortic irradiation. *Int J Radiat Oncol Biol Phys* 2001;51:261–266.
38. Hricak H, Lacey CG, Sandles LG, et al. Invasive cervical carcinoma: comparison of MR imaging and surgical findings. *Radiology* 1988;166:623–631.
39. Hricak H, Quivey J, Campos Z, et al. Carcinoma of the cervix: predictive value of clinical and magnetic resonance (MR) imaging assessment of prognostic factors. *Int J Radiat Oncol Biol Phys* 1993;27:791–801.
40. Hricak H, Phillips TL. Editorial on "The influence of tumor size and morphology on the outcome of patients with FIGO stage IB squamous cell carcinoma of the uterine cervix." *Int J Radiat Oncol Biol Phys* 1994;29:201–203.
41. Burghardt E, Hofmann HMH, Ebner F, et al. Magnetic resonance imaging in cervical cancer: a basis for objective classification. *Gynecol Oncol* 1989;33:61–67.
42. Greco A, Mason P, Leung AWL, et al. Staging of carcinoma of the uterine cervix: MRI-surgical correlation. *Clin Radiol* 1989;40:401–405.
43. Hricak H. Cancer of the uterus: the value of MRI pre- and post-irradiation. *Int J Radiat Oncol Biol Phys* 1991;21:1089–1094.
44. Subak L, Hrick H, Powell C, et al. Cervical carcinoma: computed tomography and magnetic resonance imaging for preoperative staging. *Obstet Gynecol* 1995;86:43–50.

# 5

# POSITRON EMISSION TOMOGRAPHY IMAGING FOR TARGET DETERMINATION AND DELINEATION

HOMER A. MACAPINLAC
SMITH APISARNTHANARAX
WADE L. THORSTAD
K. S. CLIFFORD CHAO

## 1. INTRODUCTION

### 1.1. Molecular Basis

- Positron emission tomography (PET)* is a functional imaging modality that detects metabolic changes within cells by using radiopharmaceuticals that are closely related to endogenous molecules.
- [18]F-fluorodeoxyglucose (FDG) is the most commonly used tracer in PET and allows us to image cancer cells on the basis of the abnormally increased glucose metabolism in tumor cells compared with nonmalignant tissue. This was initially described by Warburg et al.[1] in the 1930s, but has been used for imaging of cancer only in the past two decades.
- FDG, a glucose analog, is transported into tumor cells in abnormally increased amounts because of the upregulation of glucose transport protein 1 and hexokinase, the rate-limited enzyme in glycolysis, in malignant cells.
- Once inside the cell, FDG is phosphorylated into FDG-6-phosphate, but it does not undergo glycolysis as does glucose.
- Because most cancer cells possess low phosphatase activity, FDG-6-phosphate accumulates and subsequently becomes "trapped" within the cell.[2]
- This preferential accumulation of FDG in tumor cells allows us to image FDG-avid tumors with PET scanners.
- Bos et al.[3] have described the molecular basis for FDG accumulation in breast cancer cells, which is proposed to be caused by the presence of the hypoxia inducible factor 1 gene. The upregulation of this gene complex codes for various factors to increase the blood supply.

- PET images, therefore, are based on metabolic activity rather than anatomy. Subclinical tumor or normal sized lymph nodes may be detected with PET because of abnormal metabolism at the molecular level before changes become evident through mass effect caused by a tumor or a metastatic lymph node.

### 1.2. Rationale

- The availability of dedicated PET cameras capable of whole-body imaging has launched a revolution in imaging cancer on the basis of abnormalities in metabolism.
- Conventional imaging methods such as x-ray and computed tomography (CT) scanning are based on alterations in anatomy to detect malignancy and spread of tumor on the basis of enlargement of lymph nodes.
- Although CT is essential in radiation treatment planning, it does not provide information about tumor viability, which may be an important prognostic factor for management.
- Additional limitations of multislice CT would include difficulty in tumor delineation in the lung windows when dealing with spiculated lesions, which are commonplace in lung cancer. Tumor-related atelectasis makes it nearly impossible to assess macroscopic disease. Size-based criteria for mediastinal nodal involvement are inadequate because borderline-sized nodes may harbor metastases, and enlarged nodes may not be involved with cancer.
- FDG-PET complements some of the limitations of CT scans by improving discrimination between malignant and benign lesions, more accurately identifying cancer cells in normal-sized nodes, and excluding cancer in enlarged lymph nodes, all of which results in potentially improved staging.[4]

---

* PET refers to [18]F-FDG PET unless otherwise stated.

## 2. TECHNIQUE

### 2.1. Patient Preparation

- FDG is administered after a minimum 4-hour fast in nondiabetic patients. Fasting results in low serum glucose and insulin levels, which allows for good uptake by tumor, thereby avoiding false-negative scans.
- Patients are encouraged to drink water before the injection of FDG because this minimizes the concentration of the tracer in the urinary collecting system, and they are asked to rinse their mouth before imaging to eliminate saliva activity in the mouth.
- Diabetic patients whose diabetes is well-controlled are also asked to titrate their glucose levels to normal range at the scheduled time of injection.
- Our current protocol at the M. D. Anderson Cancer Center involves intravenous catheter placement in the antecubital fossa with the aseptic technique.
- A blood glucose sample is obtained, and then 15 to 20 mCi of FDG is injected (bolus) followed by a 10-mL saline flush. The residual activity is measured in the dose calibrator to determine the net injected dose used for calculating standardized uptake values (SUVs).
- The patient is then kept in a sitting or recumbent position and asked not to talk or drink. This minimizes FDG uptake in the muscles of the tongue and the vocalis/cricopharyngeus muscles of the larynx.

### 2.2. Image Acquisition

- After a 60- to 90-minute uptake phase, the PET/CT scan is acquired. The patient is placed in a head holder if the patient is intended for treatment planning, and a flat bed insert is installed.
- The laser positioning system is used to ensure proper and consistent positioning of the patient for subsequent treatment planning. We are currently using a Discovery ST PET/CT unit (GEMS, Milwaukee, WI) equipped with an eight-slice CT scanner at the M. D. Anderson Cancer Center.
- The CT scan is acquired with 120 kV and 220 mAs at 15 mm per rotation, which is identical for radiation treatment planning with CT alone, and with the patient at mid-inspiration while scanning over the chest to approximate the tidal breathing acquisition performed on the PET scan. The PET scan is acquired in two dimensions at 3 minutes per field of view (15 cm).
- Image acquisition from 2 cm above the orbit through the liver will ensure evaluation of the entire upper aerodigestive track to identify metastatic disease or synchronous primary cancer.
- Complete aerodigestive track imaging may also avoid misinterpreting benign pulmonary nodules for metastatic disease and serves as a baseline in the event that future imaging reveals metastatic disease or metachronous cancer.

- Attenuation correction (AC) is recommended for proper interpretation. AC corrects for apparent variability in FDG accumulation with the depth because of attenuation by normal tissue.
- Images without AC may miss superficial tumors or lymph nodes because of the edge effect distortion.
- AC also allows for semiquantitative measurement of FDG uptake through the SUV, which generally aids in differentiation of malignant from benign tissue and potentially in assessment of response to therapy.
- Diabetic patients with elevated fasting glucose levels may have poor PET images. FDG must compete for tumor uptake with abundant glucose. Diabetic patients should probably not be imaged unless the fasting glucose level is less than 150 mg/dL.
- Scalene and sternocleidomastoid muscle uptake may also be elevated in anxious patients or after neck dissection.
- Diazepam may be used to induce muscle relaxation during the FDG uptake phase.[5]
- The CT scan is used for PET reconstruction and AC. Soft tissue and lung reconstructions are performed for CT to allow adequate visualization of the appropriate structures.
- The PET/CT scans are interpreted by using vendor-provided software (Xeleris, GEMS, Waukesha, WI, USA), which allows independent viewing of the corresponding CT and PET slices with an overlay or fusion view that helps in localization of FDG activity and serves as a guide for interpretation.

## 3. CLINICAL APPLICATIONS

- Currently, PET is used for the diagnosis, staging, and restaging of non–small-cell lung cancer (NSCLC), lymphoma, melanoma, head and neck cancer, and colorectal cancer.
- More recent approval of PET for breast cancer restaging and monitoring of response to therapy, in addition to the limited approval for patients with thyroid cancer who have negative I-131 scans and elevated thyroglobulin levels, have added to the more widespread clinical use of this modality.
- A tabulation of PET in the literature by Gambhir et al.[6] of the average PET sensitivity and specificity across all oncology applications ranged from 84% to 87% (based on 18,402 patients) and 88% to 93% (based on 14,264 patients), respectively. The accuracy of PET imaging in oncology ranged from 87% to 90%.
- The following sections will focus on the current indications and uses for lung, breast, and head and neck cancers.

### 3.1. Staging and Diagnosis

- In general, PET lacks anatomic detail sufficient for determining the T stage of a tumor, whereas its strengths lie in regional nodal and distant metastatic staging.

### 3.1.1. Lung Cancer

- PET imaging in NSCLC has proven to be more accurate than CT for staging the mediastinum and identifying distant metastases.[7]
- The superior accuracy of PET in mediastinal staging was shown in prospective studies comparing PET and CT[8–19] and confirmed by multiple meta-analyses[20–23] (Table 5-1).
- According to a recent meta-analysis by Toloza et al.,[22] the pooled sensitivity and specificity for staging the mediastinum for CT scanning (20 studies with 3,438 patients) were 57% (49%–66%) and 82% (77%–86%), respectively. For PET scanning (18 studies with 1045 patients), the pooled sensitivity and specificity were 84% (78%–89%) and 89% (83%–93%), respectively.
- The meta-analysis of thirty-nine studies by Gould et al.[23] also showed similar accuracy of PET versus CT imaging. In addition, PET results were dependent on the presence or absence of enlarged mediastinal lymph nodes. PET was more sensitive but less specific for enlarged mediastinal nodes.
- When combining PET and CT, the sensitivity of the combined tests ranged from 78% to 93%, and the specificity ranged from 82% to 95%. The positive predictive value ranged from 83% to 93%, and the negative predictive value ranged from 88% to 95%.

- A preliminary study suggests that PET may also be useful for staging and evaluating small-cell lung cancer.[24]

### 3.1.2. Breast Cancer

- Several studies have shown that PET can accurately detect and stage primary breast lesions and axillary lymph node metastasis. The reported sensitivity and specificity from these studies ranged from 85% to 100% and 75% to 100%, respectively.[6,25–29]
- In the largest single-institution prospective study of 167 patients, PET had a sensitivity of 94% and specificity of 86% for detecting axillary metastases.[30]
- Compared with conventional staging methods (x-ray, ultrasound, mammography, and bone scintigraphy), PET was as accurate for primary tumor lymph node metastasis.[31,32]
- However, other studies have reported that smaller primary tumors and axillary metastases may evade PET detection, resulting in lower sensitivities.[33–38]
- Diagnostic accuracy of PET was found to be dependent on tumor size and increased from 68% to 92% for pT1 tumors and to approximately 100% for pT2 and pT3 lesions.[29]
- The first prospective multicenter study of 360 patients showed that PET possessed moderate accuracy in detecting axillary metastasis (sensitivity 61%, specificity 80%) and often failed to detect small-volume metastatic disease in the axillae.[39]

**TABLE 5-1. POSITRON EMISSION TOMOGRAPHY COMPARED WITH COMPUTED TOMOGRAPHY FOR DETECTION OF MEDIASTINAL LYMPH NODE METASTASIS IN LUNG CANCER\***

| Author/Year | No. of Patients | Sensitivity of PET (%) | Specificity of PET (%) | CT Sensitivity (%) | CT Specificity (%) |
|---|---|---|---|---|---|
| Valk et al. 1995[8] | 99 | 83 | 94 | 63 | 73 |
| Bury et al. 1996[9] | 53 | 88 | 86 | 71 | 81 |
| Vansteenkiste et al. 1997[10] | 50 | 67 | 97 | 67 | 59 |
| Vansteenkiste et al. 1998[11] | 68 | 93 | 95 | 75 | 63 |
| Vansteenkiste et al. 1998[116] | 56 | 86 | 43 | 86 | 79 |
| Berlangieri et al. 1999[13] | 50 | 80 | 97 | 65 | 90 |
| Marom et al. 1999[14] | 79 | 73 | 94 | 59 | 86 |
| Saunders et al. 1999[15] | 84 | 71 | 97 | 20 | 90 |
| Pieterman et al. 2000[16] | 102 | 91 | 86 | 75 | 66 |
| Weng et al. 2000[17] | 50 | 73 | 94 | 73 | 77 |
| Dunagan et al. 2001[18] | 72 | 52 | 88 | 50 | 87 |
| Gupta et al. 2001[19] | 77 | 87 | 91 | 68 | 61 |
| *Average* | | 79 | 89 | 64 | 76 |

CT, computed tomography; PET, positron emission tomography.
\* Includes studies with fifty or more patients.

- Compared with magnetic resonance imaging (MRI), PET was less sensitive in disclosing malignant breast lesions and less accurate in assessing multifocal disease secondary to its inferior ability to depict smaller lesions compared with PET.[40]
- In a recent study, PET was not as sensitive as sentinel lymph node (SLN) biopsy for detection of axillary metastases in early breast cancer with clinically negative axillary lymph nodes, but it was highly specific.[41] Accordingly, these authors suggested that patients with a positive axillary PET result could forgo an SLN biopsy and proceed directly to axillary lymph node dissection.
- In summary, although PET is not routinely recommended for axillary staging of newly diagnosed breast cancer and should not be substituted for histologic evaluation of axillary nodal specimens, potential uses for initial staging may include the following:

  □ Staging of patients not undergoing axillary dissection or SLN biopsy.
  □ Identification of patients who should proceed directly to axillary dissection.
  □ Staging of patients who have inconclusive conventional diagnostic results.
  □ Assessment of internal mammary nodal metastases. One study has demonstrated greater accuracy in identifying internal mammary involvement by the use of PET compared with CT.[42]

### 3.1.3. Head and Neck Cancer

- Multiple studies suggest that PET is more sensitive and specific in evaluating head and neck squamous cell carcinoma (HNSCC) lymphatic metastasis compared with anatomic modalities such as CT and MRI (Table 5-2).[43–54]
- Adams et al.[49] evaluated 1,284 lymph nodes in 60 patients with HNSCC. Sensitivity and specificity of PET were 90% and 94%, respectively, compared with values of 82% and 85% for CT, and 80% and 79% for MRI, respectively.
- Most published studies have been in selected patient groups. The study by Kau et al.[52] compared the diagnostic accuracy of PET compared with CT and MRI for metastatic lymph node detection in a routine clinical setting at an academic medical center. Sensitivity and specificity for PET were 87% and 94%, respectively, compared with values of 65% and 47% for CT, and 88% and 41% for MRI, respectively.

### 3.1.4. Unknown Primary Carcinoma Presenting with Cervical Lymph Node Metastasis

- In 1950, approximately 10% of patients with proven malignancy had no known primary site.[55]
- Improvements in diagnostic imaging and pathologic evaluation (i.e., immunohistochemical staining)

**TABLE 5-2. POSITRON EMISSION TOMOGRAPHY COMPARED WITH COMPUTED TOMOGRAPHY AND MAGNETIC RESONANCE IMAGING FOR DETECTION OF LYMPH NODE METASTASIS IN HEAD AND NECK CANCER**

| Author/Year | No. of Patients | Sensitivity of PET (%) | Specificity of PET (%) | CT/MRI Sensitivity (%) | CT/MRI Specificity (%) |
|---|---|---|---|---|---|
| Rege et al. 1994[43] | 34 | 88 | 89 | 81 (MRI) | 89 (MRI) |
| Laubenbacher et al. 1995[44] | 22 | 90 | 96 | 78 (MRI) | 71 (MRI) |
| McGuirt et al. 1995[45] | 49 | 83 | 82 | 78 (CT) | 86 (CT) |
| Benchaou et al. 1996[46] | 48 | 72 | 99 | 67 (CT) | 97 (CT) |
| Braams et al. 1997[47] | 12 | 91 | 88 | 36 (MRI) | 94 (MRI) |
| Wong et al. 1997[48] | 16 | 67 | 100 | 67 (CT/MRI) | 25 (CT/MRI) |
| Adams et al. 1998[49] | 60 | 90 | 94 | 82 (CT) | 85 (CT) |
| | | | | 80 (MRI) | 79 (MRI) |
| Myers et al. 1998[50] | 14 | 78 | 100 | 57 (CT) | 90 (CT) |
| Paulus et al. 1998[51] | 38 | 50 | 100 | 40 (CT) | 100 (CT) |
| Kau et al. 1999[52] | 70 | 87 | 94 | 65 (CT) | 47 (CT) |
| | | | | 88 (MRI) | 41 (MRI) |
| Nowak et al. 1999[53] | 71 | 80 | 92 | 80 (CT/MRI) | 84 (CT/MRI) |
| Hannah et al. 2002[54] | 48 | 82 | 100 | 81 (CT) | 81 (CT) |
| *Average* | | 80 | 95 | 70 | 76 |

MRI, magnetic resonance imaging; CT, computed tomography; PET, positron emission tomography.

**TABLE 5-3. POSITRON EMISSION TOMOGRAPHY COMPARED WITH CONVENTIONAL IMAGING FOR RECURRENCE IN BREAST CANCER**

| Author/Year | No. of Patients | Sensitivity of PET (%) | Specificity of PET (%) | CI Sensitivity (%) | CI Specificity (%) |
|---|---|---|---|---|---|
| Vranjesevic et al. 2002[64] | 61 | 93 | 84 | 79 | 68 |
| Gallowitsch et al. 2003[65] | 62 | 97 | 82 | 84 | 60 |
| Goerres et al. 2003[117] | 32 | 100 | 72 | 79 (MRI) | 94 (MRI) |

CI, conventional imaging (includes computed tomography, magnetic resonance imaging, ultrasonography, radiography, mammography, and bone scintigraphy); PET, positron emission tomography; MRI, magnetic resonance imaging.

have reduced this number to approximately 2% today.[56,57]

- Patients who present with cervical lymph node metastasis from an unknown primary tumor present difficult management decisions.
- After negative extensive workup including clinical examination, pan-endoscopy, and CT/MRI examination, 25% to 30% of these patients are found to have a primary HNSCC when evaluated with PET.[47,58–60]
- PET has been shown to change management in 33% of patients with cervical lymph node metastasis from an unknown primary site.[59]

## 3.2. Detection of Recurrence

### 3.2.1. Lung Cancer

- In a study by Bury et al.,[61] PET was more precise than CT in differentiating persistent or recurrent lesions from benign fibrosis in patients with NSCLC. PET had a sensitivity of 100% and specificity of 92%, whereas CT had a sensitivity and specificity of 71% and 95%, respectively.
- Compiled data show that average PET sensitivity and specificity for detecting lung cancer recurrence are 98% and 92%, respectively.[6]

### 3.2.2. Breast Cancer

- PET is highly accurate in restaging patients with suspected breast cancer recurrence.[62–65]
- PET had comparable or superior accuracy compared with conventional imaging (Table 5-3).
- Two studies showed that compared with combined conventional imaging, PET was more accurate for predicting outcome and diagnosing locoregional recurrence.[64,65]

### 3.2.3. Head and Neck Cancer

- The clinical outcome of patients with recurrent HNSCC is poor.
- Early identification of recurrence may therefore increase the likelihood of successful salvage treatment.
- Anatomic evaluation after surgery and irradiation or primary chemoradiotherapy is frequently inconclusive because of treatment-related disruption of normal anatomy and tissue planes.
- Several studies demonstrate that PET is superior to clinical examination and CT/MRI imaging for detecting recurrence in HNSCC (Table 5-4).[43,66–71]

**TABLE 5-4. POSITRON EMISSION TOMOGRAPHY COMPARED WITH COMPUTED TOMOGRAPHY AND MAGNETIC RESONANCE IMAGING FOR DETECTION OF RECURRENCE IN HEAD AND NECK CANCER**

| Author/Year | No. of Patients | Treatment | Time (mo)* | Sensitivity of PET (%) | Specificity of PET (%) | CT/MRI Sensitivity (%) | CT/MRI Specificity (%) |
|---|---|---|---|---|---|---|---|
| Rege et al. 1994[43] | 29 | S, RT | 44 | 93 | 86 | 70 (MRI) | 57 (MRI) |
| Lapela et al. 1995[66] | 22 | S, RT | 10 | 88 | 86 | 92 (CT) | 50 (CT) |
| Anzai et al. 1996[67] | 12 | S, RT | 10 | 88 | 100 | 25 (CT/MRI) | 75 (CT/MRI) |
| Greven et al. 1997[68] | 31 | RT | 6 | 80 | 81 | 58 (CT) | 100 (CT) |
| Greven et al. 2001[69] | 36 | RT | 1 | 46 | 100 | 40 (CT) | 100 (CT) |
| Kitagawa et al. 2003[70] | 23 | RT + CT | 1 | 100 | 90 | 75 (CT) 100 (MRI) | 59 (CT) 41 (MRI) |
| Yen et al. 2003[71]† | 67 | RT ± CT | 14 | 100 | 93 | 62 (MRI) | 44 (MRI) |

S, surgery; RT, radiotherapy; CT, chemotherapy; PET, positron emission tomography; MRI, magnetic resonance imaging.
* Median or mean time from completion of last treatment to PET scan, except for Greven et al.'s study (2001),[69] in which all patients were imaged at 1 mo.
† Nasopharyngeal carcinomas.

- The accuracy of PET in detecting recurrences, however, has shown to vary temporally according to when the images are acquired post-treatment.
- Greven et al.[69] showed that at 1 month postradiation, PET scans of various patients with HNSCC had a high incidence of false-negative interpretations (28%). At 4 months postradiation, however, none of the eighteen patients with negative scan results demonstrated local relapse (false-negative rate 0%).
- Similarly in another study, three of twenty-one PET scans (14%) completed at 2 months post-treatment had false-negative interpretations.[72]
- The appropriate timing of PET after completion of radiation therapy to assess for persistent and recurrent disease therefore remains unresolved but may be between 2 and 4 months, as suggested by the previously mentioned studies.

## 3.3. Assessment of Early Treatment Response

- Prediction of ultimate outcome early during treatment would have tremendous implications for the patient.
- Changes in FDG uptake precede changes in anatomic tumor volume and could be a more precise predictor of actual cancer cell kill or treatment response than CT.
- PET could be used to predict early response during chemotherapy and radiation therapy even potentially after only a few days of therapy.
- Early identification of nonresponders would allow physicians the benefit of avoiding overtreatment and undertreatment by discontinuing ineffective treatments and individualizing alternative treatment modalities.

### 3.3.1. Lung Cancer

- PET imaging becomes particularly valuable in situations in which lung tumors may be obscured or hidden by atelectasis, fibrosis, or inflammatory infiltrates related to radiation pneumonitis on CT.
- Studies of monitoring response after induction treatment with PET in lung cancer are limited.[12,73,74]
- After three cycles of induction chemotherapy, PET was 100% accurate in downstaging mediastinal lymph nodes in a small pilot study of nine patients with stage IIIA-N2 NSCLC.[12]
- In two other larger retrospective studies on the use of PET after induction chemoradiation, PET was found to be accurate in detecting residual tumor but not mediastinal nodal involvement. The sensitivity of PET for mediastinal disease was comparable to CT for both studies, 67% and 58%, respectively.[73,74]
- A prospective study by Mac Manus et al.[75] of seventy-three patients with NSCLC concluded that a single early post-treatment PET scan (median: 70 days) is a better predictor of survival than CT response, stage, or pretreatment performance status.

- In contrast with these studies that imaged patients after completion of therapy, Weber et al.[76] recently evaluated PET tumor response in fifty-seven patients with advanced NSCLC early during the course of therapy after the first cycle of chemotherapy. Reduction of FDG uptake was significantly correlated with the clinical outcome according to the Response Evaluation Criteria in Solid Tumors criteria.[77] Sensitivity and specificity for prediction of best response were 95% and 74%, respectively. The response rate was only 4% in patients without a metabolic response compared with 71% in those with a decrease in FDG uptake.
- Erdi et al.[78] serially scanned two patients with NSCLC by means of PET before, 8 weeks during, and after radiation therapy. The responder had a progressive reduction in all response parameters (including lesion volume by PET, average SUV, maximum SUV, and total lesion glycolysis). The nonresponder showed an initial decrease followed by a sharp increase starting at the 45-Gy level.

### 3.3.2. Breast Cancer

- PET may detect metabolic changes in breast cancer as early as 8 days after initiation of chemohormonotherapy, preceding any appreciable changes in tumor size clinically or radiographically.[79]
- Responders may be *clinically* differentiated from nonresponders after the first course of chemotherapy.[80,81]
- Jansson et al.[81] also showed that clinical response to therapy could be detected earlier than any other conventional method.
- *Pathologic* responders may also be preferentially identified by using PET.
- There was a significant difference in FDG uptake after the first course of chemotherapy between nonresponders and responders, and by the second cycle, the histopathologic response could be predicted with 91% accuracy.[82]
- For large tumors (>3 cm), PET predicts complete pathologic response after one course of chemotherapy in thirty patients with a sensitivity of 90% and specificity of 74%.[83] The mean reduction in FDG uptake in partial or complete pathologic responders was significantly greater than no response or progression.

### 3.3.3. Head and Neck Cancer

- The ability to predict the outcome of chemoradiotherapy for organ-sparing HNSCC treatment would allow early use of surgical intervention in nonresponders and more confident avoidance of surgery in those responding.
- Limited studies exist that examine the role of PET imaging during the course of therapy in HNSCC. These studies have shown that there is an association between

decline in FDG uptake during chemotherapy with or without radiation and clinical tumor response, although patient numbers in these studies were small.[84,85]

- In a larger study by Brun et al.,[86] forty-seven patients with locally advanced HNSCC who were receiving radiation and/or neoadjuvant chemotherapy metabolic rate signals after one cycle of chemotherapy or a median 24 Gy of radiation were significantly associated with favorable outcomes. Tumor response, survival, and local control were 96% and 62%, 72% and 35%, and 96% and 55%, respectively, for low and high metabolic rate of FDG.
- Studies with radiation alone, however, are more conflicting.
- Two studies demonstrated variations in FDG uptake during the course of radiation therapy. Hautzel and Muller-Gartner[87] described both increases and decreases in SUV characterized by an initial enhancement in FDG uptake after 6 Gy followed by a constant decline with increasing dose. Similarly, FDG uptake increased early during the course of radiotherapy (RT) (<20 Gy) and decreased near the completion of treatment (>45 Gy).[88] This variation in metabolic response was also shown in animal studies.[89] It has been suggested that normal tissue inflammatory changes may be responsible for these varying FDG uptake measurements that may lead to false-positive results.
- Research is ongoing to identify a PET tracer correlating early response to RT with ultimate outcome in head and neck carcinoma.

## 4. IMPACT ON RADIOTHERAPY TREATMENT PLANNING

- As a result of its ability to better assess tumor viability, PET may be used to supplement CT in the definition of the gross target volume (GTV) and its subsequent expansion to the planned treatment volume (PTV).
- It is essential to have the CT or MRI for anatomic correlation with PET because both modalities complement each other in localization of both normal and abnormal tissue.
- A complete treatment history is vital to the interpretation. For example, recent chemotherapy may cause an increase uptake in marrow uptake in the spine, and prior RT may demonstrate the reverse finding of hypometabolism in marrow.
- Postradiation changes with diminution of activity in the normal lymphoid tissues in the neck, which in turn are age dependent, should be anticipated.
- The extent of RT should be known because this may cause protracted post-treatment changes manifested as increased uptake in lungs, thyroid, and myocardium.
- In addition, intense activity in muscle flaps should be noted, and normal gastroesophageal (GE) junction activity may sometimes be pronounced in reflux esophagitis.[4]

- By using an integrated PET/CT scanner, Ciernik et al.[90] studied thirty-nine patients with various solid tumors. CT and PET were obtained in the treatment position, and coregistered images were used for treatment planning.
- Overall, in 56% of cases (22/39), the authors found that GTV delineation was significantly altered if PET imaging data were used. It is interesting that in 16% of cases, PET/CT showed distant metastases, changing the treatment strategy from curative to palliative.

### 4.1. Lung Cancer

- Many studies have reported the impact of PET on radiation treatment volumes in lung cancer, mainly by visual comparisons of PET and CT images. Subsequent series incorporated computer overlays of PET and CT data, also called image fusion (Fig. 5-1).
- Hebert et al.[91] used PET in a prospective study of twenty patients to assess the extent of disease compared with the use of chest radiography and CT. Three of twelve patients showed CT/CXR (chest x-ray) changes larger than PET, whereas two of twelve had PET volumes larger than CT/CXR.
- Kiffer et al.[92] used a simple form of graphic coregistration of each patient's coronal PET images with the anterior–posterior simulator image on which the RT volume had been marked. In this retrospective study, four of fifteen patients would have had the RT volume influenced by the PET findings.
- Nestle et al.[93] performed a retrospective analysis by using a CT-based planning with anterior–posterior portals encompassing the primary tumor and the mediastinum. PET findings would have contributed to a reduction in the radiation portals in twelve of thirty-four patients (35%).
- Munley et al.[94] conducted a study comparing single-photon emission CT lung perfusion scintigraphy (n = 104) and PET (n = 35), which were registered with the thoracic CT used to perform treatment planning. Fifty single-photon emission CT studies were judged to be "potentially useful" because of the detection of hypoperfused regions of the lungs, but they were not used during treatment planning. PET data influenced 34% (12/35) of the treatment plans examined and resulted in enlarging portions of the beam aperture.
- A theoretic study by Vanuytsel et al.[95] assessed mediastinal nodes in patients with lung cancer. The GTV was defined on the basis of CT and PET/CT data. Pathology was the gold standard for comparison (988 lymph nodes). In forty-five patients (62%), the information obtained from PET would have led to a change of the treatment volumes.
- In a prospective study of eleven patients with NSCLC, Erdi et al.[96] found an increase in PTV volume (19%) in seven cases to incorporate nodal disease. The other four patients had PTVs that decreased an average of 18% because of the exclusion of atelectasis and reduction of the

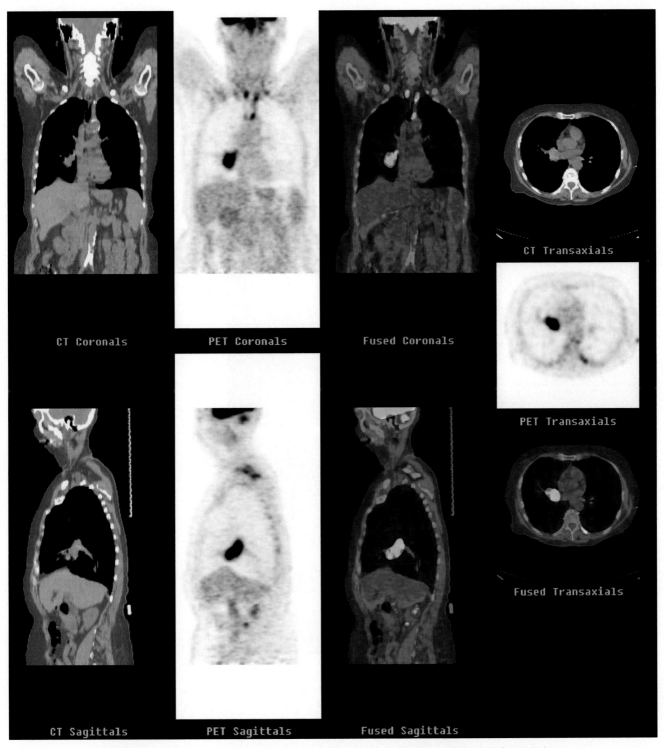

**FIGURE 5-1.** Positron emission tomography (PET) and computed tomography (CT) fusion in lung cancer depicting mediastinal metastasis. Fused coronal, sagittal, and transaxial images (*blue*).

target volume to avoid delivering higher radiation doses to critical structures.

- In summary, these various series demonstrated changes in treatment volumes ranging from 15% to 60% if PET information was used.

## 4.2. Head and Neck Cancer

- Familiarity with the normal structures in the head and neck region is crucial to interpretation and awareness

about the distribution of lymphoid tissue and thymic tissue, which is more prominent in younger patients (Fig. 5-2).

- Rahn et al.[97] evaluated thirty-four patients with primary or recurrent squamous cell carcinoma of the head and neck who underwent PET scans in addition to conventional staging procedures before treatment planning. The extent of changes of treatment strategy or target volume as the result of PET findings was analyzed. In nine of twenty-two patients with primary tumors

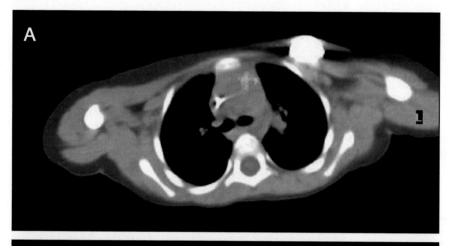

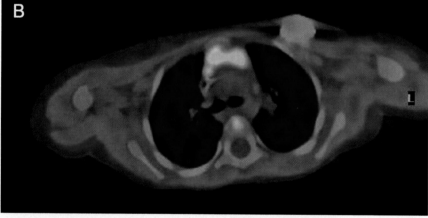

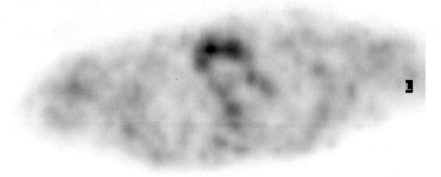

**FIGURE 5-2. A:** CT scan of the chest. Increased PET signals in the thymus must be distinguished from head and neck primary lesions; fused PET/CT image (**B**) from CT (**A**) and PET (**C**) scans.

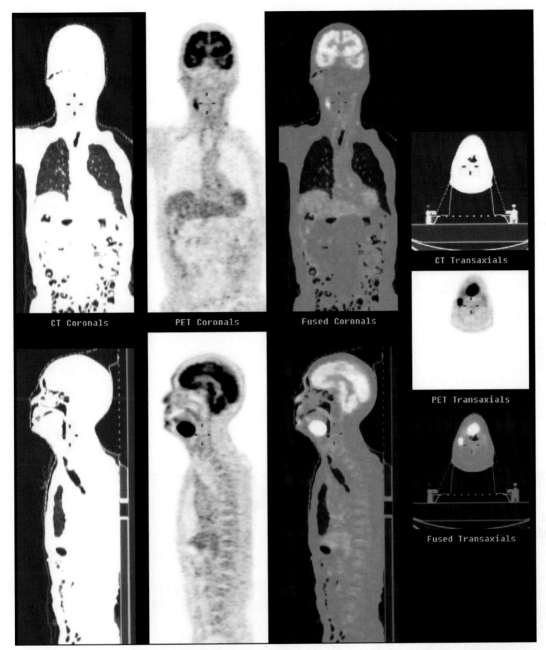

**FIGURE 5-3.**  PET/CT fusion in primary base of tongue cancer. Fused coronal, sagittal, and transaxial images (*red*).

and seven of twelve patients with recurrent disease, PET led to changes in treatment strategy or target volume.
- PET/CT images from a patient with base of tongue cancer are shown in Figure 5-3.
- A prominent variant that is pertinent to head and neck PET imaging is FDG uptake in brown fat,[98] which is responsible for cold- and diet-induced thermogenesis. It is brown in color because it is rich in mitochondria that uncouple adenosine triphosphate synthesis for heat production.

- The presence of glucose transporters in this brown fat regulates the uptake of FDG.[99] This activity is usually symmetric in the supraclavicular fat and intercostal regions. However, it can be asymmetric and can be seen in areas such as the neck, mediastinum, or pelvis.[100]

## 5. LIMITATIONS

- Despite the known advantages offered by PET imaging, it is not a perfect test because of its limited resolution and anatomic localization.

- In addition, FDG uptake is not specific only to tumor cells, and many false positives are possible secondary to active inflammation or infection.[101] Tumors such as bronchoalveolar carcinoma, particularly pure bronchioloalveolar carcinoma or well-differentiated tumors, do not demonstrate significantly increased FDG uptake and may be missed.[102]
- RT itself can cause intense FDG uptake, which may make it difficult to assess response to therapy of recurrence.
- A pilot study followed two patients with a total of eight and seven serial PET scans, respectively, through the entire course of their radiation therapy.[78] A pattern of elevated post-treatment FDG activity in the esophagus and lung along with diminished FDG activity in the bone marrow is typically seen during treatment. However, there was progressive FDG uptake subsequently in the lung parenchyma as a result of postradiation fibrosis, which becomes stable at approximately 3 months.

## 6. COST-EFFECTIVENESS

- Hollenbeak et al.[103] demonstrated the cost-effectiveness of a treatment strategy that included PET in the diagnostic workup of patients with head and neck cancer who were clinically staged N0. The incremental cost-effectiveness ratio for the PET strategy was more than $8,700 per year of lives saved or approximately $2,500 per quality-adjusted life-year.
- Valk et al.[104] demonstrated a 31% incidence of distant metastasis in a group of patients with locally advanced and recurrent head and neck cancer. The change in management from aggressive to palliative resulted in a savings-to-cost ratio of approximately 2:1.
- Larger, prospective studies are required to better assess the cost-effectiveness of PET for various clinical indications in head and neck cancer.

## 7. CLINICAL RADIOTHERAPY PLANNING WITH POSITRON EMISSION TOMOGRAPHY AND COMPUTED TOMOGRAPHY FUSION

- Anatomic and metabolic image fusion for RT treatment planning has the potential to more accurately define tumor boundaries and lymph node metastasis than anatomic imaging alone.
- Image fusion has traditionally been performed with software; accuracy and quality assurance issues regarding the "fit" of the image sets remain important concerns.
- Careful immobilization of patients with head and neck cancer with thermoplastic devices is reproducible and has been shown to allow acceptable image fusion (Figs. 5-4–5-6).[105]

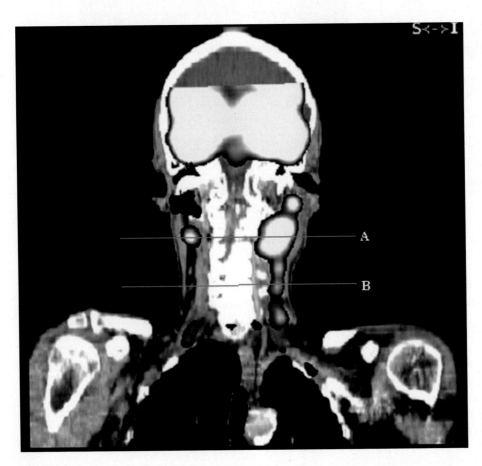

**FIGURE 5-4.** Coronal view of coregistered CT and [18]F-fluorodeoxyglucose (FDG)-PET images showing a large (3.7 × 2.8 cm) left-sided metastatic lymph node and multiple small lymph nodes on both sides of the neck in a patient with a tonsillar primary. The small lymph nodes are clearly abnormal on PET but do not meet size criteria for malignancy on CT.

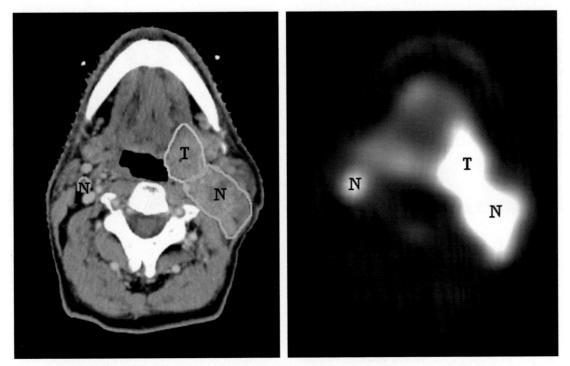

**FIGURE 5-5.** Axial CT and PET images at level **(A)** in Figure 5-3. Outlined on the left is the tonsillar primary and ipsilateral lymph node metastasis. The outlined right lymph node measures 8.3 × 8.8 × 5.6 mm on CT but is hypermetabolic on PET and pathologically involved.

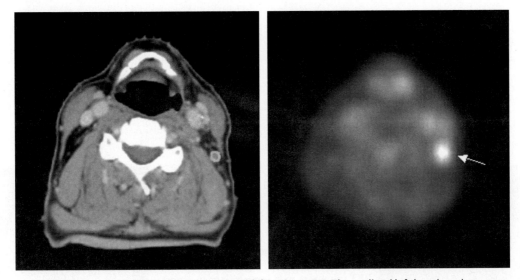

**FIGURE 5-6.** Axial CT and PET images at level **(B)** in Figure 5-3. The outlined left lymph node measures 7.0 × 6.8 × 9 mm on CT but is hypermetabolic on PET and pathologically involved.

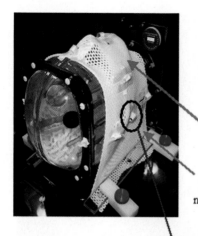

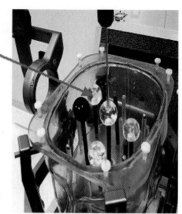

Plastic spheres and rods located
throughout the phantom

Head holder used in the study

Fiducial markers were placed on the
mask to co-register CT and PET images

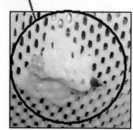

A room-in view shows plastic ampules,
serving as fiducial markers, are attached to
the surface of thermoplastic mask

**FIGURE 5-7.** An anthropomorphic head phantom developed to assess the accuracy of image registration and fusion process. Room-in-view shows a plastic ampule, serving as fiducial marker for CT-PET coregistration, attached to the surface of thermoplastic mask. (From: Chao KS, Bosch WR, Mutic S, et al. A novel approach to overcome hypoxic tumor resistance: Cu-ATSM-guided intensity-modulated radiation therapy. *Int J Radiat Oncol Biol Phys* 2001;49:1171–1182, with permission.)

- The ability to accurately immobilize patients with head and neck cancer in thermoplastic devices makes software fusion more straightforward than in other parts of the body (Figs. 5-7 and 5-8).
- New PET/CT hybrid machines are just becoming available. These hybrid-imaging units offer "hardware" fusion that should serve as a benchmark for accurate image fu-

sion and allow the synergy of excellent resolution and improved specificity.
- The acquisition of PET and CT datasets on different dates, body positions, and acquired scanners, in addition to the requirement for multiple fiducial markers and a robust image fusion program, can create a complex process.

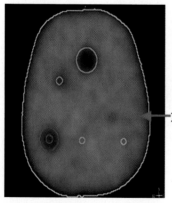

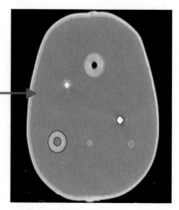

CT (phantom with immobilization mask)

PET (phantom with immobilization mask)

**FIGURE 5-8.** Validation of imaging fusion fidelity. Image registration was verified by contouring balls and rods on the primary CT scan and observing mapped contour locations on the secondary PET images. All contours were within 2 mm of their expected locations on the PET scans. (From: Chao KS, Bosch WR, Mutic S, et al. A novel approach to overcome hypoxic tumor resistance: Cu-ATSM-guided intensity-modulated radiation therapy. *Int J Radiat Oncol Biol Phys* 2001;49:1171–1182, with permission.)

- Even if PET/CT scanners are available, several issues have to be surmounted to perform radiation treatment planning with PET.
- The PET/CT unit has to be modified similarly to a CT simulation suite. The scanner should have a large bore (≥70 cm) that can accommodate the immobilization devices and comfortably fit the patient in the scanner.
- A laser positioning system and a flat bed insert should be used, and, most importantly, customized immobilization devices for head/neck and chest applications should be available.
- Image interpretation should be standardized. A prospective study by Mah et al.[106] showed significant interobserver variation; in this study, three radiation oncologists independently contoured GTVs by using CT and then PET fused with CT. The effect of PET on target definition varied with each physician, leading to a reduction in PTV in 24% to 70% of cases and an increase in 30% to 76% of cases.
- A significant portion of this problem may be attributable to image thresholding. With PET, one can vary the intensity of the scan display and may significantly artificially increase or decrease the volume of tumor. An adaptive thresholding method was developed by Erdi et al.[107] to better define the tumor volumes in PET imaging.
- Tumor motion will be a problem, particularly when respiratory motion and both breath hold and gating techniques are applied. There are several methods to account for tumor excursion and allow for more accurate definition of target volumes, including the four-dimensional (4D) method, gating method, and active breath control device.
- The 4D method is based on measuring the superior-inferior lesion motion on orthogonal radiographs or CT acquired at end-tidal inspiration and expiration to obtain a composite tumor volume within the limits of tidal breathing (Fig. 5-9).[108] The incorporation of PET into this treatment planning modality will simplify it and provide the composite 4D volume that accounts for tumor motion.
- The implementation of PET/CT would require gated PET acquisition. Nehmeh et al.[109] used a multiframe capture technique in which PET data are acquired in synchronization with respiratory motion in the respiratory gating method (Fig. 5-10). Respiratory gating showed a 28% reduction in the total lesion volume and a

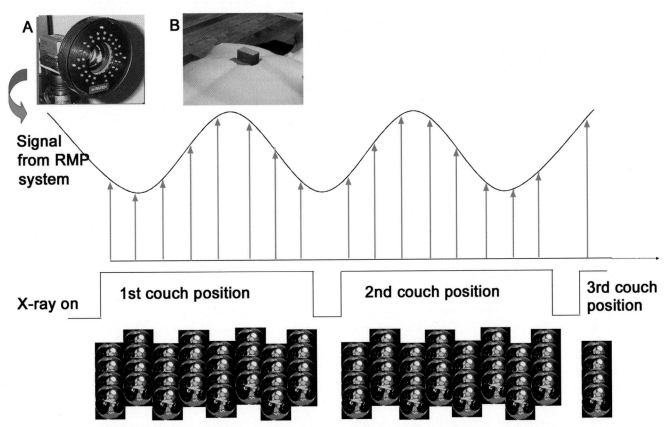

**FIGURE 5-9.** Four dimensional (4D)-CT respiratory motion tracking with retrospective gating. Respiratory motion is tracked by following a block mounted on the patient's chest **(B)** with a Varian (Cary, NC, USA) real-time position management (RPM) optical monitor **(A)**. CT images are acquired at end-tidal inspiration and expiration over complete respiratory cycles.

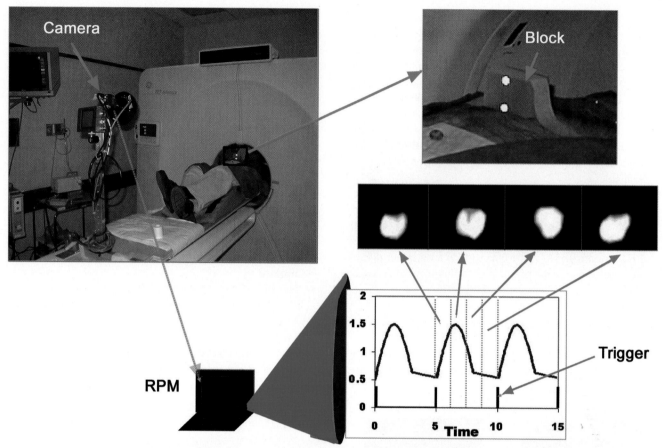

**FIGURE 5-10.** Camera-based PET respiratory gating system using RPM Respiratory Gating System (Varian). Respiratory cycles are tracked by monitoring the chest motions of the patient (represented by two passive reflective markers mounted on a block stabilized on the patient's abdomen) by using an infrared video camera on the PET table. RPM provides triggers to PET to initiate the gating cycle at selected phases or amplitudes within the breathing cycle. (From: Nehmeh SA, Erdi YE, Ling CC, et al. Effect of respiratory gating on reducing lung motion artifacts in PET imaging of lung cancer. *Med Phys* 2002;29:366–371, with permission.)

56.5% increase in the SUV. This could allow for diminution of the volume of the lung or tumor to be radiated, potentially generating greater dose delivery to the tumor and minimization of exposure of normal tissues.

## 8. FUTURE DEVELOPMENTS

- Fusion images allow the strength of anatomic imaging to compensate for the weakness of PET imaging, and vice versa.
- Emerging studies with hybrid PET/CT devices will likely demonstrate image fusion to be the new gold standard in certain cancers, such as head and neck oncologic imaging.
- Furthermore, monitoring of a therapeutic strategy during treatment may become possible, allowing a shift to a more aggressive approach in the subgroup of patients who prove to be resistant to a specific approach.

- Molecular probes for in vivo imaging of oligonucleotides, peptides, enzymes, ligands, receptors, transport substrates, tissue hypoxia, and so forth provide a biologic window with which to observe and potentially intervene in the malignant process.
- Because of the sensitivity with which radioactive events may be detected, it is possible to detect positron emitting molecular probes at tissue concentrations in the range of picomoles to femtomoles per gram.
- Although the majority of experience with imaging head and neck tumors to date is with FDG, other PET tracers have been developed to probe other important features of tumor biology.
- 11C-methionine and 11C-thymidine, precursors in DNA synthesis, have recently been used to evaluate cellular proliferation in head and neck tumors.[110,111]
- Radiopharmaceuticals that can target the hypoxic fraction of radioresistant tumors have great potential future applications.

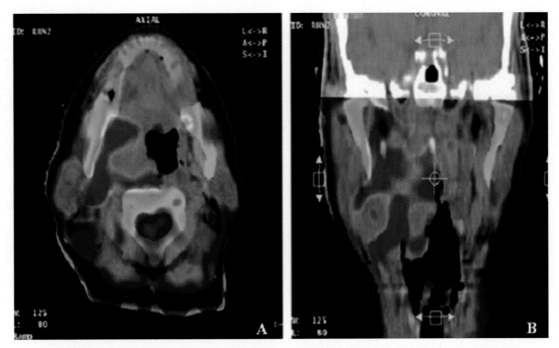

**FIGURE 5-11.** Color-washed images illustrate regions of heterogeneous [60]Cu(II)-diacetyl-bis(N[4]-methylthiosemicarbazone) ([60]Cu-ATSM) intensity within the gross tumor representing the presence of tumor hypoxia. (From: Chao KS, Bosch WR, Mutic S, et al. A novel approach to overcome hypoxic tumor resistance: Cu-ATSM-guided intensity-modulated radiation therapy. *Int J Radiat Oncol Biol Phys* 2001;49:1171–1182, with permission.)

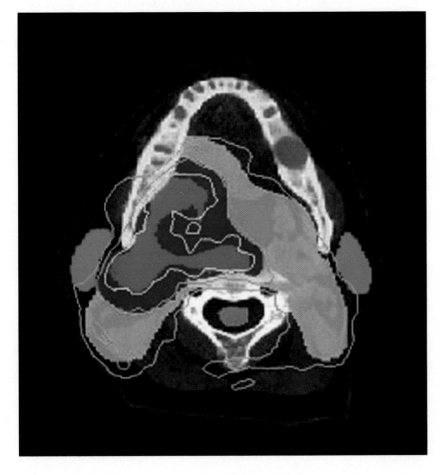

**FIGURE 5-12.** Delineation of the gross tumor volume (GTV) and its ATSM-avid fraction by PET/CT imaging fusion. (From: Chao KS, Bosch WR, Mutic S, et al. A novel approach to overcome hypoxic tumor resistance: Cu-ATSM-guided intensity-modulated radiation therapy. *Int J Radiat Oncol Biol Phys* 2001;49:1171–1182, with permission.)

- Hypoxic specific tracers including [18]F-fluoromisonida-zole and Cu(II)-diacetyl-bis(N[4]-methylthiosemicar-bazone) (Cu-ATSM) have been developed, and hypoxia in human head and neck cancers has been noninvasively imaged in vivo.[112–114]

- Dehdashti et al.[115] investigated the feasibility of clinical imaging with [60]Cu-ATSM in nineteen patients with NSCLC. The mean tumor-to-muscle ratio for [60]Cu-ATSM was significantly lower in responders ($1.5 \pm 0.4$) than in nonresponders ($3.4 \pm 0.8$) ($P = .002$). However, the mean SUV for [60]Cu-ATSM was not significantly different in responders ($2.8 \pm 1.1$) and nonresponders ($3.5 \pm 1.0$) ($P = .2$).

- Chao et al.[112] demonstrated the ability of PET to select a [60]Cu-ATSM-avid or hypoxic tumor subvolume (hGTV) in head and neck cancer. This study provided proof of principle that assessment of tumor hypoxia can be performed by using PET (Figs. 5-11 and 5-12).

## REFERENCES

1. Warburg O, Wind F, Negalein E. The metabolism of tumors in the body. *J Physiol* 1927;8:519–530.
2. Pauwels EK, McCready VR, Stoot JH, et al. The mechanism of accumulation of tumour-localising radiopharmaceuticals. *Eur J Nucl Med* 1998;25:277–305.
3. Bos R, van Der Hoeven JJ, van Der Wall E, et al. Biologic correlates of (18)fluorodeoxyglucose uptake in human breast cancer measured by positron emission tomography. *J Clin Oncol* 2002; 20:379–387.
4. Macapinlac HA, Yeung HW, Larson SM. Defining the role of FDG PET in head and neck cancer. *Clin Positron Imaging* 1999;2:311–316.
5. Barrington SF, Maisey MN. Skeletal muscle uptake of fluorine-18-FDG: effect of oral diazepam. *J Nucl Med* 1996;37:1127–1129.
6. Gambhir SS, Czernin J, Schwimmer J, et al. A tabulated summary of the FDG PET literature. *J Nucl Med* 2001;42:1S–93S.
7. Silvestri GA, Tanoue LT, Margolis ML, et al. The noninvasive staging of non-small cell lung cancer: the guidelines. *Chest* 2003;123:147S–156S.
8. Valk PE, Pounds TR, Hopkins DM, et al. Staging non-small cell lung cancer by whole-body positron emission tomographic imaging. *Ann Thorac Surg* 1995;60:1573–1581; discussion 1581–1582.
9. Bury T, Paulus P, Dowlati A, et al. Staging of the mediastinum: value of positron emission tomography imaging in non-small cell lung cancer. *Eur Respir J* 1996;9:2560–2564.
10. Vansteenkiste JF, Stroobants SG, De Leyn PR, et al. Mediastinal lymph node staging with FDG-PET scan in patients with potentially operable non-small cell lung cancer: a prospective analysis of 50 cases. Leuven Lung Cancer Group. *Chest* 1997;112:1480–1486.
11. Vansteenkiste JF, Stroobants SG, De Leyn PR, et al. Lymph node staging in non-small-cell lung cancer with FDG-PET scan: a prospective study on 690 lymph node stations from 68 patients. *J Clin Oncol* 1998;16:2142–2149.
12. Vansteenkiste JF, Stroobants SG, De Leyn PR, et al. Potential use of FDG-PET scan after induction chemotherapy in surgically staged IIIa-N2 non-small-cell lung cancer: a prospective pilot study. The Leuven Lung Cancer Group. *Ann Oncol* 1998;9:1193–1198.
13. Berlangieri SU, Scott AM, Knight SR, et al. F-18 fluorodeoxyglucose positron emission tomography in the non-invasive staging of non-small-cell lung cancer. *Eur J Cardiothorac Surg* 1999;16(Suppl 1):S25–S30.
14. Marom EM, McAdams HP, Erasmus JJ, et al. Staging non-small cell lung cancer with whole-body PET. *Radiology* 1999;212:803–809.
15. Saunders CA, Dussek JE, O'Doherty MJ, et al. Evaluation of fluorine-18-fluorodeoxyglucose whole body positron emission tomography imaging in the staging of lung cancer. *Ann Thorac Surg* 1999;67:790–797.
16. Pieterman RM, van Putten JW, Meuzelaar JJ, et al. Preoperative staging of non-small-cell lung cancer with positron-emission tomography. *N Engl J Med* 2000;343:254–261.
17. Weng E, Tran L, Rege S, et al. Accuracy and clinical impact of mediastinal lymph node staging with FDG-PET imaging in potentially resectable lung cancer. *Am J Clin Oncol* 2000;23:47–52.
18. Dunagan D, Chin R Jr., McCain T, et al. Staging by positron emission tomography predicts survival in patients with non-small cell lung cancer. *Chest* 2001;119:333–339.
19. Gupta NC, Tamim WJ, Graeber GG, et al. Mediastinal lymph node sampling following positron emission tomography with fluorodeoxyglucose imaging in lung cancer staging. *Chest* 2001;120:521–527.
20. Dwamena BA, Sonnad SS, Angobaldo JO, et al. Metastases from non-small cell lung cancer: mediastinal staging in the 1990s—meta-analytic comparison of PET and CT. *Radiology* 1999;213:530–536.
21. Hellwig D, Ukena D, Paulsen F, et al. [Meta-analysis of the efficacy of positron emission tomography with F-18-fluorodeoxyglucose in lung tumors. Basis for discussion of the German Consensus Conference on PET in Oncology 2000]. *Pneumologie* 2001;55:367–377.
22. Toloza EM, Harpole L, McCrory DC. Noninvasive staging of non-small cell lung cancer: a review of the current evidence. *Chest* 2003;123:137S–146S.
23. Gould MK, Kuschner WG, Rydzak CE, et al. Test performance of positron emission tomography and computed tomography for mediastinal staging in patients with non-small-cell lung cancer: a meta-analysis. *Ann Intern Med* 2003;139:879–892.
24. Chin R Jr., McCain TW, Miller AA, et al. Whole body FDG-PET for the evaluation and staging of small cell lung cancer: a preliminary study. *Lung Cancer* 2002;37:1–6.
25. Wahl RL, Cody RL, Hutchins GD, et al. Primary and metastatic breast carcinoma: initial clinical evaluation with PET with the radiolabeled glucose analogue 2-[F-18]-fluoro-2-deoxy-D-glucose. *Radiology* 1991;179:765–770.
26. Tse NY, Hoh CK, Hawkins RA, et al. The application of positron emission tomographic imaging with fluorodeoxyglucose to the evaluation of breast disease. *Ann Surg* 1992;216:27–34.
27. Adler LP, Crowe JP, al-Kaisi NK, et al. Evaluation of breast masses and axillary lymph nodes with [F-18] 2-deoxy-2-fluoro-D-glucose PET. *Radiology* 1993;187:743–750.
28. Utech CI, Young CS, Winter PF. Prospective evaluation of fluorine-18 fluorodeoxyclucose positron emission tomography in breast cancer for staging of the axilla related to surgery and immunocytochemistry. *Eur J Nucl Med* 1996;23:1588–1593.
29. Avril N, Dose J, Janicke F, et al. Assessment of axillary lymph node involvement in breast cancer patients with positron emission tomography using radiolabeled 2-(fluorine-18)-fluoro-2-deoxy-D-glucose. *J Natl Cancer Inst* 1996;88:1204–1209.
30. Greco M, Crippa F, Agresti R, et al. Axillary lymph node staging in breast cancer by 2-fluoro-2-deoxy-D-glucose-positron emis-

sion tomography: clinical evaluation and alternative management. *J Natl Cancer Inst* 2001;93:630–635.

31. Ohta M, Tokuda Y, Saitoh Y, et al. Comparative efficacy of positron emission tomography and ultrasonography in preoperative evaluation of axillary lymph node metastases in breast cancer. *Breast Cancer* 2000;7:99–103.

32. Schirrmeister H, Kuhn T, Guhlmann A, et al. Fluorine-18 2-deoxy-2-fluoro-D-glucose PET in the preoperative staging of breast cancer: comparison with the standard staging procedures. *Eur J Nucl Med* 2001;28:351–358.

33. van der Hoeven JJ, Hoekstra OS, Comans EF, et al. Determinants of diagnostic performance of [F-18]fluorodeoxyglucose positron emission tomography for axillary staging in breast cancer. *Ann Surg* 2002;236:619–624.

34. Avril N, Rose CA, Schelling M, et al. Breast imaging with positron emission tomography and fluorine-18 fluorodeoxyglucose: use and limitations. *J Clin Oncol* 2000;18:3495–3502.

35. Budinger TF. PET instrumentation: what are the limits? *Semin Nucl Med* 1998;28:247–267.

36. Raylman RR, Kison PV, Wahl RL. Capabilities of two- and three-dimensional FDG-PET for detecting small lesions and lymph nodes in the upper torso: a dynamic phantom study. *Eur J Nucl Med* 1999;26:39–45.

37. Guller U, Nitzsche EU, Schirp U, et al. Selective axillary surgery in breast cancer patients based on positron emission tomography with 18F-fluoro-2-deoxy-D-glucose: not yet! *Breast Cancer Res Treat* 2002;71:171–173.

38. Yang JH, Nam SJ, Lee TS, et al. Comparison of intraoperative frozen section analysis of sentinel node with preoperative positron emission tomography in the diagnosis of axillary lymph node status in breast cancer patients. *Jpn J Clin Oncol* 2001;31:1–6.

39. Wahl RL, Siegel BA, Coleman RE, et al. Prospective multicenter study of axillary nodal staging by positron emission tomography in breast cancer: a report of the staging breast cancer with PET Study Group. *J Clin Oncol* 2004;22:277–285.

40. Heinisch M, Gallowitsch HJ, Mikosch P, et al. Comparison of FDG-PET and dynamic contrast-enhanced MRI in the evaluation of suggestive breast lesions. *Breast* 2003;12:17–22.

41. Barranger E, Grahek D, Antoine M, et al. Evaluation of fluorodeoxyglucose positron emission tomography in the detection of axillary lymph node metastases in patients with early-stage breast cancer. *Ann Surg Oncol* 2003;10:622–627.

42. Eubank WB, Mankoff DA, Takasugi J, et al. 18fluorodeoxyglucose positron emission tomography to detect mediastinal or internal mammary metastases in breast cancer. *J Clin Oncol* 2001;19:3516–3523.

43. Rege S, Maass A, Chaiken L, et al. Use of positron emission tomography with fluorodeoxyglucose in patients with extracranial head and neck cancers. *Cancer* 1994;73:3047–3058.

44. Laubenbacher C, Saumweber D, Wagner-Manslau C, et al. Comparison of fluorine-18-fluorodeoxyglucose PET, MRI and endoscopy for staging head and neck squamous-cell carcinomas. *J Nucl Med* 1995;36:1747–1757.

45. McGuirt WF, Williams DW, 3rd, Keyes JW Jr., et al. A comparative diagnostic study of head and neck nodal metastases using positron emission tomography. *Laryngoscope* 1995;105:373–375.

46. Benchaou M, Lehmann W, Slosman DO, et al. The role of FDG-PET in the preoperative assessment of N-staging in head and neck cancer. *Acta Otolaryngol* 1996;116:332–335.

47. Braams JW, Pruim J, Kole AC, et al. Detection of unknown primary head and neck tumors by positron emission tomography. *Int J Oral Maxillofac Surg* 1997;26:112–115.

48. Wong WL, Chevretton EB, McGurk M, et al. A prospective study of PET-FDG imaging for the assessment of head and neck squamous cell carcinoma. *Clin Otolaryngol* 1997;22:209–214.

49. Adams S, Baum RP, Stuckensen T, et al. Prospective comparison of 18F-FDG PET with conventional imaging modalities (CT, MRI, US) in lymph node staging of head and neck cancer. *Eur J Nucl Med* 1998;25:1255–1260.

50. Myers LL, Wax MK, Nabi H, et al. Positron emission tomography in the evaluation of the N0 neck. *Laryngoscope* 1998;108:232–236.

51. Paulus P, Sambon A, Vivegnis D, et al. 18FDG-PET for the assessment of primary head and neck tumors: clinical, computed tomography, and histopathological correlation in 38 patients. *Laryngoscope* 1998;108:1578–1583.

52. Kau RJ, Alexiou C, Laubenbacher C, et al. Lymph node detection of head and neck squamous cell carcinomas by positron emission tomography with fluorodeoxyglucose F 18 in a routine clinical setting. *Arch Otolaryngol Head Neck Surg* 1999;125: 1322–1328.

53. Nowak B, Di Martino E, Janicke S, et al. Diagnostic evaluation of malignant head and neck cancer by F-18-FDG PET compared to CT/MRI. *Nuklearmedizin* 1999;38:312–318.

54. Hannah A, Scott AM, Tochon-Danguy H, et al. Evaluation of 18 F-fluorodeoxyglucose positron emission tomography and computed tomography with histopathologic correlation in the initial staging of head and neck cancer. *Ann Surg* 2002;236:208–217.

55. Abrams H, Spiro RH, Goldstein M. Metastases in carcinoma: analysis of 1000 autopsied cases. *Cancer* 1950;3:120–124.

56. Muir C. Cancer of unknown primary site. *Cancer* 1995;75:353–356.

57. Abbruzzese JL, Abbruzzese MC, Hess KR, et al. Unknown primary carcinoma: natural history and prognostic factors in 657 consecutive patients. *J Clin Oncol* 1994;12:1272–1280.

58. Kole AC, Nieweg OE, Pruim J, et al. Detection of unknown occult primary tumors using positron emission tomography. *Cancer* 1998;82:1160–1166.

59. Jungehulsing M, Scheidhauer K, Damm M, et al. 2[F]-fluoro-2-deoxy-D-glucose positron emission tomography is a sensitive tool for the detection of occult primary cancer (carcinoma of unknown primary syndrome) with head and neck lymph node manifestation. *Otolaryngol Head Neck Surg* 2000;123:294–301.

60. Johansen J, Eigtved A, Buchwald C, et al. Implication of 18F-fluoro-2-deoxy-D-glucose positron emission tomography on management of carcinoma of unknown primary in the head and neck: a Danish cohort study. *Laryngoscope* 2002;112:2009–2014.

61. Bury T, Corhay JL, Duysinx B, et al. Value of FDG-PET in detecting residual or recurrent nonsmall cell lung cancer. *Eur Respir J* 1999;14:1376–1380.

62. Moon DH, Maddahi J, Silverman DH, et al. Accuracy of whole-body fluorine-18-FDG PET for the detection of recurrent or metastatic breast carcinoma. *J Nucl Med* 1998;39:431–435.

63. Bender H, Kirst J, Palmedo H, et al. Value of 18fluoro-deoxyglucose positron emission tomography in the staging of recurrent breast carcinoma. *Anticancer Res* 1997;17:1687–1692.

64. Vranjesevic D, Filmont JE, Meta J, et al. Whole-body (18)F-FDG PET and conventional imaging for predicting outcome in previously treated breast cancer patients. *J Nucl Med* 2002;43:325–329.

65. Gallowitsch HJ, Kresnik E, Gasser J, et al. F-18 fluorodeoxyglucose positron-emission tomography in the diagnosis of tumor recurrence and metastases in the follow-up of patients with breast carcinoma: a comparison to conventional imaging. *Invest Radiol* 2003;38:250–256.

66. Lapela M, Grenman R, Kurki T, et al. Head and neck cancer: detection of recurrence with PET and 2-[F-18]fluoro-2-deoxy-D-glucose. *Radiology* 1995;197:205–211.

67. Anzai Y, Carroll WR, Quint DJ, et al. Recurrence of head and neck cancer after surgery or irradiation: prospective comparison of 2-deoxy-2-[F-18]fluoro-D-glucose PET and MR imaging diagnoses. *Radiology* 1996;200:135–141.

68. Greven KM, Williams DW 3rd, Keyes JW Jr., et al. Can positron emission tomography distinguish tumor recurrence from irradiation sequelae in patients treated for larynx cancer? *Cancer J Sci Am* 1997;3:353–357.

69. Greven KM, Williams DW 3rd, McGuirt WF Sr., et al. Serial positron emission tomography scans following radiation therapy of patients with head and neck cancer. *Head Neck* 2001;23:942–946.

70. Kitagawa Y, Nishizawa S, Sano K, et al. Prospective comparison of 18F-FDG PET with conventional imaging modalities (MRI, CT, and 67Ga scintigraphy) in assessment of combined intraarterial chemotherapy and radiotherapy for head and neck carcinoma. *J Nucl Med* 2003;44:198–206.

71. Yen RF, Hung RL, Pan MH, et al. 18-fluoro-2-deoxyglucose positron emission tomography in detecting residual/recurrent nasopharyngeal carcinomas and comparison with magnetic resonance imaging. *Cancer* 2003;98:283–287.

72. Lowe VJ, Boyd JH, Dunphy FR, et al. Surveillance for recurrent head and neck cancer using positron emission tomography. *J Clin Oncol* 2000;18:651–658.

73. Akhurst T, Downey RJ, Ginsberg MS, et al. An initial experience with FDG-PET in the imaging of residual disease after induction therapy for lung cancer. *Ann Thorac Surg* 2002;73:259–264; discussion 264–266.

74. Ryu JS, Choi NC, Fischman AJ, et al. FDG-PET in staging and restaging non-small cell lung cancer after neoadjuvant chemoradiotherapy: correlation with histopathology. *Lung Cancer* 2002;35:179–187.

75. Mac Manus MP, Hicks RJ, Matthews JP, et al. Positron emission tomography is superior to computed tomography scanning for response-assessment after radical radiotherapy or chemoradiotherapy in patients with non-small-cell lung cancer. *J Clin Oncol* 2003;21:1285–1292.

76. Weber WA, Petersen V, Schmidt B, et al. Positron emission tomography in non-small-cell lung cancer: prediction of response to chemotherapy by quantitative assessment of glucose use. *J Clin Oncol* 2003;21:2651–2657.

77. Therasse P, Arbuck SG, Eisenhauer EA, et al. New guidelines to evaluate the response to treatment in solid tumors. European Organization for Research and Treatment of Cancer, National Cancer Institute of the United States, National Cancer Institute of Canada. *J Natl Cancer Inst* 2000;92:205–216.

78. Erdi YE, Macapinlac H, Rosenzweig KE, et al. Use of PET to monitor the response of lung cancer to radiation treatment. *Eur J Nucl Med* 2000;27:861–866.

79. Wahl RL, Zasadny K, Helvie M, et al. Metabolic monitoring of breast cancer chemohormonotherapy using positron emission tomography: initial evaluation. *J Clin Oncol* 1993;11:2101–2111.

80. Bassa P, Kim EE, Inoue T, et al. Evaluation of preoperative chemotherapy using PET with fluorine-18-fluorodeoxyglucose in breast cancer. *J Nucl Med* 1996;37:931–938.

81. Jansson T, Westlin JE, Ahlstrom H, et al. Positron emission tomography studies in patients with locally advanced and/or metastatic breast cancer: a method for early therapy evaluation? *J Clin Oncol* 1995;13:1470–1477.

82. Schelling M, Avril N, Nahrig J, et al. Positron emission tomography using [(18)F] fluorodeoxyglucose for monitoring primary chemotherapy in breast cancer. *J Clin Oncol* 2000;18:1689–1695.

83. Smith IC, Welch AE, Hutcheon AW, et al. Positron emission tomography using [(18)F]-fluorodeoxy-D-glucose to predict the pathologic response of breast cancer to primary chemotherapy. *J Clin Oncol* 2000;18:1676–1688.

84. Berlangieri SU, Brizel DM, Scher RL, et al. Pilot study of positron emission tomography in patients with advanced head and neck cancer receiving radiotherapy and chemotherapy. *Head Neck* 1994;16:340–346.

85. Reisser C, Haberkorn U, Dimitrakopoulou-Strauss A, et al. Chemotherapeutic management of head and neck malignancies with positron emission tomography. *Arch Otolaryngol Head Neck Surg* 1995;121:272–276.

86. Brun E, Kjellen E, Tennvall J, et al. FDG PET studies during treatment: prediction of therapy outcome in head and neck squamous cell carcinoma. *Head Neck* 2002;24:127–135.

87. Hautzel H, Muller-Gartner HW. Early changes in fluorine-18-FDG uptake during radiotherapy. *J Nucl Med* 1997;38:1384–1386.

88. Rege S, Safa AA, Chaiken L, et al. Positron emission tomography: an independent indicator of radiocurability in head and neck carcinomas. *Am J Clin Oncol* 2000;23:164–169.

89. Humm JL, Lee J, O'Donoghue JA, et al. Changes in FDG tumor uptake during and after fractionated radiation therapy in a rodent tumor xenograft. *Clin Positron Imaging* 1999;2:289–296.

90. Ciernik IF, Dizendorf E, Baumert BG, et al. Radiation treatment planning with an integrated positron emission and computer tomography (PET/CT): a feasibility study. *Int J Radiat Oncol Biol Phys* 2003;57:853–863.

91. Hebert ME, Lowe VJ, Hoffman JM, et al. Positron emission tomography in the pretreatment evaluation and follow-up of non-small cell lung cancer patients treated with radiotherapy: preliminary findings. *Am J Clin Oncol* 1996;19:416–421.

92. Kiffer JD, Berlangieri SU, Scott AM, et al. The contribution of 18F-fluoro-2-deoxy-glucose positron emission tomographic imaging to radiotherapy planning in lung cancer. *Lung Cancer* 1998;19:167–177.

93. Nestle U, Walter K, Schmidt S, et al. 18F-deoxyglucose positron emission tomography (FDG-PET) for the planning of radiotherapy in lung cancer: high impact in patients with atelectasis. *Int J Radiat Oncol Biol Phys* 1999;44:593–597.

94. Munley MT, Marks LB, Scarfone C, et al. Multimodality nuclear medicine imaging in three-dimensional radiation treatment planning for lung cancer: challenges and prospects. *Lung Cancer* 1999;23:105–114.

95. Vanuytsel LJ, Vansteenkiste JF, Stroobants SG, et al. The impact of (18)F-fluoro-2-deoxy-D-glucose positron emission tomography (FDG-PET) lymph node staging on the radiation treatment volumes in patients with non-small cell lung cancer. *Radiother Oncol* 2000;55:317–324.

96. Erdi YE, Rosenzweig K, Erdi AK, et al. Radiotherapy treatment planning for patients with non-small cell lung cancer using positron emission tomography (PET). *Radiother Oncol* 2002;62:51–60.

97. Rahn AN, Baum RP, Adamietz IA, et al. [Value of 18F fluorodeoxyglucose positron emission tomography in radiotherapy planning of head-neck tumors]. *Strahlenther Onkol* 1998;174:358–364.

98. Hany TF, Gharehpapagh E, Kamel EM, et al. Brown adipose tissue: a factor to consider in symmetrical tracer uptake in the neck and upper chest region. *Eur J Nucl Med Mol Imaging* 2002;29:1393–1398.

99. Kawashita NH, Brito MN, Brito SR, et al. Glucose uptake, glucose transporter GLUT4, and glycolytic enzymes in brown adipose tissue from rats adapted to a high-protein diet. *Metabolism* 2002;51:1501–1505.

100. Truong M, Erasmus J, Munden R, et al. Focal FDG-uptake in mediastinal brown fat mimicking malignancy: a potential pitfall resolved on PET/CT. *Am J Roentgenol* 2004;183.

101. Shreve PD, Anzai Y, Wahl RL. Pitfalls in oncologic diagnosis with FDG PET imaging: physiologic and benign variants. *Radiographics* 1999;19:61–77; quiz 150–151.

102. Higashi K, Ueda Y, Seki H, et al. Fluorine-18-FDG PET imaging is negative in bronchioloalveolar lung carcinoma. *J Nucl Med* 1998;39:1016–1020.

103. Hollenbeak CS, Lowe VJ, Stack BC Jr. The cost-effectiveness of fluorodeoxyglucose 18-F positron emission tomography in the N0 neck. *Cancer* 2001;92:2341–2348.

104. Valk PE, Pounds TR, Tesar RD, et al. Cost-effectiveness of PET imaging in clinical oncology. *Nucl Med Biol* 1996;23:737–743.

105. Mutic S, Dempsey JF, Bosch WR, et al. Multimodality image registration quality assurance for conformal three-dimensional treatment planning. *Int J Radiat Oncol Biol Phys* 2001;51: 255–260.

106. Mah K, Caldwell CB, Ung YC, et al. The impact of (18)FDG-PET on target and critical organs in CT-based treatment planning of patients with poorly defined non-small-cell lung carcinoma: a prospective study. *Int J Radiat Oncol Biol Phys* 2002;52: 339–350.

107. Erdi YE, Mawlawi O, Larson SM, et al. Segmentation of lung lesion volume by adaptive positron emission tomography image thresholding. *Cancer* 1997;80:2505–2509.

108. Stevens CW, Munden RF, Forster KM, et al. Respiratory-driven lung tumor motion is independent of tumor size, tumor location, and pulmonary function. *Int J Radiat Oncol Biol Phys* 2001;51:62–68.

109. Nehmeh SA, Erdi YE, Ling CC, et al. Effect of respiratory gating on reducing lung motion artifacts in PET imaging of lung cancer. *Med Phys* 2002;29:366–371.

110. van Eijkeren ME, De Schryver A, Goethals P, et al. Measurement of short-term 11C-thymidine activity in human head and neck tumours using positron emission tomography (PET). *Acta Oncol* 1992;31:539–543.

111. Leskinen-Kallio S, Lindholm P, Lapela M, et al. Imaging of head and neck tumors with positron emission tomography and [11C]methionine. *Int J Radiat Oncol Biol Phys* 1994;30: 1195–1199.

112. Chao KS, Bosch WR, Mutic S, et al. A novel approach to overcome hypoxic tumor resistance: Cu-ATSM-guided intensity-modulated radiation therapy. *Int J Radiat Oncol Biol Phys* 2001;49:1171–1182.

113. Lewis JS, McCarthy DW, McCarthy TJ, et al. Evaluation of 64Cu-ATSM in vitro and in vivo in a hypoxic tumor model. *J Nucl Med* 1999;40:177–183.

114. Rasey JS, Koh WJ, Evans ML, et al. Quantifying regional hypoxia in human tumors with positron emission tomography of [18F]fluoromisonidazole: a pretherapy study of 37 patients. *Int J Radiat Oncol Biol Phys* 1996;36:417–428.

115. Dehdashti F, Mintun MA, Lewis JS, et al. In vivo assessment of tumor hypoxia in lung cancer with 60Cu-ATSM. *Eur J Nucl Med Mol Imaging* 2003;30:844–850.

116. Vansteenkiste JF, Stroobants SG, Dupont PJ, et al. FDG-PET scan in potentially operable non-small cell lung cancer: do anatometabolic PET-CT fusion images improve the localisation of regional lymph node metastases? The Leuven Lung Cancer Group. *Eur J Nucl Med* 1998;25:1495–1501.

117. Goerres GW, Michel SC, Fehr MK, et al. Follow-up of women with breast cancer: comparison between MRI and FDG PET. *Eur Radiol* 2003;13:1635–1644.

# 6

# SKULL BASE AND POSTERIOR FOSSA

## UGOROANS SELEK
## ERIC L. CHANG

---

## 1. INTRODUCTION

- Image-guided radiotherapy began to be used during the last decade in the form of three-dimensional conformal radiation therapy (3DCRT) and intensity-modulated radiation therapy (IMRT).

- Radiotherapy of the skull base and posterior fossa tumors is challenging because of the close proximity of the tumors to radiosensitive structures such as the lens, eyes, optic pathways, auditory apparatus, and brainstem.

- The limiting factor in dose delivery is the tolerance of normal tissue to radiation; the goal is to give the appropriate dose necessary to control the tumor while preserving the surrounding normal tissues within their respective tolerance doses by 3DCRT and IMRT.

- Because of the variety of tumors affecting the skull base (Table 6-1), a unified classification system has not been established. Therefore, general classifications are being based on either the location or the biologic behavior of the tumor.

- We review the complex anatomy of the skull base to serve as a guide for delineating target and normal tissue, and give several examples.

## 2. ANATOMY

- The base of the skull can be divided into the anterior, middle, and posterior cranial fossa (Fig. 6-1).

- Anterior cranial fossa (Fig. 6-1) is formed anteriorly by orbital plates of the frontal bone and the cribriform plate of the ethmoid bone, and posteriorly by the posterior edge of the lesser wing of the sphenoid bone and anterior margin of the chiasmatic groove. Below is the anterior skull base mainly separating frontal base and paranasal sinuses and involving critical structures such as the frontal lobe, orbits, and optic nerves. The planum sphenoidale is a flat region separating the cribriform area of the ethmoid bone anteriorly from the chiasmatic sulcus posteriorly. The cribriform plate transmits the olfactory nerve and anterior ethmoidal nerve.

- The chiasmatic sulcus is a linear, transversely oriented depression through which the optic canals enter the intracranial compartment at its lateral margins. Optic nerves combine at the optic chiasm, which is superior to the sella turcica in the suprasellar cistern at the base of the brain. The optic tract courses dorsolaterally around the hypothalamus and the rostral part of the cerebral peduncle.

- The middle cranial fossa (Fig. 6-1) is formed anteriorly by the posterior edge of the lesser wing of the sphenoid bone, the anterior clinoid process, and the anterior ridge of chiasmatic groove, and posteriorly by the petrous ridge of the temporal bone. The central skull base can be organized roughly into three regions. The midline is formed mainly by the sphenoid bone (sella and sphenoid sinus), covered by dura and bearing two important embryologic structures: the notochord and Rathke's pouch. Just lateral to the midline is the sagittal plane of the foramina and fissures (medial middle fossa, cavernous sinus [CS], and Meckel's cave [MC]). Further laterally is the greater wing of the sphenoid with no fissures or foramina (sphenoid wing and lateral middle fossa). This area is closely related to the pterygomaxillary region and infratemporal fossa.

- The CS and MC are the anatomic structures connecting most of the foramina. MC is a loose dural sleeve around the trigeminal nerve and the gasserian ganglion. The CS is a venous sinusoid structure located between the layers of dura, bordering the pituitary fossa and the body of the sphenoid. The CS lies superomedially to MC, extending anteriorly. The ophthalmic branch (V1) of the trigeminal nerve passes through the CS to the superior orbital fissure (SOF) as the maxillary division (V2) and with a shorter course in the CS, it enters the foramen rotundum (FR). The mandibular division of the trigeminal nerve does not truly enter the CS after exiting MC. The oculomotor (III), trochlear (IV), and abducens (VI) nerves traverse the CS to exit at the SOF. The internal carotid artery also traverses the CS after exiting the petrous carotid canal.

**TABLE 6-1. CRITICAL STRUCTURES AND VARIOUS TUMOR TYPES LOCATED IN SKULL BASE AND POSTERIOR FOSSA WITH COMMON CLINICAL SIGNS**

| | Location | Critical Structures | Tumor Type | Clinical Signs |
|---|---|---|---|---|
| Anterior | Frontobasal<br>Paranasal sinuses | Olfactory nerve<br>Frontal lobe<br>Orbit<br>Optic nerve | Meningioma<br>Esthesioneuroblastoma<br>Sinonasal malignancies | Anosmia<br>Frontal lobe<br>  dysfunction<br>Epistaxis<br>Visual changes |
| Middle | *Central:*<br>Sella<br>Sphenoid sinus | Optic nerve<br>Optic chiasm<br>Pituitary gland<br>Hypothalamus | Meningioma<br>Pituitary adenoma<br>Craniopharyngioma<br>Sinonasal malignancies<br>Sphenoid sinus carcinoma | Optic neuropathy<br>Pituitary glandular<br>  hypo/hyperfunction |
| | *Paracentral:*<br>Medial middle fossa<br>Cavernous sinus<br>Meckel's cave | Optic nerve<br>Optic chiasm<br>CN III–VI<br>Temporal lobe<br>Cavernous carotid artery | Meningioma<br>Schwannoma<br>Adenoid cystic<br>  carcinoma<br>Nasopharyngeal carcinoma | Optic neuropathy<br>Sphenocavernous<br>  syndrome |
| | *Lateral:*<br>Sphenoid wing<br>Lateral middle fossa | Temporal lobe<br>Frontal lobe<br>Trigeminal divisions<br>  2 and 3 | Meningioma<br>Schwannoma<br>Juvenile nasal<br>  angiofibroma<br>Adenoid cystic<br>  carcinoma<br>Sarcoma | Proptosis<br>Facial dysthesia<br>Facial pain<br>Trismus<br>Epistaxis |
| | Cerebellopontine angle | CN VII and VIII<br>CN V<br>Pons cerebellum | Meningioma<br>Acoustic neuroma<br>Trigeminal neuroma<br>Cholesterol granuloma<br>Epidermoid carcinoma | Hearing loss<br>Numb/weak face<br>Dysmetria ataxia<br>Brainstem signs<br>Increased pressure |
| Posterior | Petrous apex<br>  clivus | CN III–X<br>If advanced: pons,<br>  cerebellum, carotid,<br>  and basilar arteries | Meningioma<br>Trigeminal schwannoma<br>Glomus jugulare<br>Chordoma<br>Chondrosarcoma<br>Nasopharyngeal carcinoma | Abducens palsy<br>Bilateral cranial<br>  deficits<br>Brainstem signs |
| | Jugular foramen | CN IX–XI | Meningioma<br>Schwannoma<br>Paraganglioma (glomus<br>  jugulare) | Vernet's syndrome<br>(IX–XI CN palsy)<br>Collet-Sicard syndrome<br>(IX–XII CN palsy) |

CN, cranial nerve.

- The optic canal and SOF open into the orbit. Just caudal to the SOF, the FR lies in a posterior-anterior orientation through the skull base. The FR passes from the CS to the pterygopalatine fossa (PPF) (Fig. 6-2), entering the fossa at the level of the inferior orbital fissure (IOF). The V2 (maxillary) division of the trigeminal nerve, carried through the FR, crosses the upper part of the fossa and enters the orbit through the IOF. It becomes the infraorbital nerve in the floor of the orbit and exits through the infraorbital foramen to the face.

- The pterygoid canal (vidian canal) is inferomedial to the FR, transmitting the pterygoid nerve and artery from the anterior wall of foramen lacerum to the PPF.

- The foramen ovale (FO) is anterior and medial to the foramen spinosum (Fig. 6-3). The FO transmits the V3

(mandibular) division of the trigeminal nerve into the masticator space, as well as the accessory meningeal artery and the lesser superficial petrosal nerve. The foramen spinosum transmits the middle meningeal artery and recurrent branch of the mandibular nerve.

- The PPF is an important landmark that provides pathways for tumor spread by its connections: through the pterygoid canal and FR to the central skull base and middle cranial fossa; the IOF to the orbit; the pterygomaxillary fissure to the infratemporal fossa; the sphenopalatine foramen to the nasal cavity; and the pterygopalatine canals to the oral cavity.

- The posterior cranial fossa, containing the cerebellum and brainstem, is formed by the dorsum sellae and clivus of the sphenoid, occipital bone, petrous and mastoid

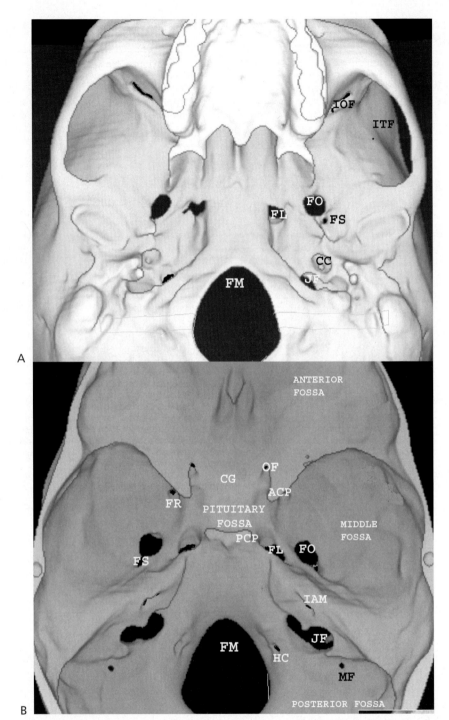

**FIGURE 6-1. A:** Exterior of the skull base. **B:** Interior of the skull base. IOF, infraorbital foramen; ITF, infratemporal fossa; FO, foramen ovale; FL, foramen lacerum; FS, foramen spinosum; CC, carotid canal; JF, jugular foramen; FM, foramen magnum; CG, chiasmatic groove; OF, optic foramen; FR, foramen rotundum; ACP, anterior clinoid process; PCP, posterior clinoid process; IAM, internal acoustic meatus; HC, hypoglossal canal; MF, mastoid foramen.

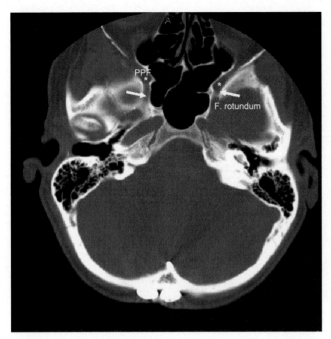

**FIGURE 6-2.** Foramen rotundum (*white arrow*) and ptery-gopalatine fossa (PPF) (*star*) demonstrated in axial computed to-mography (CT) slide with head and neck bone image resolution.

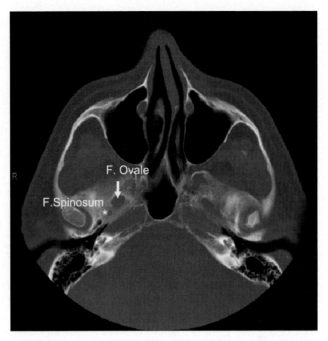

**FIGURE 6-3.** Foramen ovale (*arrow*) and foramen spinosum (*star*) demonstrated in axial CT with head and neck bone image resolution.

temporal bone, and mastoid angle of the parietal bone. Cranial nerves VII to XII exit in this fossa.

- The jugular foramen is situated between the lateral occipital bone and the petrous temporal bone (Fig. 6-1). Above the jugular foramen is the internal acoustic meatus, which transmits the facial and acoustic nerves and the internal auditory artery.

## 3. NATURAL HISTORY

### 3.1. Meningioma

- Meningiomas represent approximately 15% of primary brain tumors and occur with an annual incidence ranging from less than 1 to more than 6 per 100,000.[1,2]
- They arise from the arachnoidal cells of the meninges.[3] The peak incidence is during the sixth and seventh decades of life.
- The ratio of males to females ranges from 1:1.4 to 1:2.8.[1,4,5]
- Most meningiomas occur either along the convexities or the parasagittal plane. Six morphologic variants defined by the World Heath Organization (grade II: atypical, clear cell, and chordoid; grade III: anaplastic, papillary, and rhabdoid) are associated with aggressive clinical behavior and increased recurrence and metastasis.[6]
- Although skull base origin is infrequent, meningiomas may arise from any part of the sphenoid such as the greater wing, planum sphenoidale, tuberculum sella,

walls of the CS, petroclival, parasellar (Fig. 6-4), optic sheath, petroclinoid, or trigeminal nerve.

- Skull base meningiomas extend along the dural surfaces or intraosseously. Penetrating through bone may cause a substantial extracranial mass.
- As arachnoid cells accompany the cranial nerves, meningiomas can be found adjacent to and traversing various neural foramina.[7]

### 3.2. Esthesioneuroblastoma

- Esthesioneuroblastoma (olfactory neuroblastoma and neuroendocrine carcinoma) constitutes 1% to 5% of all malignant neoplasms of the nasal cavity.[8,9] It originates from the basal cells of the olfactory epithelium in the upper third of the nasal septum, cribriform plate, and superior turbinates (Fig. 6-5), and has a spectrum of neural and epithelial differentiation.[10,11]
- It has a fairly equal distribution between sexes, with a slight male predominance. The mean age at diagnosis is 45 years with a bimodal peak of incidence in the second and fifth decades of life.[12]
- Early symptoms are usually nasal obstruction or epistaxis. Periorbital swelling and hyposmia are also common.
- Advanced age, brain involvement, high histologic grade, and advanced Kadish stage are major prognostic factors. Polin et al.[13] reported that, in their experience at the University of Virginia, advanced Kadish stage was associated with a borderline higher rate of disease-related mortality, but not with disease-free survival.

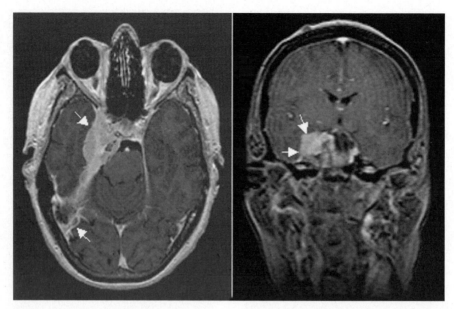

**FIGURE 6-4.** Right-sided petroclival meningioma with a characteristic dural-based tail appearance and parasellar and cavernous extension in axial and coronal T1 magnetic resonance imaging (MRI) with gadolinium.

- Synchronous cervical lymph node metastases incidence is 17% to 47%.[14]
- Distant hematogenous metastases are not usual at presentation but may occur after relapse. Metastases are mainly to lung, bone, bone marrow, or skin.[9]

### 3.3. Chordoma

- Chordomas represent approximately 1% of all malignant bone tumors and arise from remnants of the notochord.

The terminus of the notochord is in the sphenoid bone, so skull base chordomas arise in the region of the clivus (Fig. 6-6).

- Thirty-five percent of chordomas occur in the skull base, 50% occur in the sacrococcygeal region, and 15% occur in the spine.[15]
- Most chordomas in the craniovertebral area are diagnosed in persons aged 30 to 50 years, whereas sacrococcygeal chordomas have their peak incidence in persons aged 40 to 60 years.

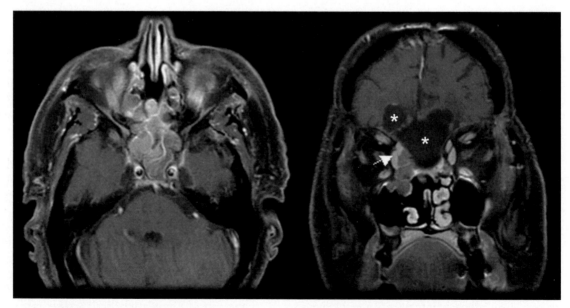

**FIGURE 6-5.** Postsurgical resection of right-sided esthesioneuroblastoma with a residual right medial orbital mass (*white arrow*) in axial and coronal T1 MRI with gadolinium. Postoperative cystic areas in coronal section (*stars*).

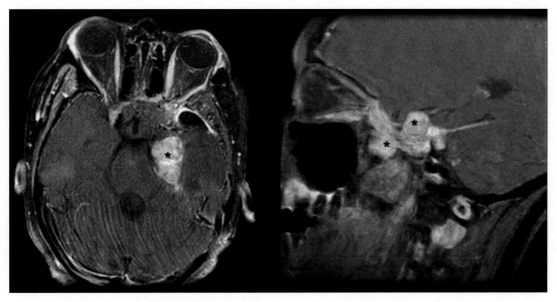

**FIGURE 6-6.** Left-sided chordoma tumor (*black stars*) with compression of brainstem in axial and coronal T1 MRI with gadolinium.

- Male predominance has been reported,[15] whereas in another series, the gender distribution was even.[16]
- The three pathologic subtypes are described as classic (most common), chondroid (mostly in the skull base), and dedifferentiated (rare, but poor prognosis).[15,17]
- Distant metastases, more common in sacral and vertebral chordomas than skull base chordomas, occur in lungs, bones, lymph nodes, liver, and skin.[18–20] Intradural metastases may appear after surgical resection of skull base chordomas, but this is rare.[21]

## 3.4. Glomus Jugulare Tumor

- Glomus jugulare tumor (GJT), also known as paraganglioma or chemodectoma, is a rare tumor with an incidence of approximately 1 per 1,000,000 persons.[22]
- GJT is the most common neoplasm of the middle ear.[23,24] It is the most commonly diagnosed neurotologic neoplasm after acoustic neuroma and originates from special neural crest elements called paraganglion cells, which, along with autonomic ganglion cells, form the paraganglia. It is composed of two types of cells: chief cells and sustentacular cells (modified Schwann cells).
- GJT is part of the diffuse neuroendocrine system. The chief cells of the glomus body are nearly identical to the chromaffin cells of the sympathetic ganglia and contain osmiophilic granules similar to those implicated in catecholamine storage.[25,26] Glomus bodies may function in a manner similar to that of the carotid body as chemoreceptors, responding to alterations in blood pH and oxygen

and carbon dioxide tensions, as well as affecting systemic blood pressure through the release of various transmitters.
- Glomus bodies have a rich blood supply and are innervated by either the tympanic branch of the glossopharyngeal nerve (Jacobson's nerve) or the auricular branch of the vagus nerve (Arnold's nerve).[25]
- Although usually benign and slow growing, GJTs are destructive. In approximately 3% of patients, the tumor is malignant.[27]
- A strong female predominance of 4:1 to 6:1 has been reported.[28,29]
- Typically, these tumors manifest themselves during the fifth and sixth decades of life.[28]
- GJTs have their epicenter in the region of the jugular bulb. Neurovascular structures within the hypoglossal canal, jugular foramen, and temporal bone can be affected (Fig. 6-7).
- Generally, patients with a GJT exhibit tinnitus; cephalgia; hyperacusis; anacusis; dizziness; or multiple injuries of cranial nerves VII, VIII, IX, X, XI, and XII.

## 3.5. Medulloblastoma

- Medulloblastoma represents 20% of childhood brain tumors. The median age at diagnosis of childhood medulloblastoma is 6 years, and approximately 25% of the diagnoses are in children younger than 3 years. Medulloblastoma in adults occurs predominantly in the third to fifth decades of life and constitutes 10% to 20% of medulloblastomas.

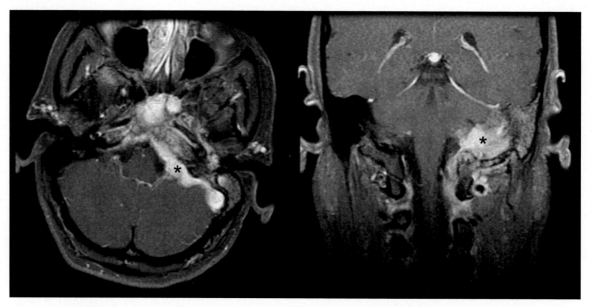

**FIGURE 6-7.** Left-sided glomus jugulare tumor (*black stars*) with extension to mastoid air cells, infratemporal fossa, cerebellopontine angle, and cavernous sinus in axial and coronal T1 MRI with gadolinium.

- Headaches, vomiting (a sign of increased intracranial pressure), and ataxia are the classic presenting triad of posterior fossa tumors.
- Most often arising in the cerebellar vermis (Fig. 6-8), the tumor grows to fill the fourth ventricle and frequently attaches to the brainstem. It has a characteristic seeding tendency associated with subarachnoid dissemination through the cerebrospinal fluid (CSF). Subarachnoid disease is detected in 20% to 25% of cases at diagnosis.[30,31]

## 4. DIAGNOSIS

### 4.1. Signs and Symptoms

- Common presenting symptoms of skull base tumors are orbitofrontal headaches because of involvement or stretching of the dura and visual disturbances because of involvement of optic nerves or neural contents of the CSs.
- Frontal base and paranasal extension may cause olfactory and frontal syndromes, such as increased intracranial pressure, seizures, or personality changes for subfrontal

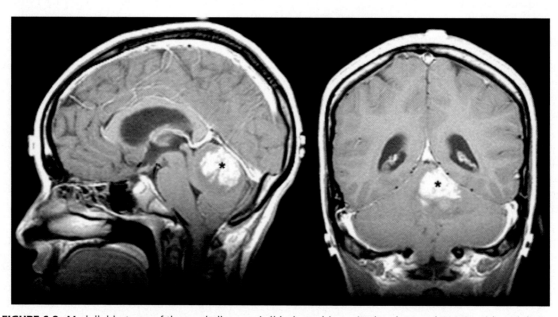

**FIGURE 6-8.** Medulloblastoma of the cerebellar vermis (*black stars*) in sagittal and coronal T1 MRI with gadolinium.

tumors, and loss of sensation of smell, nasal obstruction, rhinorrhea, or epistaxis for paranasal involvement.

- Tumors affecting the sella turcica and sphenoid sinus cause chiasmatic or hypothalamic symptoms. Chiasmatic involvement results in vision loss because of hemianopsia, either unilateral or bitemporal. Endocrinologic symptoms, such as diabetes insipidus, amenorrhea, impotence, or pituitary apoplexy, can be observed in cases of pituitary or hypothalamic involvement.
- Tumors involving the lateral middle fossa, infratemporal fossa, or sphenoid wing may extend into the orbit and induce exophthalmus, diplopia, or unilateral vision loss.
- Medial middle fossa tumors, including those of the CS and MC may present as dysfunction of one or more of the upper cranial nerves (III, IV, V1-3, or VI). Tumors in this area may encase or constrict the carotid artery in the parasellar region causing cerebral ischemia.
- Petroclival and clival involvement may result in cranial nerve deficits, cerebellar signs, corticospinal tract involvement, or increased intracranial pressure.
- Internal auditory canal or cerebellopontine angle involvement may cause hearing loss or deficits secondary to cerebellar or brainstem compression.

## 4.2. Physical Examination

- Evaluation requires clinical examination for cranial neuropathy and imaging evidence for the extent of disease in patients known to have a skull base lesion. Physical examination is based mainly on the general neurologic examination, including cranial nerves for signs of skull base lesions and basic cerebellar functions for signs of posterior fossa tumors.

## 4.3. Imaging

- Neuroimaging is critical for pretreatment planning and posttreatment surveillance.[32] Detection of differential features might predict tumor histology and help in delineation. Important features include calcification, mineralized matrix, hyperostosis, enhancement pattern, flow voids on magnetic resonance imaging (MRI), and hypervascularity on computed tomography (CT).
- CT scan and MRI are, in most cases, complementary in the diagnosis and treatment of skull base tumors.
- CT scan is superior for detecting calcification in the tumor as well as slight cortical erosion or frank bony destruction.
- MRI is better for detecting soft tissue details such as intracranial extension, compression, involvement of the neural foramina, perineural tumor spread, vascular encasement, and thrombosis.
- A slow-growing or more benign process usually presents with remodeling or pushing away bony structures. A more aggressive lesion should be favored if there is gross destruction of bone (chewed up or moth-eaten).

- Most tumors affecting bone replaces healthy bone marrow (T1 hyperintense on MRI) with isointense tumor.
- Bony hyperostosis associated with a soft-tissue tumor usually suggests meningioma and occasionally more malignant tumors, such as esthesioneuroblastoma. Hyperostosis without a soft-tissue compartment may be fibrous dysplasia, Paget's disease, or osteoblastic metastases (e.g., prostate cancer).
- Clinical correlation is required to identify extension, such as denervation (masticator musculature problems: MC or FO; ipsilateral tongue paralysis: hypoglossal canal).
- Clival tumors with gross destruction, bony fragments, and bright signal on T2-weighted MRI indicate chordoma.
- A jugular foramen origin with a moth-eaten bony pattern, with or without cranial neuropathy or tinnitus, indicates a GJT.
- Nondestructive enlargement of a neural foramen or transforaminal tumor extension indicates schwannoma or meningioma.
- An enhancing tumor in the internal auditory canal, presenting with sensorineural hearing loss (SNHL), strongly indicates acoustic schwannoma.
- Tumor involvement of the sella, parasellar region, or suprasellar cistern, with central skull base destruction, should prompt consideration of invasive pituitary adenoma.
- A review of imaging characteristics of selected tumors is given in Table 6-2.

## 4.4. Staging

- *Meningioma:* Intracranial meningiomas are generally staged according to the extent of surgical resection (Table 6-3).[33]
- *Esthesioneuroblastoma:* Kadish et al.[34] developed a staging system that has been modified by Morita et al.[12] on the basis of anatomic extension of the tumor beyond the nasal cavity (Table 6-4).
- *Chordoma:* Various classification schemes based on location have been proposed: clival, parasellar, and sellar[35]; basiocciput-caudal and basisphenoid-rostral[36]; and, of greatest help in the choice of surgical approach, superior, middle, and inferior clival.[37]
- *GJT:* Several classification systems have been proposed over the years. The most recent and widely used system is the Fisch classification[38] (Table 6-5), which was revised in 1981, and the Glasscock and Jackson classification, which is based on the site and extent of the tumor.[39]
- *Medulloblastoma:* The most widely used classification is the Chang operative staging system (Table 6-6).[40] The degree of residual tumor and presence or absence of subarachnoid or extraneural metastases determine the stage.

**TABLE 6-2. IMAGING CHARACTERISTICS OF VARIOUS TUMOR TYPES LOCATED IN SKULL BASE AND POSTERIOR FOSSA**

| Site of Origin | Tumor Type | Imaging Characteristics of Gross Tumor Volume |
|---|---|---|
| Neurovascular and meningeal structures | Meningioma | **MRI: (T1)** 60%–90% isointense, 10%–30% mildly hypointense in comparison with gray matter. **(T2)** 30%–45% increased intensity, 50% isointense to gray matter. **(Contrast)** Lesion with dural-based tail. Mostly intense homogeneous enhancement.[117–119]<br>**CT:** Isodense to slightly hyperdense to brain, good enhancement with contrast. Frequent calcification. Bone changes from hyperostosis to destructive lesion in approximately 25%.[120,121] |
| | Schwannoma | **MRI: (T1)** Intermediate intensity. **(T2)** High intensity; higher than brain but lower than CSF. **(Contrast)** Occasionally heterogeneous, marked enhancement.[122]<br>**CT:** Occasional cystic. Rare calcification and smooth bony margin with intact cortex. Contrast enhancement.[122] |
| | Glomus jugulare tumor | **MRI: (T1)** Intermediate intensity. **(T2)** Intermediate-high intensity. Flow voids. **(Contrast)** "Salt and pepper" enhancement.[123]<br>**CT:** "Moth-eaten" bony destruction with marked enhancement. |
| Cranial base | Chordoma | **MRI: (T1)** Hypointense to isointense soft tissue mass. Cystic areas, containing hemorrhage or mucoid material, may be bright. **(T2)** Hyperintense. **(Contrast)** Irregular enhancement.[124,125]<br>**CT:** Midline clival lesion with central and irregular bony destruction and soft tissue mass. Radiodensities representing remaining fragments of destroyed bone. Part of soft tissue component enhanced with contrast, but some regions with low density.[122,126] |
| | Chondrosarcoma | **MRI: (T1)** Relatively homogeneous, intermediate intensity. **(T2)** High intensity. **(Contrast)** Irregular enhancement.[127]<br>**CT:** Frequent calcified ringlets or incomplete rings (popcorn) calcification. Varied appearance with amount of chondroid matrix. Dense appearance of soft tissue component, which enhances with contrast.[122,128] |
| Subcranial with upward extension | Esthesioneuroblastoma | **MRI: (T1)** Low-intermediate, occasionally high intensity. **(T2)** Intermediate-high intensity. **(Contrast)** Homogeneous, hypervascular enhancement.<br>**CT:** Hyperostosis, destruction of cribriform plate, paranasal sinus, and orbit. |
| | Juvenile angiofibroma | **MRI: (T1)** Intermediate intensity. **(T2)** High intensity. **(Contrast)** Homogeneous intense enhancement. Flow voids representing larger high-flow vessels.[122]<br>**CT:** Pterygopalatine origin. Hypervascular, markedly enhancing tumor.[122] |
| | Adenoid cystic carcinoma | **MRI: (T1)** Intermediate intensity. **(T2)** Intermediate intensity. **(Contrast)** Irregular enhancement. Invasion along dural, periorbital, neural sheaths.<br>**CT:** Low-density tumor. |

CT, computed tomography; MRI, magnetic resonance imaging; CSF, cerebrospinal fluid.

**TABLE 6-3. SIMPSON'S CLASSIFICATION OF THE EXTENT OF RESECTION OF INTRACRANIAL MENINGIOMAS**

| | |
|---|---|
| Grade I | Gross total resection of tumor, dural attachments, and abnormal bone |
| Grade II | Gross total resection of tumor, coagulation of dural attachments |
| Grade III | Gross total resection of tumor, without resection or coagulation of dural attachments, or alternatively of its extradural extensions (e.g., invaded sinus or hyperostatic bone) |
| Grade IV | Partial resection of tumor |
| Grade V | Simple decompression (biopsy) |

**TABLE 6-4. MODIFIED KADISH STAGING OF ESTHESIONEUROBLASTOMAS**

| | |
|---|---|
| Stage A | Tumors confined to nasal cavity |
| Stage B | Tumors confined to nasal cavity and paranasal sinuses |
| Stage C | Tumors extend beyond nasal cavity and paranasal sinuses, including involvement of cribriform plate, base of skull, orbit, or intracranial cavity |
| Stage D | Tumors with metastasis to cervical lymph nodes or distant sites |

**TABLE 6-5. FISCH CLASSIFICATION OF GLOMUS TUMORS**

| | |
|---|---|
| Type A | Tumors confined to the middle ear cleft (tympanicum) |
| Type B | Tumors limited to the tympanomastoid area with no bone destruction in the infralabyrinthine compartment of the temporal bone |
| Type C | Tumors involving the infralabyrinthine compartment with extension into the petrous apex |
| Type D | Tumors with intracranial extension <2 cm in diameter |
| Type E | Tumors with intracranial extension >2 cm in diameter |

## 5. GENERAL MANAGEMENT

### 5.1. Meningioma

- The treatment of choice is complete surgical excision, but this is not always possible, because 20% to 50% of meningiomas are located in the skull base and may not be amenable to a safe surgical approach.[41]
- Recent studies report permanent cranial nerve deficits in 22% to 91% of patients undergoing surgical resection for petroclival meningiomas; an average of 54% develop new onset of neurologic symptoms after surgery.[42–46]
- To reduce the risk of neurologic deficit, a subtotal resection is often accepted. However, adjuvant therapy is usually required in these cases, because an estimated 10% to 56% of patients develop recurrence after subtotal resection.[47–49] In a number of series, fractionated radiotherapy significantly increased tumor control rates after subtotal resection of meningiomas.[50–53]
- Goldsmith et al.[51] found 5-year progression-free survival rates of 87% for benign meningiomas and 45% for malignant meningiomas in patients who were treated with radiation after subtotal resection, and a 5-year progression-free survival rate of 98% in a subset of patients with benign lesions who were treated in the era of CT/MRI-based planning.
- Smaller series looking specifically at malignant or atypical meningiomas, including data from our own institution, have also demonstrated a benefit from radiation.[54,55]
- Similarly, stereotactic radiosurgery has been used in the treatment of meningiomas. Recently, Kondziolka et al.[56] reported a 93% clinical tumor control rate in a series of ninety-nine patients with a minimum of 5 years of follow-up; they recommended gamma knife treatment for lesions less than 3 cm in diameter with regular borders that do not compress the optic chiasm.
- Adjuvant radiotherapy (3DCRT, IMRT, or stereotactic radiosurgery) is indicated for World Health Organization (WHO) grades II and III meningiomas and for WHO

**TABLE 6-6. CHANG AND HARISIADIS (LANGSTON MODIFICATION) CLASSIFICATION OF MEDULLOBLASTOMAS**

| | |
|---|---|
| T1 | Tumor < 3 cm in diameter |
| T2 | Tumor ≥ 3 cm in diameter |
| T3a | Tumor > 3 cm in diameter with extension |
| T3b | Tumor > 3 cm in diameter with unequivocal extension into the brainstem |
| T4 | Tumor > 3 cm in diameter with extension up past the aqueduct of Sylvius and/or down past the foramen magnum (i.e., beyond the posterior fossa) |
| M0 | No evidence of subarachnoid or hematogenous metastasis |
| M1 | Tumor cells in cerebrospinal fluid |
| M2 | Intracranial tumor beyond primary site (e.g., into the aqueduct of Sylvius and/or into the subarachnoid space or in the third or foramen of Luschka or lateral ventricles) |
| M3 | Gross nodular seeding in spinal subarachnoid space |
| M4 | Metastasis outside the cerebrospinal axis (especially bone marrow and bone) |

grade I tumors after subtotal resection. The recommended dose is 50.4 to 54 Gy for grade I (clinical target volume [CTV] = gross tumor volume [GTV]) and 57 to 60 Gy for grades II and III (CTV = GTV + 1–2 cm) tumors.

### 5.2. Esthesioneuroblastoma

- Preferred treatment in localized tumors is en bloc craniofacial resection of the tumor, cribriform plate, and overlying dura.[57]
- In advanced disease, preoperative radiotherapy with or without chemotherapy is preferred. An initial planned combination of surgery followed by postoperative radiotherapy may be another option.
- Cyclophosphamide, vincristine, and doxorubicin are generally preferred for concomitant radiotherapy. Platinum-based chemotherapy is preferred for advanced, high-grade tumors.
- Primary radiotherapy is preferred only in selected patients who are ineligible for surgical resection.
- Positive surgical margins are the most significant predictor of progression and decreased overall survival rates in the experience of many centers.[58–61]
- Radical surgery alone is not enough to avoid local recurrences; adjuvant postoperative high-dose radiotherapy has achieved high local control rates (92%) in recently reported series.[61–63]

- Approximately half of the recurrences occur more than 5 years after diagnosis.[64] Recurrence rates range from 30% to 70%.
- Estimated survival rates are 74% to 87% at 5 years and 54% to 60% at 10 years. Five-year survival rate after local recurrence is 82% after salvage therapy.
- We recommend as radical a surgical procedure as possible with preoperative or postoperative radiotherapy (dose ~60 Gy) and concomitant chemotherapy because aggressive, multimodality treatment is supported by the findings of many centers.[13,61,65,66]

## 5.3. Chordoma

- Wide or complete resection is the treatment of choice but is not feasible in most cases. Adjuvant radiation has been advocated for patients with positive surgical margins and residual disease.[67–69]
- Munzenrider and Liebsch[70] suggested that charged particle beams were ideal for treating skull base chordomas because such beams can deliver precise, high-dose radiation to localized areas of disease while sparing surrounding normal structures. Proton-photon therapy was recommended by both Habrand et al.[71] and Borba et al.[72] The 5-year actuarial survival rate was reported as 68%, whereas the disease-free survival rate was 63% for intracranial chordomas.
- Klekamp and Samii[73] and Romero et al.[74] produced comparable results with high-dose fractionated conventional radiotherapy. Romero et al. showed that prognosis for patients with microscopic residual disease given 48 Gy postoperative radiotherapy was better than for those who received less than 40 Gy. Klekamp and Samii reported that postoperative radiation doses of 60 to 70 Gy ensured a significantly longer recurrence-free interval in contrast with suboptimal excision without radiotherapy.
- IMRT, which can deliver precise, high-dose radiation while sparing surrounding normal structures, has not been reported to emphasize the comparison in results.
- We prefer, if possible, to prescribe 66.6 Gy in 1.8-Gy fractions given by stereotactic fractionated radiotherapy or IMRT.

## 5.4. Glomus Jugulare Tumor

- The management of jugular paraganglioma historically has shown a pendulum swing away from virtually exclusive primary surgery to more primary radiation therapy, with a recent moderating trend toward selecting treatment according to patient profile.
- The goal of surgery is complete tumor removal, whereas the goal of conventionally fractionated, external beam radiation therapy and stereotactic radiosurgery is long-term

tumor control by preventing tumor growth and regional extension that could lead to progressive symptoms and neurologic deficits.

- Local tumor control rates after total surgical removal vary from 0% to 90%.[75] Surgical removal can be associated with considerable morbidity and mortality.[76–80] In general, gross total surgical resection has been accomplished in 40% to 80% of cases in different series.[81–83]
- Progressive growth of GJTs was arrested by conventional external beam radiation therapy at rates of local control ranging from 85% to 100%, with reversal of symptoms in some patients, and complication rates ranging from 0% to 10%.[84–87]
- Despite the inherent limitations and biases of retrospective, predominantly single-institution reported series, surgery and radiation therapy seem to have similar rates of long-term local control (~90%). This is true even though patients treated with radiation therapy generally have larger or more infiltrative tumors that are not readily subject to surgical resection. Disease-related mortality is only limited to few patients with residual or recurrent tumor, irrespective of the mode of treatment. Therefore, treatment of GJTs should focus primarily on decreasing morbidity.
- A primary surgical approach is recommended for younger patients with lesions that are readily resectable without significant neurologic impairment. This approach avoids the small risk of radiation-induced second malignancy.
- Involvement of the internal carotid artery (demonstrated by balloon occlusion test), contralateral SNHL, bilateral tumors with contralateral deficits of the lower cranial nerves, concerns of venous return, or poor medical condition are common causes for inoperability and, therefore, for primary definitive radiotherapy.
- We recommend a conventionally fractionated IMRT approach for most patients whose tumors are irregularly shaped and in close proximity to radiosensitive normal structures. A dose of 45 to 50 Gy (1.8–2 Gy/fraction) is prescribed, encompassing radiographically visible tumor as CTV plus a 3-mm margin for setup uncertainty, making up the planning target volume (PTV).

## 5.5. Medulloblastoma

- The initial goal is maximal surgical resection for both treatment and reestablishment of CSF flow. Gross total resection (>90% of the tumor removed, with <1.5 cm² residual) generally is limited only by substantial invasion of the tumor into the brainstem or infiltration into the peduncle. Gross or near total resection is achieved in 90% of children older than 3 years in the United States.[88]
- Neuraxis imaging within the immediate postoperative period (1–3 days) is important to define the postoperative residual effect, which is a reliable prognostic factor.[88]

- Neuraxis staging is recommended 10 days or longer after surgery to eliminate the confusion of findings with postoperative debris. A contrast-enhanced spinal MRI and subsequent lumbar CSF cytologic studies are standard.
- Categorization of standard (or average-risk) and poor risk disease guides the treatment decision. Average risk is defined as patients older than 3 years with posterior fossa tumors who underwent total or "near-total" (<1.5 cm$^2$ of residual disease) resection with no dissemination.[40,89]
- Postoperative management currently consists of radiotherapy and chemotherapy.[90]
- Radiotherapy requires systematic inclusion of the entire subarachnoid space (craniospinal irradiation [CSI]) followed by a boost to the posterior cranial fossa. The conventional historical dose to the neuraxis has historically been 36 Gy (1.8 Gy/day). Gross total resection and postoperative CSI yield a 5- to 10-year progression-free survival rate of approximately 65%.[91–95]
- Pediatric Oncology Group and Children's Cancer Group conducted a randomized study that compared CSI at doses of 36 Gy and 23.4 Gy in average-risk meningioma, and established a standard of removing more than 90% of the tumor with less than 1.5 cm$^2$ of residual disease.[95] Reduced-dose neuraxis irradiation (23.4 Gy) is associated with increased risk of early relapse; early isolated neuraxis relapse; and lower 5-year rates of event-free survival and overall survival than standard irradiation (36 Gy). Mature analysis has confirmed these results but has showed that, with time, the differences are less pronounced (8-year analysis of event-free survival).
- The combination of reduced-dose CSI (23.4 Gy) and cisplatin-based chemotherapy has been shown to be comparable to the conventional CSI dose alone.[96] However, metastatic disease at presentation requires a dose of 36 to 39 Gy to the neuraxis.
- Boost to the posterior fossa is defined as irradiation of the entire infratentorial volume. The current effort is to use a 3DCRT approach to spare the auditory apparatus and, when possible, the pituitary hypothalamic region. The cumulative dose for boost is 54 to 55.8 Gy.
- Reduction of the boost volume from the posterior fossa to just the tumor bed is under investigation by the Children's Oncology Group.
- IMRT tumor bed boost is currently under investigation as a method to minimize ototoxicity and other morbidities associated with full posterior fossa irradiation without compromising tumor control.[97] In a previous study, Paulino et al.[98,99] compared posterior fossa boosts with tumor bed boosts by using two-dimensional radiotherapy techniques; that is, the cochlea was in the treatment field of all patients, regardless of which target volume was selected. This suggests that IMRT can decrease auditory dose rather than the size of the target volume.

- Pirzkall et al.[100] compared three different theoretic IMRT techniques with 3DCRT for particularly complex-shaped target volumes, showing that target conformality and coverage could be improved with IMRT for the subset of patients with meningiomas by averages of 10% and 36%, respectively. The conformality index improved from 1.27 for CRT to 1.12 to 1.16 for different IMRT techniques. In addition, an increased dose could be delivered with IMRT while still meeting the same constraints for adjacent organs at risk.

## 6. INTENSITY-MODULATED RADIATION THERAPY FOR SKULL BASE AND POSTERIOR FOSSA TUMORS

### 6.1. Target Volume Determination

- For IMRT, a general strategy described in the Radiation Therapy Oncology Group protocols is to encompass at least 95% of the PTV. It is also important to avoid delivering less than 93% of the prescribed dose to more than 1% of the PTV or more than 110% of the prescribed dose to more than 20% of the PTV.
- Adequate immobilization is crucial so as not to underdose the target or overdose the organs at risk because of the tight PTV for steep dose gradients.
- The suggested target volume determination for skull base tumors is summarized in Table 6-2.
- The target volume specification for definitive and postoperative IMRT in skull base tumors is summarized in Table 6-7.

### 6.2. Target Volume Delineation

- In patients receiving postoperative IMRT, CTV1 encompasses residual tumor (GTV) and the surgical bed with invasion of soft or bone tissue by the tumor. CTV2 includes primarily the prophylactically treated area or adjacent tissue whose assigned dose is lower because of tolerance constraints (e.g., the brain).
- In patients receiving definitive IMRT, CTV1 is defined as just GTV with 0- to 10-mm (occasionally 20-mm) margins based on clinical and radiologic justification. In general, because most skull base tumors are benign, including meningiomas (WHO grade I), schwannomas, GJTs, pituitary adenomas, or juvenile angiofibromas, CTV1 is equal to GTV. However, other meningiomas (WHO grades II and III), chordomas, chondrosarcomas, adenoid cystic carcinomas, or esthesioneuroblastomas are low-grade malignant tumors for which a margin over GTV is required for CTV1. CTV2 includes primarily the prophylactically treated area or an adjacent tissue whose assigned dose is lower because of tolerance constraints (e.g., the brain).

**TABLE 6-7. TARGET VOLUME SPECIFICATION FOR DEFINITIVE AND POSTOPERATIVE INTENSITY-MODULATED RADIATION THERAPY IN SKULL BASE TUMORS**

| Target | Benign Tumors* | Aggressive Tumors† |
|---|---|---|
| CTV1 | GTV, operative bed | GTV +1 cm, operative bed |
| CTV2 | Prophylactically treated area or adjacent tissue with lower assigned dose because of tolerance constraints | Prophylactically treated area or adjacent tissue with lower assigned dose because of tolerance constraints |

CTV, clinical target volume; GTV, gross tumor volume.
* Benign tumors: meningioma (World Health Organization [WHO] grade I), schwannoma, glomus jugulare, pituitary adenoma, or juvenile angiofibroma.
† Aggressive tumors: meningioma (WHO grades II and III), chordoma, chondrosarcoma, adenoid, cystic carcinoma, or esthesioneuroblastoma.

- Figure 6-9 shows CTV delineation in a 64-year-old woman with right petroclival meningioma who presented with progressive visual deficit in the right eye. MRI revealed a lesion in the right CS with multiple dura-based tails along the tentorium.
- Figure 6-10 shows CTV1 and CTV2 delineation in a 66-year-old man after surgical removal of a recurrent esthesioneuroblastoma after initial resection. The patient originally presented with headaches and a large olfactory groove tumor and underwent resection. The tumor recurred after 1.5 years at the right ethmoid and medial orbit. Although the right medial orbital mass was partially removed, a small portion of this mass remained. Adjacent brain tissue and paranasal sinuses at risk, in which the tumor did not recur, were also treated with a lower dose as CTV2.
- Figure 6-11 shows CTV delineation in 25-year-old woman with a clival chordoma who presented with headache, pain in her eyes and head, dragging of her right leg and arm, and slurred speech. She underwent a left orbital craniotomy with partial resection of the clival chordoma and decompression of the brainstem and optic nerve. She was referred for radiation therapy after tumor progression in the upper clivus involving the sella and sphenoid sinus caused marked compression and mass effect in the upper left pons.
- Figure 6-12 shows CTV delineation in a 43-year-old woman with a GJT who presented with a 20% loss of hearing in the left ear and double vision. The MRI demonstrated an expansile lesion consistent with a glomus tympanicum involving the mastoid air cells, infratemporal fossa, cerebellopontine angle, and CS.
- Figure 6-13 shows CTV1 and CTV2 delineation in a 16-year-old boy with medulloblastoma who presented with worsening headaches, neck pain, and nausea with associ-

ated symptoms of tripping easily and dropping objects. MRI defined an enhancing tumor of the cerebellar vermis with hydrocephalus for which he underwent gross total resection. CTV1 is the tumor bed after resection. CTV2 is the whole posterior fossa, which is similar to a "Mexican hat" appearance in the coronal beam eye view (Fig. 6-14).

## 6.3. Normal Tissue Delineation

- Normal tissue delineation is shown in Figures 6-14 to 6-17.
- Optic nerves are delineated starting from the eye and ending at the apex of the optic canal (Fig. 6-15).
- The optic chiasm can be difficult to delineate accurately. The oblique take-off of the chiasm posteriorly from the optic nerves must be appreciated (Fig. 6-15 and 6-16A, C). Optic pathways are delineated starting from the optic canal, extending through the infundibulum or pituitary stalk in the suprasellar cistern to the rostral part of the cerebral peduncle (Fig. 6-16B).
- The brainstem is delineated from the foramen magnum (medulla oblongata) between the basilar artery and cerebellum (pons and medulla oblongata) to the mesencephalon (cerebral peduncle) (Fig. 6-14).
- Auditory structures are delineated at the level of the internal acoustic meatus involving middle ear structures such as the cochlea (Fig. 6-17).

## 6.4. Suggested Target and Normal Tissue Doses

- All plans should be calculated with tissue homogeneity correction.

### 6.4.1. Lacrimal Gland and Cornea

- Lacrimal gland atrophy and loss of glandular function can be observed, leading to dry eye syndrome if tolerance limits are exceeded. Chronic irritation of the cornea by the eyelid may trigger corneal laceration and possible ulceration with opacification and neovascularization.
- Experience of the University of Florida with dose-response relationship for dry eye complications demonstrated no injury at doses less than 30 Gy.[101] The incidence of injury in the 30 to 40 Gy range was 5% to 25%, but it increased rapidly at doses more than 40 Gy and was 100% at doses of 57 Gy or more.
- Jiang and colleagues[102] suggested that visual impairment from corneal injury is most likely the result of a combination of radiation on the cornea and lacrimal gland injury. The 2-year incidence of visual impairment was 81% to 88% at lacrimal gland doses of 56 to 74.5 Gy and corneal doses of 31 to 41 Gy, whereas it was 17% at

*Text continues on page 97.*

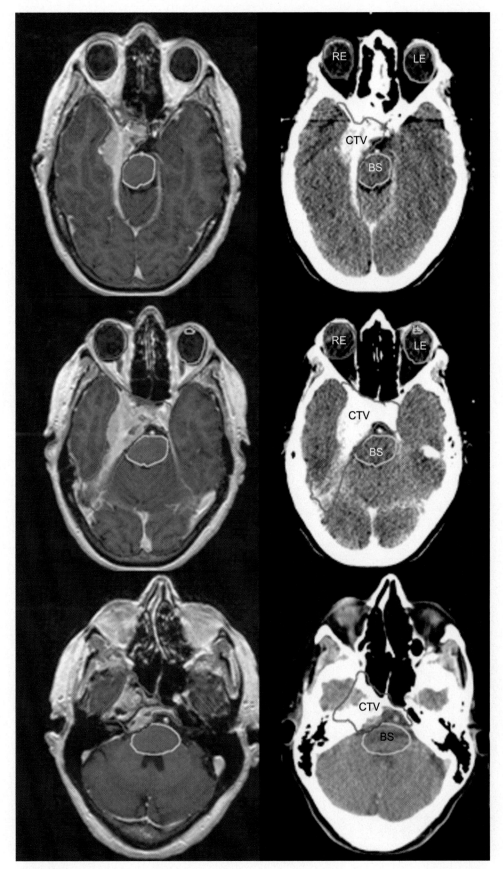

**FIGURE 6-9.** Delineation of CTV (CTV = GTV) of a petroclival World Health Organization (WHO) grade I meningioma. RE, right eye; LE, left eye; CTV, clinical target volume; BS, brainstem; GTV, gross tumor volume.

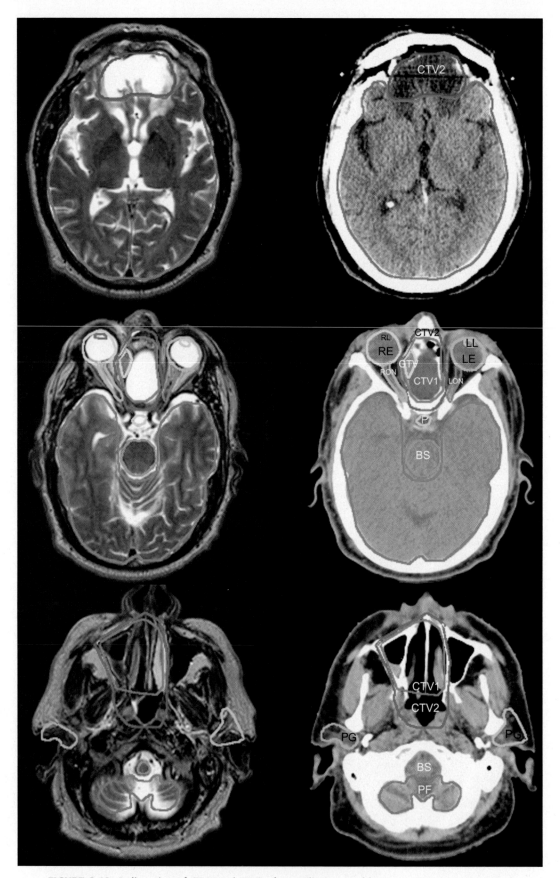

**FIGURE 6-10.** Delineation of CTV1 and CTV2 of an esthesioneuroblastoma. CTV1 is composed of residual tumor (GTV) and operative bed, which had initial recurrence. CTV2 is the area of first primary tumor before surgical resection and areas deemed at risk for recurrence. GTV, gross tumor volume; CTV, clinical target volume; RL, right lens; LL, left lens; RE, right eye; LE, left eye; RON, right optic nerve; LON, left optic nerve; P, pituitary gland; BS, brainstem; PG, parotid gland; PF, posterior fossa.

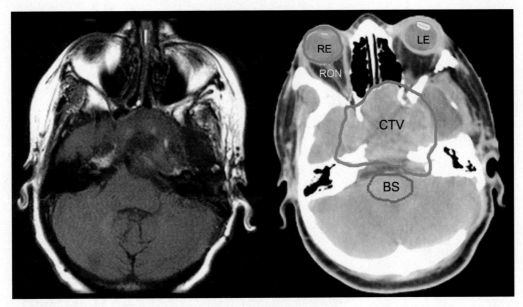

**FIGURE 6-11.** Delineation of CTV (CTV = GTV) of chordoma tumor involving clivus. CTV, clinical target volume; GTV, gross tumor volume; RE, right eye; LE, left eye; RON, right optic nerve; BS, brainstem.

lacrimal gland doses of 42 to 45 Gy and corneal doses of 23 to 30 Gy. The median time to visual injury was 9 months.

### 6.4.2. Lens

- The lens is the most radiosensitive organ in the body. It is enclosed in a capsule and consists largely of fiber cells covered anteriorly by epithelium. When there is radiation injury to the dividing cells of the lens, aberrant fibers migrate toward the posterior pole, where they constitute the beginning of a cataract.
- Cataractogenic doses were reported as 2 Gy for a single fraction, 4 Gy for multiple fractions given over a period ranging from 3 weeks to 3 months, and 5.5 Gy for multiple fractions given over a period longer than 3 months.[103] The latent period was 8 years and 7 months for doses from 2.5 to 6.5 Gy, and 4 years and 4 months for doses from 6.51 to 11.5 Gy.

### 6.4.3. Optic Pathway

- Series from the University of Texas M.D. Anderson Cancer Center revealed that visual impairment from damage to the optic nerve and chiasm occurred at a median of 27 months (range, 7–50 months) after radiotherapy.[102] At doses less than 56 Gy, optic neuropathy was not observed; the incidence remained less than 5% at 10 years with doses up to 60 Gy in fractions not exceeding 2.5 Gy. The incidence of optic neuropathy increased steeply at doses more

than 60 Gy to 34% at 10 years. Optic chiasm injury was not observed at doses less than 50 Gy, and the actuarial rate of optic chiasm complications at 10 years was only 8% for doses of 50 to 60 Gy in fractions of 2.6 Gy or less.
- The University of Florida also reported increased incidence of optic neuropathy after 60 Gy.[104] With doses of 60 Gy or more, the incidence at 15 years was 11% for fractions of less than 1.9 Gy and 47% for fractions of 1.9 Gy or more.
- The dose to the optic nerves and chiasm should be limited to less than 54 Gy, because the dose is restricted to 10 Gy for lenses. If GTV is in close proximity, the dose to the optic pathway is limited to 60 Gy with less than 10% given informed consent information regarding the risk of blindness.

### 6.4.4. Brainstem

- Debus et al.[105] reported that tolerance of fractionated radiotherapy by the brainstem seems to be a steep function of tissue volume included in the high-dose regions rather than the maximum dose of radiation to the brainstem alone. Increased risk of brainstem toxicity was significantly associated with the maximum dose to the brainstem; volume of the brainstem receiving 50 or more, 55 or more, and 60 or more Cobalt Gray equivalent (CGE); number of surgical procedures; and prevalence of diabetes or hypertension.
- The brainstem generally is restricted to a dose of no greater than 54 Gy (1 cc up to 56 Gy), if possible.

*Text continues on page 101.*

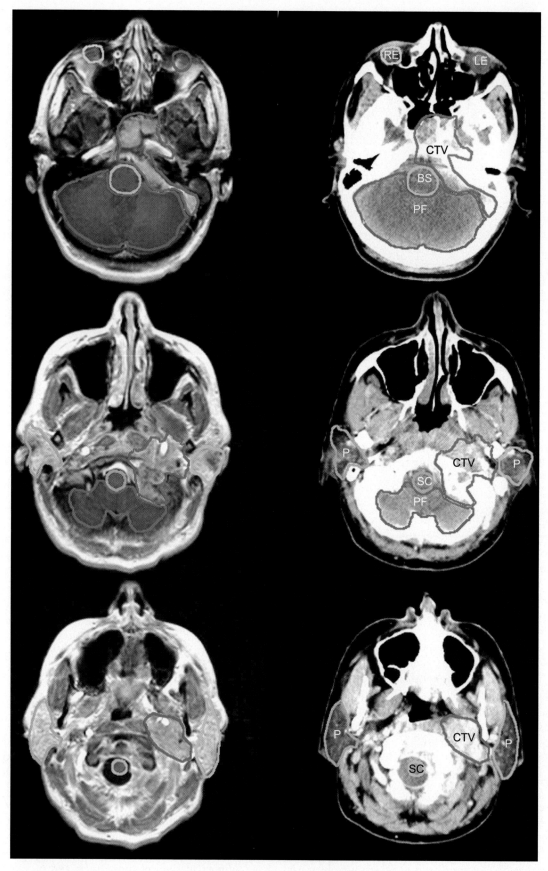

**FIGURE 6-12.** Delineation of CTV (CTV = GTV) of glomus jugulare. CTV, clinical target volume; GTV, gross tumor volume; RE, right eye; LE, left eye; BS, brainstem; P, parotid gland; PF, posterior fossa; SC, spinal cord.

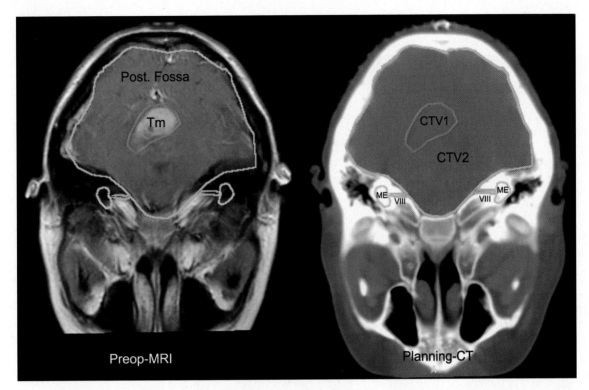

Preop-MRI

Planning-CT

**FIGURE 6-13.** Delineation of CTV1 and CTV2 of medulloblastoma. Whole posterior fossa is defined as CTV2. Surgical bed in posterior fossa, which initially contained the tumor, is defined as CTV1. CTV, clinical target volume; VIII, eighth cranial nerve; ME, middle ear apparatus.

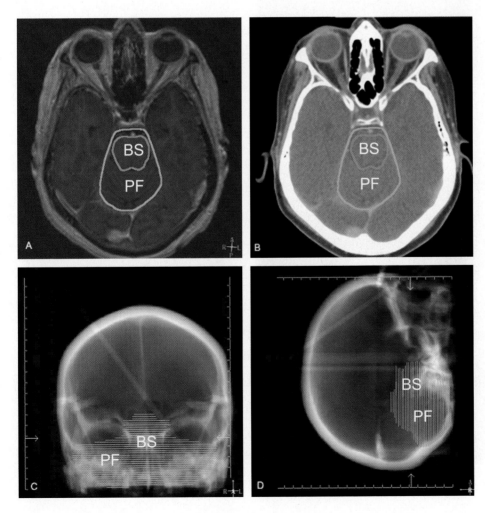

**FIGURE 6-14.** Delineation of posterior fossa (PF) and brainstem (BS).

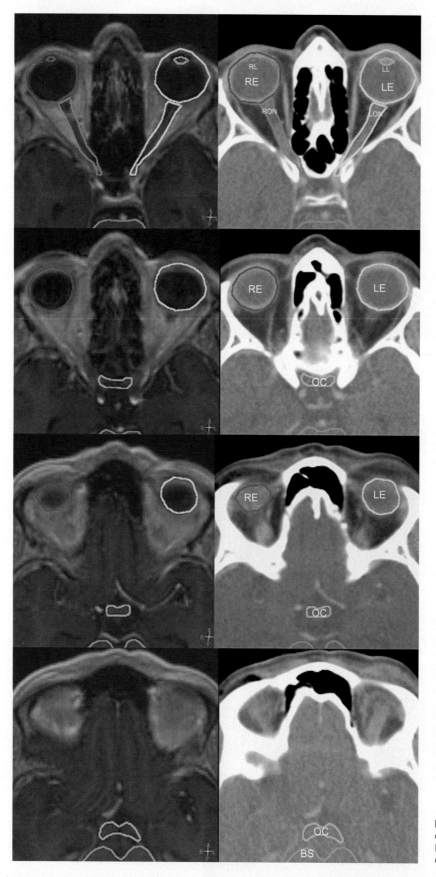

**FIGURE 6-15.** Delineation of optic nerves and chiasm. RL, right lens; LL, left lens; RE, right eye; LE, left eye; RON, right optic nerve; LON, left optic nerve; BS, brainstem; OC, optic chiasm.

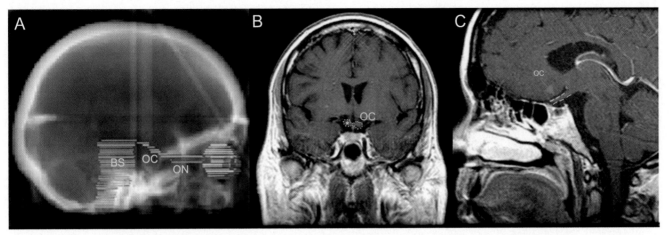

**FIGURE 6-16.** Optic tract appearance in sagittal beam eye view (OC), coronal (OC, *star* and *yellow outline*) and sagittal MRI (OC, *red arrow* and *outline*). BS, brainstem; OC, optic chiasm; ON, optic nerve.

### 6.4.5. Auditory Structures

- A dose-response relationship for radiation-induced SNHL seems to be evident. The threshold occurs at approximately 50 to 60 Gy over 5 to 6 weeks. No hearing loss was defined in children with acute leukemia after prophylactic cranial irradiation of 24 Gy in 12 fractions.[106] Evans et al.[107] detected no hearing impairment in the irradiated ear compared with the nonirradiated ear after unilateral radiotherapy of 55 to 60 Gy over 5 to 6 weeks for parotid carcinoma. However, Grau and Overgaard[108] tested hearing at baseline before irradiation and after irradiation, revealing an 8% (1/13 patients) incidence of SNHL at doses of 50 Gy or less and 44% (8/18 patients) at doses of 59 Gy or more.

- SNHL caused by radiation has been reported usually within 6 to 12 months after radiotherapy.[108] Higher hearing frequencies are affected in approximately 25% to 50% of patients after curative doses of 50 to 60 Gy or more.[109–111]

- Platinum agents also cause cumulative dose-related bilateral and irreversible ototoxicity.[112–114] High-risk criteria (i.e., young age, presence of a central nervous system tumor, and prior cranial irradiation) apply to the majority of patients with medulloblastoma. The negligible risk of hearing loss after treatment with cisplatin alone at doses of 90 to 360 mg/m$^2$ increases to 60% to 80% when combined with prior radiation.[113]

- IMRT has the advantage of sparing the cochlea and eighth cranial nerve. Huang and colleagues[97] noted that the conformal technique of IMRT delivered only 68% of the total prescribed dose (36.7 vs. 54.2 Gy) to the auditory apparatus while still delivering the full dose to the desired target volume. Their findings suggest that, de-

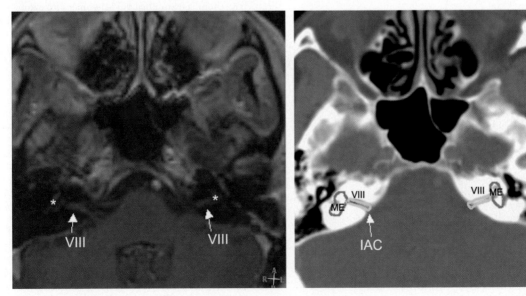

**FIGURE 6-17.** Delineation of CN VIII and middle ear apparatus including cochlea (*star*). IAC, internal acoustic canal; CN VIII, eighth cranial nerve; ME, middle ear apparatus.

spite higher doses of cisplatin and radiotherapy before cisplatin therapy, treatment with IMRT can achieve a lower rate of hearing loss.

## 6.5. Intensity-Modulated Radiation Therapy Results

- Long-term data regarding IMRT for skull base tumors are limited because of the relatively recent introduction of this technology.
- The efficacy and safety of IMRT in the treatment of meningiomas have been recently demonstrated.[115,116] Uy et al.[115] from Baylor College of Medicine revealed cumulative 5-year local control, progression-free survival, and overall survival rates of 93%, 88%, and 89%, respectively, in forty patients. Pirzkall et al.[116] also treated complex-shaped benign meningiomas of the skull base in twenty patients by using IMRT, expressing feasibility and safety with high conformality.

## REFERENCES

1. Kurland LT, Schoenberg BS, Annegers JF, et al. The incidence of primary intracranial neoplasms in Rochester, Minnesota, 1935–1977. *Ann N Y Acad Sci* 1982;381:6–16.
2. Schoenberg BS, Christine BW, Whisnant JP. The descriptive epidemiology of primary intracranial neoplasms: the Connecticut experience. *Am J Epidemiol* 1976;104:499–510.
3. Ojemann R. *Meningiomas: Clinical Features and Surgical Management.* New York: McGraw-Hill, 1985.
4. Preston-Martin S, Henderson BE, Peters JM. Descriptive epidemiology of central nervous system neoplasms in Los Angeles County. *Ann N Y Acad Sci* 1982;381:202–208.
5. Sutherland GR, Florell R, Louw D, et al. Epidemiology of primary intracranial neoplasms in Manitoba, Canada. *Can J Neurol Sci* 1987;14:586–592.
6. Radner H, Katenkamp D, Reifenberger G, et al. New developments in the pathology of skull base tumors. *Virchows Arch* 2001;438:321–335.
7. Batsakis J. *Other Neuroectodermal Tumors and Related Lesions of the Head and Neck,* 2nd ed. Baltimore: Williams & Wilkins, 1979.
8. Slevin NJ, Irwin CJ, Banerjee SS, et al. Olfactory neural tumours—the role of external beam radiotherapy. *J Laryngol Otol* 1996;110:1012–1016.
9. Stewart FM, Frieson HF. *P.A.L. Esthesioneuroblastoma.* Chichester, UK: John Wiley, 1988.
10. Taraszewska A, Czorniuk-Sliwa A, Dambska M. Olfactory neuroblastoma (esthesioneuroblastoma) and esthesioneuroepithelioma: histologic and immunohistochemical study. *Folia Neuropathol* 1998;36:81–86.
11. Hirose T, Scheithauer BW, Lopes MB, et al. Olfactory neuroblastoma. An immunohistochemical, ultrastructural, and flow cytometric study. *Cancer* 1995;76:4–19.
12. Morita A, Ebersold MJ, Olsen KD, et al. Esthesioneuroblastoma: prognosis and management. *Neurosurgery* 1993;32:706–714; discussion 714–715.
13. Polin RS, Sheehan JP, Chenelle AG, et al. The role of preoperative adjuvant treatment in the management of esthesioneuroblastoma: the University of Virginia experience. *Neurosurgery* 1998;42:1029–1037.
14. Davis RE, Weissler MC. Esthesioneuroblastoma and neck metastasis. *Head Neck* 1992;14:477–482.
15. Heffelfinger MJ, Dahlin DC, MacCarty CS, et al. Chordomas and cartilaginous tumors at the skull base. *Cancer* 1973;32:410–420.
16. O'Neill P, Bell BA, Miller JD, et al. Fifty years of experience with chordomas in southeast Scotland. *Neurosurgery* 1985;16:166–170.
17. Mitchell A, Scheithauer BW, Unni KK, et al. Chordoma and chondroid neoplasms of the spheno-occiput. An immunohistochemical study of 41 cases with prognostic and nosologic implications. *Cancer* 1993;72:2943–2949.
18. Chambers PW, Schwinn CP. Chordoma. A clinicopathologic study of metastasis. *Am J Clin Pathol* 1979;72:765–776.
19. Markwalder TM, Markwalder RV, Robert JL, et al. Metastatic chordoma. *Surg Neurol* 1979;12:473–478.
20. Volpe R, Mazabraud A. A clinicopathologic review of 25 cases of chordoma (a pleomorphic and metastasizing neoplasm). *Am J Surg Pathol* 1983;7:161–170.
21. Krol G, Sze G, Arbit E, et al. Intradural metastases of chordoma. *AJNR Am J Neuroradiol* 1989;10:193–195.
22. Thedinger BA, Glasscock ME 3rd, Cueva RA, et al. Postoperative radiographic evaluation after acoustic neuroma and glomus jugulare tumor removal. *Laryngoscope* 1992;102:261–266.
23. Spector GJ, Sobol S, Thawley SE, et al. Panel discussion: glomus jugulare tumors of the temporal bone. Patterns of invasion in the temporal bone. *Laryngoscope* 1979;89:1628–1639.
24. Spector GJ, Gado M, Ciralsky R, et al. Neurologic implications of glomus tumors in the head and neck. *Laryngoscope* 1975;85:1387–1395.
25. Gulya AJ. The glomus tumor and its biology. *Laryngoscope* 1993;103:7–15.
26. Lawson W. The neuroendocrine nature of the glomus cells: an experimental, ultrastructural, and histochemical tissue culture study. *Laryngoscope* 1980;90:120–144.
27. Gulya AJ. The glomus tumor and its biology. *Laryngoscope* 1993;103:7–15.
28. Brown JS. Glomus jugulare tumors revisited: a ten-year statistical follow-up of 231 cases. *Laryngoscope* 1985;95:284–288.
29. Woods CI, Strasnick B, Jackson CG. Surgery for glomus tumors: the Otology Group experience. *Laryngoscope* 1993;103:65–70.
30. Gajjar A, Fouladi M, Walter AW, et al. Comparison of lumbar and shunt cerebrospinal fluid specimens for cytologic detection of leptomeningeal disease in pediatric patients with brain tumors. *J Clin Oncol* 1999;17:1825–1828.
31. Fouladi M, Langston J, Mulhern R, et al. Silent lacunar lesions detected by magnetic resonance imaging of children with brain tumors: a late sequela of therapy. *J Clin Oncol* 2000;18:824–831.
32. DeMonte F, Chernov M, Fuller G, et al. Skull Base. In: Goepfert H, Ang HH, Clayman GL, et al., eds. MD Anderson Online Book: multidisciplinary care of head and neck cancer. www.headneckcancer.org; 2002.
33. Simpson D. The recurrence of intracranial meningiomas after surgical treatment. *J Neurol Neurosurg Psychiatry* 1957;20: 22–39.
34. Kadish S, Goodman M, Wang CC. Olfactory neuroblastoma. A clinical analysis of 17 cases. *Cancer* 1976;37:1571–1576.
35. Krayenbuhl H, Yasargil M. Cranial chordomas. *Prog Neurol Surg* 1975;6:380–434.
36. Raffel C, Wright DC, Gutin PH, et al. Cranial chordomas: clinical presentation and results of operative and radiation therapy in twenty-six patients. *Neurosurgery* 1985;17:703–710.
37. Sekhar LN, Sen C, Snyderman C. *Anterior, Anteriolateral, and Lateral Approaches to Extradural Petroclival Tumors.* New York: Raven Press, 1993.

38. Fisch U. Infratemporal fossa approach to tumours of the temporal bone and base of the skull. *J Laryngol Otol* 1978;92: 949–967.

39. Jackson CG, Glasscock ME 3rd, Harris PF. Glomus tumors. Diagnosis, classification, and management of large lesions. *Arch Otolaryngol* 1982;108:401–410.

40. Chang CH, Housepian EM, Herbert C Jr. An operative staging system and a megavoltage radiotherapeutic technique for cerebellar medulloblastomas. *Radiology* 1969;93:1351–1359.

41. Mathiesen T, Lindquist C, Kihlstrom L, et al. Recurrence of cranial base meningiomas. *Neurosurgery* 1996;39:2–7; discussion 8–9.

42. Samii M, Tatagiba M. Experience with 36 surgical cases of petroclival meningiomas. *Acta Neurochir (Wien)* 1992;118: 27–32.

43. Sekhar LN, Jannetta PJ. Cerebellopontine angle meningiomas. Microsurgical excision and follow-up results. *J Neurosurg* 1984; 60:500–505.

44. Olivero WC, Lister JR, Elwood PW. The natural history and growth rate of asymptomatic meningiomas: a review of 60 patients. *J Neurosurg* 1995;83:222–224.

45. Mayberg MR, Symon L. Meningiomas of the clivus and apical petrous bone. Report of 35 cases. *J Neurosurg* 1986;65: 160–167.

46. Couldwell WT, Fukushima T, Giannotta SL, et al. Petroclival meningiomas: surgical experience in 109 cases. *J Neurosurg* 1996;84:20–28.

47. Newman SA. Meningiomas: a quest for the optimum therapy. *J Neurosurg* 1994;80:191–194.

48. Levine ZT, Buchanan RI, Sekhar LN, et al. Proposed grading system to predict the extent of resection and outcomes for cranial base meningiomas. *Neurosurgery* 1999;45:221–230.

49. Condra KS, Buatti JM, Mendenhall WM, et al. Benign meningiomas: primary treatment selection affects survival. *Int J Radiat Oncol Biol Phys* 1997;39:427–436.

50. Soyuer S, Chang EL, Selek U, et al. Adjuvant or delayed radiotherapy after surgery for benign cerebral meningioma. *Radiother Oncol* 2004;71:85–90.

51. Goldsmith BJ, Wara WM, Wilson CB, et al. Postoperative irradiation for subtotally resected meningiomas. A retrospective analysis of 140 patients treated from 1967 to 1990. *J Neurosurg* 1994;80:195–201.

52. Maguire PD, Clough R, Friedman AH, et al. Fractionated external-beam radiation therapy for meningiomas of the cavernous sinus. *Int J Radiat Oncol Biol Phys* 1999;44:75–79.

53. Debus J, Wuendrich M, Pirzkall A, et al. High efficacy of fractionated stereotactic radiotherapy of large base-of-skull meningiomas: long-term results. *J Clin Oncol* 2001;19:3547–3553.

54. Milosevic MF, Frost PJ, Laperriere NJ, et al. Radiotherapy for atypical or malignant intracranial meningioma. *Int J Radiat Oncol Biol Phys* 1996;34:817–822.

55. Dziuk TW, Woo S, Butler EB, et al. Malignant meningioma: an indication for initial aggressive surgery and adjuvant radiotherapy. *J Neurooncol* 1998;37:177–188.

56. Kondziolka D, Levy EI, Niranjan A, et al. Long-term outcomes after meningioma radiosurgery: physician and patient perspectives. *J Neurosurg* 1999;91:44–50.

57. Resto VA, Eisele DW, Forastiere A, et al. Esthesioneuroblastoma: the Johns Hopkins experience. *Head Neck* 2000;22: 550–558.

58. Koka VN, Julieron M, Bourhis J, et al. Aesthesioneuroblastoma. *J Laryngol Otol* 1998;112:628–633.

59. Eich HT, Staar S, Micke O, et al. Radiotherapy of esthesioneuroblastoma. *Int J Radiat Oncol Biol Phys* 2001;49:155–160.

60. Eriksen JG, Bastholt L, Krogdahl AS, et al. Esthesioneuroblastoma—what is the optimal treatment? *Acta Oncol* 2000;39: 231–235.

61. Gruber G, Laedrach K, Baumert B, et al. Esthesioneuroblastoma: irradiation alone and surgery alone are not enough. *Int J Radiat Oncol Biol Phys* 2002;54:486–491.

62. Dulguerov P, Calcaterra T. Esthesioneuroblastoma: the UCLA experience 1970–1990. *Laryngoscope* 1992;102:843–849.

63. Chao KS, Kaplan C, Simpson JR, et al. Esthesioneuroblastoma: the impact of treatment modality. *Head Neck* 2001;23: 749–757.

64. Eden BV, Debo RF, Larner JM, et al. Esthesioneuroblastoma. Long-term outcome and patterns of failure—the University of Virginia experience. *Cancer* 1994;73:2556–2562.

65. McElroy EA Jr., Buckner JC, Lewis JE. Chemotherapy for advanced esthesioneuroblastoma: the Mayo Clinic experience. *Neurosurgery* 1998;42:1023–1027; discussion 1027–1028.

66. Levine PA, Gallagher R, Cantrell RW. Esthesioneuroblastoma: reflections of a 21-year experience. *Laryngoscope* 1999;109: 1539–1543.

67. Slater JM, Slater JD, Archambeau JO. Proton therapy for cranial base tumors. *J Craniofac Surg* 1995;6:24–26.

68. al-Mefty O, Borba LA. Skull base chordomas: a management challenge. *J Neurosurg* 1997;86:182–189.

69. Debus J, Haberer T, Schulz-Ertner D, et al. [Carbon ion irradiation of skull base tumors at GSI. First clinical results and future perspectives]. *Strahlenther Onkol* 2000;176:211–216.

70. Munzenrider JE, Liebsch NJ. Proton therapy for tumors of the skull base. *Strahlenther Onkol* 1999;175(Suppl 2):57–63.

71. Habrand JL, Mammar H, Ferrand R, et al. Proton beam therapy (PT) in the management of CNS tumors in childhood. *Strahlenther Onkol* 1999;175(Suppl 2):91–94.

72. Borba LA, Al-Mefty O, Mrak RE, et al. Cranial chordomas in children and adolescents. *J Neurosurg* 1996;84:584–591.

73. Klekamp J, Samii M. Spinal chordomas—results of treatment over a 17-year period. *Acta Neurochir (Wien)* 1996;138: 514–519.

74. Romero J, Cardenes H, la Torre A, et al. Chordoma: results of radiation therapy in eighteen patients. *Radiother Oncol* 1993; 29:27–32.

75. Reddy EK, Mansfield CM, Hartman GV. Chemodectoma of glomus jugulare. *Cancer* 1983;52:337–340.

76. Green JD Jr., Brackmann DE, Nguyen CD, et al. Surgical management of previously untreated glomus jugulare tumors. *Laryngoscope* 1994;104:917–921.

77. Patel SJ, Sekhar LN, Cass SP, et al. Combined approaches for resection of extensive glomus jugulare tumors. A review of 12 cases. *J Neurosurg* 1994;80:1026–1038.

78. Anand VK, Leonetti JP, al-Mefty O. Neurovascular considerations in surgery of glomus tumors with intracranial extensions. *Laryngoscope* 1993;103:722–728.

79. Watkins LD, Mendoza N, Cheesman AD, et al. Glomus jugulare tumours: a review of 61 cases. *Acta Neurochir* 1994; 130:66–70.

80. Springate SC, Haraf D, Weichselbaum RR. Temporal bone chemodectomas—comparing surgery and radiation therapy. *Oncology (Huntingt)* 1991;5:131–137; discussion 140, 143.

81. van der Mey AG, Frijns JH, Cornelisse CJ, et al. Does intervention improve the natural course of glomus tumors? A series of 108 patients seen in a 32-year period. *Ann Otol Rhinol Laryngol* 1992;101:635–642.

82. Gstoettner W, Matula C, Hamzavi J, et al. Long-term results of different treatment modalities in 37 patients with glomus jugulare tumors. *Eur Arch Otorhinolaryngol* 1999;256:351–355.

83. Gjuric M, Rudiger Wolf S, Wigand ME, et al. Cranial nerve and hearing function after combined-approach surgery for glomus jugulare tumors. *Ann Otol Rhinol Laryngol* 1996;105:949–954.

84. Cole JM, Beiler D. Long-term results of treatment for glomus jugulare and glomus vagale tumors with radiotherapy. *Laryngoscope* 1994;104:1461–1465.

85. Larner JM, Hahn SS, Spaulding CA, et al. Glomus jugulare tumors. Long-term control by radiation therapy. *Cancer* 1992;69: 1813–1817.

86. Schild SE, Foote RL, Buskirk SJ, et al. Results of radiotherapy for chemodectomas. *Mayo Clin Proc* 1992;67:537–540.

87. Skolyszewski J, Korzeniowski S, Pszon J. Results of radiotherapy in chemodectoma of the temporal bone. *Acta Oncol* 1991;30: 847–849.

88. Albright AL, Wisoff JH, Zeltzer PM, et al. Effects of medulloblastoma resections on outcome in children: a report from the Children's Cancer Group. *Neurosurgery* 1996;38:265–271.

89. Laurent JP, Chang CH, Cohen ME. A classification system for primitive neuroectodermal tumors (medulloblastoma) of the posterior fossa. *Cancer* 1985;56:1807–1809.

90. Kun LE, Constine LS. Medulloblastoma—caution regarding new treatment approaches. *Int J Radiat Oncol Biol Phys* 1991;20: 897–899.

91. Jenkin D, Goddard K, Armstrong D, et al. Posterior fossa medulloblastoma in childhood: treatment results and a proposal for a new staging system. *Int J Radiat Oncol Biol Phys* 1990;19: 265–274.

92. Bloom HJ, Glees J, Bell J, et al. The treatment and long-term prognosis of children with intracranial tumors: a study of 610 cases, 1950–1981. *Int J Radiat Oncol Biol Phys* 1990;18:723–745.

93. Bloom HJ, Wallace EN, Henk JM. The treatment and prognosis of medulloblastoma in children. A study of 82 verified cases. *Am J Roentgenol Radium Ther Nucl Med* 1969;105:43–62.

94. Hughes EN, Shillito J, Sallan SE, et al. Medulloblastoma at the joint center for radiation therapy between 1968 and 1984. The influence of radiation dose on the patterns of failure and survival. *Cancer* 1988;61:1992–1998.

95. Thomas PR, Deutsch M, Kepner JL, et al. Low-stage medulloblastoma: final analysis of trial comparing standard-dose with reduced-dose neuraxis irradiation. *J Clin Oncol* 2000;18:3004–3011.

96. Packer RJ, Goldwein J, Nicholson HS, et al. Treatment of children with medulloblastomas with reduced-dose craniospinal radiation therapy and adjuvant chemotherapy: a Children's Cancer Group Study. *J Clin Oncol* 1999;17:2127–2136.

97. Huang E, Teh BS, Strother DR, et al. Intensity-modulated radiation therapy for pediatric medulloblastoma: early report on the reduction of ototoxicity. *Int J Radiat Oncol Biol Phys* 2002;52:599–605.

98. Paulino AC, Saw CB, Wen BC. Comparison of posterior fossa and tumor bed boost in medulloblastoma. *Am J Clin Oncol* 2000;23:487–490.

99. Paulino AC, Narayana A, Mohideen MN, et al. Posterior fossa boost in medulloblastoma: an analysis of dose to surrounding structures using 3-dimensional (conformal) radiotherapy. *Int J Radiat Oncol Biol Phys* 2000;46:281–286.

100. Pirzkall A, Carol M, Lohr F, et al. Comparison of intensity-modulated radiotherapy with conventional conformal radiotherapy for complex-shaped tumors. *Int J Radiat Oncol Biol Phys* 2000;48:1371–1380.

101. Parsons JT, Bova FJ, Fitzgerald CR, et al. Severe dry-eye syndrome following external beam irradiation. *Int J Radiat Oncol Biol Phys* 1994;30:775–780.

102. Jiang GL, Tucker SL, Guttenberger R, et al. Radiation-induced injury to the visual pathway. *Radiother Oncol* 1994;30:17–25.

103. Merriam GSA, Focht E. The Effects of Ionizing Radiations on the Eye. In: Voeth JM, ed. *Radiation Effects and Tolerance, Normal Tissue.* Baltimore: University Park Press, 1972: 346–385.

104. Parsons JT, Bova FJ, Fitzgerald CR, et al. Radiation optic neuropathy after megavoltage external-beam irradiation: analysis of time-dose factors. *Int J Radiat Oncol Biol Phys* 1994;30: 755–763.

105. Debus J, Hug EB, Liebsch NJ, et al. Brainstem tolerance to conformal radiotherapy of skull base tumors. *Int J Radiat Oncol Biol Phys* 1997;39:967–975.

106. Thibadoux GM, Pereira WV, Hodges JM, et al. Effects of cranial radiation on hearing in children with acute lymphocytic leukemia. *J Pediatr* 1980;96:403–406.

107. Evans RA, Liu KC, Azhar T, et al. Assessment of permanent hearing impairment following radical megavoltage radiotherapy. *J Laryngol Otol* 1988;102:588–589.

108. Grau C, Overgaard J. Postirradiation sensorineural hearing loss: a common but ignored late radiation complication. *Int J Radiat Oncol Biol Phys* 1996;36:515–517.

109. Low WK, Fong KW. Long-term hearing status after radiotherapy for nasopharyngeal carcinoma. *Auris Nasus Larynx* 1998; 25:21–24.

110. Kwong DL, Wei WI, Sham JS, et al. Sensorineural hearing loss in patients treated for nasopharyngeal carcinoma: a prospective study of the effect of radiation and cisplatin treatment. *Int J Radiat Oncol Biol Phys* 1996;36:281–289.

111. Anteunis LJ, Wanders SL, Hendriks JJ, et al. A prospective longitudinal study on radiation-induced hearing loss. *Am J Surg* 1994;168:408–411.

112. Weatherly RA, Owens JJ, Catlin FI, et al. cis-platinum ototoxicity in children. *Laryngoscope* 1991;101:917–924.

113. Schell MJ, McHaney VA, Green AA, et al. Hearing loss in children and young adults receiving cisplatin with or without prior cranial irradiation. *J Clin Oncol* 1989;7:754–760.

114. McHaney VA, Thibadoux G, Hayes FA, et al. Hearing loss in children receiving cisplatin chemotherapy. *J Pediatr* 1983;102: 314–317.

115. Uy NW, Woo SY, Teh BS, et al. Intensity-modulated radiation therapy (IMRT) for meningioma. *Int J Radiat Oncol Biol Phys* 2002;53:1265–1270.

116. Pirzkall A, Debus J, Haering P, et al. Intensity modulated radiotherapy (IMRT) for recurrent, residual, or untreated skull-base meningiomas: preliminary clinical experience. *Int J Radiat Oncol Biol Phys* 2003;55:362–372.

117. Spagnoli MV, Goldberg HI, Grossman RI, et al. Intracranial meningiomas: high-field MR imaging. *Radiology* 1986;161: 369–375.

118. Zimmerman RD. *MRI of Intracranial Meningiomas.* New York: Raven Press, 1991.

119. Elster AD, Challa VR, Gilbert TH, et al. Meningiomas: MR and histopathologic features. *Radiology* 1989;170:857–862.

120. Latchaw RE, Hirsch WL. *Computerized Tomography of Intracranial Meningiomas.* New York: Raven Press, 1991.

121. Ginsberg LE. Radiology of meningiomas. *J Neurooncol* 1996; 29:229–238.

122. Curtin HD, Rabinov JD, Som PM. *Central Skull Base: Embryology, Anatomy, and Pathology. Vol 1.* St. Louis, MO: Mosby, 2003.

123. Olsen ML, Dillon WP, Kelly WM. MR imaging of paragangliomas. *AJNR Am J Neuroradiol* 1986;7:1039–1042.

124. Meyers SP, Hirsch WL Jr., Curtin HD, et al. Chordomas of the skull base: MR features. *AJNR Am J Neuroradiol* 1992;13: 1627–1636.

125. Larson TC 3rd, Houser OW, Laws ER Jr. Imaging of cranial chordomas. *Mayo Clin Proc* 1987;62:886–893.

126. Firooznia H, Pinto RS, Lin JP, et al. Chordoma: radiologic evaluation of 20 cases. *Am J Roentgenol* 1976;127:797–805.

127. Oot RF, Melville GE, New PF, et al. The role of MR and CT in evaluating clival chordomas and chondrosarcomas. *AJR Am J Roentgenol* 1988;151:567–575.

128. Brown E, Hug EB, Weber AL. Chondrosarcoma of the skull base. *Neuroimaging Clin N Am* 1994;4:529–541.

# 7

# NODAL TARGET VOLUME FOR HEAD AND NECK CANCER

**K. S. CLIFFORD CHAO**
**KIE-KIAN ANG**
**SMITH APISARNTHANARAX**
**GOKHAN OZYIGIT**

## 1. INTRODUCTION

- Promising treatment results of head and neck conformal therapy or intensity-modulated radiation therapy (IMRT) have provided significant incentives for the radiation oncology community to incorporate this imaging-based technology into daily clinical practice.

- Protecting critical normal tissue without compromising tumor target coverage requires extensive knowledge of the patterns of tumor extension and spread and the ability to accurately delineate both the tumor target volumes and the normal structures.

- Thorough understanding of the natural course of tumor spread ensures the delineation of clinical target volume (CTV) that represents the region potentially containing microscopic disease as defined in the International Commission on Radiation Units and Measurements reports 50 and 62.[1,2]

- Ideally, if an imaging modality can provide sufficient information on whether certain nodal regions contain micrometastasis, accurate determination of nodal target volume for head and neck IMRT will be possible. Unfortunately, neither physical examination nor radiologic imaging techniques used in clinical practice are proficient in detecting microscopic disease. Sako et al.[3] found that the submandibular nodes must measure at least 0.5 cm in size to be clinically detectable. Similarly, a deep cervical node located adjacent to muscles must exceed 1 cm in diameter to be clinically palpable.

- Notably, the incidence of occult nodal metastasis ranged from 25% to 60% in the 1950s to the 1960s. Even with advances in morphology-based imaging techniques, such as computed tomography (CT) or magnetic resonance imaging (MRI), determination of nodal metastasis on the basis of the size of the lymph node still underestimates between 12% and 60% of micrometastasis. Detection of micrometastasis by functional imaging is an evolving area

of research and may not be clinically applicable in the immediate future. Therefore, the current clinical practice to determine target volume for IMRT relies on historical information from surgical pathologic experiences.

- In 1948, Rouviere[4] described the anatomic details of the cervical lymphatic network (Fig. 7-1). On the basis of this description, the TNM atlas proposed a terminology that divides the head and neck lymph nodes into twelve groups according to their relationship with the adjacent muscles, vessels, and nerves.[5]

- In 1991, a Committee for Head and Neck Surgery and Oncology of the American Academy for Otolaryngology—Head and Neck Surgery postulated a classification (Robbins' classification) that divides the neck into six levels or eight nodal groups for those lymph nodes routinely removed during neck dissection.[6] These recommendations have been recently updated, with minor revisions of some boundaries by using radiologic landmarks and a better definition of sublevels of levels II and V (Table 7-1).[7]

- Lymph nodes that are not routinely dissected, such as retropharyngeal, parotid, buccal, or occipital nodes, are not included in Robbins' classification.[7] Those systems describe the boundaries of the node region on the basis of anatomic structures, such as major blood vessels, muscles, nerves, bones, and cartilage. The radiologic boundaries of these nodal levels have been summarized recently (Fig. 7-2).[8,9]

## 2. DETERMINATION OF CLINICAL TARGET VOLUMES

- Determination of CTVs was based on the incidence and location of metastatic neck nodes from various head and neck subsites, which were gathered from the published literature and summarized in Table 7-2. The distribution of nodal metastasis to different lymph node levels in the

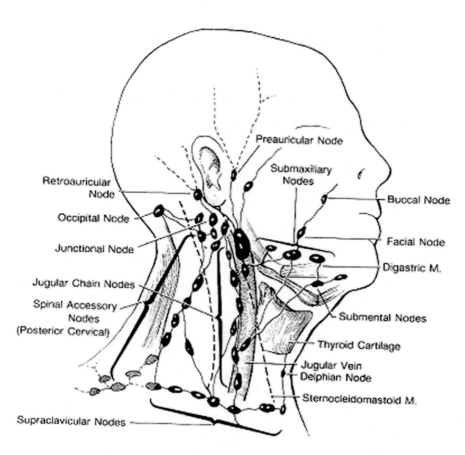

**FIGURE 7-1.** Tobias MJ (trans). Lymph nodes in the head and neck region. (Redrawn from: Rouviere H. *Anatomy of the Human Lymphatic System.* Ann Arbor, MI: Edwards Brothers, 1938:27, with permission.)

## TABLE 7-1. CLASSIFICATION AND DEFINITION OF NECK NODES

| Robbins' Classification | | Definition |
|---|---|---|
| Level | Terminology | Surgical/Anatomic Landmarks |
| Ia<br>Ib | Submental group<br>Submandibular group | Contains the submental and submandibular triangles bounded by the posterior belly of the digastric muscle, hyoid bone inferiorly, and body of the mandible superiorly. |
| II | Upper internal jugular group | Contains the upper internal jugular lymph nodes and extends from the level of the hyoid bone inferiorly to the skull base superiorly. |
| III | Middle internal jugular group | Contains the middle internal jugular lymph nodes from the hyoid bone superiorly to the cricothyroid membrane inferiorly. |
| IV | Lower internal jugular group | Contains the lower internal jugular lymph nodes from the cricothyroid membrane superiorly to the clavicle inferiorly. |
| V | Spinal accessory group | Contains the lymph nodes in the posterior triangle bounded by the anterior border of the trapezius posteriorly, the posterior border of the sternocleidomastoid muscle anteriorly, and the clavicle inferiorly.<br>(For descriptive purposes, level V may be further subdivided into upper, middle, or lower levels corresponding to the superior and inferior planes that define levels II, III, and IV.) |
| VI | Anterior compartment group | Contains the lymph nodes of the anterior compartment from the hyoid bone superiorly to the suprasternal notch inferiorly. On each side, the lateral border is formed by the medial border of the carotid sheath. |
| VII | Upper mediastinal group | Contains the lymph nodes inferior to the suprasternal notch in the upper mediastinum. |

Other groups: retropharyngeal, buccinator (facial), intraparotid, preauricular, postauricular, and suboccipital.

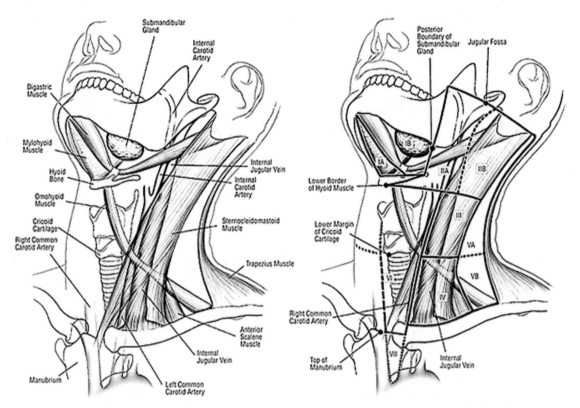

**FIGURE 7-2.** Left anterior view of neck. Pertinent anatomy that relates to the nodal classification (*left*); outline of the levels of the classification (*right*). Note that the line of separation between levels I and II is the posterior margin of the submandibular gland. The separation between levels II and III and level V is the posterior edge of the sternocleidomastoid muscle. However, the line of separation between levels IV and V is an oblique line extending from the posterior edge of the sternocleidomastoid muscle to the posterior edge of the anterior scalene muscle. The posterior edge of the internal jugular vein separates level IIA and IIB nodes. The top of the manubrium separates levels VI and VII. (From: Som PM, Curtin HD, Mancuso AA. An imaging-based classification for the cervical nodes designed as an adjunct to recent clinically based nodal classifications. *Arch Otolaryngol Head Neck Surg* 1999;125:388–396, with permission.)

head and neck region varies by primary tumor subsite. The number under each column represents the percentage of lymph node metastasis in patients with squamous cell carcinoma arising from various head and neck subsites. Because metastatic nodes may manifest in more than one nodal level at presentation, the summation of percentage from all nodal levels (regions) may exceed 100%, especially in the N+ group.

- Treatment of the contralateral neck remains controversial because there are few data on the patterns of pathologic node distribution in the contralateral neck. Treatment also likely results from clinical judgment rather than from scientific evidence. However, contralateral nodal regions should be included especially in tumors that tend to spread to the contralateral neck nodes or those that arise from or invade a midline structure, such as the soft palate, base of tongue (BOT), posterior pharyngeal wall, or nasopharynx. For example, nodal metastasis exists in 85% to 90% of patients with nasopharyngeal carcinoma, and approximately 50% of them have

bilateral disease; therefore, both sides of the neck should be treated for this particular disease.

- Table 7-3 shows that macroscopic or microscopic bilateral nodal metastases present with more than 30% of tumor residing in the BOT, pharyngeal wall, and pyriform sinus.

- The probability of contralateral nodal metastasis can be predicted with better accuracy if these tumor characteristics are taken into account. Table 7-4 shows the tumor factors for oral cavity carcinoma that could influence the incidence of contralateral nodal metastasis.

- On the other hand, tumors arising from the true vocal cord, paranasal sinuses, and middle ear have a low risk of lymph node metastasis, so only the ipsilateral neck should be included in the IMRT field.

- If a tumor arises from the buccal mucosa and retromolar trigone, which have a lower chance of contralateral neck node metastasis, especially when the primary tumor size is small and no involvement of the ipsilateral neck node is evident, the contralateral neck may not require treatment.

**TABLE 7-2. INCIDENCE AND DISTRIBUTION OF METASTATIC DISEASE IN CLINICALLY NEGATIVE (N−) AND POSITIVE (N+) NECK NODES (%)**

| Clinical Presentation | Radiologically Enlarged Retropharyngeal Nodes | | Pathologic Nodal Metastasis | | | | | | | | | |
|---|---|---|---|---|---|---|---|---|---|---|---|---|
| | | | Level I | | Level II | | Level III | | Level IV | | Level V | |
| | N− | N+ | N− | N+ | N− | N+ | N− | N+ | N− | N+ | N− | N+ |
| Nasopharynx | 40 | 86 | — | — | — | — | — | — | — | — | — | — |
| Oral cavity | | | | | | | | | | | | |
| Oral tongue | — | — | 14 | 39 | 19 | 73 | 16 | 27 | 3 | 11 | 0 | 0 |
| Floor of mouth | — | — | 16 | 72 | 12 | 51 | 7 | 29 | 2 | 11 | 0 | 5 |
| Alveolar ridge and RMT | — | — | 25 | 38 | 19 | 84 | 6 | 25 | 5 | 10 | 1 | 4 |
| Oropharynx | | | | | | | | | | | | |
| BOT | 0 | 6 | 4 | 19 | 30 | 89 | 22 | 22 | 7 | 10 | 0 | 18 |
| Tonsil | 4 | 12 | 0 | 8 | 19 | 74 | 14 | 31 | 9 | 14 | 5 | 12 |
| Hypopharynx | | | | | | | | | | | | |
| Pharyngeal wall | 16 | 21 | 0 | 11 | 9 | 84 | 18 | 72 | 0 | 40 | 0 | 20 |
| Pyriform sinus | 0 | 9 | 0 | 2 | 15 | 77 | 8 | 57 | 0 | 23 | 0 | 22 |
| Larynx | | | | | | | | | | | | |
| Supraglottic larynx | 0 | 4 | 6 | 2 | 18 | 70 | 18 | 48 | 9 | 17 | 2 | 16 |
| Glottic larynx | — | — | 0 | 9 | 21 | 42 | 29 | 71 | 7 | 24 | 7 | 2 |

RMT, retromolar trigone; BOT, base of tongue.
Compiled with permission from: McLaughlin MP, Mendenhall WM, Mancuso AA, et al. Retropharyngeal adenopathy as a predictor of outcome in squamous cell carcinoma of the head and neck. *Head Neck* 1995;17:190–198.[28] Candela FC, Kothari K, Shah JP. Patterns of cervical node metastases from squamous carcinoma of the oropharynx and hypopharynx. *Head Neck* 1990;12:197–203.[29] Shah JP, Candela FC, Poddar AK. The patterns of cervical lymph node metastases from squamous carcinoma of the oral cavity. *Cancer* 1990;66:109–113.[30] Bataini JP, Bernier J, Brugere J, et al. Natural history of neck disease in patients with squamous cell carcinoma of oropharynx and pharyngolarynx. *Radiother Oncol* 1985;3:245–255.[31] Byers RM, Wolf PF, Ballantyne AJ. Rationale for elective modified neck dissection. *Head Neck Surg* 1988;10:160–167.[32] Lindberg R. Distribution of cervical lymph node metastases from squamous cell carcinoma of the upper respiratory and digestive tracts. *Cancer* 1972;29:1446–1449.[33]
From: Chao KS, Wippold FJ, Ozyigit G, et al. Determination and delineation of nodal target volumes for head-and-neck cancer based on patterns of failure in patients receiving definitive and postoperative IMRT. *Int J Radiat Oncol Biol Phys* 2002;53:1174–1184, with permission.[9]

**TABLE 7-3. INCIDENCE OF CONTRALATERAL OR BILATERAL NECK NODE METASTASIS BY PRIMARY TUMOR SITE**

| | cN+, Bilateral | cN+, Contralateral Only | cN−, pN+ Bilateral |
|---|---|---|---|
| Oral tongue | 12% | — | 33% |
| FOM | 27% | — | 21% |
| BOT | 37% | — | 55% |
| Tonsil | 16% | 2% | — |
| Pharyngeal wall | 50% | — | 37% |
| Pyriform sinus | 49% | 6% | 59% |
| Supraglottis | 39% | 2% | 26% |
| Glottic larynx | — | — | 15% |

BOT, base of tongue; FOM, floor of mouth.
Compiled with permission from: Bataini JP, Bernier J, Brugere J, et al. Natural history of neck disease in patients with squamous cell carcinoma of oropharynx and pharyngolarynx. *Radiother Oncol* 1985;3:245–255.[31] Byers RM, Wolf PF, Ballantyne AJ. Rationale for elective modified neck dissection. *Head Neck Surg* 1988;10:160–167.[32] Northrop M, Fletcher GH, Jesse RH, et al. Evolution of neck disease in patients with primary squamous cell carcinoma of the oral tongue, floor of mouth, and palatine arch, and clinically positive neck nodes neither fixed nor bilateral. *Cancer* 1972;29:23–30.[34] Woolgar JA. Histological distribution of cervical lymph node metastases from intraoral/oropharyngeal squamous cell carcinomas. *Br J Oral Maxillofac Surg* 1999;37:175–180.[35] Buckley JG, MacLennan K. Cervical node metastases in laryngeal and hypopharyngeal cancer: a prospective analysis of prevalence and distribution. *Head Neck* 2000;22:380–385.[36]
From: Chao KS, Wippold FJ, Ozyigit G, et al. Determination and delineation of nodal target volumes for head-and-neck cancer based on patterns of failure in patients receiving definitive and postoperative IMRT. *Int J Radiat Oncol Biol Phys* 2002;53:1174–1184, with permission.[9]

**TABLE 7-4. FACTORS INFLUENCING CONTRALATERAL LYMPH NODE METASTASIS IN ORAL CANCER**

| Variable | RR of Contralateral LN Metastasis | 95% CI |
|---|---|---|
| Tumor site | | |
| Tongue | 1.0 | Ref. |
| FOM | 1.5 | 0.9–2.6 |
| RMT | 0.3 | 0.1–1.1 |
| Distance from midline | | |
| >1 cm | 1.0 | Ref. |
| Cross <1 cm | 2.8 | 1.1–7.5 |
| Cross >1 cm | 12.7 | 5.6–29.1 |
| Tumor stage | | |
| T1 | 1.0 | Ref. |
| T2, T3 | 2.2 | 0.7–5.5 |
| T4 | 5.8 | 2.0–16.3 |

RMT, retromolar trigone; FOM, floor of mouth; LN, lymph node; RR, relative risk; CI, confidence interval.
Modified with permission from: Kowalski LP, Medina JE. Nodal metastases: predictive factors. *Otolaryngol Clin North Am* 1998;31:621–637.[37]

- Previously, we defined two CTVs: CTV1 for the high-risk region and CTV2 for the low-risk region or prophylactically treated neck.[9–11] Generous CTVs were used mainly to avoid undesirable marginal failure. Recently, we reported the patterns of failure among 126 patients who underwent head and neck IMRT.[10] The majority of failures occurred within CTV1, which was the high-risk region and received the full-prescribed dose. We have also observed that quality of life was worse with an increase of CTV size (Chao KS, 2004).
- On the basis of this observation and clinical outcome analysis, we currently adopted a revised strategy for tar-

get volume specification (Table 7-5).[12] In these guidelines, three CTVs are now defined.

- CTV1 for patients receiving definitive IMRT is defined as gross tumor volume (GTV) or nodal GTV with margins based on clinical and radiologic justification (see next section for further details on CTV margin recommendations).
- CTV1 for postoperative patients encompasses the preoperative GTV plus 1- to 2-cm margin including the resection bed with soft tissue invasion by the tumor or extracapsular extension (ECE) by metastatic neck nodes. Preoperative CT imaging, surgical defects, or postsurgical changes seen on postoperative CT scan determine the surgical bed.
- CTV2 for patients receiving definitive IMRT encompasses the CTV1 and the region adjacent to CTV1 but with no direct tumor involvement based on clinical findings and CT or MRI imaging. Radiologically or clinically involved neck node is also included in CTV2 with 1-cm margins truncating air and bone.
- CTV2 for postoperative patients primarily includes the clinically/radiologically or pathologically uninvolved cervical lymph nodes, deemed as elective nodal regions, or prophylactically treated neck.
- CTV3 for patients receiving definitive IMRT include the clinically/radiologically or pathologically uninvolved cervical lymph nodes, deemed as elective nodal regions, or prophylactically treated neck (previously classified as CTV2).

- Our approach to selective neck treatment is similar to the recommendations proposed by Gregoire et al.[13] These target volume specifications were integrated with the published clinical data shown in Table 7-2. On the basis of these historical data, we proposed that a treatment of

**TABLE 7-5. TARGET VOLUME SPECIFICATION FOR DEFINITIVE AND POSTOPERATIVE INTENSITY-MODULATED RADIATION THERAPY**

| Target | Definitive IMRT | High-Risk Postoperative IMRT | Intermediate-Risk Postoperative IMRT |
|---|---|---|---|
| CTV1 | Gross tumor (primary and enlarged nodes) with margins based on clinical and radiologic justification*† | Surgical bed with soft-tissue involvement or nodal region with extracapsular involvement | Surgical bed without soft-tissue involvement or nodal region without capsular extension |
| CTV2 | Soft tissue and nodal regions adjacent to the CTV1† | Elective nodal regions‡ | Elective nodal regions‡ |
| CTV3 | Elective nodal regions‡ | | |

IMRT, intensity-modulated radiation therapy; CTV, clinical target volume.
* Margins of 1 cm based on extracapsular extension pathologic data from: Apisarnthanarax S, Elliott D, El Naggar AK, et al. Determination of the magnitude of clinical target volume margins based on pathological examination of microscopic extracapsular extension of metastatic neck nodes. *Int J Radiat Oncol Biol Phys* (submitted 2004); with permission. Margins of 2 to 3 cm for muscle involvement.
† No skin involvement or risk for microscopic extension: 2- to 3-mm sparing of dermal structures.
‡ Suggested guidelines for elective nodal regions are shown in Table 7-6.

the N0 neck is warranted if the probability of occult cervical metastasis is higher than 5%.

- The CTV (CTV1, CTV2, and CTV3) determination guidelines for various head and neck tumor subsites for postoperative and definitive IMRT are divided into separate recommendations for node negative and node positive neck, which are summarized in Tables 7-6 and 7-7, respectively. These suggested recommendations represent consensus guidelines from the M. D. Anderson Cancer Center.[14]

- IMRT is applied to the upper neck for salivary sparing. The lower neck is treated with a conventional AP lower neck port if indicated. The standard superior border for the lower neck field is at the level of the thyroid notch. In patients with a tumor or metastatic lymph node extending below this level, the junction line is adjusted to avoid bisecting gross disease.

## 3. DELINEATION OF CLINICAL TARGET VOLUME

- Because the definition of neck node level and the anatomic boundaries described in Robbins' Classification were designed on the basis of specific soft tissue landmarks for surgical procedures and are not easily seen on CT and MRI slices, we implemented modified guidelines for the delineation of the various node levels in the neck. We supplemented Robbins' classification with a retropharyngeal nodal group to assist readers in better understanding of the nodal target volume determination and delineation for head and neck IMRT. Our recommendations for the radiologic boundaries of these nodal levels are summarized in Table 7-8.

  □ Level Ia:
  - Contains the submental nodes.
  - Drain the skin of chin, mid-lower lip, tip of the tongue, and anterior floor of the mouth.
  - Greatest risk of harboring metastases from the lower lip, floor of the mouth, anterior oral tongue, and anterior alveolar mandibular ridge.

  □ Level Ib:
  - Contains the submandibular nodes.
  - Drain the medial canthus, lower nasal cavity, hard and soft palate, maxillary and alveolar ridges, cheek, upper and lower lips, and most of the anterior tongue. It also receives efferent lymphatics from the submental nodes.

## TABLE 7-6. SUGGESTED CLINICAL TARGET VOLUME DETERMINATION GUIDELINES FOR NODE NEGATIVE (N0) NECK

| Tumor Site | Clinical Presentation | CTV1 | CTV2[@] | CTV3 |
|---|---|---|---|---|
| **Nasopharynx** | Any T N0 | GTVp | Optional | IN+CN (I$_b$–V, RPLN) |
| **Maxillary sinus** | T1, T2 N0 | GTVp | — | — |
| | T3, T4 N0 | GTVp | Optional | IN (I and II, RPLN) |
| **Oral cavity** | | | | |
| Buccal, RMT | T1, T2 N0 | GTVp | — | IN*(I–III) |
| Oral tongue | T3, T4 N0 | GTVp | Optional | IN+CN (I–V) |
| FOM | Any T N0 | GTVp | Optional | IN+CN (I–V) |
| **Oropharynx** | | | | |
| Tonsil | T1, T2 N0 | GTVp | — | IN+CN* (I$_b$–D) |
| BOT | T3, T4 N0 | GTVp | Optional | IN+CN (I$_b$, RPLN) |
| Soft palate | Any T N0 | GTVp | Optional | IN+CN (I$_b$, RPLN) |
| **Hypopharynx†** | Any T N0 | GTVp | Optional | IN+CN (II–V, RPLN) |
| **Larynx** | | | | |
| Glottic | T1, T2 N0 | GTVp | — | — |
| | T3, T4 N0 | GTVp | Optional | IN+CN (II–V) |
| Supraglottic | Any T N0 | GTVp | Optional | IN+CN (II–V) |

CTV, clinical target volume; RMT, retromolar trigone; FOM, floor of mouth; BOT, base of tongue; GTVp, primary gross tumor volume; IN, ipsilateral nodal levels; CN, contralateral nodal levels; RPLN, retropharyngeal lymph node.
Roman numerals represent neck nodal levels.
* CN optional for locally advanced tonsil cancer.
† Hypopharynx includes pyriform sinus and pharyngeal wall.
Suggested IMRT dose schedule for chemoradiation: CTV1 = 70 Gy/35 fx or 70 Gy/33 fx; CTV2 = 63 Gy/35 fx or 59.4 Gy/33 fx; CTV3 = 56 Gy/35 fx or 54 Gy/33 fx. For small oropharyngeal tumors (T1-2 N0-1 M0) or when definitive IMRT is used without concomitant chemotherapy, suggested doses are: CTV1 = 66 Gy/30 fx; CTV2 = 60 Gy/30Gy; CTV3 = 54 Gy/30 fx.
[@] Optional margins around CTV1.
Guidelines based on consensus reached within M. D. Anderson Cancer Center.[14]

## TABLE 7-7. SUGGESTED CLINICAL TARGET VOLUME DETERMINATION GUIDELINES FOR NODE POSITIVE (N+) NECK

| Tumor Site | Clinical Presentation | CTV1 | CTV2 | CTV3 |
|---|---|---|---|---|
| Nasopharynx<br>Maxillary sinus<br>Oral cavity<br>Oropharynx<br>Hypopharynx<br>Larynx | Any T N+ | GTVp+n | IN (adjacent LNs*) | IN+CN+RPLN†<br>(remaining LNs) |

GTVp, primary gross tumor volume; n, nodal gross tumor volume; IN, ipsilateral nodal levels; CN, contralateral nodal levels; RPLN, retropharyngeal lymph nodes; CTV, clinical target volume.
Oral cavity: buccal, retromolar trigone, oral tongue, floor of mouth; Oropharynx: base of tongue, tonsil, soft palate; Hypopharynx: pyriform sinus, pharyngeal wall; Larynx: supraglottic, glottic.
* Immediate adjacent nodal level or 3 to 4 cm from CTV1 nodal basin.
† Include RPLN for midline and more advanced tumors.
Suggested IMRT dose schedule for chemoradiation: CTV1 = 70 Gy/35 fx or 70 Gy/33 fx; CTV2 = 63 Gy/35 fx or 59.4 Gy/33 fx; CTV3 = 56 Gy/35 fx or 54 Gy/33 fx. For small oropharyngeal tumors (T1-2 N0-1 M0) or when definitive IMRT is used without concomitant chemotherapy, suggested doses are: CTV1 = 66 Gy/30 fx; CTV2 = 60 Gy/30Gy; CTV3 = 54 Gy/30 fx.
Guidelines based on consensus reached within M. D. Anderson Cancer Center.[14]

## TABLE 7-8. RECOMMENDATIONS FOR RADIOLOGIC BOUNDARIES OF NECK NODE REGIONS

| Level | Recommended Boundaries |
|---|---|
| I | • Cranial: mylohyoid muscle, cranial edge of submandibular gland; Caudal: hyoid bone<br>• Anterior: symphysis menti; Posterior: posterior edge of submandibular gland<br>• Lateral: medial edge of mandible; Medial: lateral edge of anterior belly of digastric muscle |
| II | • Cranial: caudal edge of lateral process of C1 vertebrae (N0 cases) or cranial base (N+ cases); Caudal: cranial edge of hyoid bone<br>• Anterior: posterior margin of submandibular gland; Posterior: the posterior edge of SCM<br>• Lateral: medial edge of SCM; Medial: medial edge of vessel bundle,* paraspinal muscle |
| III | • Cranial: bottom edge of hyoid bone; Caudal: lower margin of cricoid cartilage<br>• Anterior: posterolateral edge of sternohyoid muscle; Posterior: the posterior edge of SCM<br>• Lateral: medial edge of SCM; Medial: medial edge of vessel bundle,* paraspinal muscle |
| IV | • Cranial: lower margin of cricoid cartilage; Caudal: 2 cm cranial to sternoclavicular joint (N0 cases) or sternoclavicular joint (N+ cases)<br>• Anterior: posterolateral edge of SCM muscle; Posterior: the anterior edge of paraspinal muscle<br>• Lateral: lateral border of SCM; Medial: medial border of vessel bundle, lateral border of thyroid |
| V | • Cranial: cranial base; Caudal: transverse cervical vessels, cranial border of clavicle (non-contrast CT)<br>• Anterior: posterior edge of SCM; Posterior: anterior edge of trapezius muscle<br>• Lateral: platysma muscle, skin; Medial: paraspinal muscle |
| Retropharyngeal | • Cranial: base of skull; Caudal: cranial edge of the body of hyoid bone<br>• Anterior: levator veli palatini; Posterior: prevertebral muscles<br>• Lateral: medial edge of vessel bundle; Medial: midline |

SCM, sternocleidomastoid muscle.
* Vessel bundle: internal carotid artery and internal jugular vein.
Modified with permission from: Chao KS, Wippold FJ, Ozyigit G, et al. Determination and delineation of nodal target volumes for head-and-neck cancer based on patterns of failure in patients receiving definitive and postoperative IMRT. *Int J Radiat Oncol Biol Phys* 2002;53:1174–1184.[9]

- Greatest risk of harboring metastases from the oral cavity, anterior nasal cavity, soft tissue structures of the mid-face, and submandibular gland.

□ Level IIa:

- Contains upper one-third of jugular lymph nodes anterior to the jugular vein.
- Receives efferent lymphatics from the face; parotid gland; and submandibular, submental, and retropharyngeal lymph nodes. It also directly drains from the nasal cavity, pharynx, larynx, external auditory canal, middle ear, and sublingual and submandibular glands.
- Greatest risk of harboring metastases from the oral cavity, nasal cavity, nasopharynx, oropharynx, hypopharynx, larynx, and major salivary glands.

□ Level IIb:

- Contains upper one-third of jugular lymph nodes posterior to the jugular vein.
- Greatest risk of harboring metastases from the oropharynx and nasopharynx, and less likely from the oral cavity, larynx and hypopharynx.

□ Level III:

- Contains middle jugular lymph nodes.
- Drains from the BOT, tonsils, larynx, hypopharynx, and thyroid gland. Receives efferent lymphatics from levels II and V and some from the retropharyngeal, pretracheal, and recurrent laryngeal nodes.
- Greatest risk of harboring metastases from the oropharynx, nasopharynx, oral cavity, larynx, and hypopharynx.

□ Level IV:

- Contains the lower jugular lymph nodes.
- Receives efferent lymphatics from levels III and V, and some from the retropharyngeal, pretracheal, and recurrent laryngeal nodes.
- Greatest risk of harboring metastases from the larynx, hypopharynx, and cervical esophagus.

□ Level V:

- Contains the posterior cervical lymph nodes.
- Drains from the occipital scalp, postauricular and nuchal regions, skin of the lateral and posterior neck, nasopharynx, and oropharynx (tonsil and BOT).
- Greatest risk of harboring metastases from the nasopharynx, oropharynx, subglottic larynx, apex of pyriform sinus, cervical esophagus, and thyroid gland.

□ Retropharyngeal nodes:

- Contains the lymph nodes that lie within the retropharyngeal space.

- Greatest risk of harboring metastases from the nasopharynx, oropharynx, soft palate, hypopharynx, and pharyngeal tumors with positive neck nodes in other levels.

■ In view of the differences observed between recent guidelines, a multidisciplinary working party including members of both groups was created to try to elaborate a unique set of recommendations for the delineation of the various levels in the node negative neck. Subsequently, the party was extended to representatives of American and European cooperative groups.

■ The general principles that guided the activities of the panel were to translate as accurately as possible the surgical guidelines into a set of radiologic guidelines by using axial CT sections and to minimize differences in interpretation of the guidelines by defining less ambiguous boundaries than previously described.

■ As a result of this consensus meeting, a complete atlas of contrast-enhanced CT sections depicting the various node levels from the base of the skull to the level of the sternoclavicular joint for the node negative neck has been posted on the websites of the Danish Head and Neck Cancer Study Group (http://www.dshho.suite.dk/dahanca/guidelines.html), European Organization for Research and Treatment of Cancer (http://groups.eortc.be/radio/ATLAS.html), and Radiation Therapy Oncology Group (http://www.rtog.org/hnatlas/main.html).

■ The recent recommendations proposed by several authors on the locations of the surgical neck levels are also in good agreement with our system.[8,13,15]

■ According to our guidelines, all margins of each specific neck node level could be demarcated on axial CT sections without contrast (Fig. 7-3A and B).

■ Figure 7-4 illustrates an example of sequential steps in delineating the CTVs.

■ One significant pathologic factor to take into consideration for target volume delineation is the presence of ECE. The probability of tumor extending outside of the nodal capsule increases as a function of tumor size. When metastatic nodal disease expands and ruptures the capsule of cervical lymph nodes, the incidence of local recurrence increases.

■ Huang et al.[16] demonstrated a higher tumor recurrence in patients with ECE (+) neck, whereas postoperative radiation therapy improved local regional control. Peters et al.[17] defined the resected neck into high- and low-risk groups to which different radiation doses were recommended.

■ Therefore, when delineating target volume in the postoperative neck, inclusion of generous soft tissue margins around the tumor bed is imperative. If the information regarding which lymph node levels containing ECE (+) nodes is not available pathologically, a preoperative imaging study (CT or MRI) can assist in determining which regions require a more generous soft tissue margin for CTV1 and CTV2 delineation.

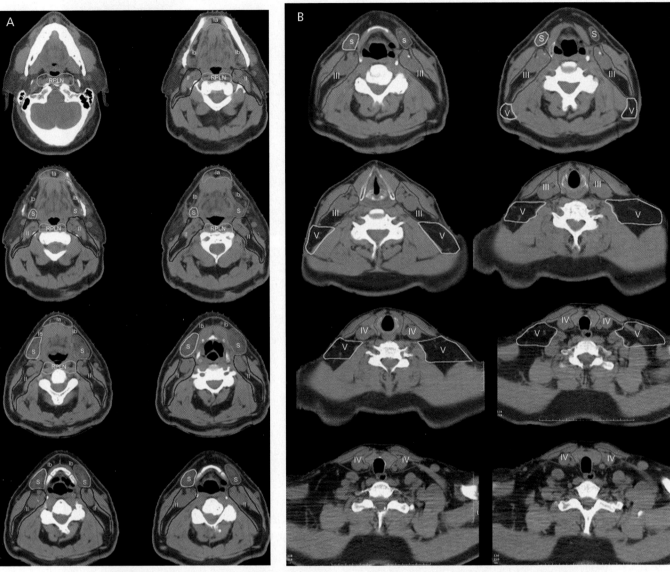

**FIGURE 7-3.** An atlas of the delineation of the clinical target volumes (CTVs) for head and neck squamous cell carcinoma with N0 neck in noncontrast axial computed tomography (CT) slices. **A:** Levels I and II. **B:** Levels III and IV.

- Figure 7-5 differentiates ECE (+) and ECE (−) necks in patients receiving postoperative IMRT. In the ECE (+) neck, soft tissues are more generously included, and the CTV1 and CTV2 should extend close to the skin surface, especially in the region or level of the ECE (−) node(s) specified by the pathologic findings.

- When postoperative IMRT is required for the ECE (−) neck, the target volume should avoid skin surface to decrease acute dermal toxicity. In our experience, sparing 2 to 3 mm of dermal structures in target volume design (Fig. 7-5) clearly results in much better radiation tolerance, less treatment breaks, and no compromise in locoregional control.

- Although the lower neck was treated with conventional techniques in the majority of patients, similar principles were applied to depict CTV delineation in the lower neck region for readers' reference in Figures 7-4 to 7-6.

- Also, it should be emphasized that margins for organ motion or patient set-up error are not included in delineating the target volume because they are determined by the individual institutions implementing head and neck IMRT programs. With the use of reinforced thermoplastic mask for immobilization, our experience indicated that 3 mm margins were required for IMRT plan computation to count for patient set-up uncertainty.[18,19]

- The dilemma comes when definitive IMRT is used to treat an undissected neck, and no pathologic information is available to determine whether metastatic disease has extended outside the lymph node capsules. In this case, we seek surgical pathologic experience for guidance.

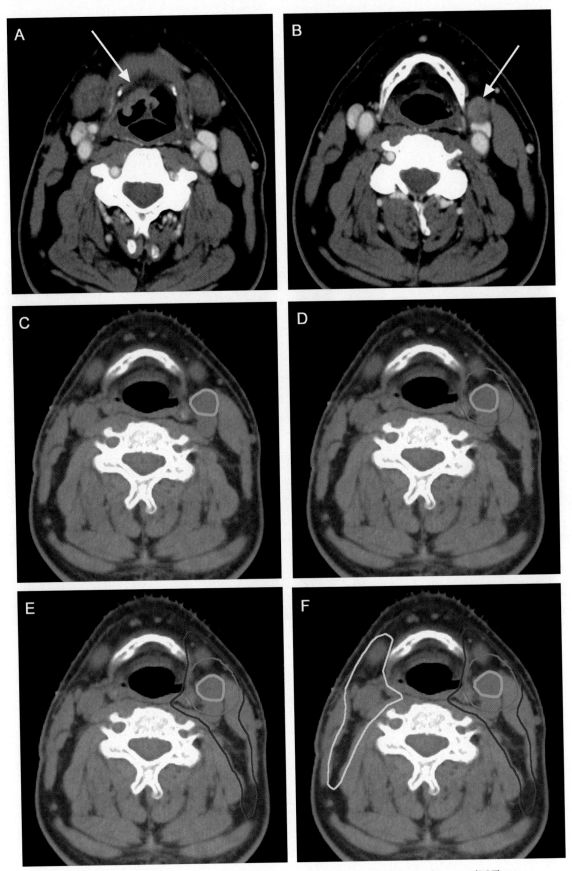

**FIGURE 7-4. A–E:** Steps to delineate the CTVs in a patient with a T1N1 base of tongue (BOT) cancer for definitive intensity-modulated radiation therapy (IMRT). Successive steps in the treatment planning process. **A:** Diagnostic head and neck CT shows primary T1 BOT lesion (*arrow*) on right side. **B:** A 1.5-cm enlarged left jugulodigastric lymph node (*arrow*). **C:** Primary nodal target volume (*outlined in green*). **D:** CTV1 (*outlined in red*). **E:** CTV2 outlines (*blue*) adjacent lymph nodes, including level V nodes. **F:** CTV3 outlines (*yellow*) elective contralateral nodes.

Table 7-9 summarizes the incidence of ECE in various sizes of lymph nodes that contain metastatic disease. When nodal size is as small as 1 cm, 17% to 40% may have broken through the capsule. When the size of the metastatic node exceeds 3 cm, more than 75% have ECE. This information is pertinent to target volume design because additional soft tissue margins around the whole nodal level where grossly enlarged nodes reside should be included in CTV1, which usually provides margins around the gross disease truncating air and bone (Fig. 7-5). The CTVs that we used are, for the most part, generous and likely contributive to the high control rates. Because head and neck IMRT is still in its infancy, we elected to be generous in target volume delineation to avoid undesirable marginal failure.

- To address this uncertainty of CTV margins, a retrospective pathologic-imaging correlation study was performed at M. D. Anderson Cancer Center.[20] The ECE of forty-seven neck lymph node samples from the neck dissections of twenty-three patients with squamous head and neck cancer were measured and correlated with CT imaging. The median size of lymph nodes was 1.1 cm (0.4–4 cm), and the median ECE was 1.8 mm (0.4–9 mm). As shown in the scatter plot in Figure 7-7, approximately 96% of the lymph nodes had an ECE of 6 mm or less. No lymph node had an ECE that extended beyond 1 cm from the lymph node capsule. Although preliminary, these data indicate that 5-mm and 10-mm margins beyond the GTV would be able to cover 90% and 100% of microscopic nodal extension, respectively. These recommendations will continue to be adjusted according to future prospective pathologic-imaging studies.
- Sparing salivary gland function is important in preserving the quality of life of patients. The literature has shown a dose response of parotid gland function after radiation treatment.[21–24] We elected not to spare the deep lobe of the parotid gland to prevent marginal failure in the parapharyngeal space. Therefore, only the superficial lobes of parotid glands were demarcated.

## 4. DOSE PRESCRIPTION FOR HEAD AND NECK INTENSITY-MODULATED RADIATION THERAPY

- Conventional radiation techniques sequentially deliver various amounts of radiation dose to different target volumes on the basis of the rank of "risk." Usually, several plans will be generated for a full course of treatment to first cover the whole region with a lower dose followed by a cone-down boost to the areas with higher risk of containing gross or microscopic disease.
- In contrast, IMRT delivers a single plan throughout the course of radiotherapy. Although we have the option to generate two or more IMRT plans simulating conven-

tional scheme, it may require more resources and manpower in contouring and data processing.
- The options for dose prescription are:

1. Set the dose prescription to the low-dose target at 1.8 to 2 Gy and increase daily fraction size (reduce total dose) to the high-dose region.
2. Keep the daily fraction size at 2 Gy to the high-dose region and increase total dose to the low-dose region to compensate for lower daily fraction size (1.7–1.6 Gy). Currently, there are various examples in implementing IMRT dose prescription within these two categories (Table 7-10).

- Mohan and colleagues[25] examined IMRT fractionation strategies based on radiobiologic considerations and defined the term "simultaneous integrated boost" to describe IMRT treatments designed to synchronously deliver different dose levels to different tissues of the head and neck region.
- Butler and colleagues[26] used an inverse-planning IMRT-based accelerated fractionation schedule for the treatment of head and neck cancer and named it "Simultaneous Modulated Accelerated Radiation Therapy" (SMART).
- SMART used higher daily doses (2.4 Gy) to high-dose target to shorten the overall treatment time to 5 weeks without requiring multiple daily doses. Dose limits to critical structures were adjusted to compensate for the larger fraction size.
- This IMRT dose scheme tries to limit the high-dose volume and reduce the risk of late complications associated with larger fraction size. However, critical normal tissues such as muscle, mucosa, blood vessels, and nerves are still embedded within target volumes. The long-term quality of life data are not yet available with this approach.
- The ongoing Radiation Therapy Oncology Group study H-0022 adopted a strategy to accommodate the fraction size differences and deliver a higher than standard fraction dose to the GTV of early stage oropharyngeal cancer (T1, T2, or N1) and standard fraction doses to the CTVs. The GTV received a total of 66 Gy in thirty fractions at 2.2 Gy per fraction. High-risk CTVs received 60 Gy, and low-risk CTVs received 54 Gy at 2 Gy and 1.8 Gy per fraction, respectively. Thus, the GTV received a normalized total dose of 70 Gy in 2-Gy fractions within 6 weeks.
- This approach may be suitable for patients with early stage head and neck cancer (smaller high-dose target volume) who are to receive definitive radiation without concurrent chemotherapy. The short- and long-term toxicity profiles are unknown.
- We presented therapeutic results and toxicity data by using the approach of maintaining daily fraction size at 2 Gy to the high-dose region and increasing the total dose to the low-dose region to compensate for the lower daily fraction.[12]

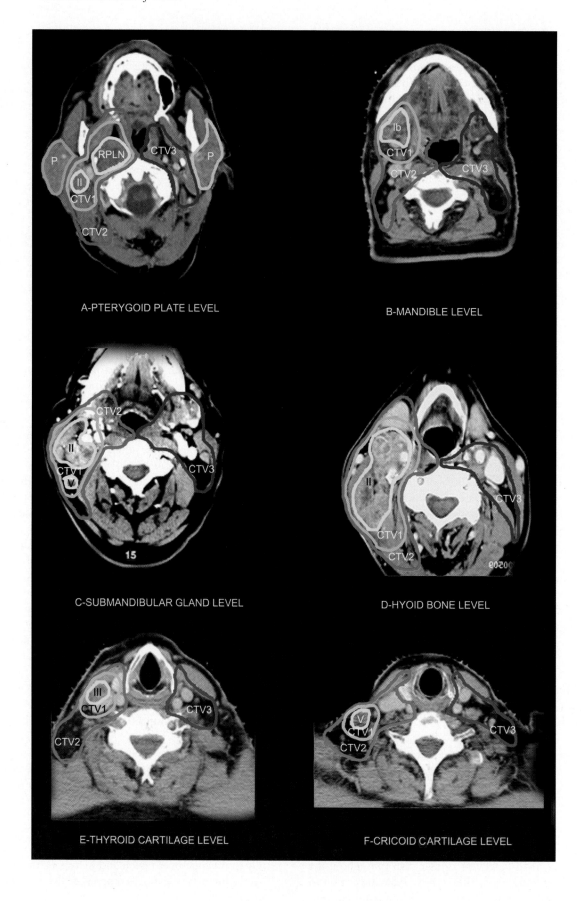

A-PTERYGOID PLATE LEVEL

B-MANDIBLE LEVEL

C-SUBMANDIBULAR GLAND LEVEL

D-HYOID BONE LEVEL

E-THYROID CARTILAGE LEVEL

F-CRICOID CARTILAGE LEVEL

☐ The concern that lower fraction size to the prophylactically treated areas may result in a higher local failure rate was addressed because we have not observed an increase in tumor recurrence.

☐ Further, IMRT prescription is usually normalized to 90% to 80% isodose line, which will create hot spots within the high-dose target.

☐ In addition, the majority of patients receiving definitive IMRT in the current series were also treated with concurrent chemotherapy. To avoid unforeseen detrimental late complications, we elected to limit daily fraction size to the high-dose region at no more than 2 Gy per day. Grade 3 or above late complications with this approach were less than 2.5%.

■ The observation that patients treated with less than 2 Gy per day to the high-dose target had inferior disease-free survival requires further confirmation.[27] This could be associated with the learning curve of early implementation of the techniques.

■ Daily fraction size to CTV has been found to be associated with locoregional control rate in our experience. Patients receiving 2-Gy fraction doses to primary target volume (CTV1) showed better 2-year disease-free survival (94% vs. 78%, $P = .05$).[27] Because we have not noticed a significant difference in treatment tolerance in patients treated with less than 2 Gy versus 2 Gy per fraction, the 2 Gy per fraction is our preferred dose prescription scheme.

■ Table 7-11 summarizes the corresponding dose prescriptions for CTV1, CTV2, and CTV3. CTV1 is considered a higher risk volume; a higher dose is given to this target volume.

## 5. CLINICAL RESULTS OF HEAD AND NECK INTENSITY-MODULATED RADIATION THERAPY

■ Between February 1997 and December 2000, 126 patients were treated for head and neck cancer with curative intent.[10,12]

■ The primary tumor was located in the nasopharynx in 12 patients, paranasal sinuses or nasal cavity in 9 patients, oral cavity in 15 patients, oropharynx in 63 patients, supraglottic larynx in 8 patients, hypopharynx in 8 patients, unknown primary in 9 patients, and other regions of the head and neck in 3 patients.

■ A total of 52 patients received definitive IMRT (4 with stage II disease, 9 with stage III disease, and 39 with stage IV tumor). The clinical/radiologic nodal status of these 52 patients was N0 in 12 patients, N1 in 9 patients, N2 in 24 patients (N2a in 9, N2b in 11, N2c in 4), and N3 in 7 patients. Among them, 17 refused chemotherapy and were treated with RT alone, whereas the remaining 35 were treated with concurrent chemotherapy per an intramural protocol. Chemotherapy was cisplatin-based regimens in all cases.

■ A total of 74 patients received postoperative IMRT (5 with stage I disease, 4 with stage II disease, 17 with stage III disease, 39 with stage IV disease, and 9 with unknown primaries). The pathologic nodal status of these 74 patients was N0 in 18 patients, N1 in 13 patients, N2 in 37 patients (N2a in 10, N2b in 19, N2c in 8), and N3 in 6 patients.

■ ECE was present in thirty-two patients. Chemotherapy was not routinely given in the postoperative setting; however, five patients with extensive nodal involvement in the lower neck received adjuvant cisplatin-based chemotherapy at the treating physician's discretion.

■ According to our guidelines, the radiation dose (mean ± standard deviation) for fifty-two patients receiving definitive IMRT was 70.23 ± 3.44 Gy to CTV1 and 60.15 ± 2.87 Gy to CTV2. The mean dose to CTV1 and CTV2 in seventy-four postoperative cases was 65.05 ± 4.21 Gy and 57.78 ± 5.58 Gy, respectively.

■ The median follow-up was 26 months (range, 12–55 months). Persistent disease was defined as the histopathologically proven residual disease within 6 months after the completion of definitive IMRT.

■ Dose-volume histograms of failures within the IMRT field (excluding low neck recurrence) were calculated on an 8-mm³ isotropic voxel grid by using a commercial data analysis software (Matlab, MathWorks, Novi, MI) to analyze treatment failures and categorize the failures as "in-field" if more than 95% of disease volume was within either CTV1 or CTV2, "marginal" if 20% to 95% of disease volume was within CTV1 or CTV2, or "out-field" if less than 20% of disease volume was within either CTV1 or CTV2.

**FIGURE 7-5.** CTV target delineation of clinically N+/N− necks in BOT cancers receiving definitive IMRT. Axial enhanced CT scans at the level of pterygoid plates **(A)**, mandible **(B)**, submandibular gland **(C)**, hyoid bone **(D)**, thyroid cartilage **(E)**, and cricoid cartilage **(F)** in a patient with metastatic head and neck cancer. CTVs with the presence of metastatic lymphadenopathy are compared with those without radiologic evidence of metastatic neck node. The gross tumor was operatively demarcated to provide readers visual assistance in understanding the location of gross nodal disease and corresponding target volume. CTV1 (*red line*); CTV2 (*blue line*); Ib, level Ib node; II, level II node; III, level III node; V, level V node; N+, positive nodes; N−, negative nodes; NR, nodes of Rouviere; GTV, gross tumor volume (grossly enlarged lymph node). (Adapted from: Chao KS, Wippold FJ, Ozyigit G, et al. Determination and delineation of nodal target volumes for head-and-neck cancer based on the patterns of failure in patients receiving definitive and postoperative IMRT. *Int J Radiat Oncol Biol Phys* 2002;53:1174–1184, with permission.)

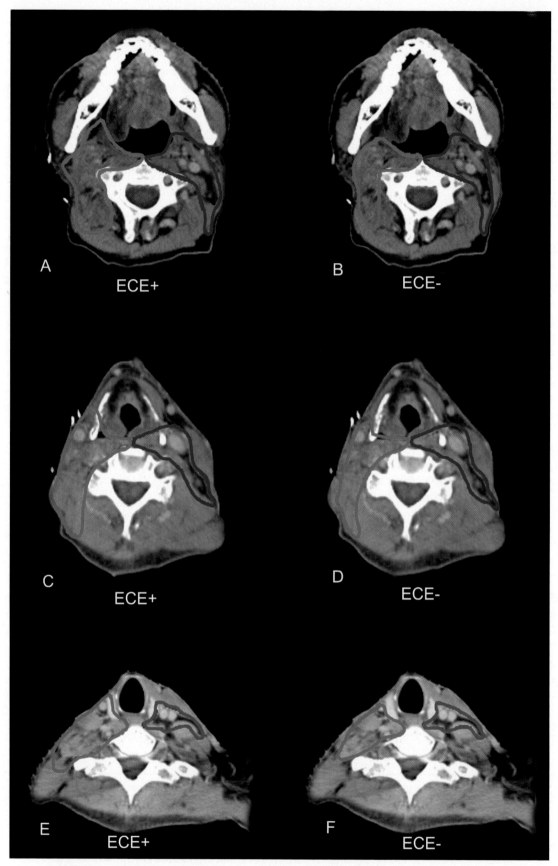

**FIGURE 7-6.** CTV delineation of pathologically extracapsular extension (ECE)± necks in BOT cancers receiving postoperative IMRT. Axial enhanced postoperative CT scans at the level of mandible **(A, B)**, thyroid cartilage **(C, D)**, and thyroid gland **(E, F)** in a patient with metastatic head and neck cancer. CTVs with the presence of ECE+ **(A, C, E)** are compared with ECE− volumes **(B, D, F)**. CTV1 (*red line*); CTV2 (*blue line*); ECE+, presence of extracapsular extension; ECE−, absence of ECE; GTV, gross tumor volume (grossly enlarged lymph node). (Adapted from: Chao KS, Wippold FJ, Ozyigit G, et al. Determination and delineation of nodal target volumes for head-and-neck cancer based on the patterns of failure in patients receiving definitive and postoperative IMRT. *Int J Radiat Oncol Biol Phys* 2002;53:1174–1184, with permission.)

## TABLE 7-9. INCIDENCE OF EXTRACAPSULAR EXTENSION OF METASTATIC NECK NODE BY SIZE

| Author | Node Size (cm) | | |
|--------|:---:|:---:|:---:|
| | <1 | 1–3 | >3 |
| Johnson et al.[38] | — | 65 | 75 |
| Snow et al.[39] | 22 | 52 | 74 |
| Synderman et al.[40] | — | 38 | 67 |
| Carter et al.[41] | 17 | 83 | 95 |
| Hirabayashi et al.[42] | 43 | — | 81 |

From: Apisarnthanarax S, Elliott D, El Naggar AK, et al. Determination of the magnitude of clinical target volume margins based on pathological examination of microscopic extracapsular extension of metastatic neck nodes. *Int J Radiat Oncol Biol Phys* (submitted 2004) with permission.

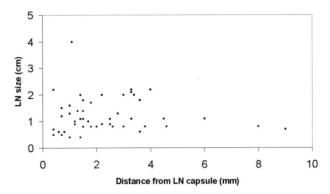

**FIGURE 7-7.** Pathologic extent of ECE of forty-seven ECE+ dissected neck nodes from twenty-three patients with head-and-neck cancer. (Modified from: Apisarnthanarax S, Elliott D, El Naggar AK, et al. Determination of the magnitude of clinical target volume margins based on pathological examination of microscopic extracapsular extension of metastatic neck nodes. *Int J Radiat Oncol Biol Phys* (submitted 2004) with permission.

## TABLE 7-10. HEAD AND NECK INTENSITY-MODULATED RADIATION THERAPY TARGET DOSE SPECIFICATIONS FROM PREVIOUSLY PUBLISHED LITERATURE

| Author | Concurrent Chemotherapy | Sites | Fraction Number | CTV1 (70/2 Gy)† | CTV2 (60/2 Gy)† | CTV3 (50/2 Gy)† |
|--------|:---:|--------|:---:|:---:|:---:|:---:|
| Butler et al.[26] | No | All sites | 25 | 60/2.4 Gy | — | 50/2 Gy |
| RTOG H-0022* | No | Oropharynx (early stage) | 30 | 66/2.2 Gy | 60/2 Gy | 54/1.8 Gy |
| Lee et al.[43] | Yes | Nasopharynx | 33 | 70/2.12 Gy | 59.4/1.8 Gy | — |
| Chao et al.[9] | Yes | All sites | 35 | 70/2 Gy | 63/1.8 Gy | 56/1.6 Gy |

CTV, clinical target volume; RTOG, Radiation Therapy Oncology Group.
* http://www.rtog.org/members/protocols/h0022/main.html.
† Conventional prescription.

## TABLE 7-11. INTENSITY-MODULATED RADIATION THERAPY CLINICAL TARGET VOLUME AND NORMAL TISSUE DOSE SPECIFICATION WITH BIOLOGIC EQUIVALENT DOSE CORRECTION FOR HEAD AND NECK CANCER

| Target Volume | Definitive RT Conventional Technique | IMRT | | | |
|:---:|:---:|:---:|:---:|:---:|:---:|
| | | Definitive with Chemotherapy (35 Fractions) | Definitive without Chemotherapy (30 Fractions) | High-Risk Postoperative* (30 Fractions) | Intermediate-Risk Postoperative† (30 Fractions) |
| CTV1 | 70/2 Gy | 70/2 Gy | 66/2.2 Gy | 63/2.1 Gy | 60/2 Gy |
| CTV2 | 60/2 Gy | 63/1.8 Gy | 60/2 Gy | 54/1.8 Gy | 54/1.8 Gy |
| CTV3 | 50/2 Gy | 56/1.6 Gy | 54/1.8 Gy | — | — |

CTV, clinical target volume; IMRT, intensity-modulated radiation therapy.
* Microscopic positive margin.
† Negative surgical margin, extracapsular extension, and multiple lymphadenopathies.
Normal tissue tolerance for IMRT prescription: optic nerve and optic chiasm 55 Gy, retina 45 Gy, brainstem 50–55 Gy, spinal cord 45–48 Gy, parotid gland 20–30 Gy, mandible 70 Gy.

**TABLE 7-12. REPORTED OUTCOMES OF SELECT PUBLISHED HEAD AND NECK INTENSITY-MODULATED RADIATION THERAPY SERIES**

| Author | N | Subsite | LC (%) | LRC (%) | OS (%) |
|---|---|---|---|---|---|
| Butler et al.[26] | 20 | Multiple | NA | 85* | NA |
| Dawson et al.[44] | 58 | Multiple | NA | 79 (2-yr) | |
| | | | | 75 (5-yr) | NA |
| Lee et al.[43] | 67 | NPC | 97 (4-yr) | 98 (4-yr) | 88 (4-yr) |
| Chao et al.[10] and Ozyigit et al.[12] | 126 | Multiple | 92 (3-yr) | 83 (3-yr) | 85 (3-yr) |

N, number of patients; LC, local control; LRC, locoregional control; OS, overall survival; NA, not available; NPC, nasopharyngeal carcinoma.
* Locoregional control includes one patient with persistent disease. Mean follow-up in this series was 15.2 months.
Modified with permission from: Ozyigit G, Thorsdat WL, Chao KS. Toxicity profile of intensity-modulated radiation therapy for head and neck carcinoma and potential role of amifostine. *Semin Oncol* 2003;30(suppl 6):101–108.

- Persistent or recurrent nodal disease was found in 6 of 52 patients (12%) receiving definitive IMRT; 4 treatment failures were "in-field" to the CTV1, and 2 treatment failures were in the lower neck outside of the IMRT volume.

- Postoperative IMRT in the nodal region failed in 7 of 74 patients (9%). One treatment failure was "marginal" to the CTV1 but "in-field" to the CTV2; 2 treatment failures were marginal to the CTV2; 2 treatment failures were in the lower neck and outside of the IMRT field; and 2 treatment failures were in the CTV1, but there was also lower neck failure in one of these, which was outside of the IMRT field.

- Predominant "in-field" failure denotes the urgent requirement to discern the radioresistant tumor, such as hypoxic tumor, by functional imaging or molecular markers.

- Three-year local control and locoregional control rates were 92% and 83%, respectively. Three-year overall survival was 85%.

- Table 7-12 summarizes recently reported therapeutic outcomes of published head and neck IMRT series.

## REFERENCES

1. International Commission on Radiation Units (ICRU). International Commission on Radiation Units and Measurements Report #62: Prescribing, recording, and reporting photon beam therapy (supplement to ICRU Report 50). Washington, DC: ICRU, 1999.
2. International Commission on Radiation Units (ICRU). Prescribing, recording, and reporting photon beam therapy. Washington, DC: ICRU, 1993.
3. Sako K, Bradier RN, Marchetta FC, et al. Fallibility of palpation in the diagnosis of metastases to cervical nodes. *Surg Gynecol Obstet* 1964;118:989–990.
4. Rouviere H. *Anatomie Humaine Descriptive et Topographique, 6th ed.* Paris: Masson et Cie, 1948.
5. Spiessl B, Beahrs OH, Hermanek P. Head and neck tumors. In: Spiessl B, ed. *TNM Atlas. Illustrated Guide to the TNM/pTNM Classification of Malignant Tumours, 2nd revision.* Berlin: Springer, 1992:4–5.
6. Robbins KT, Medina JE, Wolfe GT, et al. Standardizing neck dissection terminology. Official report of the Academy's committee for head and neck surgery and oncology. *Arch Otolaryngol Head Neck Surg* 1991;117:601–605.
7. Robbins KT, Clayman G, Levine PA, et al. Neck dissection classification update: revisions proposed by the American Head and Neck Society and the American Academy of Otolaryngology—Head and Neck Surgery. *Arch Otolaryngol Head Neck Surg* 2002;128:751–758.
8. Som PM, Curtin HD, Mancuso AA. An imaging-based classification for the cervical nodes designed as an adjunct to recent clinically based nodal classifications. *Arch Otolaryngol Head Neck Surg* 1999;125:388–396.
9. Chao KS, Wippold FJ, Ozyigit G, et al. Determination and delineation of nodal target volumes for head-and-neck cancer based on patterns of failure in patients receiving definitive and postoperative IMRT. *Int J Radiat Oncol Biol Phys* 2002;53:1174–1184.
10. Chao KS, Ozyigit G, Tran BN, et al. Patterns of failure in patients receiving definitive and postoperative IMRT for head-and-neck cancer. *Int J Radiat Oncol Biol Phys* 2003;55:312–321.
11. Ozyigit G, Chao KS. Clinical experience of head-and-neck cancer IMRT with serial tomotherapy. *Med Dosim* 2002;27:91–98.
12. Ozyigit G, Thorsdat WL, Chao KS. Outcome of intensity-modulated radiation therapy in organ function preservation for head and neck carcinoma and potential role of amifostine. *Semin Oncol* (in press).
13. Gregoire V, Coche E, Cosnard G. Selection and delineation of lymph node target volumes in head and neck conformal radiotherapy. Proposal for standardizing terminology and procedure based on the surgical experience. *Radiother Oncol* 2000;56:135–150.
14. Chao KS, Morrison WH, Ang KK, et al. M.D. Anderson consensus guidelines for head and neck target volume determination and delineation. *Int J Radiat Oncol Biol Phys* (submitted).
15. Nowak PJ, Wijers OB, Lagerwaard FJ, et al. A three-dimensional CT-based target definition for elective irradiation of the neck. *Int J Radiat Oncol Biol Phys* 1999;45:33–39.
16. Huang DT, Johnson CR, Schmidt-Ullrich R, et al. Postoperative radiotherapy in head and neck carcinoma with extracapsular lymph node extension and/or positive resection margins: a comparative study. *Int J Radiat Oncol Biol Phys* 1992;23:737–742.
17. Peters LJ, Goepfert H, Ang KK, et al. Evaluation of the dose for postoperative radiation therapy of head and neck cancer: first report of a prospective randomized trial. *Int J Radiat Oncol Biol Phys* 1993;26:3–11.
18. Chao KS, Low DA, Perez CA, et al. Intensity-modulated radiation therapy in head and neck cancers: the Mallinckrodt experience. *Int J Cancer* 2000;90:92–103.
19. Low DA, Chao KS, Mutic S, et al. Quality assurance of serial tomotherapy for head and neck patient treatments. *Int J Radiat Oncol Biol Phys* 1998;42:681–692.

20. Apisarnthanarax S, Elliott D, El Naggar AK, et al. Determination of the magnitude of clinical target volume margins based on pathological examination of microscopic extracapsular extension of metastatic neck nodes. *Int J Radiat Oncol Biol Phys* (submitted 2004).

21. Emami B, Lyman J, Brown A, et al. Tolerance of normal tissue to therapeutic irradiation. *Int J Radiat Oncol Biol Phys* 1991;21: 109–122.

22. Eisbruch A, Ten Haken RK, Kim HM, et al. Dose, volume, and function relationships in parotid salivary glands following conformal and intensity-modulated irradiation of head and neck cancer. *Int J Radiat Oncol Biol Phys* 1999;45:577–587.

23. Chao KS, Deasy JO, Markman J, et al. A prospective study of salivary function sparing in patients with head-and-neck cancers receiving intensity-modulated or three-dimensional radiation therapy: initial results. *Int J Radiat Oncol Biol Phys* 2001;49:907–916.

24. Chao KS, Majhail N, Huang C, et al. Intensity-modulated radiation therapy reduces late salivary toxicity without compromising tumor control in patients with oropharyngeal carcinoma: a comparison with conventional techniques. *Radiother Oncol* 2001;61: 275–280.

25. Mohan R, Wu Q, Manning M, et al. Radiobiological considerations in the design of fractionation strategies for intensity-modulated radiation therapy of head and neck cancers. *Int J Radiat Oncol Biol Phys* 2000;46:619–630.

26. Butler EB, Teh BS, Grant WH 3rd, et al. Smart (simultaneous modulated accelerated radiation therapy) boost: a new accelerated fractionation schedule for the treatment of head and neck cancer with intensity modulated radiotherapy. *Int J Radiat Oncol Biol Phys* 1999;45:21–32.

27. Lin M, Ozyigit G, Chao K. Impact of tumor stage and radiation fraction size on tumor control and treatment toxicity in head and neck cancer patients treated with IMRT. Proceedings in American Society for Therapeutic Radiation and Oncology 44th annual meeting. New Orleans, LA: 2002.

28. McLaughlin MP, Mendenhall WM, Mancuso AA, et al. Retropharyngeal adenopathy as a predictor of outcome in squamous cell carcinoma of the head and neck. *Head Neck* 1995;17:190–198.

29. Candela FC, Kothari K, Shah JP. Patterns of cervical node metastases from squamous carcinoma of the oropharynx and hypopharynx. *Head Neck* 1990;12:197–203.

30. Shah JP, Candela FC, Poddar AK. The patterns of cervical lymph node metastases from squamous carcinoma of the oral cavity. *Cancer* 1990;66:109–113.

31. Bataini JP, Bernier J, Brugere J, et al. Natural history of neck disease in patients with squamous cell carcinoma of oropharynx and pharyngolarynx. *Radiother Oncol* 1985;3:245–255.

32. Byers RM, Wolf PF, Ballantyne AJ. Rationale for elective modified neck dissection. *Head Neck Surg* 1988;10:160–167.

33. Lindberg R. Distribution of cervical lymph node metastases from squamous cell carcinoma of the upper respiratory and digestive tracts. *Cancer* 1972;29:1446–1449.

34. Northrop M, Fletcher GH, Jesse RH, et al. Evolution of neck disease in patients with primary squamous cell carcinoma of the oral tongue, floor of mouth, and palatine arch, and clinically positive neck nodes neither fixed nor bilateral. *Cancer* 1972;29:23–30.

35. Woolgar JA. Histological distribution of cervical lymph node metastases from intraoral/oropharyngeal squamous cell carcinomas. *Br J Oral Maxillofac Surg* 1999;37:175–180.

36. Buckley JG, MacLennan K. Cervical node metastases in laryngeal and hypopharyngeal cancer: a prospective analysis of prevalence and distribution. *Head Neck* 2000;22:380–385.

37. Kowalski LP, Medina JE. Nodal metastases: predictive factors. *Otolaryngol Clin North Am* 1998;31:621–637.

38. Johnson JT, Barnes EL, Myers EN, et al. The extracapsular spread of tumors in cervical node metastasis. *Arch Otolaryngol* 1981;107:725–729.

39. Snow GB, Annyas AA, van Slooten EA, et al. Prognostic factors of neck node metastasis. *Clin Otolaryngol* 1982;7:185–192.

40. Snyderman NL, Johnson JT, Schramm VL, Jr., et al. Extracapsular spread of carcinoma in cervical lymph nodes. Impact upon survival in patients with carcinoma of the supraglottic larynx. *Cancer* 1985;56:1597–1599.

41. Carter RL, Bliss JM, Soo KC, et al. Radical neck dissections for squamous carcinomas: pathological findings and their clinical implications with particular reference to transcapsular spread. *Int J Radiat Oncol Biol Phys* 1987;13:825–832.

42. Hirabayashi H, Koshii K, Uno K, et al. Extracapsular spread of squamous cell carcinoma in neck lymph nodes: prognostic factor of laryngeal cancer. *Laryngoscope* 1991;101:502–506.

43. Lee N, Xia P, Quivey JM, et al. Intensity-modulated radiotherapy in the treatment of nasopharyngeal carcinoma: an update of the UCSF experience. *Int J Radiat Oncol Biol Phys* 2002;53:12–22.

44. Dawson LA, Anzai Y, Marsh L, et al. Patterns of local-regional recurrence following parotid-sparing conformal and segmental intensity-modulated radiotherapy for head and neck cancer. *Int J Radiat Oncol Biol Phys* 2000;46:1117–1126.

# 8

# PARANASAL SINUSES AND NASAL CAVITY

ANGEL BLANCO
GOKHAN OZYIGIT
K. S. CLIFFORD CHAO

## 1. ANATOMY

- The nasal cavity begins at the limen nasi and ends at the posterior nasal choanae. The bony partitions between the nasal cavity, sinuses, and orbits are thin and offer little resistance to cancer spread.
- The posterior choanae communicate directly with the nasopharynx. The nasal cavity is located between the base of the cranium superiorly and the hard palate inferiorly. It is divided into right and left halves by a midline septum. The bones and cartilages that compose the roof and sides of the external nose are shown in Figure 8-1.
- The vomer extends from the body of sphenoid and makes the lower and posterior portion of the septum. The upper and anterior parts of the septum are continuous with the cribriform plate, which is paper thin and has no real barrier to tumor invasion. The septum is usually deflected to one side.
- Lateral walls of the nasal cavity are composed of three turbinates that form the roof of a passage or meatus that communicates with the nasal cavity: the inferior, middle, and superior concha (Fig. 8-2).
- The nasolacrimal duct enters the nasal cavity through the inferior meatus. The frontal sinus and anterior and middle ethmoidal cells communicate to the nasal cavity through the middle meatus. The superior meatus receives the opening of the posterior ethmoid air cells.
- The pterygopalatine fossa is situated inferiorly to the inferior orbital fissure, and the infraorbital nerve is located superior to this fossa as it enters the foramen rotundum (Fig. 8-3).
- The ethmoid sinus cells are composed of air cells, which are located between the medial walls of the orbit and the lateral walls of the nasal cavity (Fig. 8-2). These air cells are divided into three groups: anterior, middle, and posterior. The partition between these cavities is thin and gives no resistance to tumor spread. A thin, incomplete

bone called the lamina papyracea is also penetrated easily by tumors.
- The posterior ethmoidal cells are closely related to the optic canal and optic nerve. The lacrimal bone covers the anterior cells laterally. The roof of the ethmoid sinuses relates to the cranial fossa. The fovea ethmoidalis is the part of the frontal bone that comprises the roof of the anterosuperior ethmoidal cells.
- The olfactory nerve merges with the nasal cavity from the cribriform plate of the ethmoid bone and innervates the upper one-third of the septum. Branches of the olfactory nerve that penetrate the cribriform plate provide a route of tumor invasion and spread to the floor of the anterior cranial fossa (Fig. 8-2).
- The sphenoid sinus is a midline structure in the body of the sphenoid bone. The hypophysis and optic chiasm are located superiorly, the cavernous sinuses are located laterally, the nasal cavity and ethmoid sinuses are located anteriorly, and the nasopharynx is located inferiorly. The clivus and brainstem are situated posteriorly. Each sinus connects with the nasal cavity in the sphenoethmoid recess by an aperture in the upper part of its anterior wall.
- The right and left sphenoid sinuses are also divided by a septum and are considered as one. Because the septum is often incomplete or, at best, very thin, the septum is rarely in the anatomic midline.
- Each maxillary sinus has four walls: nasal, orbital, facial, and infratemporal. The nasal wall forms the base, and the apex extends into the zygomatic process of the maxilla. The sections of maxillary antrum are shown in Figures 8-2 and 8-3.
- The roots of the first and second molar teeth, and occasionally other teeth, often project into the floor of sinus. The nasal wall has openings to the meatal meatus under the middle turbinate. The floor of maxillary sinus is usually caudal to the floor of the nasal cavity in adults and older children.

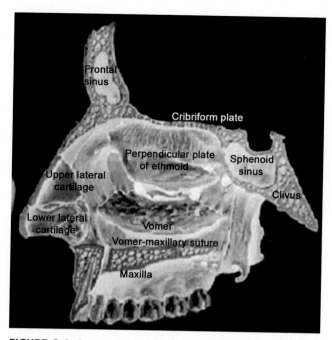

**FIGURE 8-1.** Bones and cartilage that compose the roof and sides of the external nose, nasal cavity, and paranasal sinuses.

- Two irregular air cavities separated by a bony septum form the frontal sinuses. The posterior wall of frontal sinuses that separates them from the anterior cranial fossa is usually thick, whereas they are separated from the anterior ethmoid cells by thin, bony walls.

## 2. NATURAL HISTORY

- Most lesions are advanced and commonly involve several adjacent sinuses, the nasal cavity, and often the nasopharynx.
- There is often orbital invasion from maxillary sinus or ethmoid sinus cancers. Orbital invasion from nasal cavity tumors occurs late.
- The anterior cranial fossa is invaded by way of the cribriform plate and roof of the ethmoid sinuses. The middle cranial fossa is invaded by way of the infratemporal fossa, pterygoid plates, or lateral extension from the sphenoid sinus.
- Lesions involving the olfactory region tend to destroy the septum and may invade through the nasal bone, producing expansion of the nasal bridge and eventually skin invasion.

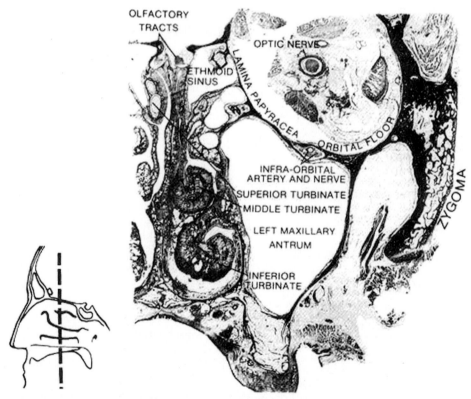

**FIGURE 8-2.** Coronal section through the maxillary antrum. (From: Bridger MWM, van Nostrand AWP. The nose and paranasal sinuses: applied surgical anatomy—a histologic study of whole organ sections in three planes. *J Otolaryngol* 1978;7[Suppl 6]:14, with permission.)

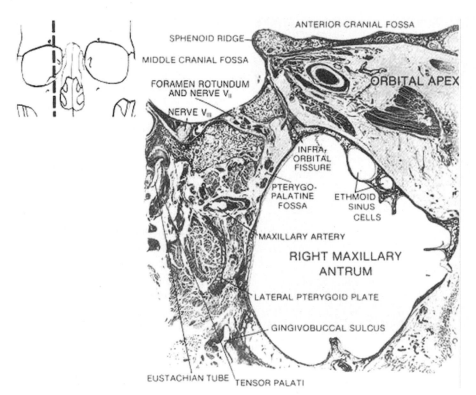

**FIGURE 8-3.** Sagittal section through the antrum and apex of the orbit. (From: Bridger MWM, van Nostrand AWP. The nose and paranasal sinuses: applied surgical anatomy—a histologic study of whole organ sections in three planes. *J Otolaryngol* 1978;7[Suppl 6]:18, with permission.)

- Lesions of the anterolateral infrastructure of the maxillary sinus commonly extend through the lateral inferior wall and appear in the oral cavity, where they erode through the maxillary gingiva or into the gingivobuccal sulcus (Fig. 8-4). Tumor that extends posteriorly from the maxillary sinus has immediate access to the base of the skull.
- Lymph node metastases generally do not occur until the tumor has extended to areas that contain abundant capillary lymphatics (Table 8-1). The submandibular and subdigastric lymph nodes are most commonly involved.

## 3. DIAGNOSIS AND STAGING SYSTEM

### 3.1. Signs and Symptoms

- History of recurrent nasal obstruction and recently worsened sinusitis are the common symptoms. Minor and intermittent epistasis may be observed. The mass may protrude from the nose.
- Obstruction of the nasolacrimal system may cause epiphora. Frontal headache, aberration or loss of smell, diplopia, and proptosis secondary to invasion of the orbit are other signs and symptoms that can be observed in paranasal sinus and nasal cavity tumors.

### 3.2. Physical Examination

- The nasal cavity is inspected by a nasal speculum. A fiber optic nasoscope can also be used.
- Cranial nerve examination is very important in paranasal and nasal cavity tumors to evaluate the extension of tumor.

### 3.3. Imaging

- Sinonasal computed tomography (CT) and magnetic resonance imaging (MRI) should be performed in both the axial and the coronal planes. The anterior skull base, floor of orbit, and cavernous sinus are evaluated on coronal sections. The orbital apex, pterygopalatine fossa, infratemporal fossa, and face are studied on axial sections. Sections must be 3 mm thick or less.
- The lymph nodes are not routinely studied in sinonasal cancer. If there is soft tissue, nasopharynx mucosa involvement, or high-grade lesions, the neck is examined.
- The absence of bone on CT is not necessarily an indication of bone invasion because most of the bony parts are very thin in this region.
- Because of the conical shape of the orbit, the maxillary antrum projects into the posteromedial floor of the orbit on axial images.

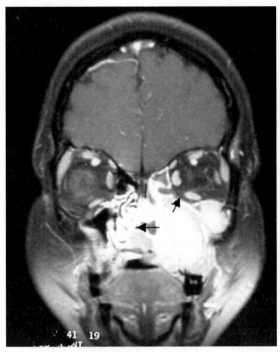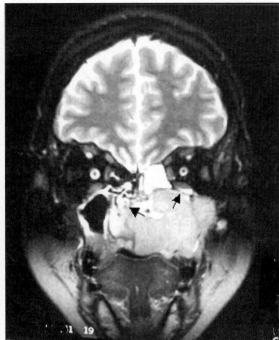

**FIGURE 8-4.** Magnetic resonance imaging (MRI) of patient with T4N0 maxillary adenocystic carcinoma. An extensive soft tissue mass in the left maxillary sinus extending into the ethmoid and orbit with bone destruction (*arrows*).

- Normal perineural enhancement should not be confused with pathologic enhancement of the nerve when evaluating perineural spread of the tumor along the infraorbital nerves.
- CT can detect intracranial invasion by detecting the bony erosion at the sinodural interface. The overlying dura often appears thickened and is enhanced by tumor invasion.
- The earliest sign of orbital invasion is erosion of cortical bone and displacement of extraconal orbital fat. Tumor spread to the infratemporal fossa can be detected by erosion of the cortical bone along the posterior wall of the

maxillary antrum. This is often seen near the groove of the posterior superior alveolar neurovascular bundle.

## 3.4. Staging

- The latest staging system of the American Joint Committee on Cancer can be applied to both paranasal sinus and nasal cavity carcinomas (Table 8-2).[1]
- The University of Florida staging system[2] can also be used for tumors of the nasal cavity and the ethmoid and sphenoid sinuses:
- Stage I: limited to site of origin.
- Stage II: extension to adjacent sites (e.g., orbit, nasopharynx, paranasal sinuses, skin, and pterygomaxillary fossa).
- Stage III: base of skull or pterygoid plate destruction; intracranial extension.

## 4. PROGNOSTIC FACTORS

- Massive tumor extension into the base of the skull, nasopharynx, posterior wall, roof of the sphenoid sinus, or cavernous sinus significantly increases surgical morbidity and decreases the likelihood of obtaining clear surgical margins.
- Tumor extension through the periorbital region usually requires sacrifice of the eye.
- The prognostic significance of lymph node metastases has been addressed in a number of recent studies. A ret-

**TABLE 8-1. INCIDENCE OF LYMPH NODE METASTASIS AT PRESENTATION IN PARANASAL SINUS CARCINOMAS**

| Author | No. of Patients | LN (+) in Percentage |
|---|---|---|
| Blanco et al.[3] | 106 | 7 |
| Cheng and Wang[10] | 66 | 22 |
| Jiang et al.[11] | 73 | 8 |
| Kurohara et al.[12] | 924 | 21 |
| Le et al.[4] | 97 | 11 |
| Myers et al.[5] | 141 | 4 |
| Paulino et al.[13] | 42 | 10 |

LN, lymph node.

**TABLE 8-2. AMERICAN JOINT COMMITTEE ON CANCER STAGING SYSTEM FOR CARCINOMA OF THE PARANASAL SINUSES**

**Primary tumor (T)**

TX   Primary tumor cannot be assessed

T0   No evidence of primary tumor

Tis   Carcinoma *in situ*

**Maxillary sinus**

T1   Tumor limited to antral mucosa with no erosion or destruction of bone

T2   Tumor causing bone erosion or destruction including extension into hard plate or middle nasal meatus, except extension to posterior wall of maxillary sinus and pterygoid plates.

T3   Tumor invades any of the following: bone of posterior wall of maxillary sinus, subcutaneous tissues, floor of medial wall of orbit, pterygoid fossa, or ethmoid sinuses

T4a   Tumor invades anterior orbital contents, skin of cheek, pterygoid plates, infratemporal fossa, cribriform plate, or sphenoid or frontal sinuses

T4b   Tumor invades any of the following: orbital apex, dura, brain, middle cranial fossa, cranial nerves other than maxillary division of trigeminal nerve V2, nasopharynx, or clivus

**Nasal cavity and ethmoid sinus**

T1   Tumor restricted to any one subsite, with or without bony invasion

T2   Tumor invading two subsites in a single region or extending to involve an adjacent region within the nasoethmoidal complex, with or without bony invasion

T3   Tumor extends to invade the medial wall or floor of orbit, maxillary sinus, palate, or cribriform plate

T4a   Tumor invades any of the following: anterior orbital contents, skin of nose or cheek, minimal extension to anterior cranial fossa, pterygoid plates, or sphenoid or frontal sinuses

T4b   Tumor invades any of the following: orbital apex, dura, brain, middle cranial fossa, cranial nerves other than V2, nasopharynx, or clivus.

**Regional lymph nodes (N)**

NX   Regional lymph nodes cannot be assessed

N0   No regional lymph node metastasis

N1   Metastasis in a single ipsilateral lymph node ≤ 3 cm in greatest dimension

N2   Metastasis in a single ipsilateral lymph node > 3 cm but not > 6 cm in greatest dimension; in multiple ipsilateral lymph nodes none > 6 cm in greatest dimension; or in bilateral or contralateral lymph nodes none > 6 cm in greatest dimension

N2a   Metastasis in a single ipsilateral lymph node > 3 cm but not > 6 cm in greatest dimension

N2b   Metastasis in multiple ipsilateral lymph nodes none > 6 cm in greatest dimension

N2c   Metastasis in bilateral or contralateral lymph nodes none > 6 cm in greatest dimension

N3   Metastasis in a lymph node > 6 cm in greatest dimension

**Distant metastases (M)**

MX   Presence of distant metastasis cannot be assessed

M0   No distant metastasis

M1   Distant metastasis

*Stage grouping*

| Stage | T | N | M |
|---|---|---|---|
| Stage 0 | Tis | N0 | M0 |
| Stage I | T1 | N0 | M0 |
| Stage II | T2 | N0 | M0 |
| Stage III | T3 | N0 | M0 |
|  | T1 | N1 | M0 |
|  | T2 | N1 | M0 |
|  | T3 | N1 | M0 |
| Stage IVA | T4a | N0–2 | M0 |
|  | T1–3 | N2 | M0 |
| Stage IVB | T4b | Any N | M0 |
|  | Any T | N3 | M0 |
| Stage IVC | Any T | Any N | M1 |

From: Greene FL, American Joint Committee on Cancer, American Cancer Society. *AJCC Cancer Staging Manual, 6th ed.* New York: Springer, 2002, with permission.

rospective review of the Washington University experience identified nodal involvement at diagnosis as a significant predictor of decreased locoregional control and disease-free survival.[3]

- Similar findings were reported by investigators at Stanford University, who observed a significant decrease in distant relapse among patients who achieved nodal control in the neck compared with those who experienced a neck relapse (29% vs. 81% at 5 years). There was also a trend for decreased survival with nodal relapse.[4]

- Likewise, in a review of the long-term experience with the treatment of paranasal sinus malignancies at the University of Michigan, Myers et al.[5] identified nodal positivity as an adverse prognostic factor for survival. Together,

these data indicate a possible role for prophylactic treatment of the ipsilateral cervical lymph nodes in patients presenting with locally advanced, high-grade tumors.

## 5. GENERAL MANAGEMENT

- Meta-analysis data showing the cross-tabulation of site, T stage, and treatment modality according to changes in decades are summarized in Table 8-3.

- Actuarial locoregional control and disease-specific actuarial survival rates according to treatment modality in patients with nasal cavity and paranasal sinus carcinoma are shown in Table 8-4.

## TABLE 8-3. META-ANALYSIS DATA: CROSS-TABULATION OF SITE, T STAGE, AND TREATMENT MODALITY

| | Decade (%) | | | |
|---|---|---|---|---|
| | 1960s | 1970s | 1980s | 1990s |
| *Site* | | | | |
| Maxillary sinus | 26 | 31 | 39 | 45 |
| Ethmoid sinus | 27 | 37 | 56 | 51 |
| Nasal cavity | 63 | 54 | 59 | 66 |
| *T stage* | | | | |
| T1 | 28 | 83 | 87 | 90 |
| T2 | 22 | 53 | 62 | 70 |
| T3 | 10 | 28 | 44 | 44 |
| T4 | 0 | 18 | 19 | 28 |
| *Treatment* | | | | |
| Surgery | 36 | 54 | 57 | 70 |
| Surgery and RT | 33 | 42 | 54 | 56 |
| RT | 21 | 19 | 28 | 33 |
| Chemotherapy* | 0 | 21 | 34 | 42 |
| **Number of patients** | **3,137** | **3,877** | **5,966** | **3,416** |

RT, radiotherapy.
* Chemotherapy data include patients who received chemotherapy as part of their treatment, usually combined with other treatment modalities.
Modified from: Dulguerov P, Jacobsen MS, Allal AS, et al. Nasal cavity and paranasal sinus carcinoma: are we making progress? A series of 220 patients and a systematic review. *Cancer* 2001;92:3012–3029, with permission.

- Blanco et al.[3] reported the results of 106 patients with paranasal sinus carcinoma who were treated with curative intent at Washington University. Five-year local tumor control, locoregional tumor control, disease-free survival, and overall survival rates were 61%, 41%, 35%, and 29%, respectively.

- Primary surgery followed by postoperative irradiation to a lesser dose than used for irradiation alone is preferred to reduce the risk of unilateral or bilateral optic nerve injury.[6] In most cases, postoperative doses are limited to 60 Gy; 66 to 68 Gy is administered for positive margins.

## TABLE 8-4. ACTUARIAL LOCOREGIONAL CONTROL AND DISEASE-SPECIFIC SURVIVAL RATES ACCORDING TO TREATMENT MODALITY IN PATIENTS WITH NASAL CAVITY AND PARANASAL SINUS CARCINOMA

| Treatment | N | Survival (%) | | |
|---|---|---|---|---|
| | | 2-Yr | 5-Yr | 10-Yr |
| *ALRC* | | | | |
| Surgery | 44 | 74 | 70 | 70 |
| Surgery and radiotherapy | 113 | 70 | 63 | 57 |
| Radiotherapy | 61 | 47 | 40 | 38 |
| *CSAS* | | | | |
| Surgery | 44 | 84 | 79 | 76 |
| Surgery and radiotherapy | 113 | 82 | 66 | 60 |
| Radiotherapy | 61 | 59 | 57 | 33 |

ALRC, actuarial locoregional control; CSAS, carcinoma-specific actuarial survival.
Modified from: Dulguerov P, Jacobsen MS, Allal AS, et al. Nasal cavity and paranasal sinus carcinoma: are we making progress? A series of 220 patients and a systematic review. *Cancer* 2001;92:3012–3029, with permission.

- For unresectable lesions, high-dose irradiation remains the only alternative with either once per day fractionation of 1.8 to 2.0 Gy to a total dose of 70 Gy or twice-daily treatment (1.1–1.2 Gy per fraction with a 6-hour interfraction interval) to total doses of 74 to 79 Gy.[7]

## 5.1. Nasal Cavity

- Traditional intranasal excision, the Caldwell-Luc procedure, and ethmoidectomy result in a high recurrence rate.
- In 45 patients with nasal cavity cancers (18 treated with definitive irradiation and 27 treated with surgery and irradiation), the 5-year disease-specific and overall survival rates were 83% and 75%, respectively.[8]
- No clear role for chemotherapy has been defined.

## 5.2. Ethmoid Sinus

- If the tumor is resectable, surgery is usually performed first. Postoperative irradiation is advised, even if resection margins are negative.
- Removal requires medial maxillectomy and en bloc ethmoidectomy. If the tumor extends superiorly to involve the fovea ethmoidalis or cribriform plate, a combined craniofacial approach is required.

## 5.3. Maxillary Sinus

- Most malignancies require radical maxillectomy including the entire maxilla and ethmoid sinus through a Weber-Fergusson incision. The globe and orbital floor are preserved for inferiorly located tumors.
- Orbital exenteration is indicated when the tumor has spread through the periorbita.
- If the ethmoid roof is involved, craniofacial resection is required.
- Early infrastructure lesions are often cured by surgery alone, but in most cases of maxillary sinus cancer, irradiation is given postoperatively, even if the margins are clear.
- Massive tumor extension to the base of the skull, nasopharynx, or sphenoid sinus may contraindicate surgery.
- Borderline resectable lesions are sometimes treated with full-dose external-beam irradiation, followed by surgery if technically feasible.
- It is reasonable to expect 5-year survival rates of approximately 60% to 70% for T1 and T2 lesions and 30% to 40% for T3 and T4 lesions, respectively, after resection and postoperative irradiation.[6] For advanced, unresectable disease, average 5-year survival rates of 10% to 15% are achieved with high-dose irradiation alone.[6]

## 5.4. Sphenoid Sinus

- Irradiation is usually the treatment by default. See "General Management" for a description of radiation dose guidelines.

## 5.5. Neck

- Patients with recurrent or poorly differentiated cancers and tumors that extend to an area with dense capillary lymphatics (nasopharynx, oropharynx, and oral cavity) have a higher risk of metastasis and are often given elective neck irradiation of 50 Gy over 5 to 6 weeks, administered in 1.8- to 2-Gy daily fractions.

## 6. INTENSITY-MODULATED RADIATION THERAPY IN NASAL CAVITY AND PARANASAL SINUS CARCINOMAS

### 6.1. Target Volume Determination

- If chemotherapy was delivered before radiation, the targets should be outlined on the planning CT according to their pre-chemotherapy extent.
- The target volume specification for definitive and postoperative intensity-modulated radiation therapy (IMRT) in paranasal sinus and nasal cavity cancers is summarized in Table 7-5.
- Suggested target volume determination for paranasal sinus and nasal cavity cancers is summarized in Table 8-5.

### 6.2. Target Volume Delineation

- In patients receiving postoperative IMRT, clinical target volume (CTV)1 encompasses the residual tumor and the region adjacent to it but not directly involved by the tumor, the surgical bed with soft tissue invasion by the tumor, or extracapsular extension by metastatic neck nodes. CTV2 includes primarily the prophylactically treated neck.
- In patients receiving definitive IMRT, CTV1 encompasses the gross tumor (primary and enlarged nodes) and the region adjacent to it but not directly involved by the tumor. CTV2 includes primarily the prophylactically treated neck.
- CTV1 and CTV2 delineation in a patient with clinically T2N0M0 squamous cell carcinoma of ethmoid sinus who received definitive IMRT is shown in Figure 8-5. The patient presented with a headache, which was initially thought to be sinusitis pain. But further studies revealed a mass in the ethmoid sinus extending into the nasal cavity. Biopsy of this mass showed a squamous cell carcinoma. There was no palpable adenopathy in the neck. Only the primary site was treated with definitive IMRT.

**TABLE 8-5. CLINICAL TARGET VOLUME DETERMINATION GUIDELINES FOR MAXILLARY SINUS TUMORS**

| Clinical Presentation | CTV1 | CTV2 | CTV3 |
|---|---|---|---|
| T1 and T2N0 | GTVp | — | — |
| T3 and T4N0 | GTVp | Optional@ | IN (I and II, RPLN) |
| Any T N+ | GTVp+n | IN (adjacent LNs*) | IN+CN+RPLN† (remaining LNs) |

N0, node negative neck; N+, node positive neck; GTVp, primary gross tumor volume; n, nodal gross tumor volume; IN, ipsilateral nodal levels; CN, contralateral nodal levels; RPLN, retropharyngeal lymph node; CTV, clinical target volume; LN, lymph node; IMRT, intensity-modulated radiation therapy. Roman numerals represent neck nodal levels.
* Two to 3 cm from CTV1 nodal basin.
@ Optional margins around CTV
† Include RPLN for advanced tumors
Suggested IMRT dose schedule for chemoradiation: CTV1 = 70 Gy/35 fx or 70 Gy/33 fx; CTV2 = 63 Gy/35 fx or 59.4 Gy/33 fx; CTV3 = 56 Gy/35 fx or 54 Gy/33 fx. For small oropharyngeal tumors (T1-2N0-1M0) and when definitive IMRT is used without concomitant chemotherapy, suggested doses are: CTV1 = 66 Gy/30 fx; CTV2 = 60 Gy/30 fx; CTV3 = 54 Gy/30 fx.

- CTV1 and CTV2 delineation in a patient with clinically T4N2bM0 squamous cell carcinoma of nasal cavity who received definitive IMRT is shown in Figure 8-6. The patient presented with a nasal mass. CT showed a tumoral lesion originating from the nasal cavity, extending into the orbital cavity and maxillary sinus. On physical examination, there was evidence of skin involvement on the nose and a palpable lymph node at the junction of levels II and I on the right side of the neck. Both the primary site and the bilateral neck were treated with definitive IMRT.

- CTV1 and CTV2 delineation in a patient with clinically T4aN0M0 poorly differentiated carcinoma of sinonasal region receiving definitive IMRT is shown in Figure 8-7. The patient presented with a history of left facial numbness, left eye proptosis, and left-sided tooth pain. CT showed a destructive mass in the left nasal ethmoid region with destruction of the left maxillary sinus and involvement of the medial orbital wall, extending into the orbit. The patient received two cycles of neoadjuvant chemotherapy consisting of VP-16 and carboplatin. After chemotherapy, proptosis completely resolved, and MRI showed striking improvement in the patient's lesion in the nasal cavity and the ethmoid region. However, he still had persistent disease. The primary site was treated with definitive IMRT to spare orbital functions and the lacrimal gland. Bilateral upper jugular nodes were prophylactically treated because of the advanced stage. The gross disease received 70 Gy, whereas pre-chemotherapy tumor volume was treated with 60 Gy. Reduced radiaton dose to pre-cheotherapy tumor volume can be considered to optimize the critical normal tissue (optic nerve, optic chiasm, or brain stem) spairing. However, physicians may elect to carry pre-chemotherapy tumor volume to full dose.

## 6.3. Normal Tissue Delineation

- Normal tissue delineation is shown in Figure 8-8.

### 6.4. Suggested Target and Normal Tissue Doses

- See Chapter 7 for suggested target and normal tissue doses (Table 7-11).
- To avoid excessive risk of damage to vision, fraction dose to CTV1 may be reduced to 1.8 or 1.9 Gy if CTV1 is in the close proximity of the optic nerve or optic chiasm.

### 6.5. Intensity-Modulated Radiation Therapy Results

- A total of 9 patients with paranasal and nasal cavity carcinoma were treated with IMRT between February 1997 and December 2000 at Washington University[8]: 3 patients were treated postoperatively, and 6 patients were treated with definitive IMRT. The T stages were T1 (1 patient), T3 (1 patient), and T4 (7 patients). The N stages were N0 (6 patients), N1 (1 patient), and N2 (2 patients) (American Joint Committee on Cancer staging: stage I [1 patient], stage II [1 patient], and stage IV [7 patients]). The median follow-up time was 36 months (range 13–42 months). We observed no locoregional recurrence or distant metastasis. All patients are alive, except 1 who died of intercurrent disease.
- Gastrostomy tube placement was required in 2 patients during the course of IMRT. Grade III late xerostomia developed in 1 patient. Altered vision (2 patients) and otitis requiring tympanostomy tube (1 patient) were other serious late complications of IMRT.

*Text continues on page 133.*

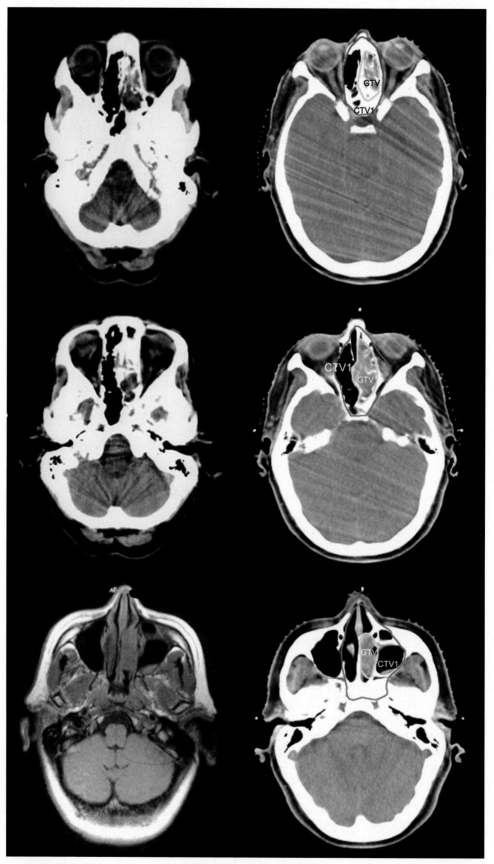

**FIGURE 8-5.** Clinical target volume (CTV) delineation in a patient with T2N0M0 ethmoid sinus carcinoma who received definitive intensity-modulated radiation therapy (IMRT). CTV1 (*red line*); gross tumor volume (GTV) (*yellow line*).

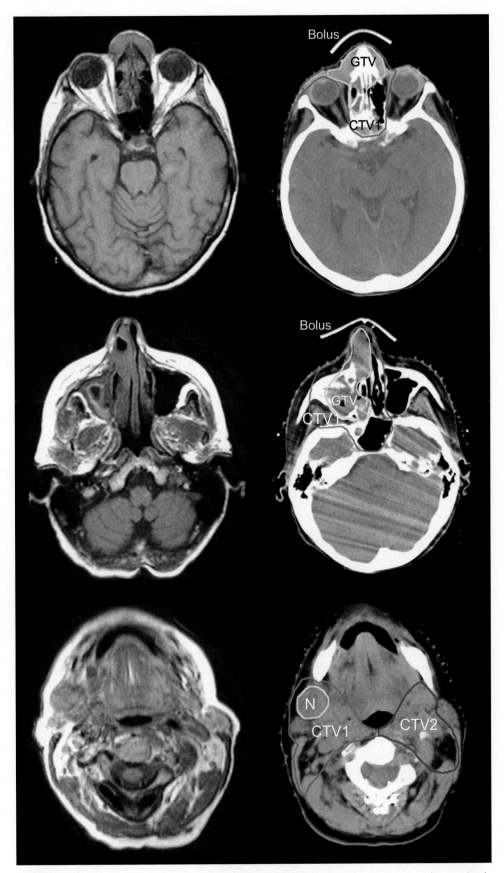

**FIGURE 8-6.** CTV delineation in a patient with T4N2bM0 nasal cavity carcinoma who received definitive IMRT. Bolus was used because of skin involvement by tumor. CTV1 (*red line*); CTV2 (*dark blue line*); gross tumor volume (GTV) and lymph node (N) (*yellow lines*).

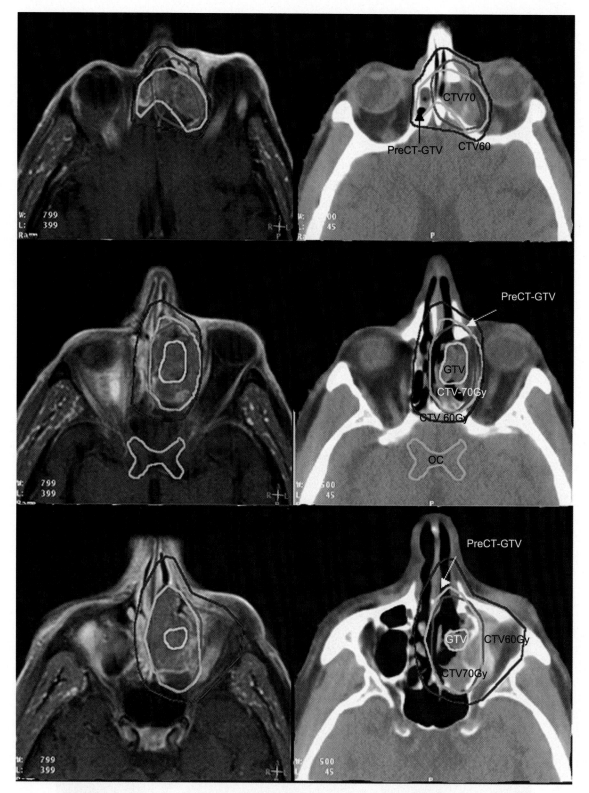

**FIGURE 8-7.** CTV delineation in a patient with T4aN0M0 sinonasal carcinoma receiving definitive IMRT after two courses of neoadjuvant chemotherapy. Pre-chemotherapy gross tumor volume extent was determined by the pre-chemotherapy MRI fusion study (*left*). CTV-70Gy (*red line*) is the persistent disease after chemotherapy with 70 Gy administered; CTV-60Gy (*dark blue line*) is the region covering the pre-chemotherapy gross tumor volume (GTV). Persistent tumor (*yellow line*).

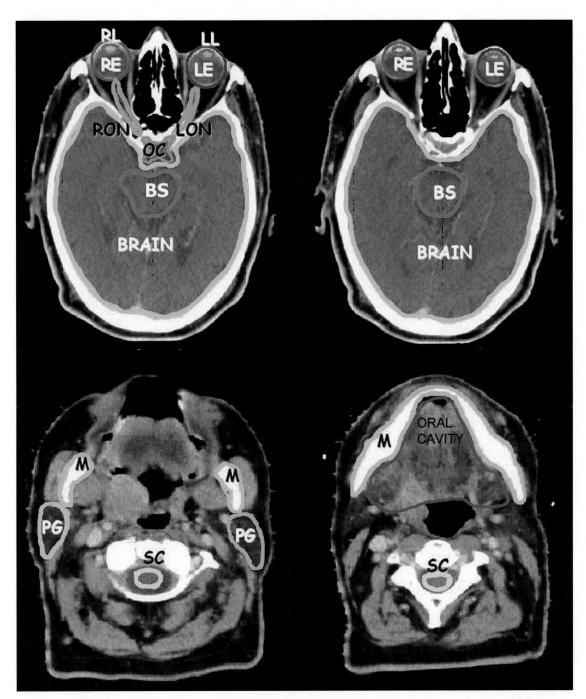

**FIGURE 8-8.** Normal tissue delineation. RL, right lens; LL, left lens; RE, right eye; LE, left eye; RON, right optic nerve; LON, left optic nerve; OC, optic chiasm; M, mandible; PG, parotid gland; SC, spinal cord; BS, brainstem.

## REFERENCES

1. Greene FL, American Joint Committee on Cancer, American Cancer Society. *AJCC Cancer Staging Manual, 6th ed.* New York: Springer, 2002.
2. Cassisi NJ, Million RR. *Management of Head and Neck Cancer: A Multidisciplinary Approach, 2nd ed.* Philadelphia: Lippincott, 1994.
3. Blanco AI, Chao KS, Ozyigit G, et al. Carcinoma of the paranasal sinuses: long-term outcomes with radiation therapy. *Int J Radiat Oncol Biol Phys* 2004;59:51–58.
4. Le QT, Fu KK, Kaplan MJ, et al. Lymph node metastasis in maxillary sinus carcinoma. *Int J Radiat Oncol Biol Phys* 2000;46: 541–549.
5. Myers LL, Nussenbaum B, Bradford CR, et al. Paranasal sinus malignancies: an 18-year single institution experience. *Laryngoscope* 2002;112:1964–1969.
6. Parsons JT, Bova FJ, Fitzgerald CR, et al. Radiation optic neuropathy after megavoltage external-beam irradiation: analysis of time-dose factors. *Int J Radiat Oncol Biol Phys* 1994;30: 755–763.

7. Parsons JT, Bova FJ, Fitzgerald CR, et al. Radiation optic neuropathy after megavoltage external-beam irradiation: analysis of time-dose factors. *Int J Radiat Oncol Biol Phys* 1994;30:755–763.

8. Ang KK, Jiang GL, Frankenthaler RA, et al. Carcinomas of the nasal cavity. *Radiother Oncol* 1992;24:163–168.

9. Chao KS, Ozyigit G, Tran BN, et al. Patterns of failure in patients receiving definitive and postoperative IMRT for head-and-neck cancer. *Int J Radiat Oncol Biol Phys* 2003;55:312–321.

10. Cheng VS, Wang CC. Carcinomas of the paranasal sinuses: a study of sixty-six cases. *Cancer* 1977;40:3038–3041.

11. Jiang GL, Ang KK, Peters LJ, et al. Maxillary sinus carcinomas: natural history and results of postoperative radiotherapy. *Radiother Oncol* 1991;21:193–200.

12. Kurohara SS, Webster JH, Ellis F, et al. Role of radiation therapy and of surgery in the management of localized epidermoid carcinoma of the maxillary sinus. *Am J Roentgenol Radium Ther Nucl Med* 1972;114:35–42.

13. Paulino AC, Fisher SG, Marks JE. Is prophylactic neck irradiation indicated in patients with squamous cell carcinoma of the maxillary sinus? *Int J Radiat Oncol Biol Phys* 1997;39:283–289.

# 9

# NASOPHARYNX

**NANCY Y. LEE**
**K. S. CLIFFORD CHAO**

## 1. ANATOMY

- The nasopharynx is roughly cuboidal; its borders are the posterior choanae anteriorly, the body of the sphenoid superiorly, the clivus and first two cervical vertebrae posteriorly, and the soft palate inferiorly (Fig. 9-1).
- The lateral and posterior walls are composed of the pharyngeal fascia, which extends outward bilaterally along the undersurface of the apex of the petrous pyramid just medial to the carotid canal. The roof of the nasopharynx slopes downward and is continuous with the posterior wall.
- The eustachian tube opens into the lateral wall; the posterior portion of the eustachian tube is cartilaginous and protrudes into the nasopharynx, making a ridge just posterior to the torus tubarius. Just posterior to the torus is a recess called Rosenmüller fossa.
- The roof and the posterior wall of the nasopharynx consist of the clivus and basisphenoid, which are the foundation of the central skull base and cavernous sinus; the bony portion of the eustachian tube lies lateral to the carotid canal.
- Many foramina and fissures are located in the base of the skull, through which several structures pass (Table 9-1). Some are potential routes of spread of nasopharyngeal carcinoma (Fig. 9-2).
- The jugular fossa, which lies just posterior to the carotid foramen, is usually larger on the right side. The jugular spur separates the pars nervosa from the pars venosum of the fossa.
- Cranial nerve IX lies within pars nervosa of the jugular fossa, whereas cranial nerves X through XII lie within the pars venosum along with the jugular vein.
- The base of the pterygoid plates is part of the basisphenoid; the pterygopalatine fossa lies between the pterygoid processes and the maxillary sinus and is contiguous with the inferior orbital fissure superiorly and the infratemporal fossa laterally. The foramen rotundum can be seen just above the base of the pterygoid processes.
- The upper pharyngeal musculature attaches to the basisphenoid and styloid process. Levator and tensor veli palatini muscles attachments are visualized along the inferior petrous apex and basisphenoid, respectively.
- An extensive submucosal capillary lymphatic plexus exists in the nasopharyngeal region. This can explain the high incidence of neck node metastasis at initial presentation of patients. The tumor initially spreads to the retropharyngeal, junctional, and jugulodigastric lymph nodes, and then along the internal jugular and spinal accessory chain. Incidence and distribution of clinically positive neck nodes in nasopharyngeal carcinoma are shown in Table 9-2.[1]
- Lymphatics of the nasopharyngeal mucosa run in an anteroposterior direction to meet in the midline; from there, they drain into a small group of nodes lying near the base of the skull in the space lateral and posterior to the parapharyngeal or retropharyngeal space. This group lies close to cranial nerves IX, X, XI, and XII, which run through the parapharyngeal space.
- The retropharyngeal lymph nodes are an important route of spread. The lateral retropharyngeal lymph nodes are located in the retropharyngeal space near the lateral border of the posterior pharyngeal wall and medial to the carotid artery. Directly behind them (Rouviere nodes) are the lateral masses of the atlas (C1). Usually one node occurs in each side, but occasionally two and very rarely three are found, and they can be found even at the level of the hyoid bone (C3). These nodes atrophy with age and may be absent unilaterally, but are rarely absent entirely. Incidence of retropharyngeal lymphadenopathy in nasopharyngeal cancers is shown in Table 9-3.
- Clinically involved lymph nodes of the parotid area may also be involved. This route of spread is possible from the lymphatics of the eustachian tube, which may drain by way of the lymph vessels of the tympanic membrane and external auditory canal to the peri-parotid lymph nodes.
- Another lymphatic pathway from the nasopharynx leads to the deep posterior cervical node at the confluence of the spinal accessory and jugular lymph node chains.[2]
- A third pathway is to the jugulodigastric node, which is frequently involved in nasopharyngeal carcinoma, according to Lederman.[3]

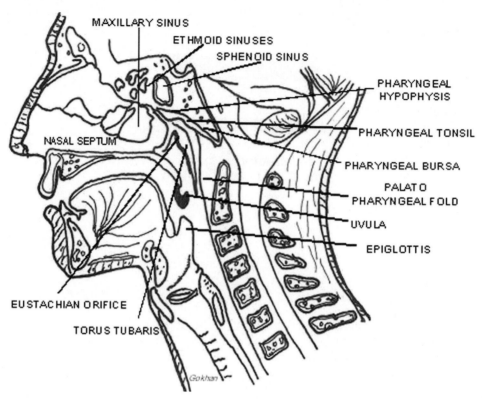

**FIGURE 9-1.** Nasopharynx and related structures in the midsagittal section of the head.

## TABLE 9-1. FORAMINA OF THE BASE OF SKULL AND ASSOCIATED ANATOMIC STRUCTURES

| Foramen | Structures |
|---|---|
| Cribriform plate (ethmoid) | Olfactory nerve and anterior ethmoidal nerve |
| Optic foramen | Optic nerve and ophthalmic artery |
| Superior orbital fissure | Third (oculomotor), fourth (trochlear), and sixth (abducent) nerves, and ophthalmic division of fifth (trigeminal) nerve; ophthalmic vein; orbital branch of middle meningeal and recurrent branch of lacrimal arteries; sympathetic plexus; some filaments from carotid plexus |
| Foramen rotundum | Maxillary division of trigeminal nerve to pterygopalatine fossa |
| Foramen ovale | Mandibular division of trigeminal nerve, accessory meningeal artery, lesser superficial petrosal nerve |
| Foramen lacerum | Upper portion: internal carotid, sympathetic carotid plexus<br>Lower portion: vidian nerve, meningeal branch of ascending pharyngeal artery, emissary vein |
| Foramen spinosum | Middle meningeal artery and vein, recurrent branch of mandibular nerve |
| Internal acoustic meatus | Seventh (facial) and eighth (auditory) nerves, internal auditory artery from basilar artery |
| Jugular foramen | Anterior portion: inferior petrosal sinus<br>Posterior portion: transverse sinus, meningeal branches from occipital and ascending pharyngeal arteries<br>Intermediate portion: ninth (glossopharyngeal), tenth (vagus), and eleventh (spinal accessory) nerves |
| Hypoglossal canal | Hypoglossal nerve, meningeal branch of ascending pharyngeal artery |
| Foramen magnum | Spinal cord, spinal accessory nerve, vertebral vessels, anterior and posterior spinal vessels |

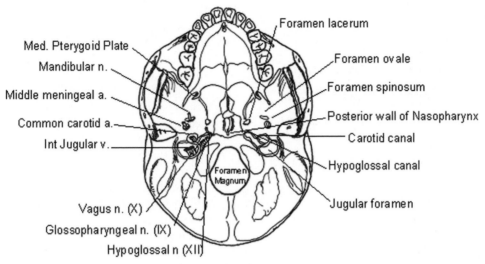

**FIGURE 9-2.** Superior view of the base of skull showing the main foramina and associated anatomical structures.

**TABLE 9-2. INCIDENCE AND DISTRIBUTION OF METASTATIC DISEASE IN CLINICALLY POSITIVE (N+)\* NECK NODES (%) IN THE NASOPHARYNX (MIR DATA)**

| | Clinical Nodal Metastasis | | | | | | |
|---|---|---|---|---|---|---|---|
| | Patients with N+ (%) | Level I | Level II | Level III | Level IV | Level V | Other† |
| Nasopharynx | 115/164 (70%) | 10/115 (8%) | 67/115 (58%) | 11/115 (9%) | 11/115 (9%) | 36/115 (31%) | 3/115 (2%) |

\* Bilateral neck node metastasis was found in 28% and only contralateral neck node metastasis was found in 3% at presentation.
† Parotid, postauricular, and buccal nodes.
Modified from: Perez C, Venkata R, Victor M, et al. Carcinoma of the nasopharynx: Factors affecting prognosis. *Int J Radiat Oncol Biol Phys* 1991;23:271–280.

**TABLE 9-3. INCIDENCE OF RETROPHARYNGEAL LYMPHADENOPATHY IN NASOPHARYNGEAL CANCERS (AFTER CT ERA)**

| Author | Incidence of Retropharyngeal Lymph Nodes (Percentage of the Total Number of Patients) | | |
|---|---|---|---|
| | Total | N0 Neck\* | N+ Neck† |
| McLaughlin et al.[28] | 14/19 (74%) | 2/5 (40%) | 12/14 (86%) |
| Chua et al.[29] | 106/364 (29%) | 21/134 (16%) | 85/230 (37%) |
| Chong et al.[9] | No data | No data | 59/91 (65%) |
| **TOTAL** | 120/383 (31%) | 23/139 (17%) | 156/335 (47%) |

\* Clinically negative nodes in levels I–V.
† Clinically positive nodes in levels I–V.

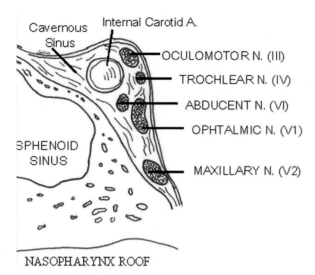

**FIGURE 9-3.** Coronal section through the sphenoid sinus and roof of nasopharynx showing the relative positions of cranial nerves III to VI.

## 2. NATURAL HISTORY

- Carcinoma of the nasopharynx frequently arises from the lateral wall, with a predilection for the fossa of Rosenmüller and the roof of the nasopharynx.
- Tumor may involve the mucosa or grow predominantly in the submucosa, invading adjacent tissues including the nasal cavity. In approximately 5% of patients, tumor extends into the posterior or medial walls of the maxillary antrum and ethmoids.
- In more advanced stages, tumor may involve the oropharynx, particularly the lateral or posterior wall.
- Upward extension of tumor through the foramen lacerum results in cranial nerve involvement and destruction of the middle fossa (Figs. 9-2 and 9-3).
- Approximately 90% of patients develop lymphadenopathy, which is present in 60% to 85% at initial diagnosis.

About 50% of patients have bilateral lymph node involvement.[4]

- The T and N stage distribution of nasopharyngeal carcinoma patients at initial presentation according to the American Joint Commission on Cancer (AJCC) 1988 staging system is shown in Table 9-4. This data is also summarized in Table 9-5 according to the AJCC 1997 staging system.
- The incidence of distant metastasis is not related to the stage of the primary tumor, but correlates strongly with degree of cervical lymph node involvement. In 63 patients with N0 necks, 11 (17%) developed metastatic disease in contrast to 69 of 93 (74%) with N3 cervical lymphadenopathy.[5] The most common site of distant metastasis is bone, followed by lung and liver.[6]

## 3. DIAGNOSIS AND STAGING SYSTEM

### 3.1. Signs and Symptoms

- Tumor growth into the posterior nasal fossa can produce nasal stuffiness, discharge, or epitaxis. Occasionally, the voice will have a nasal twang.
- The orifice of the eustachian tube can be obstructed by a relatively small tumor; ear pain or a unilateral decrease in hearing can occur. Sometimes blockage of the eustachian tube produces a middle ear transudate.
- Headache or pain in the temporal or occipital region can occur. Proptosis sometimes results from direct extension of tumor into the orbit.
- Sore throat can occur when tumor involves the oropharynx.
- Although a neck mass elicits medical attention in only 18% to 66% of cases, clinical involvement of cervical lymph nodes on examination at presentation ranges from 60% to 87%.[3,7]
- Some patients present with cranial nerve involvement. In 218 patients, 26% had cranial nerve involvement, but it

**TABLE 9-4. T AND N STAGE DISTRIBUTION OF NASOPHARYNGEAL CARCINOMA PATIENTS AT INITIAL PRESENTATION ACCORDING TO AMERICAN JOINT COMMITTEE ON CANCER 1988**

| Author | T1 | T2 | T3 | T4 | N0 | N1 | N2 | N3 |
|---|---|---|---|---|---|---|---|---|
| Chua et al.[30] | 92 | 89 | 153 | — | 27 | 46 | 196 | 63 |
| Jian et al.[19] | 5 | 13 | 9 | 13 | 8 | 6 | 20 | 6 |
| Ozyar et al.* | 11 | 23 | 32 | 24 | 18 | 17 | 38 | 17 |
| Wang[31] | 46 | 102 | 46 | 65 | 92 | 23 | 128 | 16 |
| Mesic et al.[32] | 31 | 102 | 45 | 70 | 35 | 30 | 59 | 114 |
| Lee et al.* | 565 | 1,076 | 648 | 2,225 | 1,261 | 600 | 2,403 | 250 |
| Perez et al.[1] | 21 | 33 | 26 | 63 | 48 | 23 | 63 | 8 |
| TOTAL | 771 (14%) | 1,438 (26%) | 959 (17%) | 2,460 (43%) | 1,489 (27%) | 745 (13%) | 2,907 (51%) | 474 (9%) |

* Unpublished data.

**TABLE 9-5. T AND N STAGE DISTRIBUTION OF NASOPHARYNGEAL CARCINOMA PATIENTS AT INITIAL PRESENTATION ACCORDING TO AMERICAN JOINT COMMITTEE ON CANCER 1997**

| Author | T1 | T2 | T3 | T4 | N0 | N1 | N2 | N3 |
|---|---|---|---|---|---|---|---|---|
| Ozyar et al.* | 34 | 32 | 7 | 17 | 18 | 27 | 25 | 20 |
| Lee et al.* | 1,641 | 648 | 1,229 | 996 | 1,261 | 1,404 | 785 | 1,064 |
| Chien et al.[33] | 55 | 29 | 14 | 19 | 45 | 40 | 6 | 26 |
| **TOTAL** | 1,730 (37%) | 709 (15%) | 1,250 (26%) | 1,032 (22%) | 1,324 (28%) | 1,471 (31%) | 816 (17%) | 1,110 (24%) |

* Unpublished data.

was present at initial diagnosis in only 3% of patients.[3] Leung et al. reported a 12% incidence of cranial nerve involvement in 564 patients with primary nasopharyngeal carcinoma; it was higher in patients staged with computed tomography (CT) (52 of 177, 29%).[8]

- Cranial nerves III through VI are involved by extension of tumor up through the foramen lacerum to the cavernous sinus. Cranial nerves VII, VIII, and I are rarely involved (Fig. 9-4).

## 3.2. Physical Examination

- Fiber optic nasoscopes and laryngoscopes are the main tools for examination of the nasopharyngeal region. Early lesions mostly occur on the lateral walls or roof. The site of origin is almost never the nasopharyngeal surface of the soft palate, nor is often invaded secondarily, even by advanced tumors. In early cases, only slight fullness in the Rosenmüller fossa, or a submucosal bulge or asymmetry in the roof may be the only lesions that can be seen. Lymphomas and minor salivary gland tumors have a tendency to remain submucosal until large.

- Nasoscopes may aid us by showing tumor growth into the anterior and superior nasal cavity. Tumor may be seen submucosally infiltrating along the posterior tonsillar pillars and occasionally down the posterior pharyngeal wall.

- The evaluations of cranial nerves are essential. The fifth and sixth cranial nerves are most commonly involved. Otitis media and decreased hearing can be found on ear examination. Table 9-6 summarizes functions of the cranial nerves, which should be examined during the initial consultation.

## 3.3. Imaging

- Imaging is required for both staging and treatment planning in all nasopharyngeal carcinomas as well as in the follow-up of patients.

- The main imaging tools of the nasopharyngeal region are CT and magnetic resonance imaging (MRI).

- The normal anatomy of the nasopharynx as seen on CT is shown in Figure 9-5.

- MRI is the preferred primary examination for disease in

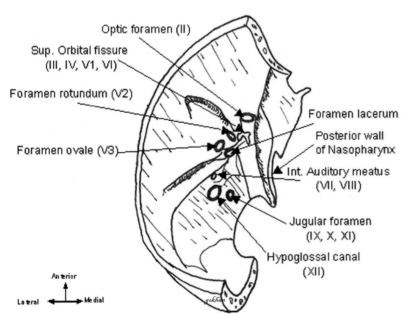

**FIGURE 9-4.** Superomedial view of the base of the skull showing the relations of nasopharynx to foramina of passage of cranial nerves.

**TABLE 9-6. FUNCTIONS OF THE CRANIAL NERVES**

| Cranial Nerve | Function | Abnormality |
|---|---|---|
| **I. Olfactory** | Smell | Decreased smell sensation |
| **II. Optic** | Vision | Unilateral amaurosis |
| **III. Oculomotor** | Eye movement<br>Innervates the striated muscles of the eyelid<br>Papillary constriction and accommodation of lens for near vision | Ophthalmoplegia<br>Ptosis<br>Loss of accommodation |
| **IV. Trochlear** | Innervates superior oblique muscle | Limitation in down and inward gazing |
| **V. Trigeminal** | V1, V2: cutaneous and proprioceptive sensation from skin, muscles, and joints in face and mouth, and sensory innervation of teeth<br>V3: innervates muscle of mastication, sensory innervation of mandibular region of face | Pain and anesthesia in supraorbital and maxillary regions of face<br>Pain and anesthesia in mandibulary regions of face |
| **VI. Abducens** | Innervates lateral rectus muscle | Diplopia, limitation of lateral gaze |
| **VII. Facial** | Innervates muscles of facial expression<br>Taste sensation from anterior ⅔ of tongue | Shadowing of nasolabial sulcus<br>Impairment of facial expression<br>Loss of taste in anterior ⅔ of tongue |
| **VIII. Vestibulocochlear** | Audition<br>Equilibrium, postural reflexes, orientation of head in spaces | Decreased audition<br>Vertigo, dizziness |
| **IX. Glossopharyngeal** | Swallowing<br>Innervates the carotid body<br>Innervates taste buds in posterior ⅓ of tongue | Dysphagia<br>Aberrant sense of taste in posterior ⅓ of the tongue |
| **X. Vagus** | Innervates striated muscles in larynx and pharynx and controls speech<br>Visceral sensation from pharynx, larynx, thorax, and abdomen | Hypoesthesia of mucous membranes in soft palate, pharynx and larynx<br>Loss of gag reflex<br>Aspiration symptoms |
| **XI. Spinal accessory** | Motor innervation of trapezius, sternocleidomastoid muscles | Paralysis of trapezius, sternocleidomastoid muscles |
| **XII. Hypoglossal** | Motor innervation of intrinsic muscles of tongue | Unilateral paralysis and atrophy of tongue |

the nasopharynx, parapharyngeal space, infratemporal fossa, and for skull base invasion (Fig. 9-6).

- The neck is always included when CT is performed. Both axial and coronal sections should be performed regardless of whether CT or MRI is the primary examination method.
- The torus tubarius, eustachian tube orifice, and fossa of Rosenmüller are often asymmetric in appearance. Lymphoid tissue has a tendency to atrophy with age, which can be responsible for superficial contour variation of the nasopharyngeal region. Lymphoid tissue is better visualized with MRI.
- The carotid artery and jugular veins should always be clearly visible in the poststyloid parapharyngeal space, along with at least some surrounding fatty tissue. The intervening cranial nerves IX through XII and the sympathetic chain can sometimes be seen in high-resolution MRI.

- The retropharyngeal lymph nodes are visible on MRI medial to the carotid artery at the border between the poststyloid parapharyngeal and retropharyngeal spaces (Fig. 9-7). The nodes are normally 3 to 5 mm in size in adults and 10 to 15 mm in infants and children.
- The fifth nerve ganglion, within Meckel's cave, and its branches both inside and outside the cavernous sinus, are easily recognized on good-quality MRI and CT.
- The third, fourth, and sixth cranial nerves, along with the first division of the trigeminal nerve, are best visualized on coronal MRI as they go through the wall of the cavernous sinus.
- The fat within nasopharyngeal spaces is normally symmetric, although the size of vessels coursing through the spaces may vary slightly; obliteration of fat is a sign of pathologic involvement in MRI or CT.
- The third division of trigeminal nerve often is seen on MRI exiting the foramen ovale.

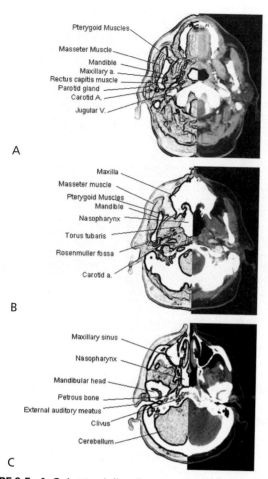

A

B

C

**FIGURE 9-5. A–C:** Anatomic line diagrams showing the different levels of nasopharyngeal region, to correlate with the accompanying CT images at the same level.

- Perineural enhancement within the cranial nerve exit, the foramina, and prominent enhancement of venous plexuses just below the skull base are normal variants.

### 3.4. Staging

- The multiplicity of staging systems makes comparison of results from different institutions extremely difficult.
- The comparison of stage distribution of nasopharyngeal carcinoma patients according to AJCC 1988 and AJCC 1997 staging systems is shown in Table 9-7. Substantial down-staging was noted with the 1997 staging system, especially for more advanced disease.
- The latest AJCC 2002 staging system, which did not change from AJCC 1997, is shown in Table 9-8.

### 4. PROGNOSTIC FACTORS

- *Epidemiological factors:* Race, age, and gender have prognostic significance.[9] Perez et al. found that patients younger than 50 years had better survival and local control.[1] Sham and Choy found similar results in their retrospective analysis of 759 patients.[10]
- *Stage:* Sham and Choy, and Perez et al. showed stage as a significant factor determining survival and local control.[1,10]
- *Cranial nerve involvement:* This was significantly associated with decreased survival in several series. Lee et al., Sham and Choy, and Perez et al. found it to be a significant prognostic factor. [1,10,11] However, Chu et al. did not found it as a prognostic factor.[12]

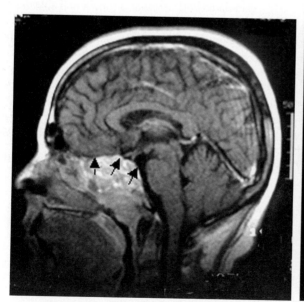

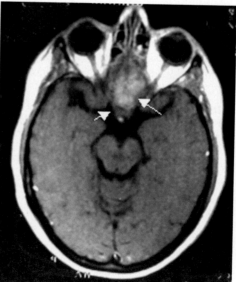

**FIGURE 9-6.** Coronal and sagittal MRI sections showing a T4 nasopharyngeal carcinoma invading the base of the skull (*arrows*).

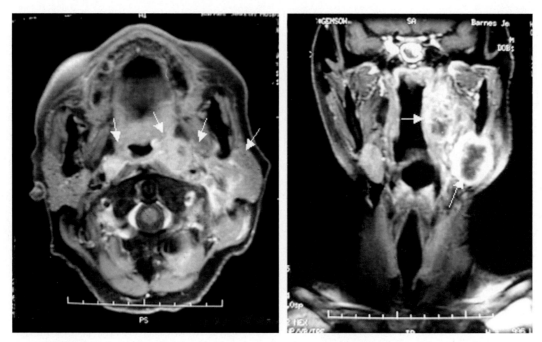

**FIGURE 9-7.** Coronal and sagittal MRI sections showing tumor extent in a nasopharyngeal carcinoma patient.

- *Lymph node metastasis:* Survival decreases as cervical lymph node involvement progresses from the upper to the middle and lower nodes.[4]
- *Bilateral cervical lymph node involvement:* Bilateral neck node metastasis was found to be an ominous prognostic factor by Lee et al., demonstrating that bilaterality was associated with a higher risk of nodal failure.[11] However, Sham and Choy did not find bilaterality to be a prognostic factor.[10]
- *Histology:* In 122 patients with localized nasopharyngeal carcinoma, histology was the most important prognostic factor for survival; the relative risk of death was 3.4 and 3.2 times greater for nonkeratinizing and squamous cell carcinoma, respectively, compared with undifferentiated carcinoma.[13] On the other hand, others noted no difference in survival or incidence of distant metastasis between keratinizing and nonkeratinizing squamous cell carcinoma.[1,11]

## 5. GENERAL MANAGEMENT

- Because the nasopharynx is immediately adjacent to the base of the skull, surgical resection with an acceptable margin is often not achievable. Radiation therapy has been the sole treatment for carcinoma of the nasopharynx. Studies showing the incidence of failure at primary site correlated with T stage are summarized in Table 9-9.
- Rarely, radical neck dissection has been performed for treatment of neck node metastasis, but it is not superior to irradiation alone. The incidence of failure in the neck correlated with N stage is shown in Table 9-10.
- A randomized phase III Intergroup trial that compared chemoradiotherapy versus radiotherapy alone in patients with stage III and IV nasopharyngeal cancers revealed the advantage of chemotherapy.[14] Radiotherapy was administered in both arms for a total dose of 70 Gy by conven-

## TABLE 9-7. MIGRATION OF PATIENT DISTRIBUTION BASED ON AMERICAN JOINT COMMITTEE ON CANCER 1988 AND 1997 STAGING SYSTEMS OF NASOPHARYNGEAL CANCER PATIENTS (LITERATURE REVIEW)

| Center | Stage I 1988 | Stage I 1997 | Stage II 1988 | Stage II 1997 | Stage III 1988 | Stage III 1997 | Stage IV 1988 | Stage IV 1997 |
|---|---|---|---|---|---|---|---|---|
| Cooper et al.[34] | 7 | 19 | 12 | 33 | 13 | 23 | 75 | 32 |
| Cheng et al.[16] | — | — | — | 32 | 12 | 44 | 95 | 31 |
| Ozyar et al.[35] | 2 | 8 | 6 | 21 | 13 | 26 | 69 | 35 |
| Lee et al.[11]* | 156 | 439 | 283 | 929 | 488 | 1,369 | 3,587 | 1,777 |
| **TOTAL** | 165 3% | 466 10% | 301 6% | 1,015 21% | 526 12% | 1,462 30% | 3,826 79% | 1,875 39% |

* Figures were estimated from percentages in the original publication.

**TABLE 9-8. COMPARISON OF AMERICAN JOINT COMMITTEE ON CANCER 1988 AND 2002 STAGING SYSTEMS FOR NASOPHARYNGEAL CARCINOMA**

| AJCC 1988 | AJCC 2002* |
|---|---|
| **Primary Tumor** | |
| TX Primary tumor cannot be assessed | Primary tumor cannot be assessed |
| T0 No evidence of primary tumor | No evidence of primary tumor |
| Tis Carcinoma *in situ* | Carcinoma in situ |
| T1 Tumor confined to the one side of nasopharynx | Tumor confined to the nasopharynx |
| T2 Tumor cofined to more than one side of nasopharyx | Tumor extends to soft tissues of oropharynx and/or nasal fossa |
| T2a — | Without parapharyngeal extension |
| T2b — | With parapharyngeal extension |
| T3 Tumor extends to nasal cavity or oropharynx. | Tumor invades bony structures and/or paranasal sinuses |
| T4 Bony erosion, intracranial extension, cranial nerve involvement | Tumor with intracranial extension and/or involvement of cranial nerves, infratemporal fossa, hypopharynx, orbit, or masticator space |
| **Neck Nodes** | |
| Nx Regional lymph nodes cannot be assessed | Regional lymph nodes cannot be assessed |
| N0 No regional lymph node metastasis | No regional lymph node metastasis |
| N1 Unilateral metastasis in lymph node(s), ≤3 cm in greatest dimension. | Unilateral metastasis in lymph node(s), ≤6 cm in greatest dimension, above the supraclavicular fossa |
| N2 a: Unilateral, single, >3 cm but ≤6 cm<br>b: Unilateral, multiple, <6 cm | Bilateral metastasis in lymph node(s), ≤6 cm in greatest dimension, above the supraclavicular fossa |
| c: Bilateral but ≤6 cm | Metastasis in a lymph node(s): |
| N3 Metastasis in a lymph node(s): >6 cm in dimension | |
| N3a — | >6 cm in dimension |
| N3b — | Extension to the supraclavicular fossa |
| **Metastases** | |
| MX Distant metastasis cannot be assessed | Distant metastasis cannot be assessed |
| M0 No distant metastasis | No distant metastasis |
| M1 Distant metastasis present | Distant metastasis present |

From: Greene FL, American Joint Committee on Cancer, American Cancer Society. *AJCC cancer staging manual*, 6th ed. New York: Springer; 2002.

**TABLE 9-9. NASOPHARYNGEAL CARCINOMA: INCIDENCE OF FAILURE AT PRIMARY SITE CORRELATED WITH T STAGE (AMERICAN JOINT COMMITTEE ON CANCER, 1988)**

| Author | T STAGE (%) | | | |
|---|---|---|---|---|
| | T1 | T2 | T3 | T4 |
| Chu et al.[12] | 24 | 21 | 63 | 45 |
| Hoppe et al.[36] | 13 | 6 | 32 | 56 |
| Kajanti and Mäntylä[37] | 13 | 17 | 58 | 100 |
| Lee et al.[38] | 26 | 28 | 39 | — |
| Mesic et al.[32] | 3 | 15 | 26 | 28 |
| Petrovich et al.[5] | 20 | 32 | 50 | 88 |
| Perez et al.[1] | 20 | 24 | 44 | 60 |
| **AVERAGE** | 25 | 26 | 40 | 69 |

**TABLE 9-10. NASOPHARYNGEAL CARCINOMA: INCIDENCE OF FAILURE IN THE NECK CORRELATED WITH N STAGE (AMERICAN JOINT COMMITTEE ON CANCER, 1988)**

| Author | Nodal Stage* | | |
|---|---|---|---|
| | N1 | N2 | N3 |
| Hoppe et al.[36] | 8% (25) | 13% (15) | 11% (18) |
| Kajanti and Mäntylä[37] | 22% (76) | 30% (61) | 0% (63) |
| Perez et al.[1] | 12% (28) | 25% (74) | 22% (13) |
| **RANGE** | 8%–22% | 13%–30% | 0%–22% |

* Parenthesis indicate number of patients.

**TABLE 9-11. OVERALL SURVIVAL RATES AT 3 YEARS BASED ON AMERICAN JOINT COMMITTEE ON CANCER 1997 SYSTEM (LITERATURE REVIEW)**

| Center | N | RT | CT | Stage I | Stage II | Stage III | Stage IV |
|---|---|---|---|---|---|---|---|
| Cooper et al.[34] | 107 | 70 Gy | — | 70% | 65% | 61% | 56% |
| Cheng et al.[16]* | 107 | 70 Gy | + | — | 100% | 93% | 69% |
| Ozyar et al.[35]† | 90 | 66 Gy | + | 100% | 72% | 65% | 55% |
| Lee et al.[11]‡ | 4,514 | 60 Gy | + | 94% | 83% | 76% | 50% |
| Chien et al.[33]§ | 117 | | + | 88% | 86% | 61% | 48% |
| | 4,935 | 60–70 Gy | | 70%–100% | 65%–100% | 61%–93% | 48%–69% |

N, number of patients; RT, radiotherapy; CT, chemotherapy.
* Concomitant CDDP+5-FU followed by two cycles of CDDP+5-FU in Stage II, III, IV.
† Neoadjuvant or concomitant cisplatin in N2–N3 patients.
‡ Chemotherapy in patients with advanced disease and incomplete remission after radiotherapy.
§ Three cycles of adjuvant cisplatin and 5-FU in stage III–IV patients.

tional techniques. The investigational arm received chemotherapy with cisplatin 100 mg/m$^2$ on days 1, 22, and 43 during radiotherapy. After completion of radiotherapy, patients received additional post-radiotherapy and chemotherapy with cisplatin 80 mg/m$^2$ on day 1 and fluorouracil 1,000 mg/m$^2$/d on days 1 to 4 every 4 weeks for three courses. The 3-year progression-free survival rate was 24% versus 69% in favor of the chemotherapy arm ($P < 0.001$). The 3-year overall survival rate was 47% versus 78%, respectively ($P = 0.005$).

- There are only a few articles available showing their treatment results according to the AJCC 1997 staging system. Overall survival rates of some studies at 3 years based on the new AJCC 1997 system is shown in Table 9-11.
- Neoadjuvant or adjuvant chemotherapy has been used to treat primary or recurrent nasopharynx cancer with complete response rates of 10% to 20% and partial response

rates of 40%. Recently, significant impact on long-term survival has been reported.

- The results of a recent randomized phase III study showed that adjuvant chemotherapy in advanced nasopharyngeal carcinoma patients has no benefit for overall survival or relapse-free survival.[15]
- Cheng et al. demonstrated that concurrent chemotherapy followed by radiation therapy produced effective treatment in advanced nasopharyngeal cancer: an 84% 5-year overall survival rate, a 74% disease-free survival rate, and 90% locoregional control rate. The experience of this study substantiates the Intergroup trial's conclusion.[16]
- The results of some phase III combined chemotherapy and radiotherapy studies are summarized in Table 9-12.
- These phase III studies showed that concurrent chemotherapy followed by adjuvant chemotherapy

**TABLE 9-12. PHASE III COMBINED CHEMOTHERAPY AND RADIOTHERAPY STUDIES (LITERATURE REVIEW)**

| Center | Stage (AJCC 1988) | Treatment | No. of Patients | LRR (%) | DFS (%) | Years |
|---|---|---|---|---|---|---|
| Milan[39] | I–IV | RT 60 Gy | 116 | 27 | 56 | 4 |
| | | RT+6 cycles VCA | 113 | 24 | 58 | |
| INSG[40,41] | IV | RT 70 Gy | 168 | 23 | 31 | 3 |
| | | 3 cycles BEP+RT 70 Gy | 171 | 15 | 47 | |
| Hong Kong[42] | N size ≥4 cm or N3 | RT (66 Gy+Boost) | 40 | 15 | 78 | 2 |
| | | 2 cycles PF+RT+3 cycles PF | 37 | 16 | 68 | |
| AOCOA[30] | N size ≥3 cm, N2–N3 or T3 | RT 66–74 Gy | 134 | 31 | 46 | 3 |
| | | 2–3 cycles PE+RT | 152 | 25 | 58 | |
| Intergroup study[14] | III–IV | RT 70 Gy | 69 | 41 | 24 | 3 |
| | | RT and 3 cycles P+3 cycles PF | 78 | 14 | 69 | |

AJCC, American Joint Committee on Cancer; LRR, locoregional recurrence; DFS, disease-free survival; RT, radiotherapy; VCA, vincristine, cyclophosphamide, and doxorobucin; INSG, International Nasopharynx Group; BEP, bleomycin, epirubicin, and cisplatin; PF, cisplatin and 5-fluorouracil; AOCOA, Asian-Oceanian Clinical Oncology Association; PE, cisplatin and epirubicin; P, platin.

yielded better therapeutic results in advanced nasopharyngeal carcinoma. Another important conclusion is that concurrent use of cisplatin during radiotherapy is essential, and chemotherapy, which is given either neoadjuvant or adjuvant to radiotherapy, has only little or no benefit in advanced nasopharyngeal carcinoma if given without concomitant cisplatin.

- A meta-analysis of 1,528 patients from six randomized trials has shown that the addition of chemotherapy to standard radical radiation therapy for locoregionally advanced nasopharyngeal cancer increases both disease-free/progression-free and overall survival by 19% to 40% at 2 to 4 years after treatment.[17]
- Two recently published meta-analyses, only in abstract forms, also demonstrated the benefit of chemotherapy as an addition to radiotherapy in terms of overall survival and disease-free survival.[17,18] One analysis of ten randomized trials has shown that the addition of chemotherapy offers a small but significant effect on the overall survival, and the largest effect was noted with the use of concurrent chemoradiotherapy.[18]

## 6. INTENSITY-MODULATED RADIATION THERAPY IN NASOPHARYNGEAL CARCINOMA

### 6.1. Target Volume Determination

- If chemotherapy was delivered before radiation, the targets should be outlined on the planning CT according to their prechemotherapy extent.
- Because of the high likelihood of cervical metastases, most authors recommend electively treating all of the cervical lymphatics in N0 patients. Contrary to this universal philosophy is a randomized study by Ho showing that survival of N0 patients having prophylactic irradiation of the cervical lymphatics was not better than that of N0 patients without receiving neck irradiation.[19] However, Lee et al.

reported that in 384 patients with clinically negative necks patients, 11% (44 patients) of those receiving elective neck irradiation had regional failure compared with 40% (362 of 906) of those not electively treated.[7] This study strongly supports elective irradiation of the neck in patients with clinically negative neck nodes.

- Lymph node groups at risk in the nasopharyngeal region include the following:

  a. Submandibular nodes (surgical level I): if level II node is involved.
  b. Upper deep jugular (junctional, parapharyngeal) nodes: all cases.
  c. Subdigastric (jugulodigastric) nodes, midjugular, lower neck, and supraclavicular nodes (levels II through IV): all cases, bilaterally.
  d. Posterior cervical nodes (level V): all cases, bilaterally.
  e. Retropharyngeal nodes: all cases.

- The target volume specification for definitive and postoperative intensity-modulated radiation therapy (IMRT) in nasopharyngeal cancer is summarized in Table 7-5.
- Suggested target volume determination for nasopharyngeal carcinoma is shown in Table 9-13.

### 6.2. Clinical Target Volume Delineation

- CTV1 and CTV2 delineation in a patient with clinically T2N1 (AJCC 1997) squamous cell carcinoma of nasopharynx receiving definitive IMRT is shown in Figure 9-8.
- CTV1 and CTV2 delineation in a patient with clinically T2bN0 (AJCC 1997) squamous cell carcinoma of the nasopharynx receiving definitive IMRT concurrent with chemotherapy. For this patient, an MRI as well as positron emission tomography (PET) fusion was done, as shown in Figure 9-9.

*Text continues on page 148.*

### TABLE 9-13. TARGET VOLUME DETERMINATION GUIDELINES FOR NASOPHARYNGEAL TUMORS

| Clinical Presentation | CTV1 | CTV2 | CTV3 |
|---|---|---|---|
| Any TN0 | GTVp | Optional@ | IN+CN (Ib-V, RPLN) |
| Any TN+ | GTVp+n | IN (adjacent LNs*) | IN+CN+RPLN† (remaining LNs) |

Roman numerals represent neck nodal levels.
CTV, clinical target volume; N0, node negative neck; N+, node positive neck; GTVp, primary gross tumor volume; N, nodal gross tumor volume; IN, ipsilateral nodal levels; CN, contralateral nodal levels; RPLN, retropharyngeal lymph nodes.
* 2–3 cm from CTV1 nodal basin
† Includes RPLN for midline and more advanced tumors
@ Optional margins around CTVI. If the risk of nodal metastasis is high, can consider just CTV2 to encompass all lymph node regions and omit CTV3.
Suggested IMRT dose schedule for chemoradiation: CTV1 = 70 Gy/35 fx or 70 Gy/33 fx; CTV2 = 63 Gy/35 fx or 59.4 Gy/33 fx; CTV3 = 56 Gy/35 fx or 54 Gy/33 fx. When definitive IMRT is used without concomitant chemotherapy, suggested doses are: CTV1 = 66 Gy/30 fx; CTV2 = 60 Gy/30 Gy; CTV3 = 54 Gy/30 fx.

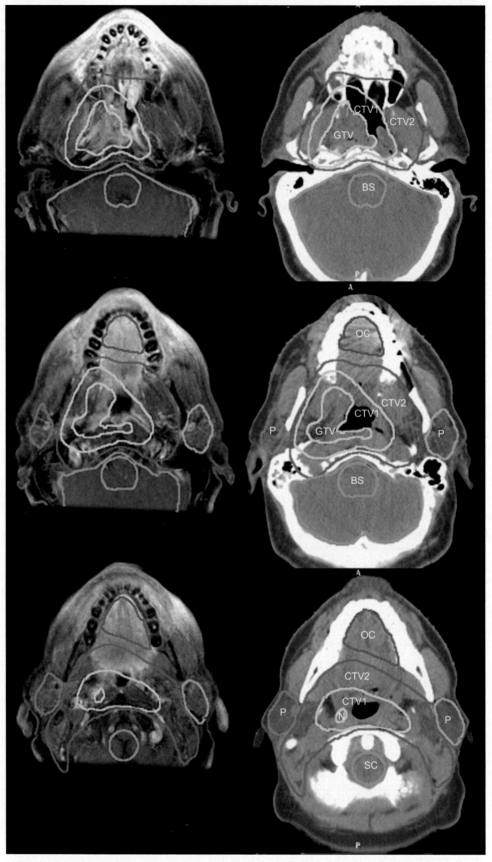

**FIGURE 9-8.** CTV (clinical target volume) delineation in a patient with a T2N1M0 (AJCC 1997) nasopharyngeal carcinoma receiving definitive IMRT. CTV1, *gold;* CTV2, *red;* gross tumor volume (GTV), *yellow line;* right parotid gland (P), *rust line;* left parotid gland, *aqua line;* oral cavity, *magenta line;* spinal cord (SC), *green line.*

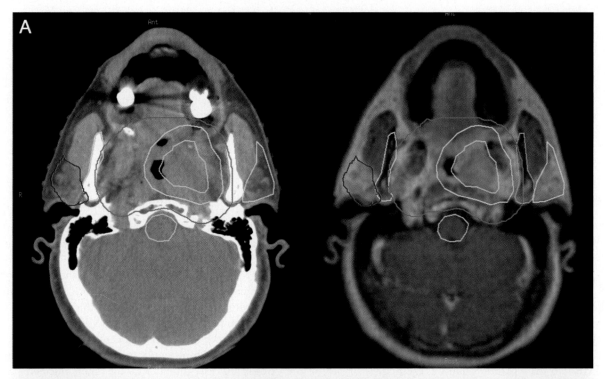

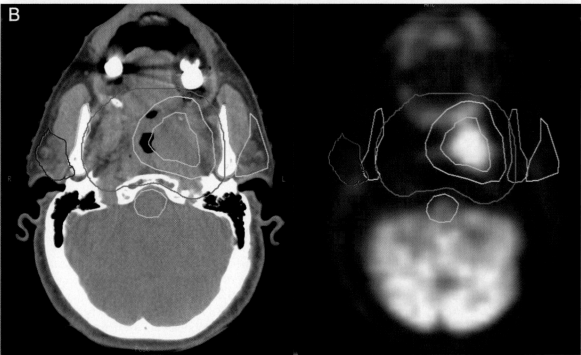

**FIGURE 9-9.** CTV (clinical target volume) delineation using MRI and PET fusion in a patient with a T2bN0M0 (AJCC 1997) nasopharyngeal carcinoma receiving definitive IMRT. **A:** CT-MRI fusion. **B:** CT-PET fusion. Gross tumor volume (GTV), *light blue volume;* CTV1, *yellow volume;* CTV2, *red volume.* (Courtesy of physics staff: S. Tener and M. Bevilacqua)

- CTV1 and CTV2 delineation in a patient with clinically T4N2 (AJCC 1997) squamous cell carcinoma of nasopharynx receiving definitive IMRT is shown in Figure 9-10.

## 6.3. Normal Tissue Delineation

- See Chapter 8 for normal tissue delineation (Fig. 8-8).

## 6.4. Suggested Target and Normal Tissue Doses

- See Chapter 7 for suggested target and normal tissue doses (Table 7-11).

## 6.5. IMRT Results

- Cheng et al. showed that target coverage of the primary tumor was maintained and nodal coverage was improved in 17 nasopharyngeal carcinoma patients, as compared with conventional beam arrangements.[20] Also, the ability of IMRT to spare parotid gland was exciting.
- Hunt et al. reported similar results with twenty-three primary nasopharyngeal carcinoma patients.[21] However, no attempt to spare the parotids was done in their series and the mean parotid dose was quite high at 60.5 Gy. Substantial improvements in terms of inputting the proper constraints for the normal tissues have been done since then.
- Xia et al. compared the treatment plans involving IMRT for nasopharyngeal carcinoma. In their series, the coverage to the GTV as well as the CTV was superior with the inverse-planned IMRT plans. In addition, when using proper dose constraints to the normal structures, inverse-planned IMRT plans achieved the least dose delivered to the brain stem, chiasm, optic structures, as well as the parotid. There was substantial reduction of the mean parotid dose to as low as 21.4 Gy.[22]
- An update of the UCSF experience in the treatment of nasopharyngeal carcinoma by Lee et al. showed that in 87 patients treated with IMRT, the 4-year local progression-free survival, regional progression-free survival, distant metastases recurrence-free survival, and overall survival were 94%, 98%, 66%, and 73%, respectively, with a median follow-up of 31 months.[23] Excellent locoregional control for nasopharyngeal carcinoma was achieved with intensity-modulated radiotherapy. IMRT provided excellent tumor target coverage and allowed

the delivery of a high dose to the target with significant sparing of the salivary glands and other nearby critical normal tissues.

- Kwong et al. presented the preliminary experience from Queen Mary Hospital in Hong Kong of fifty T1-2N0-1M0 nasopharyngeal cancer patients who underwent IMRT. With a median time of 14 months after the completion of radiotherapy, the 2-year nasopharynx, neck, and distant failure-free survival rates were 100%, 94.1%, 94%, respectively.[24]
- These single institution IMRT results for nasopharyngeal cancer are very promising. Therefore, a phase II RTOG study on the use of IMRT for nasopharyngeal carcinoma is currently ongoing to test the transportability of a single-institution's IMRT experience to a multi-institutional setting. [25]
- Chao and associates previously presented results from Washington University-Mallinckrodt.[26] One hundred and three patients were treated with conventional external beam radiation therapy only (MIR-RT). Twenty-two patients received external beam irradiation with concomitant chemotherapy according to the Intergroup Study 0099 regimen. Among them, thirteen patients were treated by conventional beam arrangement (MIR-CRT), and nine patients were treated with IMRT (MIR-IMRT). Three-year progression-free survival for radiation therapy alone was 51% for MIR patients as compared with 24% in IGS ($P < 0.05$). Progression-free survival at 3 years after chemo-radiotherapy was 90% for MIR patients and 69% in IGS ($P < 0.05$).
- In an updated report, 12 nasopharyngeal carcinoma patients were treated with IMRT between February 1997 and December 2000.[27] The T stages were one T1, three T2, three T3, and five T4. The N stages were one N0, three N1, four N2, and four N3 (AJCC staging: two stage II, two stage III, eight stage IV). Patients received chemotherapy according to the Intergroup 0099 regimen. Median follow-up time was 31 months (range 19–52 months). We observed one neck recurrence. Three patients developed distant metastasis. One patient died of distant metastasis. No patient failed at the nasopharynx.
- Figure 9-11 shows pre- and post-IMRT MRI sections of a T4N3 nasopharyngeal carcinoma patient showing the complete regression of the tumor.
- G-tube was placed in two patients during the course of IMRT. We observed no grade 3-4 late complications in our patients treated with IMRT. Six grade II and four grade I late xerostomia were observed. Decreased hearing was common with cisplatin chemotherapy.

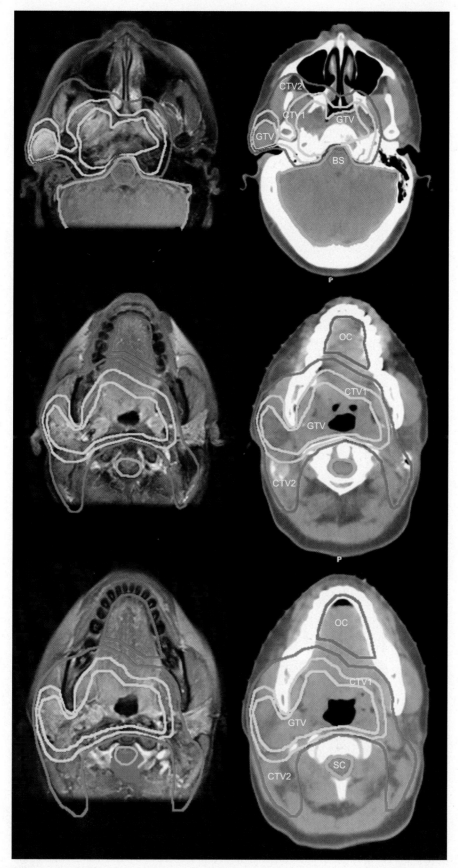

**FIGURE 9-10.** CTV (clinical target volume) delineation in a patient with a T4N2M0 (AJCC 1997) nasopharyngeal carcinoma receiving definitive IMRT. CTV1, *gold;* CTV2, *red;* gross tumor volume (GTV), *yellow line;* oral cavity, *magenta line.*

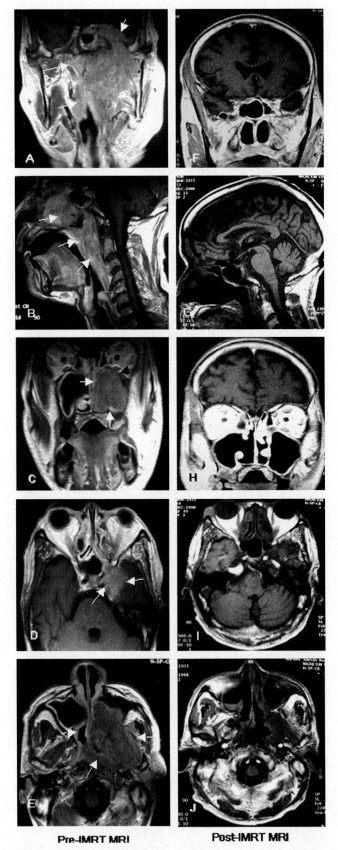

Pre-IMRT MRI                    Post-IMRT MRI

**FIGURE 9-11.** Pre-IMRT (**A–E**) and post-IMRT (**F–J**) MRI sections of a patient with T4N3 nasopharyngeal carcinoma showing complete regression of the tumor after a total IMRT dose of 70.3 Gy with concurrent platinum-based chemotherapy.

# REFERENCES

1. Perez C, Venkata R, Victor M, et al. Carcinoma of the nasopharynx: Factors affecting prognosis. *Int J Radiat Oncol Biol Phys* 1991;23:271–280.
2. Fletcher G, Healey JJ, McGraw J, et al. Nasopharynx. In: Fletcher G, ed. *Cancer of the head and neck*. Baltimore: Williams & Wilkins;1967:152–178.
3. Lederman M. Cancer of the nasopharynx: its natural history and treatment. Springfield, IL: Charles C Thomas;1961.
4. Qin D, Hu Y, Yan J, et al. Analysis of 1379 patients with nasopharyngeal carcinoma treated with radiation. *Cancer* 1988;61: 1117–1124.
5. Petrovich Z, Cox J, Middleton R, et al. Advanced carcinoma of the nasopharynx. II. Pattern of failure in 256 patients. *Radiother Oncol* 1985;4:15–20.
6. Valentini V, Balducci M, Ciarniello V, et al. Tumors of the nasopharynx: review of 132 cases. *Rays* 1987;12:77–88.
7. Fletcher G, Million R. *Nasopharynx*, 3rd ed. Philadelphia: Lea & Febiger;1980.
8. Leung S, Tsao S, Teo P, et al. Cranial nerve involvement by nasopharyngeal carcinoma: response to treatment and clinical significance. *Clin Oncol* 1990;2:138–141.
9. Chong V, Fan V, Khoo J. Retropharyngeal lymphadenopathy in nasopharyngeal carcinoma. *Eur J Radiol* 1995;21:100–105.
10. Sham J, Choy D. Prognostic factors of nasopharyngeal carcinoma: a review of 759 patients. *Br J Radiol* 1990;63:51–58.
11. Lee A, Foo W, Law S, et al. Staging of nasopharyngeal carcinoma: from Ho's to the new UICC system. *Int J Cancer* 1999;84:179–187.
12. Chu A, Flynn M, Achino E, et al. Irradiation of nasopharyngeal carcinoma: correlations with treatment factors and stage. *Int J Radiat Oncol Biol Phys* 1984;10:2241–2249.
13. Kaasa S, Kragh-Jensen E, Bjordal K, et al. Prognostic factors in patients with nasopharyngeal carcinoma. *Acta Oncol* 1993;32: 531–536.
14. Al-Sarraf M, LeBlanc M, Giri PGS, et al. Chemoradiotherapy versus radiotherapy in patients with advanced nasopharyngeal cancer: phase III randomized intergroup study 0099. *J Clin Oncol* 1998;16:1310–1317.
15. Chi K, Change Y, Guo W. Phase III study of adjuvant chemotherapy in advanced nasopharyngeal carcinoma patients. *Int J Radiat Oncol Biol Phys* 2002;52:1238–1244.
16. Cheng S, Jian J, Tsai S, et al. Long-term survival of nasopharyngeal carcinoma following concomitant radiotherapy and chemotherapy. *Int J Radiat Oncol Biol Phys* 2000;48:1323–1330.
17. Huncharek M, Kupelnick B. Combined chemoradiation versus radiation therapy alone in locally advanced nasopharyngeal carcinoma: results of a meta-analysis of 1,528 patients from six randomized trials. *Am J Clin Oncol* 2002;25:219–223.
18. Thephamongkhol K, Browman G, Hodson I, et al. Does the addition of chemotherapy to radiotherapy improve the survival of patients with locally advanced nasopharyngeal cancer? A systematic review and meta-analysis of randomized controlled trials. *Int J Radiat Oncol Biol Phys* 2003;57:S247–S248.
19. Jian J, Cheng S, Prosnitz L, et al. T classification and clivus margin as risk factors for determining locoregional control by radiotherapy of nasopharyngeal carcinoma. *Cancer* 1998;82:261–267.
20. Cheng JCH, Chao KSC, Low D. Comparison of IMRT techniques for nasopharyngeal carcinoma. *Int J Cancer* 2001;96:126–132.
21. Hunt MA, Zelefsky MJ, Wolden S, et al. Treatment planning and delivery of intensity-modulated radiation therapy for primary nasopharynx cancer. *Int J Radiat Oncol Biol Phys* 2001;49: 623–632.
22. Xia P, Fu KK, Wong GW, et al. Comparison of treatment plans involving intensity-modulated radiotherapy for nasopharyngeal carcinoma. *Int J Radiat Oncol Biol Phys* 2000;48: 329–337.
23. Lee N, Xia P, Quivey JM, et al. Intensity-modulated radiotherapy in the treatment of nasopharyngeal carcinoma: an update of the UCSF experience. *Int J Radiat Oncol Biol Phys* 2002;53: 12–22.
24. Kwong DL, Pow E, McMillan A, et al. Intensity-modulated radiotherapy for early stage nasopharyngeal carcinoma: preliminary results on parotid sparing. *Int J Radiat Oncol Biol Phys* 2003; 57:S303.
25. Sultanem K, et al. Three-dimensional intensity-modulated radiotherapy in the treatment of nasopharyngeal carcinoma: the University of California-San Francisco experience. *Int J Radiat Oncol Biol Phys* 2000;48:711–722.
26. Chao K, Cengiz M, Perez C. Intensity-modulated radiotherapy (IMRT) yields superior functional outcome in locally advanced nasopharyngeal carcinoma–comparison with intergroup study 0099. Proceedings in American Society of Clinical Oncology 36th annual meeting. New Orleans, LA; 2000.
27. Ozyigit G, Chao K. Clinical experience of head-and-neck cancer IMRT with serial tomotherapy. *Med Dosim* 2002;27:91–98.
28. McLaughlin M, Mendelhall W, Mancuso A, et al. Retropharyngeal adenopathy as a predictor of outcome in squamous cell carcinoma of the head and neck. *Head Neck* 1995;17: 190–198.
29. Chua D, Sham J, Kwong D. Retropharyngeal lymphadenopathy in patients with nasopharyngeal carcinoma. A computed tomography based study. *Cancer* 1997;79:869–877.
30. Chua D, Sham J, Choy D, et al. Preliminary report of the Asian-Oceanian clinical oncology association randomized trial comparing cisplatin and epirubicin followed by radiotherapy versus radiotherapy alone in the treatment of patients with locoregionally advanced nasopharyngeal carcinoma. *Cancer* 1998;83: 2270–2283.
31. Wang C. Carcinoma of the oropharynx. In: Wang C, ed. *Radiation therapy for head and neck neoplasms*. New York: Wiley-Liss;1997.
32. Mesic J, Fletcher G, Goepfert H. Megavoltage irradiation of epithelial tumors of the nasopharynx. *Int J Radiat Oncol Biol Phys* 1981;7:447–453.
33. Chien C, Chen S, Hsieh C, et al. Retrospective comparison of the AJCC 5th edition classification for nasopharyngeal carcinoma with the AJCC 4th edition: an experience in Taiwan. *Jpn J Clin Oncol* 2001;31:363–369.
34. Cooper J, Cohen R, Stevens R. A comparison of staging systems for nasopharyngeal carcinoma. *Cancer* 1998;83:213–219.
35. Ozyar E, Yildiz F, Akyol F, et al. Comparison of AJCC 1988 and 1997 classifications for nasopharyngeal carcinoma. *Int J Radiat Oncol Biol Phys* 1999;44:1079–1087.
36. Hoppe R, Goffinet D, Bagshaw M. Carcinoma of the nasopharynx: eighteen years' experience with megavoltage radiation therapy. *Cancer* 1976;37:2605–2612.
37. Kajanti M, Mäntylä M. Carcinoma of the nasopharynx: a retrospective analysis of treatment results in 125 patients. *Acta Oncol* 1990;29:611–614.
38. Lee A, Law S, Foo W, et al. Nasopharyngeal carcinoma: local control by megavoltage irradiation. *Br J Radiol* 1993;66:528–536.
39. Rossi A, Molinari R, Borracchi P, et al. Adjuvant chemotherapy with vincristine, cyclophosphamide and doxorubicin after

radiotherapy in local-regional nasopharyngeal cancer: results of a 4-year multicenter randomized trial. *J Clin Oncol* 1988;6: 1401–1410.

40. Cvitkovic E. Neoadjuvant chemotherapy with epirubicin, cisplatin, bleomycin in undifferentiated nasopharyngeal cancer: preliminary results of international phase III trial (abst). *Proceed Am Soc Clin Oncol* 1994;13:283.

41. Group INCS. Preliminary results of a randomized trial comparing neoadjuvant chemotherapy (cisplatin, epirubicin, beomycin) plus radiotherapy versus radiotherapy alone in stage IV (>or=N2, M0) undifferentiated nasopharyngeal carcinoma. A positive effect on progression free survival. International Nasopharynx Cancer Study Group. VUMCA I trial. *Int J Radiat Oncol Biol Phys* 1996;35:463–469.

42. Chan A, Teo P, TWT L, et al. A prospective randomized study of chemotherapy adjunctive to definitive radiotherapy in advanced nasopharyngeal carcinoma. *Int J Radiat Oncol Biol Phys* 1995;33: 569–577.

# 10

# ORAL CAVITY

**GOKHAN OZYIGIT**
**UGOROANS SELEK**

## 1. ANATOMY

- The *oral cavity* consists of the upper and lower lips, gingivobuccal sulcus, buccal mucosa, upper and lower gingiva (including alveolar ridge), hard palate, floor of the mouth, and anterior two-thirds of the mobile tongue.
- The *lips* are composed of the orbicularis muscle, which is covered by skin and mucous membrane on the inner surface; the transitional area between the two is the vermilion border. The blood supply comes from the labial artery, a branch of the facial artery. The motor nerve branches come from the facial nerve. The sensory nerves to the upper and lower lips are the infraorbital branch of the maxillary nerve and branches of the mental nerve, respectively, which originates in the inferior alveolar nerve. The commissure is partially innervated by the buccal branch of the mandibular nerve.
- The *alveolar ridge of the maxilla,* which is covered by mucosa and the teeth and continues medially with the hard palate, forms the upper gingiva. The *lower gingiva* covers the mandible from the gingivobuccal sulcus to the mucosa of the floor of the mouth. It continues posteriorly with the retromolar trigone and superiorly with the maxillary tuberosity. There are no minor salivary glands in the mucous membrane over the alveolar ridges.
- The *buccal mucosa* is made up of the mucous membrane covering the internal surface of the lips and cheeks (buccinator muscle), extending from the line of attachment of the upper and lower alveolar ridges to the point of contact of the lips posteriorly and the orbicularis anteriorly. The masseter muscle lies posteriorly and laterally to the buccinator muscle. The blood supply comes from the facial artery. The buccal nerve, a branch of the mandibular nerve, supplies sensory fibers. The motor nerve to the buccinator muscle is derived from the facial nerve.
- The *floor of the mouth*, bounded by the lower gingiva anteriorly and laterally, extends to the insertion of the anterior tonsillar pillar into the tongue posteriorly (Fig. 10-1). It is divided into halves by the lingual frenulum and is covered by a mucous membrane with stratified squamous epithelium.

- The *sublingual glands* lie below the mucous membrane and are separated by the midline genioglossus and geniohyoid muscles. The genial tubercles are bony protuberances occurring at the point of insertion of these two muscle groups on the symphysis. Muscles include the mylohyoid and digastric muscles.
- The *submaxillary glands* are located on the external surface of the mylohyoid muscle between its insertion to the mandible. The submaxillary duct (Wharton's duct) is approximately 5 cm long and courses between the sublingual gland and genioglossus muscle; its orifice is in the anterior floor of the mouth, near the midline. The sensory nerve is the lingual nerve, a branch of the submaxillary nerve. The arterial supply is the lingual artery, a branch of the external carotid artery.
- The *tongue* is a muscular organ composed of the styloglossus, hyoglossus, and hyoid muscles. It is covered by a mucous membrane with stratified squamous epithelium. The circumvallate papillae, situated posteriorly with a V-shaped configuration, separate the base of the tongue from the mobile tongue. The *oral tongue* consists of the tip, dorsum, lateral borders, and undersurface. The blood supply is the lingual artery, a branch of the external carotid artery. The sensory nerve is the lingual nerve, a branch of the maxillary nerve. The hypoglossal nerve is the motor nerve. The chorda tympani branch of the sensory root of the facial nerve innervates the taste buds.

## 2. NATURAL HISTORY

- Floor of the mouth cancers mostly originate within 2 cm of the anterior midline. They invade early beneath the mucosa into the sublingual gland and the midline genioglossus and geniohyoid muscles. The mylohyoid muscles act as a barrier in early stages. Even small and early lesions may extend into the periosteum, but mandible invasion occurs late in the course of the disease. Submandibular ducts may be obstructed by the tumor.
- Oral tongue cancers mainly originate from the lateral and undersurfaces of the tongue. They tend to remain in the

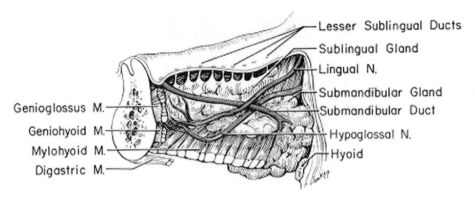

**FIGURE 10-1.** Floor of the oral cavity. (From: Million RR, Cassisi NJ, Clark JR. Cancer of the Head and Neck. In: DeVita VT Jr., Hellman S, Rosenberg SA, eds. *Cancer: Principles and Practice of Oncology, 2nd ed.* Philadelphia: JB Lippincott, 1985:431, with permission.)

tongue in early stages. Perineural invasion is rare. Tip of the tongue cancers are diagnosed in the early stages. Advanced lesions invade the floor of the mouth and root of the tongue, producing fixation. Posterior lesions usually grow into the musculature of the tongue, anterior tonsillar pillar, base of the tongue, and mandible.

- Most of the buccal mucosa lesions develop on the lateral walls. Advanced lesions invade the underlying muscles and eventually penetrate to the skin and infratemporal fossa. Advanced lesions may also involve the parotid gland and facial nerve.
- The lesions of the retromolar trigone spread early to the adjacent buccal mucosa, anterior tonsillar pillar, lower gum, and maxilla. Invasion of the periosteum of the mandible may be seen early, but invasion of the underlying mandible tends to be a late manifestation. The cortex of the mandible is dense, which explains the infrequent bone invasion in the region of the retromolar trigone. Mandibular involvement was noted in 14% of 110 patients with primary retromolar trigone carcinomas.[1]
- Retromolar trigone lesions have an overall metastatic rate of approximately 45%.[2]

## 3. DIAGNOSIS AND STAGING SYSTEM

### 3.1. Signs and Symptoms

- A lump in the floor of the mouth is first noticed for early stage floor of mouth tumors. Bleeding, loose teeth, halitosis, a painful mass in the submandibular region, and change in speech are other symptoms that can be seen in advanced lesions.
- Irritation and the sensation of a lump are the most frequent symptoms in tongue cancer. The pain becomes progressively worse and may be referred to the external ear canal. Bleeding is uncommon. Speech and swallowing may be affected in advanced lesions.
- Leukoplakia is present in half of the cases in buccal mucosa tumors. Obstruction of Stensen's duct may cause

swelling of the parotid gland. Extension into pterygoids, masseter, or buccinator muscles may cause trismus. Intermittent bleeding may be seen during chewing.
- Retromolar trigone lesions can produce local pain and referred pain to the external auditory canal and preauricular area. Trismus may be seen if the lesion invades pterygoid muscles. Hyperesthesia may indicate perineural invasion.

### 3.2. Physical Examination

- The extent of disease in oral cavity lesions is determined by visual examination and palpation. Topical anesthesia may be required for examination.
- Bimanual palpation determines the extent of induration and degree of fixation to the periosteum. Large lesions bulge into the submental or submandibular space. The submandibular duct and gland as well as parotid duct and gland are evaluated by bimanual palpation.

### 3.3. Imaging

#### 3.3.1. Floor of the Mouth

- The floor of the mouth is seen as fat-containing space lying between the paired bellies of the genioglossus and geniohyoid muscles on computed tomography (CT) and magnetic resonance imaging (MRI) of axial sections.
- The mylohyoid muscle is seen better on coronal sections because it extends from the mylohyoid line of the mandible to the hyoid.
- The sublingual spaces are usually symmetric. The submandibular space is separated from the floor of the mouth by the mylohyoid muscle and is located in the suprahyoid part of the neck. Because these spaces contain glandular and fat tissue, they are easily distinguished from adjacent muscles on both CT and MRI. The lingual vessel bundle is seen coursing these spaces. The hypoglossal and lingual nerves are normally invisible.

- The hyoglossus muscle is visible on axial and coronal images coursing within the glandular and fatty tissue of the sublingual space.
- The small space lying between the digastric muscles next to their insertion on the mandible is the submental space. The submandibular space contains the submandibular gland, facial vessels, and lymph nodes, which are normally small (<5 mm) in the submental space.

### 3.3.2. Oral Tongue

- It is difficult to differentiate the zone between the floor of the mouth and the ventral surface of the oral tongue in axial images. This is much easier on coronal or sagittal sections of MRI or coronal CT sections. In the sagittal plane of MRI, various intrinsic muscle bundles and fat tissue can easily be seen. The styloglossus muscle interdigitates with the hyoglossus muscle within the posterior aspect of the tongue.
- The muscles and spaces medial and lateral to the styloglossus muscle are potential places of tumor spread toward the skull base from the floor of the mouth and tongue base.

- Although CT and MRI cannot detect microscopic spread beyond the palpable margins of the tumor, they can help to map the gross tumor boundary before surgical or radiation therapy.

### 3.3.3. Retromolar Trigone

- CT is the choice of imaging because a detailed study of bony structures, soft tissues, and regional nodes is required. Spread to the lingual muscles can be recognized better on MRI than on CT. Occult spread anteriorly along the attachment of the mylohyoid muscle may be visible on CT or MRI when not palpable or visible by clinical examination. Supplemental MRI may be useful in looking for such perineural spread and determining extension into the nasal cavity or soft palate.

## 3.4. Staging

- Table 10-1 shows the American Joint Committee on Cancer staging system for carcinoma of the oral cavity.[3]

**TABLE 10-1. TNM CLASSIFICATION FOR CARCINOMA OF THE ORAL CAVITY**

**Primary tumor (T)**

| | |
|---|---|
| TX | Primary tumor cannot be assessed |
| T0 | No evidence of primary tumor |
| Tis | Carcinoma *in situ* |
| T1 | Tumor ≤ 2 cm in greatest dimension |
| T2 | Tumor > 2 cm but not > 4 cm in greatest dimension |
| T3 | Tumor > 4 cm in greatest dimension |
| T4a | Tumor invades through cortical bone into deep extrinsic muscle of tongue (genioglossus, hyoglossus, palatoglossus, and styloglossus), maxillary sinus, or skin of face |
| T4b | Tumor involves masticator space, pterygoid plates, or skull base and/or encases external carotid artery |

**Regional lymph nodes (N)**

| | |
|---|---|
| NX | Regional lymph nodes cannot be assessed |
| N0 | No regional lymph node metastasis |
| N1 | Metastasis in a single ipsilateral lymph node, ≤ 3 cm in greatest dimension |
| N2 | Metastasis in a single ipsilateral lymph node, > 3 cm but not > 6 cm in greatest dimension; in multiple ipsilateral lymph nodes, none > 6 cm in greatest dimension; or in bilateral or contralateral lymph nodes, none > 6 cm in greatest dimension |
| N2a | Metastasis in a single ipsilateral lymph node > 3 cm but not > 6 cm in greatest dimension |
| N2b | Metastasis in multiple ipsilateral lymph nodes, none > 6 cm in greatest dimension |
| N2c | Metastasis in bilateral or contralateral lymph nodes, none > 6 cm in greatest dimension |
| N3 | Metastasis in a lymph node > 6 cm in greatest dimension |

**Distant metastases (M)**

| | |
|---|---|
| MX | Presence of distant metastasis cannot be assessed |
| M0 | No distant metastasis |
| M1 | Distant metastasis |

*Stage grouping*

| | | | |
|---|---|---|---|
| Stage 0 | Tis | N0 | M0 |
| Stage I | T1 | N0 | M0 |
| Stage II | T2 | N0 | M0 |
| Stage III | T3 | N0 | M0 |
| | T1 | N1 | M0 |
| | T2 | N1 | M0 |
| | T3 | N1 | M0 |
| Stage IVA | T4a | N0 or N1 | M0 |
| | Any T | N2 | M0 |
| Stage IVB | Any T | N3 | M0 |
| | T4b | Any N | M0 |
| Stage IVC | Any T | Any N | M1 |

From: Greene FL, American Joint Committee on Cancer, American Cancer Society. *AJCC Cancer Staging Manual, 6th ed.* New York: Springer, 2002, with permission.

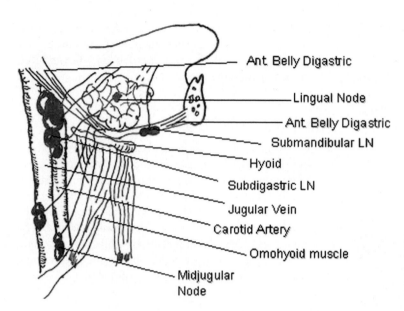

**FIGURE 10-2.** Lymphatics of the tongue. (Adapted from: Rouviere H. Lymphatics of the tongue and of the salivary gland. In: Tobias MJ, ed. *Anatomy of the Human Lymphatic System.* Ann Arbor, MI: Edwards Brothers, 1938:44, with permission.)

## 4. RISK FACTORS FOR NODAL METASTASIS

- Lymphatics of the upper lip drain mostly to the submandibular lymph nodes; the periauricular and parotid lymph nodes occasionally receive lymphatic channels from the upper lip. Lower lip lymphatics drain to the submandibular and posteriorly to the subdigastric lymph nodes. Lymphatics of the lower gingiva drain to the submandibular and subdigastric lymph nodes.
- The first echelon of lymph node drainage of the floor of the mouth is to the submandibular and subdigastric lymph nodes.
- Primary lymphatic drainage in the oral tongue is to the subdigastric and submandibular lymph nodes. Rouviere and Tobias[4] described the lymphatic trunks that bypass this primary lymphatic drainage and go directly to the midjugular lymph nodes, which probably accounts for the relative frequency of metastatic lymph nodes in these locations (Fig. 10-2).
- Lymphatic drainage of the buccal mucosa is primarily to the submandibular and subdigastric lymph nodes.
- Clinically detected nodal metastases on admission by T stage vary according to subsites of the oral cavity (Table 10-2). The incidence and distribution of metastatic disease in clinically negative and positive neck nodes also change according to subsites of cancer in the oral cavity (Tables 10-3–10-5).
- There are several factors influencing contralateral nodal metastasis in oral cavity cancer (Table 10-6). Except for lesions arising from the tip of the tongue or extending across the midline, metastatic disease usually occurs in the ipsilateral cervical lymph nodes.[5]
- Approximately 30% to 65% of patients with oral tongue and floor of mouth cancer have clinically positive neck nodes on presentation.[5]

- The distribution of pathologically positive neck nodes after elective modified neck dissection in patients with carcinomas in the oral tongue, floor of the mouth, and retromolar trigone is shown in Figures 10-3, 10-4, and 10-5, respectively.
- Byers et al.[6] reported the incidence of nodal metastasis by T stage and subsite in oral cavity cancer after elective nodal dissection (Table 10-7).
- The incidence of bilateral lymph node involvement is relatively high for floor of mouth cancers because many lesions are near or cross the midline;[5,6] 5% to 10% of oral tongue cancers have bilateral lymph node metastases.[5,6]

## TABLE 10-2. CLINICALLY DETECTED NODAL METASTASES (%) ON ADMISSION BY T STAGE

| | N0 | N1 | N2, N3 |
|---|---|---|---|
| **Oral tongue** | | | |
| T1 | 86 | 10 | 4 |
| T2 | 70 | 19 | 11 |
| T3 | 52 | 16 | 31 |
| T4 | 24 | 10 | 66 |
| **Floor of mouth** | | | |
| T1 | 89 | 9 | 2 |
| T2 | 71 | 18 | 10 |
| T3 | 66 | 20 | 24 |
| T4 | 46 | 10 | 43 |
| **Retromolar trigone or ant tonsillar pillar** | | | |
| T1 | 88 | 2 | 9 |
| T2 | 62 | 18 | 20 |
| T3 | 46 | 21 | 33 |
| T4 | 32 | 18 | 50 |

Compiled from the data of M. D. Anderson Cancer Center.[5]

**TABLE 10-3. INCIDENCE AND DISTRIBUTION OF METASTATIC DISEASE IN CLINICALLY NEGATIVE (N−) AND POSITIVE (N+) NECK NODES (IN PERCENTAGE)**

| | Radiologically Enlarged Retropharyngeal Nodes | | Pathologic Nodal Metastasis | | | | | | | | | |
| | | | Level I | | Level II | | Level III | | Level IV | | Level V | |
| Clinical presentation | N− | N+ | N− | N+ | N− | N+ | N− | N+ | N− | N+ | N− | N+ |
|---|---|---|---|---|---|---|---|---|---|---|---|---|
| Oral tongue | — | — | 14 | 39 | 19 | 73 | 16 | 27 | 3 | 11 | 0 | 0 |
| Floor of mouth | — | — | 16 | 72 | 12 | 51 | 7 | 29 | 2 | 11 | 0 | 5 |
| Alveolar ridge and retromolar trigone | — | — | 25 | 38 | 19 | 84 | 6 | 25 | 5 | 10 | 1 | 4 |

Modified from: Chao KS, Wippold FJ, Ozyigit G, et al. Determination and delineation of nodal target volumes for head-and-neck cancer based on the patterns of failure in patients receiving definitive and postoperative IMRT. *Int J Radiat Oncol Biol Phys* 2002;53:1174–1184, with permission.

**TABLE 10-4. INCIDENCE OF NECK NODE METASTASES BY PRIMARY TUMOR SITE**

| Tumor Site | cN+ at Presentation (%) | cN0, pN+ Pathologically (%) | cN−, N+ with N0 Neck Treatment (%) |
|---|---|---|---|
| FOM | 30–59 | 21–50 | 20–35 |
| Gingiva | 18–52 | 12–19 | 17 |
| Hard palate | 13–24 | No data | 22 |
| Buccal mucosa | 9–31 | 0/10 | 16 |
| Oral tongue | 34–65 | 25–54 | 38–52 |

FOM, floor of mouth; C, clinical; P, pathologic.
Modified from: Chao KS, Wippold FJ, Ozyigit G, et al. Determination and delineation of nodal target volumes for head-and-neck cancer based on the patterns of failure in patients receiving definitive and postoperative IMRT. *Int J Radiat Oncol Biol Phys* 2002;53:1174–1184, with permission.

**TABLE 10-5. INCIDENCE OF CONTRALATERAL OR BILATERAL NECK NODE METASTASES BY PRIMARY TUMOR SITE**

| Tumor Site | cN+, Bilateral (%) | cN+, Contralateral Only (%) | cN−, pN+ Bilateral (%) |
|---|---|---|---|
| Oral tongue | 12% | — | 33% |
| FOM | 27% | — | 21% |

FOM, floor of mouth; C, clinical; P, pathologic.
Modified from: Chao KS, Wippold FJ, Ozyigit G, et al. Determination and delineation of nodal target volumes for head-and-neck cancer based on the patterns of failure in patients receiving definitive and postoperative IMRT. *Int J Radiat Oncol Biol Phys* 2002;53:1174–1184, with permission.

**TABLE 10-6. FACTORS INFLUENCING CONTRALATERAL LYMPH NODE METASTASIS IN ORAL CANCER**

| Variable | RR of Contralateral Metastasis | 95% CI |
|---|---|---|
| **Tumor Site** | | |
| Tongue | 1.0 | Ref. |
| FOM | 1.5 | 0.9–2.6 |
| RMT | 0.3 | 0.1–1.1 |
| **Distance from midline** | | |
| >1 cm | 1.0 | Ref. |
| Cross < 1 cm | 2.8 | 1.1–7.5 |
| Cross > 1 cm | 12.7 | 5.6–29.1 |
| **Tumor stage** | | |
| T1 | 1.0 | Ref. |
| T2, T3 | 2.2 | 0.7–5.5 |
| T4 | 5.8 | 2.0–16.3 |

RMT, retromolar trigone; FOM, floor of mouth; RR, relative risk; CI, confidence interval.
Compiled from the data of: Kowalski LP, Medina JE. Nodal metastases: predictive factors. *Otolaryngol Clin North Am* 1998;31:621–637, with permission.[16]

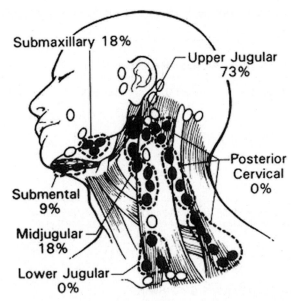

**FIGURE 10-3.** Distribution of pathologically positive neck nodes after elective modified neck dissection in forty-eight patients with oral tongue carcinoma. (From: Byers RM, Wolf PF, Ballantyne AJ. Rationale for elective modified neck dissection. *Head Neck Surg* 1988;10:162, with permission.)

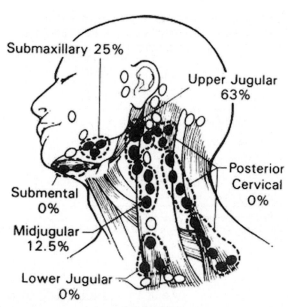

**FIGURE 10-5.** Distribution of pathologically positive neck nodes after elective modified neck dissection in patients with retromolar trigone carcinoma. (From: Byers RM, Wolf PF, Ballantyne AJ. Rationale for elective modified neck dissection. *Head Neck Surg* 1988;10:163, with permission.)

## 5. GENERAL MANAGEMENT

- A variety of therapeutic measures are available for managing localized carcinomas of the oral cavity, including surgery, radiation therapy, laser excision, and combinations of these methods.

### 5.1. Buccal Mucosa

- Primary surgery is effective for small, superficial T1 lesions without involvement of the commissure. The procedure removes the malignancy and eradicates any adjacent leukoplakia.

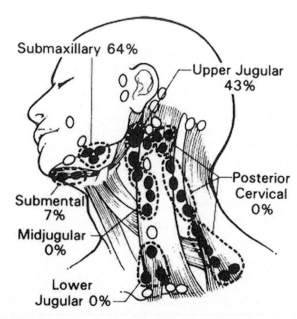

**FIGURE 10-4.** Distribution of pathologically positive neck nodes after elective modified neck dissection in sixty-two patients with floor of mouth carcinoma. (From: Byers RM, Wolf PF, Ballantyne AJ. Rationale for elective modified neck dissection. *Head Neck Surg* 1988;10:162, with permission.)

**TABLE 10-7. ELECTIVE NODAL DISSECTION: INCIDENCE OF NODAL METASTASIS BY T CLASSIFICATION AND SITE IN ORAL CANCER**

| Primary Site | Tx, T1, T2 | T3, T4 | Total |
|---|---|---|---|
| Oral tongue | 21% | 32% | 25% |
| Floor of mouth | 19% | 26% | 21% |
| Lower gum | 12% | 13% | 12% |
| Buccal mucosa | 0% | 0% | 0% |
| Retromolar trigone | 36% | 33% | 35% |

Modified from: Byers RM, Wolf PF, Ballantyne AJ. Rationale for elective modified neck dissection. *Head Neck Surg* 1988;10:165, with permission.

- For intermediate T2 lesions and those involving the commissure, irradiation, which produces a high cure rate with good functional and cosmetic results, is preferred.
- For T1 and most T2 lesions without nodal involvement, results with irradiation are best when photon or electron beam therapy is combined with interstitial implant or intraoral cone therapy.
- For T3 and T4 tumors with deep muscular invasion, cure rates after radiation therapy are poor. These lesions are usually treated with radical surgery, reconstruction, and postoperative irradiation.
- For moderately advanced lesions, with or without positive nodes, appropriate radiation therapy must include the primary site and regional lymph nodes. This is best achieved with external-beam irradiation through ipsilateral and anterior wedged-pair fields for a tumor dose of 55 to 60 Gy in 6 weeks, followed by boost irradiation that spares the mandible and an interstitial implant, intraoral cone, or electron beam for an additional 20 Gy.
- Table 10-8 summarizes the treatment result for carcinoma of the buccal mucosa.

## 5.2. Oral Tongue

- Management of carcinoma of the oral tongue is difficult and controversial and depends on the primary lesion's size, location, and growth pattern and the nodal status in the neck.

### 5.2.1. T1 and T2 Tongue Lesions

- Although surgery or irradiation is effective in controlling small cancers, it is not unreasonable to consider transoral surgical resection for small, well-defined le-

sions involving the tip and anterolateral border of the tongue.[7] These lesions can be cured by resection without risk of functional morbidity, particularly in aged and feeble patients.

- Radiation therapy (60–65 Gy in 6–7 weeks) is preferred for small, posteriorly situated, ill-defined lesions inaccessible for surgical excision through the oral route.
- Superficial, exophytic T1 and T2 lesions with little muscle involvement are amenable to successful treatment with irradiation (70 Gy in 7 weeks).
- For moderately advanced, medium-sized T2 tumors involving the adjacent floor of the mouth, surgical treatment must include partial glossectomy, partial mandibulectomy, and radical neck dissection. As an alternative to surgery, comprehensive irradiation (70–75 Gy in 7–8 weeks) with progressively decreasing fields to the primary site and neck nodes can be used, and surgery is reserved for salvage of residual or recurrent disease.

### 5.2.2. T3 and T4 Tongue Lesions

- Advanced disease with deep muscle invasion, often associated with cervical lymph node metastases, is unlikely to be cured with irradiation alone.
- These lesions are best managed by planned combined irradiation (50–60 Gy in 5–6 weeks) and surgery.
- Excisional biopsy is usually inadequate for carcinoma of the oral tongue, even for small lesions.
- Wide local excision is the treatment of choice for well-circumscribed lesions that can be excised transorally with at least 1-cm margins.
- Wide local excision of lesions of the posterior part of the mobile tongue is difficult, and without reconstruction can result in serious functional deficits in swallowing and

## TABLE 10-8. TREATMENT RESULTS: BUCCAL MUCOSA

| Author | No. of Patients | Treatment | Local Control (%) | | 5-Yr Cause-Specific Survival Rate (%) | |
|---|---|---|---|---|---|---|
| Bloom and Spiro[17] | 121 | S | — | | Stage I | 77 |
| | | | | | Stage II | 65 |
| | | | | | Stage III | 27 |
| | | | | | Stage IV | 18 |
| Urist et al.[18] | 105 | S | | | Stage I | 95 |
| | | | | | Stages II and III | 80 |
| | | | | | Stage IV | 55 |
| MacComb and Fletcher[19] | 115 | RT±S | Stage I | 90 | | |
| | | | Stages II and III | 88 | | |
| | | | Stage IV | 38 | | |
| Wang[20] | 60 | RT | | | 45% (3-yr NED) | |

S, surgery; RT, radiation therapy; NED, no evidence of disease.

speech. External irradiation combined with interstitial implant may be used for these patients.

- The extent of surgery for larger lesions is usually hemi- or total glossectomy.
- Postoperative irradiation is recommended for larger lesions, close or positive margins, and perineural invasion. It is also recommended for patients with initially positive surgical margins, who later have negative surgical margins on re-excision.[7,8]
- Treatment results for carcinoma of the oral tongue are summarized in Table 10-9.

## 5.3. Floor of the Mouth

- When the tumor is small or limited to the mucosa, it is highly curable by surgery or irradiation alone.
- Very small superficial lesions can be treated with interstitial implant (60–65 Gy) or intraoral cone (45 Gy over 3 weeks) alone.
- T1 and early T2 lesions must be treated with external-beam irradiation and various boost techniques, such as interstitial implant (45 Gy external plus 25 Gy with implant) or intraoral cone (45 Gy external plus 20 Gy intraoral cone).
- In floor of mouth lesions that are tethered or fixed to the mandible, resection of the inner table is often recommended, which results in reasonable speech and swallowing.
- Postoperative irradiation is usually recommended because of associated negative prognostic factors.
- For advanced lesions as the result of bone invasion, wide local excision of tumor along with segmental resection of the mandible is often followed by reconstruction of the floor of the mouth and mandible.
- For very advanced disease involving the floor of the mouth, tongue, and mandible and massive neck disease, the chance of cure with any aggressive treatment is low and often associated with formidable complications; a course of irradiation should strongly be considered.

- For extensive, infiltrative T3 and T4 lesions with marked involvement of the adjacent muscle of the tongue and mandible, radical surgery followed by plastic closure and postoperative irradiation is the procedure of choice.
- For advanced T3 and T4 lesions, external-beam irradiation is given through large opposing lateral portals with equal loading covering the primary lesion and nodal areas to a dose of approximately 45 Gy in 4.5 to 5 weeks, followed by two- or three-step reduced fields to a total dose of 70 to 74 Gy.
- The treatment results for floor of mouth carcinoma are summarized in Table 10-10.

## 5.4. Management of Neck Nodes

- In patients with small lesions resected with adequate margins and thickness of less than 2 mm without poor prognostic factors, no further elective treatment is required if the neck is clinically and radiographically negative.
- The neck should be treated in patients who have resected primary lesions of the oral tongue or floor of the mouth more than 2- to 3-mm thick or poor prognostic factors such as perineural or perilymphatic invasion.
- Any form of bilateral neck dissection has worse cosmetic results than a moderate dose of irradiation (45–50 Gy).
- If neck dissection reveals only one positive node with no extracapsular extension, we usually recommend no radiation therapy to the neck.[9] If neck dissection shows more than one node, and especially metastases at more than one nodal station or extracapsular extension of a single or multiple nodes, a course of postoperative irradiation to the neck is indicated.
- In patients with clinically or radiographically positive neck nodes (by CT scan with contrast), the treatment of choice for the neck is ipsilateral neck dissection followed by bilateral postoperative neck irradiation.

## TABLE 10-9. TREATMENT RESULTS: ORAL TONGUE

| Author | No. of Patients | | Treatment | Local Control (%) | | 5-Yr Cause-Specific Survival Rate (%) | |
|---|---|---|---|---|---|---|---|
| | T1, T2 | T3, T4 | | T1, T2 | T3, T4 | T1, T2 | T3, T4 |
| Cassisi and Million[21] | 45 | 29 | I+E | 8/10, 60 | 42, 0/5 | 7/9, 76 | 42,* 20 |
| Decroix and Ghossein[22,23] | 382 | 220 | E+I | 86, 78 | 71 -† | 80, 56 | 25 -† |
| Gilbert et al.[24] | 20 | 36 | I+E | 91, 63 | 36 -† | 73, 37 | 19 -† |
| Wang[20] | 116 | 87 | E | 86, 43 | 17, 18 | 64, 36 | 19, 5 (3-yr NED) |

I, interstitial; E, external radiotherapy; NED, no evidence of disease.
* Stage III.
† No T4 data.

## TABLE 10-10. TREATMENT RESULTS: FLOOR OF MOUTH

| Author | No. of Patients T1, T2 | No. of Patients T3, T4 | Treatment | Local Control (%) T1, T2 | Local Control (%) T3, T4 | 5-Yr Cause-Specific Survival Rate (%) T1, T2 | 5-Yr Cause-Specific Survival Rate (%) T3, T4 |
|---|---|---|---|---|---|---|---|
| Wang[20] | 174 | 61 | RT | 90, 72 | 23, 24 | 85, 56 | 7, 13 |
| Rodgers et al.[25] | 73 | 25 | RT | 86, 69 | 55, 40 | 96, 70 | 67, 1/5 |
| | 22 | 2 | S | 90, 75 | 62 | 83, 66 | — |
| Fu et al.[26] | 153 | — | RT | 90, 81 | 67, -* | 83, 71 | 43, 10 |
| Nason et al.[27] | 114 | 75 | S | — | — | 69, 64 | 46, 26 |
| Gilbert et al.[24] | 40 | 15 | RT | 85, 50 | 20, -* | 73, 37 | 25, -* |

S, surgery, RT, external radiotherapy.
* No T4 data.

- Contralateral prophylactic neck dissection is a serious disservice to the patient.[9]

## 5.5. Chemotherapy

- Clinical trials for advanced tumors evaluating the use of chemotherapy preoperatively, before radiation therapy, as an adjuvant therapy after surgery, or as a part of combined modality therapy have not clarified the appropriate treatment scheme.
- A recent randomized, multicenter trial enrolling 198 patients with a resectable stage T2 to T4 (>3 cm), N0 to N2, M0 untreated, squamous cell carcinoma of the oral cavity showed that neoadjuvant chemotherapy was unable to improve survival but had a role in reducing the number of patients who underwent mandibulectomy (31% vs. 52%) or radiation therapy (33% vs. 46%).[10]
- A meta-analysis of sixty-three randomized prospective trials published between 1965 and 1993 showed an 8% absolute survival advantage in the subset of patients receiving concomitant chemotherapy and radiation therapy.[11] Patients receiving adjuvant or neoadjuvant chemotherapy had no survival advantage in this meta-analysis.
- Eighteen ongoing trials may further clarify the role of concomitant chemotherapy and radiation therapy in the management of oral cavity cancer.

## 6. INTENSITY-MODULATED RADIATION THERAPY IN ORAL CAVITY CANCERS

### 6.1. Target Volume Determination

- If chemotherapy was delivered before radiation, the targets should be outlined on the planning CT according to their pre-chemotherapy extent.

- Lymph node groups at risk in the oral cavity include the following:
  a. Submandibular nodes (surgical level Ib): all cases.
  b. Upper deep jugular (junctional and parapharyngeal) nodes: all cases (at the neck side ipsilateral to the primary tumor).
  c. Subdigastric (jugulodigastric) nodes, midjugular, lower neck, and supraclavicular nodes (levels II–IV): all cases, bilaterally.
  d. Posterior cervical nodes (level V): all cases, at the neck side where there is an evidence of jugular nodal metastases.
  e. Retropharyngeal nodes: all cases, if there is an evidence of jugular nodal metastases.
- The target volume specification for definitive and postoperative intensity-modulated radiation therapy (IMRT) in oral cavity cancer is summarized in Table 7-5.
- The suggested target volume determination for oral cavity carcinoma is summarized in Table 10-11.

### 6.2. Target Volume Delineation

- In patients receiving postoperative IMRT, clinical target volume (CTV)1 encompasses the residual tumor and the region adjacent to it but not directly involved by the tumor, the surgical bed with soft tissue invasion by the tumor, or the extracapsular extension by metastatic neck nodes. CTV2 primarily includes the prophylactically treated neck.
- In patients receiving definitive IMRT, CTV1 is defined as a gross tumor (primary and enlarged nodes) with 5- to 20-mm margins based on clinical and radiologic justification. CTV2 includes the region adjacent to the CTV1 (i.e., ipsilateral upper neck of the involved tumor site). Prophylactically treated neck (classified as CTV2 in postoperative IMRT) is termed as CTV3.

**TABLE 10-11. TARGET VOLUME DETERMINATION GUIDELINES FOR ORAL CAVITY TUMORS**

| Tumor Site | Clinical Presentation | CTV1 | CTV2 | CTV3 |
|---|---|---|---|---|
| **Buccal, RMT** | T1, T2 N0 | GTVp | — | IN* (I–III) |
| | T3, T4 N0 | GTVp | optional | IN+CN (I–V) |
| | Any T N+ | GTVp+n | IN (adjacent LNs†) | IN+CN+RPLN‡ (remaining LNs) |
| **Oral tongue, FOM** | Any T N0 | GTVp | optional | IN+CN (I–V) |
| | Any T N+ | GTVp+n | IN (adjacent LNs†) | IN+CN+RPLN‡ (remaining LNs) |

RMT, retromolar trigone; FOM, floor of mouth; N0, node negative neck; N+, node positive neck; GTVp, primary gross tumor volume; N, nodal gross tumor volume; IN, ipsilateral nodal levels; CN, contralateral nodal levels; RPLN, retropharyngeal lymph nodes; IMRT, intensity-modulated radiation therapy; CTV, clinical target volume.
Roman numerals represent neck nodal levels.
* CN optional for local extension.
† Two to 3 cm from CTV1 nodal basin.
‡ Include optional RPLN for more advanced tumors invading midline structure such as soft palate or posterior pharangeal wall. Chance of RPLN metastasis is low.
Suggested IMRT dose schedule for chemoradiation: CTV1 = 70 Gy/35 fx or 70 Gy/33 fx; CTV2 = 63 Gy/35 fx or 59.4 Gy/33 fx; CTV3 = 56 Gy/35 fx or 54 Gy/33 fx. When definitive IMRT is used without concomitant chemotherapy, suggested doses are: CTV1 = 66 Gy/30 fx; CTV2 = 60 Gy/30Gy; CTV3 = 54 Gy/30 fx.
@ optional margin around CTV,

- CTV1 and CTV2 delineation in a patient with clinically T3N2bM0 squamous cell carcinoma of the retromolar trigone who received definitive IMRT is shown in Figure 10-6. The patient presented with an ulcerative right-sided mass in the retromolar trigone. The lesion was not fixed to the mandible. There were also multiple, palpable level II and III lymph nodes on physical examination. Biopsy revealed a squamous cell carcinoma of the retromolar trigone. The patient was treated with definitive IMRT.

- CTV1 and CTV2 delineation in a patient with pathologic T2N2bM0 squamous cell carcinoma of the tongue receiving postoperative IMRT is shown in Figure 10-7. The patient presented with an ulcerative 2 × 3 cm lesion on the left side of his tongue. On physical examination, there were multiple, palpable level II lymph nodes on the right side of the neck. The patient underwent hemiglossectomy with right modified neck dissection. Pathology specimen revealed a squamous cell carcinoma. Two of thirteen lymph nodes were positive without extracapsular extension. The patient was treated with postoperative IMRT.

## 6.3. Normal Tissue Delineation

- See Chapter 8 for normal tissue delineation (Fig. 8-9).

## 6.4. Suggested Target and Normal Tissue Doses

- See Chapter 7 for suggested target and normal tissue doses (Table 7-11).

## 6.5. Intensity-Modulated Radiation Therapy Results

- A total of 15 patients with oral cavity carcinoma were treated with IMRT between February 1997 and December 2000 at Washington University[12]; 2 patients were treated postoperatively, and 13 patients were treated with definitive IMRT. The T stages were T1 (3 patients), T2 (5 patients), T3 (3 patients), and T4 (4 patients). The N stages were N0 (5 patients), N1 (2 patients), and N2 (8 patients) (according to the American Joint Committee on Cancer staging system: stage I [2 patients], stage II [2 patients], stage III [2 patients], and stage IV [9 patients]). We observed 5 locoregional recurrences, and distant metastasis developed in 1 patient.[13,14] All patients are alive except 2 who died of the cancer.

- A gastrostomy tube was temporarily placed in two patients during treatment. No grade 3 or 4 late complications were seen. Radiation Therapy Oncology Group grades 1 and 2 xerostomia were observed as late sequelae in five and three patients, respectively.

- Claus et al.[15] reported results of eight patients with oral cavity cancer who were treated with IMRT. The majority of patients had recurrent tumor and in-field relapses within 4 months after the end of the IMRT, with a median overall survival of 7 months. Acute toxicity as the result of radiation was acceptable. Dysphagia and pain were the predominant acute toxicities. In regard to late complications, no myelitis, carotid rupture, or cranial nerve palsy was observed. Osteoradionecrosis of the mandible developed in one patient, and feeding-tube dependency occurred in one patient. No fatal late complications were observed in this group.

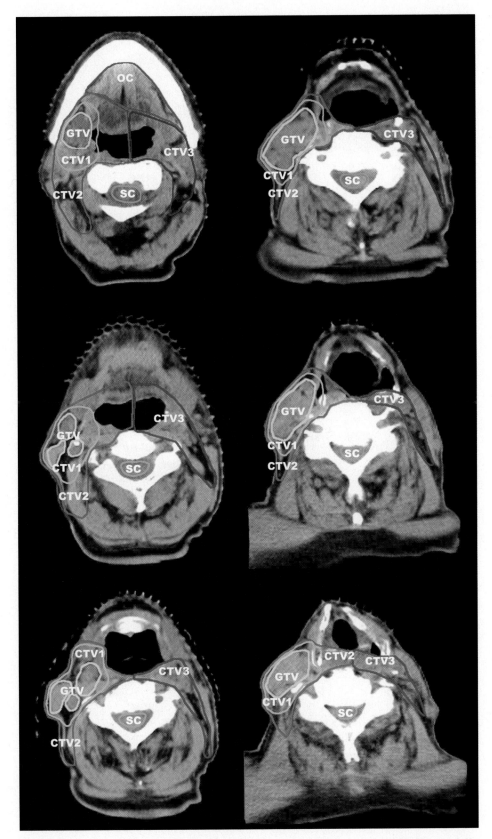

**FIGURE 10-6.** Clinical target volume (CTV) delineation in a patient with T3N2bM0 retromolar trigone carcinoma who received definitive IMRT. CTV1 (*gold yellow line*); CTV2 (*red line*); CTV3 (*dark blue line*); gross tumor volume (GTV) (*yellow line*); oral cavity (OC) (*magenta line*); spinal cord (SC) (*green line*).

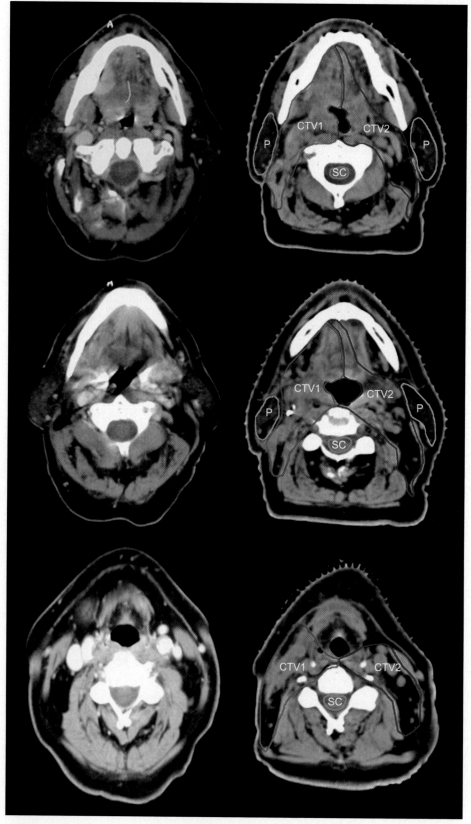

**FIGURE 10-7.** CTV delineation in a patient with T2N2bM0 oral tongue carcinoma who received postoperative IMRT. CTV1 (*red line*); CTV2 (*dark blue line*); right parotid (P) gland (*rust line*); left parotid gland (*aqua line*); spinal cord (SC) (*green line*).

# REFERENCES

1. Byers RM, Anderson B, Schwarz EA, et al. Treatment of squamous carcinoma of the retromolar trigone. *Am J Clin Oncol* 1984;7:647–652.
2. Perez CA. Tonsillar Fossa and Faucial Arc. In: Brady LW, ed. *Principles and Practice of Radiation Oncology, 3rd ed.* Philadelphia: Lippincott-Raven, 1998:1003–1032.
3. Greene FL, American Joint Committee on Cancer, American Cancer Society. *AJCC Cancer Staging Manual, 6th ed.* New York: Springer, 2002.
4. Rouviere H, Tobias MJ. *Anatomy of the Human Lymphatic System.* Ann Arbor, MI: Edwards Brothers, 1938.
5. Lindberg R. Distribution of cervical lymph node metastases from squamous cell carcinoma of the upper respiratory and digestive tracts. *Cancer* 1972;29:1446–1449.
6. Byers RM, Wolf PF, Ballantyne AJ. Rationale for elective modified neck dissection. *Head Neck Surg* 1988;10:160–167.
7. Spiro RH, Spiro JD, Strong EW. Surgical approach to squamous carcinoma confined to the tongue and the floor of the mouth. *Head Neck Surg* 1986;9:27–31.
8. Scholl P, Byers RM, Batsakis JG, et al. Microscopic cut-through of cancer in the surgical treatment of squamous carcinoma of the tongue. Prognostic and therapeutic implications. *Am J Surg* 1986;152:354–360.
9. Emami B. Oral Cavity. In: Brady LW, ed. *Principles and Practice of Radiation Oncology, 3rd ed.* Philadelphia: Lippincott-Raven, 1998:981–1002.
10. Licitra L, Grandi C, Guzzo M, et al. Primary chemotherapy in resectable oral cavity squamous cell cancer: a randomized controlled trial. *J Clin Oncol* 2003;21:327–333.
11. Pignon JP, Bourhis J, Domenge C, et al. Chemotherapy added to locoregional treatment for head and neck squamous-cell carcinoma: three meta-analyses of updated individual data. MACH-NC Collaborative Group. Meta-Analysis of Chemotherapy on Head and Neck Cancer. *Lancet* 2000;355:949–955.
12. Chao KS, Wippold FJ, Ozyigit G, et al. Determination and delineation of nodal target volumes for head-and-neck cancer based on patterns of failure in patients receiving definitive and postoperative IMRT. *Int J Radiat Oncol Biol Phys* 2002;53:1174–1184.
13. Chao KS, Ozyigit G, Tran BN, et al. Patterns of failure in patients receiving definitive and postoperative IMRT for head-and-neck cancer. *Int J Radiat Oncol Biol Phys* 2003;55:312–321.
14. Ozyigit G, Chao KS. Clinical experience of head-and-neck cancer IMRT with serial tomotherapy. *Med Dosim* 2002;27:91–98.
15. Claus F, Duthoy W, Boterberg T, et al. Intensity modulated radiation therapy for oropharyngeal and oral cavity tumors: clinical use and experience. *Oral Oncol* 2002;38:597–604.
16. Kowalski LP, Medina JE. Nodal metastases: predictive factors. *Otolaryngol Clin North Am* 1998;31:621–637.
17. Bloom ND, Spiro RH. Carcinoma of the cheek mucosa. A retrospective analysis. *Am J Surg* 1980;140:556–559.
18. Urist MM, O'Brien CJ, Soong SJ, et al. Squamous cell carcinoma of the buccal mucosa: analysis of prognostic factors. *Am J Surg* 1987;154:411–414.
19. MacComb WS, Fletcher GH. Intra-oral cavity. In: MacComb WS, Fletcher GH, eds. *Cancer of the Head and Neck.* Baltimore: Williams & Wilkins, 1967:179–212.
20. Wang CC. Radiation therapy for head and neck cancers. *Cancer* 1975;36:748–751.
21. Cassisi NJ, Million RR, Mancuso AA, et al. Oral Cavity. In: Million RR, ed. *Management of Head and Neck Cancer: A Multidisciplinary Approach. 2nd ed.* Philadelphia: Lippincott, 1994:321–400.
22. Decroix Y, Ghossein NA. Experience of the Curie Institute in treatment of cancer of the mobile tongue: II. Management of the neck nodes. *Cancer* 1981;47:503–508.
23. Decroix Y, Ghossein NA. Experience of the Curie Institute in treatment of cancer of the mobile tongue: I. Treatment policies and result. *Cancer* 1981;47:496–502.
24. Gilbert EH, Goffinet DR, Bagshaw MA. Carcinoma of the oral tongue and floor of mouth: fifteen years' experience with linear acceleration therapy. *Cancer* 1975;35:1517–1524.
25. Rodgers LW Jr., Stringer SP, Mendenhall WM, et al. Management of squamous cell carcinoma of the floor of mouth. *Head Neck* 1993;15:16–19.
26. Fu KK, Lichter A, Galante M. Carcinoma of the floor of mouth: an analysis of treatment results and the sites and causes of failures. *Int J Radiat Oncol Biol Phys* 1976;1:829–837.
27. Nason RW, Sako K, Beecroft WA, et al. Surgical management of squamous cell carcinoma of the floor of the mouth. *Am J Surg* 1989;158:292–296.

# 11

# OROPHARYNX

## K. S. CLIFFORD CHAO
## GOKHAN OZYIGIT

## 1. ANATOMY

- The oropharynx is the posterior continuation of the oral cavity; it communicates with the nasopharynx above and the laryngopharynx below. It can be subdivided into the palatine (faucial) arch and oropharynx proper.

## 1.1. Tonsillar Fossa and Faucial Arc

- The palatine arch, a junctional area between the oral cavity and the laryngopharynx, is formed by the soft palate and the uvula superiorly, the anterior tonsillar pillar and glossopalatine sulcus laterally, and the glossopharyngeal sulcus and the base of the tongue (BOT) inferiorly.
- Figure 11-1 shows a coronal section of the oropharynx with relationships in the parapharyngeal regions.
- The retromolar trigone has been included in the structures of the faucial arch, although it is actually located within the oral cavity. Its apex is in line with the tuberosity of the maxilla (behind the last upper molar); the lateral border extends upward into the buccal mucosa; medially, it blends with the anterior tonsillar pillar; and its base is formed by the distal surface of the last lower molar and the adjacent gingivolingual sulcus.
- The lateral walls of the oropharynx are limited posteriorly by the tonsillar fossa and posterior tonsillar pillar (pharyngopalatine folds). These pillars are folds of mucous membrane that cover the underlying glossopalatine and pharyngopalatine muscles. Deep to the lateral wall of the tonsillar fossa are the superior constrictor muscles of the pharynx, upper fibers of the middle constrictor, pharyngeus and stylopharyngeus muscles, and glossopalatine and pharyngopalatine muscles. The tonsillar fossa continues into the lateral and posterior pharyngeal walls.
- The tonsillar fossa and faucial arch have a rich submucosal lymphatic network that is laterally grouped in four to six lymphatic ducts that drain into the subdigastric, upper cervical, and parapharyngeal lymph nodes. Sub-

maxillary lymph nodes may be affected in lesions involving the retromolar trigone, the buccal mucosa, or even the BOT.

## 1.2. Base of Tongue

- The BOT is bounded anteriorly by the circumvallate papillae, laterally by the glossopharyngeal sulci and oropharyngeal walls, and inferiorly by the glossoepiglottic fossae or valleculae and the pharyngoepiglottic fold.
- The vallecula is the transition zone between the BOT and the epiglottis and is considered a part of the BOT.
- The surface of the tongue is irregular because of the submucosal lymphoid follicles, but the mucous membrane is smooth when compared with the dorsum of the oral tongue. The lymphoid tissue at the BOT does not penetrate the intrinsic tongue muscles.
- The BOT is almost parallel to the posterior pharyngeal wall. Its musculature is continuous with that of the oral tongue and the floor of the mouth anteriorly. The genioglossus fibers fan out in the tongue to interdigitate with the intrinsic tongue musculature (Fig. 11-2). The tongue base also is continuous with the preepiglottic space.

## 2. NATURAL HISTORY

## 2.1. Tonsil

- Many tonsillar tumors are keratinizing squamous cell carcinomas, which can be graded I to IV, depending on the degree of differentiation.
- Carcinomas arising in the faucial arch tend to be keratinizing and more differentiated than those of the tonsillar fossa.
- Tonsillar fossa lesions tend to be infiltrative, often involving the adjacent retromolar trigone, soft palate, and BOT. Perez[1] reported that the primary tumor was confined to the tonsillar fossa in only 5.4% of 384 patients;

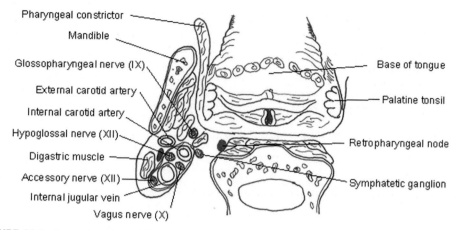

**FIGURE 11-1.** Coronal section of the oropharynx showing relationships in the parapharyngeal regions.

65% had involvement of the soft palate, and 41% had extension into the BOT.

- Tumors of the faucial arch can be superficially spreading, exophytic, ulcerative, or infiltrative; the last two types are frequently combined. They become extensive and involve the adjacent hard palate or buccal mucosa in less than 20% of patients.[1]
- Tumors of the tonsillar fossa have a high incidence of lymph node metastases (60%–70%); most are in the subdigastric lymph nodes, midjugular chain, and submaxillary lymph nodes (in lesions extending anteriorly); 5% to 10% involve the posterior cervical lymph nodes (Table 11-1).[1]

- Metastases in the low cervical chain occur in approximately 5% to 15% of patients with upper cervical lymph node involvement.[1]
- The incidence of metastatic lymph nodes in the neck increases with tumor stage. Less than 10% of T1 lesions, 30% of T2 lesions, and 65% to 70% of T3 and T4 lesions have metastatic cervical lymph nodes.[1]
- Contralateral lymphadenopathy in tonsillar tumors is noted in 10% to 15% of patients with positive ipsilateral lymph nodes, more frequently if the primary tumor extends to or beyond the midline (Table 11-2).[1]
- Tonsillar pillar and soft palate lesions have an overall metastatic rate of approximately 45%. Initially, the most

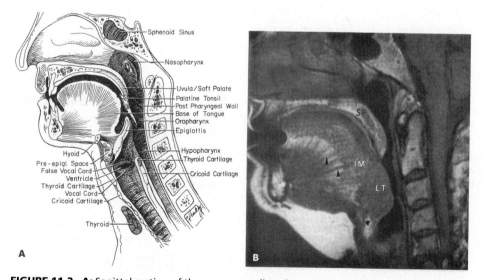

**FIGURE 11-2. A:** Sagittal section of the upper aerodigestive tract. **B:** Sagittal magnetic resonance imaging (MRI). Lymphoid tissue (*LT*) at the tongue base does not penetrate the intrinsic tongue muscles (*IM*); it is limited to the surface. Genioglossus fibers fan out in the tongue (*arrowheads*) to finally interdigitate with the intrinsic tongue musculature. The tongue base is continuous with the preepiglottic space (*arrow*). Areas of high signal intensity within soft palate (*SP*) are the result of its fatty content. (From: Million RR, Cassisi NJ, Mancuso AA. Oropharynx. In: Million RR, Cassisi NJ, eds. *Management of Head and Neck Cancer: A Multidisciplinary Approach, 2nd ed.* Philadelphia: JB Lippincott, 1994:402, with permission.)

**TABLE 11-1. INCIDENCE AND DISTRIBUTION OF METASTATIC DISEASE IN NEGATIVE (N−) AND POSITIVE (N+) NECK NODES (%)**

| Clinical presentation | Radiologically Enlarged Retropharyngeal Nodes | | Pathologic Nodal Metastasis | | | | | | | | | |
|---|---|---|---|---|---|---|---|---|---|---|---|---|
| | | | Level I | | Level II | | Level III | | Level IV | | Level V | |
| | N− | N+ | N− | N+ | N− | N+ | N− | N+ | N− | N+ | N− | N+ |
| Tonsil | 4 | 0 | 19 | 14 | 9 | 5 | 4 | 0 | 19 | 14 | 9 | 5 |
| Base of tongue | 0 | 6 | 4 | 19 | 30 | 89 | 22 | 22 | 7 | 10 | 0 | 18 |

Modified from: Chao KS, Wippold FJ, Ozyigit G, et al. Determination and delineation of nodal target volumes for head and neck cancer based on the patterns of failure in patients receiving definitive and postoperative IMRT. *Int J Radiat Oncol Biol Phys* 2002;53:1174–1184, with permission.

frequent site of nodal involvement is the jugulodigastric lymph nodes. Approximately 10% of patients have submaxillary lymph node involvement. Tumors of the retromolar trigone, anterior faucial pillar, and soft palate rarely metastasize to the posterior cervical lymph nodes. Contralateral spread is infrequent (10%).[1]

## 2.2. Base of Tongue

- Squamous cell carcinoma of the BOT tends to have early, silent, and deep infiltration; therefore, it is difficult to estimate tumor extension by clinical examination. However, tumors originating from the peripheral regions usually remain there.[2–4]
- BOT cancers have little tendency to spread to the palatine tonsils, whereas tonsillar cancers tend to invade the BOT.
- Vallecular lesions are often exophytic and invade along the mucosa to the lingual surface of the epiglottis, laterally along the pharyngoepiglottic fold, and then to the lateral pharyngeal wall and anterior wall of the pyriform sinus.
- The first echelon nodes are the subdigastric (level II nodes), then along the jugular chain to the midjugular

and lower jugular nodes. If anterior extension into the oral tongue or massive upper neck disease is present, then the submandibular lymph nodes may be involved. The posterior cervical lymph nodes are often involved, but submental spread is rare.
- Bilateral and contralateral lymphatic spread is common (Fig. 11-3). Retrograde spread to retropharyngeal lymph nodes has been reported particularly in advanced lesions.[2–4]
- The deeply infiltrating nature of BOT cancers correlates with the high frequency of lymphatic metastases at presentation (80% of patients overall, with bilateral spread in 37%–55%).[2–6]
- The incidence of clinically positive neck node at presentation is approximately 50% to 83% (Table 11-3).
- The incidence of pathologically positive neck node in clinical N0 neck is approximately 22% to 33%. Contralateral lymphatic metastasis at presentation is 37% (Table 11-2).[2–4] Table 11-1 shows the percentage of the incidence and distribution of metastatic disease in clinically negative and positive neck nodes in BOT cancers.

## 3. DIAGNOSIS AND STAGING SYSTEM

### 3.1. Signs and Symptoms

#### 3.1.1. Tonsil

- Sore throat is the most frequent symptom. Asymptomatic lesions are frequently found on routine examination.
- Dysphagia or otalgia is related to the anastomotic-tympanic nerve of Jacobson.
- Trismus may be a late manifestation if the masseter or pterygoid muscle is involved.
- Invasion of the tongue will eventually limit tongue mobility. Ulceration at the junction of the anterior tonsillar pillar and oral tongue can cause a great deal of pain.
- Tumors of the tonsillar fossa have similar signs and symptoms, except that the lesions tend to be larger before symptoms develop. Ipsilateral sore throat and otalgia are the hallmarks of these lesions.

**TABLE 11-2. INCIDENCE OF CONTRALATERAL OR BILATERAL NECK NODE METASTASES BY PRIMARY TUMOR SITE**

| Tumor Site | cN+, Bilateral | cN+, Contralateral Only | cN−, pN+ Bilateral |
|---|---|---|---|
| Tonsil | 16% | 2% | — |
| Base of tongue | 37% | — | 55% |

c, clinical; p, pathologic.
Modified from: Chao KS, Wippold FJ, Ozyigit G, et al. Determination and delineation of nodal target volumes for head and neck cancer based on the patterns of failure in patients receiving definitive and postoperative IMRT. *Int J Radiat Oncol Biol Phys* 2002;53:1174–1184, with permission.

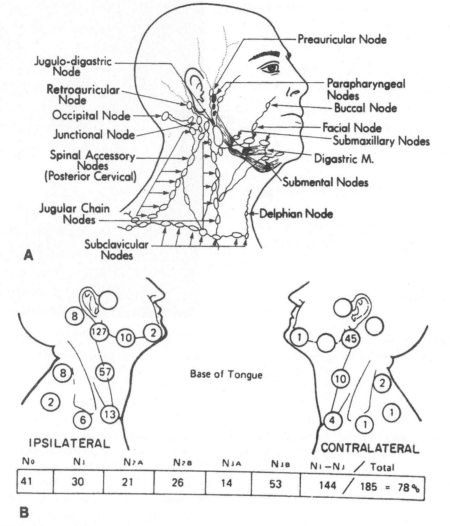

**FIGURE 11-3. A:** Lymphatics of head and neck. Both deep *(shaded)* parapharyngeal and superficial nodes (jugulodigastric) are commonly involved. (From: Base of tongue. In: Chao KS, Perez CA, Brady LW, eds. *Radiation Oncology: Management Decisions, 1st ed.* Philadelphia: Lippincott-Raven, 1999:246.) **B:** Distribution of nodal involvement at presentation of squamous cell carcinoma of base of the tongue (BOT). (From: Lindberg RD. Distribution of cervical lymph node metastases from squamous cell carcinoma of the upper respiratory and digestive tract. *Cancer* 1972;29:1446–1449, with permission.)

**TABLE 11-3. CLINICALLY DETECTED NODAL METASTASES (%) ON ADMISSION BY T STAGE OF BASE OF TONGUE CARCINOMAS (2,328 PATIENTS)**

|  | N0 | N1 | N2, N3 |
|---|---|---|---|
| T1 | 26–30 | 15–28 | 46–55 |
| T2 | 26–29 | 14–36 | 38–56 |
| T3 | 26–30 | 23 | 47–52 |
| T4 | 16–24 | 8–26 | 50–76 |

Compiled from the data of the Curie Institute,[5] Memorial Sloan-Kettering Cancer Center,[6] and M. D. Anderson Cancer Center.[3]

- Lymphomas of the tonsil tend to be large submucosal masses but may ulcerate and appear similar to carcinomas.

### 3.1.2. Base of Tongue

- The BOT is visualized only by indirect mirror examination, so earlier diagnosis is rare. The earliest symptom is mild sore throat. Many of the early lesions are asymptomatic and relatively silent, and a subdigastric neck mass is frequently the first sign.
- Necrosis and internal bleeding may cause sudden enlargement and mild tenderness.

- Dysphagia, a nasal quality to the voice, and deep-seated otalgia occur with enlargement of the mass. Otalgia is associated with tumor involvement of the retropharyngeal space.
- Hypoglossal nerve invasion is rare but can cause unilateral paralysis and atrophy of the tongue when it does occur.

## 3.2. Physical Examination

### 3.2.1. Tonsil

- Indirect mirror examination and digital palpation are required for diagnosis.
- In addition to a complete history and physical examination, a complete examination of the head and neck is mandatory.

### 3.2.2. Base of Tongue

- Early lesions are usually submucosal and relatively soft. Because the surface of the BOT is irregular, it is difficult to palpate the mass. Rigid or flexible endoscopes permit examination in some patients.
- Palpation through the lateral floor of the mouth can be helpful to detect anterior extension.
- Fullness in the soft tissue around the hyoid bone may be a sign of inferior penetration through the valleculae.
- Fixation of the tongue causes incomplete protrusion to the site that is fixed.

## 3.3. Imaging

- The main imaging tools of the oropharyngeal region are computed tomography (CT) and magnetic resonance imaging (MRI).
- CT is better for the lymph nodes and bone detail, so it is the preferred initial study. MRI is used adjunctively.
- Evaluation of the BOT should include slices from the nasopharynx to the lower neck. Axial sections are often sufficient; however, coronal sections may be required when lesions invade the base of the skull. Sagittal MRI is necessary for detection of early preepiglottic space invasion.
- CT and MRI sections of this region require injection of contrast media. Contiguous 3- to 4-mm slices should be used through the primary tumor and neck. It is important to keep the field of view small so that the pictures are magnified and spatial resolution is optimized. Evaluation of the BOT must include a complete CT study of the cervical and retropharyngeal nodes (Fig. 11-4).
- CT and MRI are excellent for showing the deep structures surrounding the pharynx. The deep tissue planes are generally symmetric, and obliteration of the deep fat spaces, such as the parapharyngeal space or invasion of

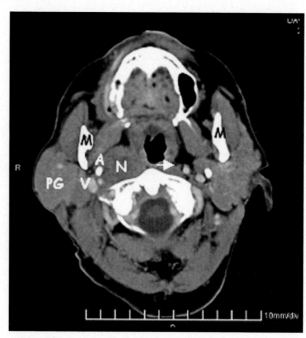

**FIGURE 11-4.** Computed tomography (CT) study shows an enlarged retropharyngeal lymph node (*N*). The node lies medial to the carotid artery (*A*), parotid gland (*PG*), and jugular vein (*JV*). A more normal-sized retropharyngeal node (*arrow*) is present on the opposite side. *M*, mandible.

deep musculature, is a sign of invasion. Such spread is frequently not expressed as signs and symptoms or detected by physical examination. The pharyngeal wall becomes tightly surrounded by musculature, and the intervening fat planes are less visible lower in the oropharynx, making diagnosis of invasion more difficult.

- Lymphoid tissue is present throughout the oropharynx and is responsible for most of the variation seen in the surface contours on CT and MRI. Inexperienced interpreters may frequently misinterpret various bumps and bulges on the mucosal surfaces for tumors. These regions should either be ignored or be used as prompts to look for adjacent deep infiltration as a sign of pathology. These surfaces are best evaluated by physical examination, not by CT or MRI. There are no findings that can distinguish lymphoid tissue and other benign mucosal lesions from cancer other than infiltration of the deeper structures.
- Any tumor that is suspicious for deep infiltration should be studied primarily with CT. A significant portion of MRI studies in this area will be of low quality because of motion artifacts. In general, MRI is preferred for the evaluation of the parapharyngeal space.
- The relationship of tumor margins to both lingual neurovascular bundles can be anticipated on imaging with far greater precision than on physical examination. Occasionally, retrograde spread of tumor out of the tongue along the lingular neurovascular bundles to the external carotid artery will be visible.

- Tumors in the region may also grow onto the styloid musculature. Inferior growth along the mylohyoid and hyoglossus muscles may bring the tumor to the insertion of these muscles on the hyoid bone, and there may be direct extension into the soft tissues of the suprahyoid and infrahyoid neck at that point. Occult spread from the BOT to the preepiglottic space may also be visualized.

## 3.4. Staging

- The American Joint Committee on Cancer staging system for carcinoma of the oropharynx is shown in Table 11-4.[7]

## 4. PROGNOSTIC FACTORS

### 4.1. Tonsil

- *Stage:* The stage of primary tumor and presence of involved cervical lymph nodes have a significant correlation with local control and survival.[8–11]
- *Treatment-related factors:* External-beam dose and fractionation schedule also significantly influence local control.[11] Cause-specific survival rate is influenced by planned neck dissection.[11]
- *Histologic differentiation:* Multivariate analysis revealed that survival was significantly influenced by histologic differentiation.[11]

### TABLE 11-4. TNM CLASSIFICATION FOR CARCINOMA OF THE OROPHARYNX

**Primary tumor (T)**

| | |
|---|---|
| TX | Primary tumor cannot be assessed |
| T0 | No evidence of primary tumor |
| Tis | Carcinoma *in situ* |
| T1 | Tumor ≤2 cm in greatest dimension |
| T2 | Tumor >2 cm but not >4 cm in greatest dimension |
| T3 | Tumor >4 cm in greatest dimension |
| T4a | Tumor invades the larynx, deep extrinsic muscle of tongue, medial pterygoid, mandible, and hard palate |
| T4b | Tumor invades lateral the pterygoid muscle, pterygoid plates, lateral nasopharynx, or skull base or encases carotid artery |

**Regional lymph nodes (N)**

| | |
|---|---|
| NX | Regional lymph nodes cannot be assessed |
| N0 | No regional lymph node metastasis |
| N1 | Metastasis in a single ipsilateral lymph node, ≤3 cm in greatest dimension |
| N2 | Metastasis in a single ipsilateral lymph node, >3 cm but not >6 cm in greatest dimension; in multiple ipsilateral lymph nodes, none >6 cm in greatest dimension; or in bilateral or contralateral lymph nodes, none >6 cm in greatest dimension |
| N2a | Metastasis in a single ipsilateral lymph node >3 cm but not >6 cm in greatest dimension |
| N2b | Metastasis in multiple ipsilateral lymph nodes, none >6 cm in greatest dimension |
| N2c | Metastasis in bilateral or contralateral lymph nodes, none >6 cm in greatest dimension |
| N3 | Metastasis in a lymph node >6 cm in greatest dimension |

**Distant metastases (M)**

| | |
|---|---|
| MX | Presence of distant metastasis cannot be assessed |
| M0 | No distant metastasis |
| M1 | Distant metastasis |

*Stage grouping*

| | | | |
|---|---|---|---|
| Stage 0 | Tis | N0 | M0 |
| Stage I | T1 | N0 | M0 |
| Stage II | T2 | N0 | M0 |
| Stage III | T3 | N0 | M0 |
| | T1 | N1 | M0 |
| | T2 | N1 | M0 |
| | T3 | N1 | M0 |
| Stage IVA | T4a | N0 or N1 | M0 |
| | T1–T4a | N2 | M0 |
| Stage IVB | T4b | Any N | M0 |
| | Any T | N3 | M0 |
| Stage IVC | Any T | Any N | M1 |

From: Greene FL, American Joint Committee on Cancer, American Cancer Society. *AJCC Cancer Staging Manual, 6th ed.* New York: Springer, 2002, with permission.

## 4.2. Base of Tongue

- *Tumor size and extent:* BOT cancers have a worse prognosis than those in the oral tongue because of greater size at diagnosis, more frequent spread to adjacent structures, and higher rate of lymphatic spread. However, stage for stage, they may have a prognosis similar to that of oral tongue cancers.[12]
- *Stage:* One of the most dominant prognostic factors is tumor stage.[12]
- *Overall treatment time:* Survival and locoregional control become worse when overall treatment time increases.[12]
- *Histopathologic grade:* Poorly differentiated or undifferentiated carcinomas are shown to have better survival and local control rates.[5]
- *Other:* Other prognosticators include age (better survival >45 years) and extension to both epilarynx and endolarynx (associated with poor survival).[5,13]

## 5. GENERAL MANAGEMENT

- Surgery or radiation is equally successful in controlling early stage oropharyngeal cancer. Radiation may be the preferred modality where the functional deficit will be great, such as the tongue base or tonsil. A total of 175 patients with American Joint Committee on Cancer (AJCC) stage I and II oropharyngeal carcinoma were treated with external beam radiotherapy at M. D. Anderson Cancer Center.[14] The actuarial 5-year locoregional control and disease-free survival rates were 81% and 77%, respectively.

- The management of advanced stage carcinomas of the oropharynx requires a multidisciplinary approach to establish optimal treatment. In general, the preferred treatment has been to combine surgery with postoperative radiation therapy. This approach has become the standard in this specific grouping whenever it can be applied. Aggressive radiation therapy alone will give equivalent control rates to surgery for cancers originating in the tonsil.

## 5.1. Tonsillar Fossa and Faucial Arc

### 5.1.1. Tumors of Tonsillar Fossa

- Tables 11-5 and 11-6 show the initial local control rates for carcinoma of the tonsil according to T stages with different treatment strategies.
- Table 11-7 summarizes the disease-specific survival of patients with carcinoma of the tonsil.
- T1 or T2 lesions can be treated with irradiation or surgery alone.
- T1, T2, and T3 tumors are treated with irradiation alone (60–75 Gy in 6–8 weeks, depending on stage). Regional lymph nodes are treated with 50 Gy (subclinical disease) to 75 Gy depending on nodal involvement. Interstitial brachytherapy has been used to deliver an additional dose (25–30 Gy) to the primary tumor.[15]
- In T3 and T4 tumors, a combination of irradiation and surgery has been advocated because of the higher incidence of recurrences with either modality alone.[9,10,16] These lesions are treated with radical tonsillectomy with ipsilateral neck dissection followed by irradiation (50–60 Gy), depending on the status of the surgical margins and extent of cervical lymph node involvement.[17]

**TABLE 11-5. CARCINOMA OF THE TONSIL: INITIAL LOCAL CONTROL ACCORDING TO T STAGES WITH IRRADIATION ALONE**

| Author | Stage | | | | | | | |
|---|---|---|---|---|---|---|---|---|
| | T1 | | T2 | | T3 | | T4 | |
| | N | % | N | % | N | % | N | % |
| Amornmarn et al.[36] | 4/4 | 100 | 7/8 | 88 | 21/38 | 55 | 5/20 | 25 |
| Bataini et al.[8] | 32/36 | 89 | 78/93 | 84 | 111/173 | 64 | 77/163 | 47 |
| Dubois et al.[37] | 34/49 | 69 | 39/84 | 46 | 7/82 | 9 | — | — |
| Fayos and Lampe[38] | 8/10 | 80 | 36/47 | 77 | 12/31 | 39 | 4/14 | 29 |
| Lusinchi et al.[39] | 42/48 | 88 | 114/145 | 79 | — | — | — | — |
| Mantravadi et al.[40] | 3/3 | 100 | 16/21 | 76 | 20/61 | 33 | 1/9 | 11 |
| Mendenhall et al.[41] | 4/4 | 100 | 17/18 | 94 | 23/31 | 74 | 5/12 | 42 |
| Perez et al.[42] | 14/16 | 87 | 26/41 | 63 | 31/41 | 76 | 19/36 | 53 |
| Total | 141/170 | 83 | 333/457 | 73 | 225/457 | 50 | 111/254 | 44 |

**TABLE 11-6. CARCINOMA OF THE TONSIL: LOCAL CONTROL ACCORDING TO T STAGES**

| | Treatment | N | T1 | T2 | T3 | T4 | Overall |
|---|---|---|---|---|---|---|---|
| | | | Local Control Rates (%) | | | | |
| Perez et al.[42] | S+RT | 230 | 80 | 71 | 65 | 58 | 68 |
| Foote et al.[16] | S±RT | 72 | 78 | 76 | 44 | — | 71 |
| Pernot et al.[43] | RT-Ir192 | 361 | 89 | 85 | 67 | — | 80 |
| Bataini et al.[8] | RT | 465 | 90 | 84 | 64 | 47 | 64 |
| Wong et al.[44] | RT | 150 | 94 | 81 | 67 | 63 | 75 |
| Perez et al.[42] | RT | 154 | 76 | 63 | 59 | 33 | 56 |
| Amornmarn et al.[36] | RT | 185 | 94 | 80 | 51 | 19 | 58 |
| Mendenhall et al.[41] | RT | 400 | 83 | 81 | 74 | 60 | 76 |

S, surgery; RT, radiation therapy; N, number of patients.

## 5.1.2. Tumors of Faucial Arch

- T1 lesions less than 1 cm in diameter are treated with wide surgical resection or irradiation alone (60–65 Gy in 6–7 weeks).[18,19]
- T2 tumors require more extensive surgical procedures, including partial resection of the mandible if there is bone involvement.[20] Because of the tendency of these tumors to extend to the midline, the site of lymph node metastasis is less predictable; therefore, neck dissection should be performed only in patients with palpable cervical lymph nodes.
- T2 tumors can also be treated with irradiation alone (65–70 Gy). Irradiation has the advantage of treating subclinical disease in the neck (50 Gy total dose).[18,21]
- Interstitial brachytherapy (20–30 Gy) in the primary tumor has been combined with external irradiation (50 Gy).
- In more extensive lesions, preoperative or postoperative irradiation can be used in doses similar to those used in the tonsil.

## 5.2. Base of Tongue

- Exophytic or surface tumors respond well to irradiation alone. Ulcerative, endophytic cancers that are partly or completely fixed require surgery.[22,23]
- When all stages are considered, overall treatment results for BOT cancer seem to be most optimal for combinations of surgery and irradiation when compared with conventional irradiation alone.

### 5.2.1. Surgical Management

- Radical neck dissection yields information to determine whether postoperative irradiation is required, which is recommended for patients with disease more extensive than stage N1 or with extracapsular extension.
- Thawley et al.[24] reported that 47% of patients treated with combined surgery and preoperative irradiation had the mandible preserved.
- Tumors of the lower BOT that involve the valleculae and extend inferiorly to the supraglottic larynx and pyriform

**TABLE 11-7. TONSIL CARCINOMA: DISEASE-SPECIFIC SURVIVAL RATES**

| | Treatment | No. of Patients | Stage IV Disease (%) | 5-Yr Cause-Specific Survival Rate |
|---|---|---|---|---|
| Givens et al.[9] | S+RT | 22 | 68 | 32 |
| Pernot et al.[43] | RT-Ir192 | 361 | 8 | 63 |
| Wong et al.[44] | RT | 150 | — | 70 |
| Gwozdz et al.[45] | RT | 83 | 53 | 71 |
| Garrett et al.[46] | RT | 372 | 54 | 54 |
| Amornmarn et al.[36] | RT | 185 | 46 | 42 |
| Mendenhall et al.[41] | RT | 400 | 56 | 70 |

S, surgery; RT, radiation therapy.

**TABLE 11-8. BASE OF TONGUE: LOCAL CONTROL RESULTS CORRELATED WITH T STAGE (IRRADIATION ALONE)**

| | Local Control by T Stage | | | |
| --- | --- | --- | --- | --- |
| | **T1** | **T2** | **T3** | **T4** |
| Puthawala et al.[47] | 2/2 (100%) | 14/16 (88%) | 30/40 (75%) | 8/12 (67%) |
| Crook et al.[22] | 11/13 (85%) | 25/35 (71%) | No data | No data |
| Spanos et al.[48] | 29/32 (91%) | 35/49 (71%) | 50/64 (78%) | 15/29 (52%) |
| Foote et al.[49] | 8/9 (89%) | 27/30 (90%) | 25/31 (81%) | 5/14 (36%) |
| Wang[50] | 35/40 (89%) | 55/69 (79%) | 37/78 (48%) | 8/37 (21%) |
| Brunin et al.[5] | 27/29 (93%) | 35/56 (63%) | 42/95 (44%) | 8/36 (23%) |
| Harrison et al.[6] | 14/17 (87%) | 29/31 (93%) | 14/18 (82%) | 2/2 (100%) |
| Chao et al.[51] | 10/18 (55%) | 14/23 (61%) | 8/16 (50%) | 5/11 (45%) |
| **Total** | **136/160 (85%)** | **234/309 (76%)** | **206/342 (60%)** | **51/141 (36%)** |

sinus may be controlled by partial glossectomy and subtotal supraglottic laryngectomy or partial laryngopharyngectomy with preservation of voice.[24,25]

- Prerequisites for a subtotal supraglottic laryngectomy include no gross involvement of pharyngoepiglottic fold, preservation of one lingual artery, resection of less than 80% of the BOT, pulmonary function suitable for supraglottic laryngectomy, and medical condition suitable for a major operation.
- Locoregional control is approximately 48% with surgery alone.[26]

### 5.2.2. Irradiation Alone

- Doses to the primary tumor and palpable lymph nodes range from 65 to 75 Gy delivered in 6.5 to 7.5 weeks. Doses for elective irradiation of subclinical, microscopic lymphatic metastases should be at least 50 Gy.
- Small T1 and T2 BOT tumors without significant infiltration and surface or exophytic T2 and T3 lesions of the glossopharyngeal sulcus (glossopalatine sulcus) are controlled by high-dose radiation, with locoregional control of 70%.[22]

- Large, unresectable BOT cancers that cross the midline, infiltrate, and fix the tongue are often irradiated palliatively to achieve as much tumor regression as possible.
- Local control results correlated with T and N stage, and disease-specific survival rates according to T and N stage in the literature are summarized in Tables 11-8, 11-9, and 11-10, respectively.

### 5.2.3. Combined Surgery and Irradiation

- Surgery combined with irradiation is best suited for larger tumors that extend beyond the BOT or infiltrate and partially fix the tongue.
- Adjuvant irradiation should be routinely used for resectable T3 and T4 BOT cancers to reduce the likelihood of recurrence.[24]
- Bilateral fields covering the primary site and upper necks are necessary because of the significant primary tumor burden and high rate of contralateral and bilateral lymphatic spread.
- To eradicate residual microscopic disease, doses of 56 to 60 Gy (66 Gy for positive margins or extracapsular ex-

**TABLE 11-9. BASE OF TONGUE: LOCAL CONTROL RESULTS CORRELATED WITH N STAGE (IRRADIATION ALONE)**

| | Local Control by N Stage (%) | | |
| --- | --- | --- | --- |
| | **N0** | **N1** | **N2–3** |
| Brunin et al.[5] | 39/68 (57%) | 25/56 (46%) | 47/92 (51%) |
| Harrison et al.[6] | 6/10 (60%) | 21/24 (87%) | 31/32 (96%) |
| Wang[50] | 53/75 (71%) | 23/42 (55%) | 59/107 (55%) |
| Chao et al.[51] | 21/23 (91%) | 7/10 (70%) | 24/35 (68%) |
| **Total** | **119/176 (64%)** | **69/122 (68%)** | **161/266 (61%)** |

**TABLE 11-10. BASE OF TONGUE: DISEASE-SPECIFIC SURVIVAL RATES CORRELATED WITH T AND N STAGE (IRRADIATION ALONE)**

|  | Massachusetts General Hospital[50] | | Curie Institute[5] | | Washington University[51] | |
|---|---|---|---|---|---|---|
|  | DSS | N | DSS | N | DSS | N |
| T1 | 78% | 40 | 60% | 29 | 18 | 61% |
| T2 | 76% | 69 | 42% | 56 | 23 | 65% |
| T3 | 40% | 78 | 29% | 95 | 16 | 39% |
| T4 | 16% | 37 | 20% | 36 | 11 | 42% |
| N0 | 67% | 75 | 48% | 68 | 23 | 59% |
| N1 | 56% | 42 | 32% | 56 | 10 | 50% |
| N2–3 | 42% | 107 | 27% | 92 | 35 | 41% |

DSS, disease-specific survival; N, number of patients.

tension) may be delivered to the primary tumor bed and necks beginning 4 to 6 weeks after surgery.
- Locoregional control ranges from 57% to 84% with the combined approach (Table 11-11).

## 5.3. Chemotherapy

- In a meta-analysis of 63 trials (10,741 patients), locoregional treatment with chemotherapy yielded a pooled hazard ratio of death of 0.90 (95% CI 0.85–0.94, $P <$ .0001), corresponding to an absolute survival benefit of 4% at 2 and 5 years compared with patients receiving no chemotherapy.[27] There was no significant benefit associated with adjuvant or neoadjuvant chemotherapy in this analysis; however, the potential benefit should be further evaluated.
- Chemotherapy given concomitantly with radiotherapy demonstrated significant benefits that were revealed in several randomized trials.[28–31] In a multi-institutional study, Calais et al.[30] demonstrated improved 3-year locoregional control (66% vs. 47%) and overall survival (51% vs. 31%) in the concomitant chemoradiation arm

in 226 patients with oropharyngeal cancer by using 70 Gy conventional radiation with carboplatin and 5-FU starting on days 1, 22, and 43 versus radiotherapy alone.
- Altered fractionation schemes with concurrent chemotherapy were also shown to be effective in improving survival. Jeremic et al.[31] established 5-year survival of 46% (vs. 25%) by using 77 Gy (1.1 Gy twice/day) with cisplatin (6 mg/m$^2$/d).
- Newer drug combinations, usually containing cisplatin, have shown high complete response rates in nonkeratinizing head and neck cancers and may improve results of treatment.[32–34] Currently, Radiation Therapy Oncology Group phase III trial H-0129 is retrieving patients with advanced head and neck cancer for concurrent chemoradiation to determine whether intensification of radiation with concomitant boost schedule, relative to conventional fractionation plus cisplatin in the combined therapy setting, can further improve overall survival.
- Agents that selectively enhance the effects of irradiation in the tumor are under investigation, such as hypoxic cell sensitizers, chemical modifiers, hyperthermia, and high linear energy transfer irradiation.

**TABLE 11-11. LOCOREGIONAL CONTROL AND DISEASE-SPECIFIC SURVIVAL RATES FOR POSTOPERATIVE RADIOTHERAPY SERIES**

|  | Primary Site | Neck | Disease-Specific Survival |
|---|---|---|---|
| Goffinet et al.[52] | 64% (9/14) | 50% (7/14) | NA (6/14)* |
| Kraus et al.[53] | 80% (50/63) | 82% (52/63) | 61% |
| Chao et al.[51] | 85% (79/93) | 89% (83/93) | 57% |
| **Total** | **82% (164/201)** | **84% (168/201)** | **57%–64%** |

NA, not available.
*Of fourteen patients, six died of disease.

## 6. INTENSITY-MODULATED RADIATION THERAPY IN OROPHARYNX CANCER

### 6.1. Target Volume Determination

- Gross tumor volume for oropharyngeal carcinoma is the volume seen on CT or MRI.
- If chemotherapy was delivered before radiation, the targets should be outlined on the CT planning according to their pre-chemotherapy extent.
- Lymph node groups at risk in the oropharyngeal region include the following:

  a. Submandibular nodes (surgical level I): all cases.
  b. Upper deep jugular (junctional, parapharyngeal) nodes: all cases.
  c. Subdigastric (jugulodigastric) nodes, midjugular, lower neck, and supraclavicular nodes (levels II–IV): all cases.
  d. Posterior cervical nodes (level V): when levels II and III are involved.
  e. Retropharyngeal nodes: all cases.

- The target volume specification for definitive and postoperative intensity-modulated radiation therapy (IMRT) in oropharyngeal cancer is summarized in Table 7-5.
- Suggested target volume determination for oropharyngeal carcinoma is shown in Table 11-12.

### 6.2. Target Volume Delineation

#### 6.2.1. Tonsil

- Clinical target volume (CTV)1 and CTV2 delineation in a patient with clinically T1N2bM0 squamous cell carcinoma of the tonsil who received definitive IMRT is shown in Figure 11-5. This patient presented with a palpable sore throat and a right-sided neck mass in which squamous cell of the right tonsil was discovered. The tumor was confined in the right tonsillar fossa, not extending to the BOT or pharyngeal wall. There were two lymph nodes noted: one in the right level II area (measuring 3 × 3 cm) and one in the junction of the level III and level V area. He was given concomitant chemotherapy and definitive IMRT.
- CTV1 and CTV2 delineation in a patient with clinically T1N0M0 squamous cell carcinoma of the tonsil who received ipsilateral postoperative IMRT is shown in Figure 11-6. The patient presented with an enlarged right tonsil. CT showed an enlarged tonsil, and no lymphadenopathy was seen. The patient underwent bilateral tonsillectomy, and the final diagnosis was confirmed as squamous cell carcinoma. The patient was treated with postoperative IMRT. The contralateral neck was not treated.
- CTV1 and CTV2 delineation in a patient with clinically T2N2a squamous cell carcinoma of the tonsil who received postoperative IMRT is shown in Figure 11-7. The

*Text continues on page 180.*

**TABLE 11-12. TARGET VOLUME DETERMINATION GUIDELINES FOR OROPHARYNGEAL TUMORS**

| Tumor Site | Clinical Presentation | CTV1 | CTV2 | CTV3 |
|---|---|---|---|---|
| **Tonsil** | T1 and T2 N0 | GTVp | — | IN* (I_b–V) |
| | T3 and T4 N0 | GTVp | Optional@ | IN+CN (I_b–V, RPLN) |
| | Any T N+ | GTVp+n | IN (adjacent LNs†) | IN+CN+RPLN‡ (remaining LNs) |
| **BOT** | Any T N0 | GTVp | Optional@ | IN+CN (I_b–V, RPLN)‡ |
| **Soft palate** | Any T N+ | GTVp+n | IN (adjacent LNs†) | IN+CN+RPLN‡ (remaining LNs) |

BOT, base of tongue; N0, node negative neck; N+, node positive neck; GTVp, primary gross tumor volume; n, nodal gross tumor volume; IN, ipsilateral nodal levels; CN, contralateral nodal levels; RPLN, retropharyngeal lymph node; CTV, clinical target volume.
Roman numerals represent neck nodal levels.
*CN optional for local extension.
†Two to 3 cm from CTV1 nodal basin.
‡Include RPLN for midline and more advanced tumors.
Suggested IMRT dose schedule for chemoradiation: CTV1 = 70 Gy/35 fx or 70 Gy/33 fx; CTV2 = 63 Gy/35 fx or 59.4 Gy/33 fx; CTV3 = 56 Gy/35 fx or 54 Gy/33 fx. For small oropharyngeal tumors (T1–2, N0–1, M0) or when definitive IMRT is used without concomitant chemotherapy, suggested doses are: CTV1 = 66 Gy/30 fx; CTV2 = 60 Gy/30Gy; CTV3 = 54 Gy/30 fx.
@Optional margins around CTV1.

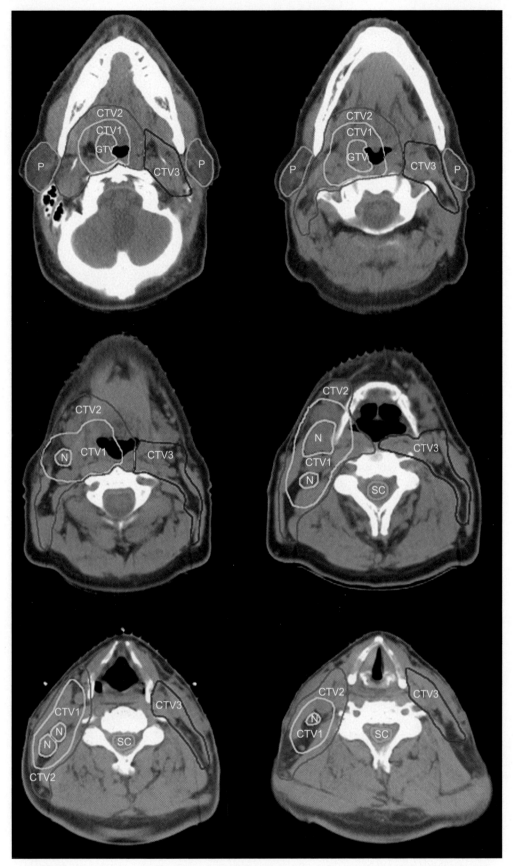

**FIGURE 11-5.** Clinical target volume (CTV) delineation of a patient with T1N2b tonsil carcinoma who is receiving definitive intensity-modulated radiation therapy (IMRT). Gross tumor volume (GTV) (*yellow line*); CTV1 (*gold yellow line*); CTV2 (*red line*); CTV3 (*dark blue line*); P, parotid gland; right parotid gland (*rust line*); left parotid gland (*aqua line*); spinal cord (SC) (*green line*).

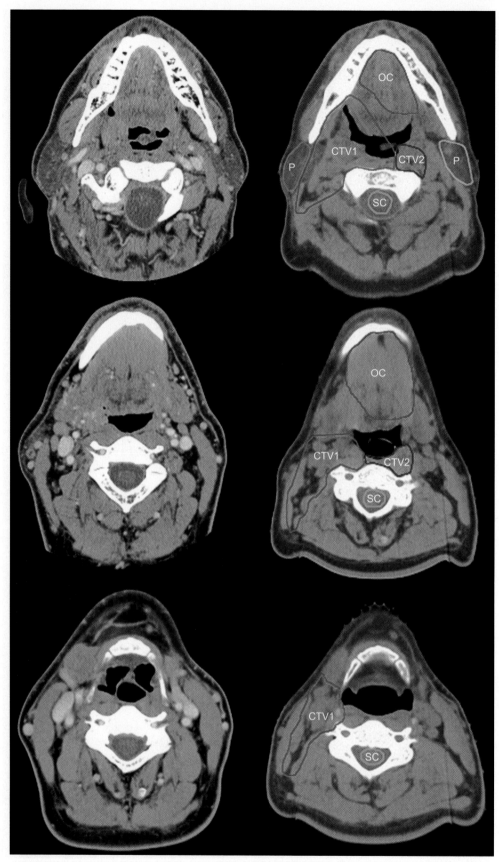

**FIGURE 11-6.** CTV delineation of a patient with T1N0M0 tonsil carcinoma who is receiving ipsilateral postoperative IMRT. GTV (*yellow line*); CTV1 (*gold yellow line*); CTV2 (*dark blue line*); P, parotid gland; right parotid gland (*rust line*); left parotid gland (*aqua line*); oral cavity (OC) (*magenta line*); spinal cord (SC) (*green line*).

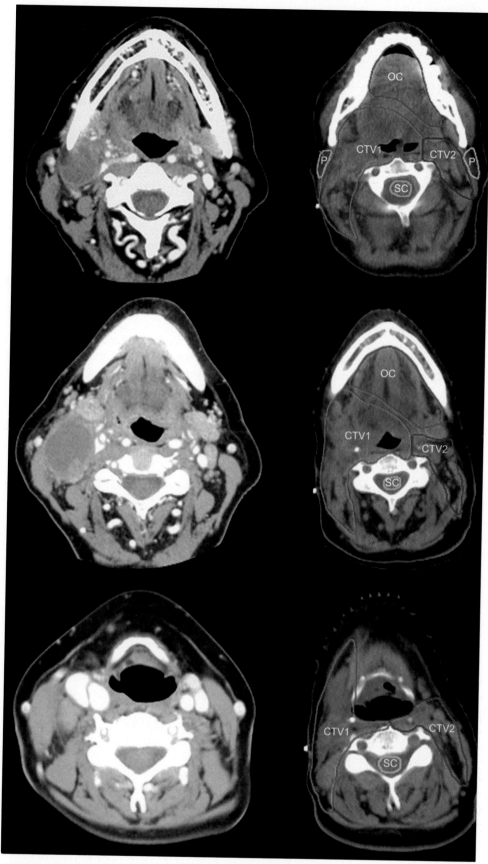

**FIGURE 11-7.** CTV delineation of a patient with T2N2a tonsil carcinoma who is receiving postoperative IMRT. CTV1 (*red line*); CTV2 (*dark blue line*); P, parotid gland; right parotid gland (*rust line*); left parotid gland (*aqua line*); oral cavity (OC) (*magenta line*); spinal cord (SC) (*green line*).

patient presented with a right-sided neck mass. CT imaging confirmed a right-sided neck mass and showed a right tonsillar mass. The patient underwent a right tonsillectomy and a right modified radical neck dissection. Both confirmed a squamous cell carcinoma diagnosis. One of thirteen lymph nodes were positive at level 2 with focal extranodal extension. The patient was treated with postoperative IMRT to the tumor bed and bilateral neck.

### 6.2.2. Base of Tongue

- In patients receiving definitive IMRT, CTV1 encompasses the gross tumor (primary and enlarged nodes) and the region adjacent to it but not directly involved with it. CTV2 includes primarily the prophylactically treated neck.
- CTV1 and CTV2 delineation in a patient with a clinical T4N2bM0 squamous cell carcinoma of BOT who received definitive IMRT is shown in Figure 11-8. The patient presented with a left-sided neck mass. CT showed a BOT lesion and left-sided neck lymphadenopathies. Biopsy of the left side of the BOT confirmed the diagnosis of squamous cell carcinoma.
- In patients receiving postoperative IMRT, CTV1 encompasses the residual tumor and the region adjacent to it but not directly involved with it, the surgical bed with soft tissue invasion by the tumor, or the extracapsular extension by metastatic neck nodes. CTV2 includes primarily the prophylactically treated neck.
- CTV1 and CTV2 delineation in a patient with pathologic T3N2bM0 squamous cell carcinoma of BOT who received definitive IMRT is shown in Figure 11-9. The patient presented with a history of dysphagia as the result of a tumor arising from the right side of the BOT metastasizing to the level II and III lymph nodes on the right side of the neck. The tumor was staged clinically and radiologically T3N2bM0. Concomitant chemotherapy was given with definitive IMRT.
- CTV1 and CTV2 delineation in a patient with pathologic T3N2bM0 squamous cell carcinoma of BOT who received definitive IMRT is shown in Figure 11-10. The patient presented with a history of throat pain, otalgia, and hoarseness as the result of a tumor arising from the left side of the BOT metastasizing to the level II and III lymph node on the right side of the neck. Positron emission tomography study showed increased pathologic activity in the left side of the BOT and left side of the neck as well as normal physiologic accumulation in the right side of the BOT and sublingual glands. The tumor was staged clinically and radiologically T3N2bM0. Concomitant chemotherapy was given with definitive IMRT.

### 6.3. Normal Tissue Delineation

- See Chapter 8 for normal tissue delineation (Fig. 8-8).
- Caution on sparing nontarget normal tissue cannot be overstated. Because IMRT will deliver radiation through multiple gantry angles, many nontarget normal tissues will be in the way of either the entrance or exit beams. In oropharyngeal cancer, it is critical to impose dose constraints to these normal tissues to avoid unnecessary toxicity, such as mucositis. Figure 11-11 depicts the importance and consequences of omitting radiation dose constraints to the lips and oral cavity (aiming for <30 Gy).

### 6.4. Suggested Target and Normal Tissue Doses

- See Chapter 7 for suggested target and normal tissue doses (Table 7-11).

### 6.5. Intensity-Modulated Radiation Therapy Results

- Following these guidelines, we treated 74 patients with oropharyngeal carcinoma by using IMRT between February 1997 and December 2001 at Washington University.[35] The primary site was the tonsil in 50 patients, BOT in 18 patients, and soft palate in 6 patients. A total of 43 patients were treated postoperatively, and 31 patients were treated with definitive IMRT. The T stages were T1 (16 patients), T2 (25 patients), T3 (14 patients), and T4 (19 patients). The N stages were N0 (12 patients), N1 (16 patients), N2 (42 patients), and N3 (4 patients) (AJCC staging: stage I [2 patients], stage II [3 patients], stage III [14 patients], and stage IV [43 patients]). The median follow-up time was 33 months (9–60 months); 10 locoregional recurrences were observed. Distant metastasis developed in 6 patients, 6 patients died of disease, and 3 patients died of concurrent disease.
- A gastrostomy tube was placed in 17 patients during the course of IMRT. We observed no grade 3 or 4 late complications in the patients who were treated with IMRT. Grade I late xerostomia was observed in 32 patients, grade II late xerostomia was observed in 9 patients, and grade I late mucositis was observed in 3 patients. In addition, trismus was observed in 3 patients after radiotherapy.
- Figure 11-12 shows pre- and posttreatment CT slices of a patient with T2N2bM0 tonsil cancer who received definitive IMRT.
- In a comparison study of acute and late toxicity between conventional radiation therapy beam techniques (conformal radiation therapy [CRT]) and IMRT, 430 patients with oropharyngeal cancer (260 with tonsil primary tumors and 170 with BOT primary tumors) were treated with preoperative CRT, postoperative CRT, definitive CRT, postoperative IMRT, or definitive IMRT at Washington University.[51] The AJCC stages were stage I (24 patients), stage II (88 patients), stage III (128 patients), and stage IV (190 patients). Median follow-up time was 3.9 years (1–23 years). Side effects were scored according to the Radiation Therapy Oncology Group radiation morbidity criteria.

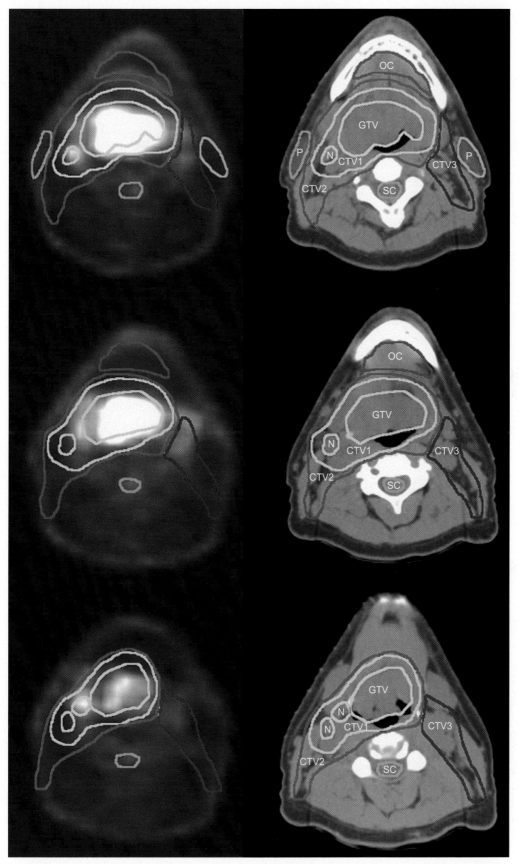

**FIGURE 11-8.** CTV delineation in a patient with T4N2bM0 squamous cell carcinoma of the BOT who is receiving definitive IMRT. Positron emission tomography fusion study (*left*). GTV (*yellow line*); CTV1 (*gold yellow line*); CTV2 (*red line*); CTV3 (*dark blue line*); P, parotid gland; right parotid gland (*rust line*); left parotid gland (*aqua line*); oral cavity (OC) (*magenta line*); spinal cord (SC) (*green line*).

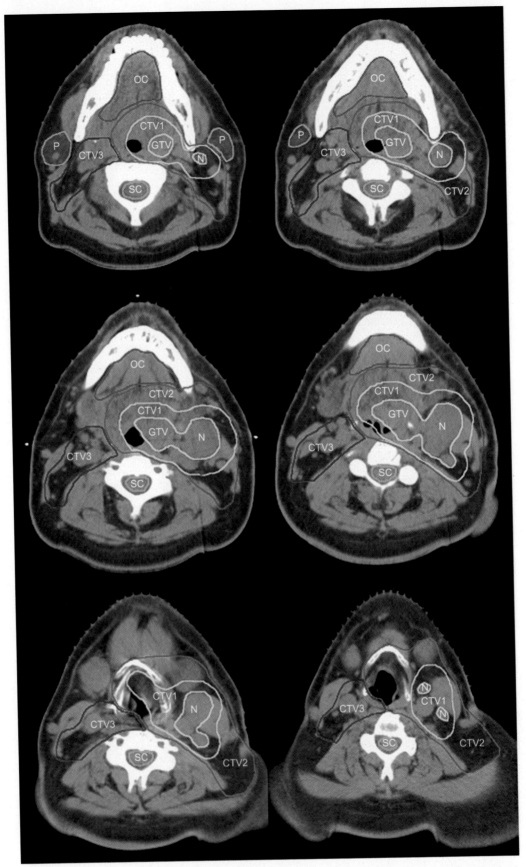

**FIGURE 11-9.** CTV delineation in a patient with T3N2bM0 squamous cell carcinoma of the BOT who is receiving definitive IMRT. GTV (*yellow line*); CTV1 (*gold yellow line*); CTV2 (*red line*); CTV3 (*dark blue line*); P, parotid gland; right parotid gland (*rust line*); left parotid gland (*aqua line*); oral cavity (OC) (*magenta line*); spinal cord (SC) (*green line*).

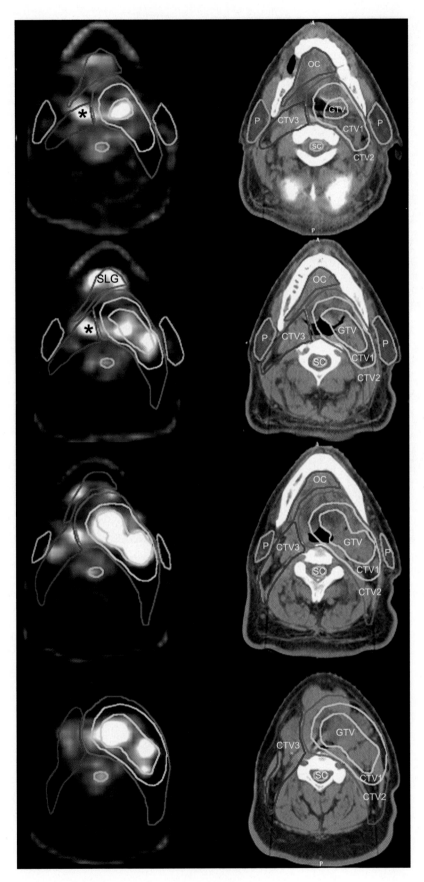

**FIGURE 11-10.** CTV delineation in a patient with T3N2bM0 squamous cell carcinoma of the BOT who is receiving definitive IMRT. Positron emission tomography fusion study (*left*). Note the physiologic hyperactivity in the right side of the BOT (*) and in sublingual glands (SLGs). GTV (*yellow line*); CTV1 (*gold yellow line*); CTV2 (*red line*); CTV3 (*dark blue line*); P, parotid gland; right parotid gland (*rust line*); left parotid gland (*aqua line*); oral cavity (OC) (*magenta line*); spinal cord (SC) (*green line*).

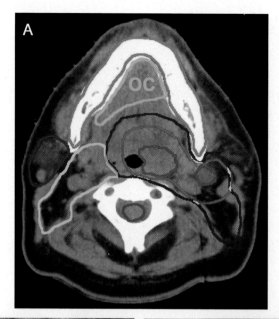

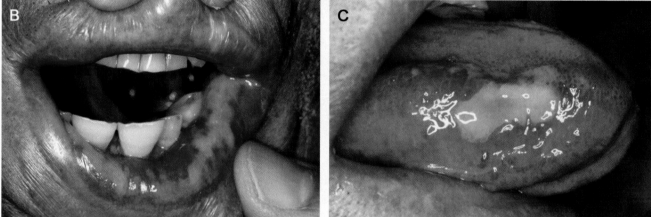

**FIGURE 11-11. A:** After completing CTV contouring, the oral cavity (OC) should be delineated to avoid excessive entrance or exit beam dose. **B** and **C:** Patients with excessive mucosal reaction on lips **(B)** and oral tongue **(C)** after 3 weeks of treatment when dose constraints were not imposed on these nontarget normal tissues.

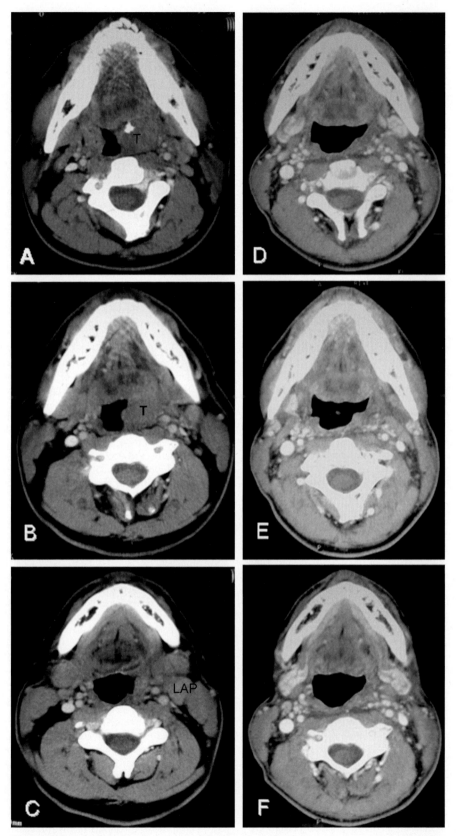

**FIGURE 11-12.** Pre-IMRT **(A–C)** and post-IMRT **(D–F)** CT sections of a patient with T2N2bM0 tonsil carcinoma showing complete regression of the tumor after a total IMRT dose of 70 Gy. T, tumor; LAP, lymphadenopathy.

- A significant reduction in late xerostomia was observed in patients who were treated with IMRT, based on parotid-sparing dosimetric advantages. When treated with CRT, 78% to 84% of patients experienced grade 2 or higher late salivary toxicity, compared with only 17% to 30% in patients who were treated with IMRT ($P <$ .0001).

## REFERENCES

1. Perez CA. Tonsillar Fossa and Faucial Arc. In: Perez CA, Brady LW, eds. *Principles and Practice of Radiation Oncology, 3rd ed.* Philadelphia: Lippincott-Raven, 1998:1003–1032.
2. Fletcher GH. *Textbook of Radiotherapy, 3rd ed.* Philadelphia: Lea & Febiger, 1980.
3. Lindberg R. Distribution of cervical lymph node metastases from squamous cell carcinoma of the upper respiratory and digestive tracts. *Cancer* 1972;29:1446–1449.
4. Chao KSC, Ozyigit G. *Intensity Modulated Radiation Therapy for Head-and-Neck Cancer.* Philadelphia: Lippincott Williams & Wilkins, 2003.
5. Brunin F, Mosseri V, Jaulerry C, et al. Cancer of the base of the tongue: past and future. *Head Neck* 1999;21:751–759.
6. Harrison LB, Lee HJ, Pfister DG, et al. Long term results of primary radiotherapy with/without neck dissection for squamous cell cancer of the base of tongue. *Head Neck* 1998;20:668–673.
7. Greene FL, American Joint Committee on Cancer, American Cancer Society. *AJCC Cancer Staging Manual, 6th ed.* New York: Springer, 2002.
8. Bataini JP, Asselain B, Jaulerry C, et al. A multivariate primary tumour control analysis in 465 patients treated by radical radiotherapy for cancer of the tonsillar region: clinical and treatment parameters as prognostic factors. *Radiother Oncol* 1989;14:265–277.
9. Givens CD Jr., Johns ME, Cantrell RW. Carcinoma of the tonsil. Analysis of 162 cases. *Arch Otolaryngol* 1981;107:730–734.
10. Perez CA, Patel MM, Chao KS, et al. Carcinoma of the tonsillar fossa: prognostic factors and long-term therapy outcome. *Int J Radiat Oncol Biol Phys* 1998;42:1077–1084.
11. Mendenhall WM, Amdur RJ, Stringer SP, et al. Radiation therapy for squamous cell carcinoma of the tonsillar region: a preferred alternative to surgery? *J Clin Oncol* 2000;18:2219–2225.
12. Mendenhall WM, Stringer SP, Amdur RJ, et al. Is radiation therapy a preferred alternative to surgery for squamous cell carcinoma of the base of tongue? *J Clin Oncol* 2000;18:35–42.
13. Iidstad ST, Bigelow ME, Remensnyder JP. Squamous cell carcinoma of the tongue: a comparison of the anterior two thirds of the tongue with its base. *Am J Surg* 1983;146:456–461.
14. Selek U, Garden AS, Morrison WH, et al. Results of radiation for early stage carcinoma of the oropharynx. *Int J Radiat Oncol Biol Phys* 2003;57(suppl2):S404.
15. Behar RA, Martin PJ, Fee WE Jr., et al. Iridium-192 interstitial implant and external beam radiation therapy in the management of squamous cell carcinomas of the tonsil and soft palate. *Int J Radiat Oncol Biol Phys* 1994;28:221–227.
16. Foote RL, Schild SE, Thompson WM, et al. Tonsil cancer. Patterns of failure after surgery alone and surgery combined with postoperative radiation therapy. *Cancer* 1994;73:2638–2647.
17. Kramer S, Gelber RD, Snow JB, et al. Combined radiation therapy and surgery in the management of advanced head and neck cancer: final report of study 73-03 of the Radiation Therapy Oncology Group. *Head Neck Surg* 1987;10:19–30.
18. Horton D, Tran L, Greenberg P, et al. Primary radiation therapy in the treatment of squamous cell carcinoma of the soft palate. *Cancer* 1989;63:2442–2445.
19. Lo K, Fletcher GH, Byers RM, et al. Results of irradiation in the squamous cell carcinomas of the anterior faucial pillar-retromolar trigone. *Int J Radiat Oncol Biol Phys* 1987;13:969–974.
20. Leemans CR, Engelbrecht WJ, Tiwari R, et al. Carcinoma of the soft palate and anterior tonsillar pillar. *Laryngoscope* 1994;104:1477–1481.
21. Keus RB, Pontvert D, Brunin F, et al. Results of irradiation in squamous cell carcinoma of the soft palate and uvula. *Radiother Oncol* 1988;11:311–317.
22. Crook J, Mazeron JJ, Marinello G, et al. Combined external irradiation and interstitial implantation for T1 and T2 epidermoid carcinomas of base of tongue: the Creteil experience (1971–1981). *Int J Radiat Oncol Biol Phys* 1988;15:105–114.
23. Parsons JT, Million RR, Cassisi NJ. Carcinoma of the base of the tongue: results of radical irradiation with surgery reserved for irradiation failure. *Laryngoscope* 1982;92:689–696.
24. Thawley SE, Simpson JR, Marks JE, et al. Preoperative irradiation and surgery for carcinoma of the base of the tongue. *Ann Otol Rhinol Laryngol* 1983;92:485–490.
25. Rollo J, Rozenbom CV, Thawley S, et al. Squamous carcinoma of the base of the tongue: a clinicopathologic study of 81 cases. *Cancer* 1981;47:333–342.
26. Foote RL, Olsen KD, Davis DL, et al. Base of tongue carcinoma: patterns of failure and predictors of recurrence after surgery alone. *Head Neck* 1993;15:300–307.
27. Pignon JP, Bourhis J, Domenge C, et al. Chemotherapy added to locoregional treatment for head and neck squamous-cell carcinoma: three meta-analyses of updated individual data. MACH-NC Collaborative Group. Meta-Analysis of Chemotherapy on Head and Neck Cancer. *Lancet* 2000;355:949–955.
28. Wendt TG, Grabenbauer GG, Rodel CM, et al. Simultaneous radiochemotherapy versus radiotherapy alone in advanced head and neck cancer: a randomized multicenter study. *J Clin Oncol* 1998;16:1318–1324.
29. Brizel DM, Albers ME, Fisher SR, et al. Hyperfractionated irradiation with or without concurrent chemotherapy for locally advanced head and neck cancer. *N Engl J Med* 1998;338:1798–1804.
30. Calais G, Alfonsi M, Bardet E, et al. Randomized trial of radiation therapy versus concomitant chemotherapy and radiation therapy for advanced-stage oropharynx carcinoma. *J Natl Cancer Inst* 1999;91:2081–2086.
31. Jeremic B, Shibamoto Y, Milicic B, et al. Hyperfractionated radiation therapy with or without concurrent low-dose daily cisplatin in locally advanced squamous cell carcinoma of the head and neck: a prospective randomized trial. *J Clin Oncol* 2000;18:1458–1464.
32. Merlano M, Benasso M, Corvo R, et al. Five-year update of a randomized trial of alternating radiotherapy and chemotherapy compared with radiotherapy alone in treatment of unresectable squamous cell carcinoma of the head and neck. *J Natl Cancer Inst* 1996;88:583–589.
33. Pfister DG, Harrison LB, Strong EW, et al. Organ-function preservation in advanced oropharynx cancer: results with induction chemotherapy and radiation. *J Clin Oncol* 1995;13:671–680.
34. Pfister DG. Chemotherapy in locally advanced, squamous cell head and neck cancer: limitations, lessons learned, and evolving standards of care. *Cancer Invest* 1995;13:134–136.
35. Chao KS, Ozyigit G, Blanco AI, et al. Intensity-modulated radiation therapy for oropharyngeal carcinoma: impact of tumor volume. *Int J Radiat Oncol Biol Phys* 2004;59:43–50.
36. Amornmarn R, Prempree T, Jaiwatana J, et al. Radiation management of carcinoma of the tonsillar region. *Cancer* 1984;54:1293–1299.
37. Dubois JB, Broquerie JL, Delard R, et al. Analysis of the results of irradiation in the treatment of tonsillar region carcinomas. *Int J Radiat Oncol Biol Phys* 1983;9:1195–1203.

38. Fayos JV, Lampe I. Radiation therapy of carcinoma of the tonsillar region. *Am J Roentgenol Radium Ther Nucl Med* 1971;111:85–94.

39. Lusinchi A, Wibault P, Marandas P, et al. Exclusive radiation therapy: the treatment of early tonsillar tumors. *Int J Radiat Oncol Biol Phys* 1989;17:273–277.

40. Mantravadi RV, Liebner EJ, Ginde JV. An analysis of factors in the successful management of cancer of tonsillar region. *Cancer* 1978;41:1054–1058.

41. Mendenhall WM, Parsons JT, Cassisi NJ, et al. Squamous cell carcinoma of the tonsillar area treated with radical irradiation. *Radiother Oncol* 1987;10:23–30.

42. Perez CA, Carmichael T, Devineni VR, et al. Carcinoma of the tonsillar fossa: a nonrandomized comparison of irradiation alone or combined with surgery: long-term results. *Head Neck* 1991; 13:282–290.

43. Pernot M, Malissard L, Hoffstetter S, et al. Influence of tumoral, radiobiological, and general factors on local control and survival of a series of 361 tumors of the velotonsillar area treated by exclusive irradiation (external beam irradiation+brachytherapy or brachytherapy alone). *Int J Radiat Oncol Biol Phys* 1994;30: 1051–1057.

44. Wong CS, Ang KK, Fletcher GH, et al. Definitive radiotherapy for squamous cell carcinoma of the tonsillar fossa. *Int J Radiat Oncol Biol Phys* 1989;16:657–662.

45. Gwozdz JT, Morrison WH, Garden AS, et al. Concomitant boost radiotherapy for squamous carcinoma of the tonsillar fossa. *Int J Radiat Oncol Biol Phys* 1997;39:127–135.

46. Garrett PG, Beale FA, Cummings BJ, et al. Carcinoma of the tonsil: the effect of dose-time-volume factors on local control. *Int J Radiat Oncol Biol Phys* 1985;11:703–706.

47. Puthawala AA, Syed AM, Eads DL, et al. Limited external beam and interstitial 192iridium irradiation in the treatment of carcinoma of the base of the tongue: a ten year experience. *Int J Radiat Oncol Biol Phys* 1988;14:839–848.

48. Spanos WJ Jr., Shukovsky LJ, Fletcher GH. Time, dose, and tumor volume relationships in irradiation of squamous cell carcinomas of the base of the tongue. *Cancer* 1976;37:2591–2599.

49. Foote RL, Parsons JT, Mendenhall WM, et al. Is interstitial implantation essential for successful radiotherapeutic treatment of base of tongue carcinoma? *Int J Radiat Oncol Biol Phys* 1990;18: 1293–1298.

50. Wang CC. Carcinoma of the oropharynx. In: Wang CC, ed. *Radiation Therapy for Head and Neck Neoplasms, 3rd ed.* New York: Wiley-Liss, 1997:387.

51. Chao KS, Majhail N, Huang CJ, et al. Intensity-modulated radiation therapy reduces late salivary toxicity without compromising tumor control in patients with oropharyngeal carcinoma: a comparison with conventional techniques. *Radiother Oncol* 2001; 61: 275–280.

52. Goffinet DR, Fee WE, Jr., Wells J, et al. 192Ir pharyngoepiglottic fold interstitial implants. The key to successful treatment of base tongue carcinoma by radiation therapy. *Cancer* 1985;55: 941–948.

53. Kraus DH, Vastola AP, Huvos AG, et al. Surgical management of squamous cell carcinoma of the base of the tongue. *Am J Surg* 1993;166:384–388.

# 12

# HYPOPHARYNX AND LARYNX

**K. S. CLIFFORD CHAO**
**ADAM S. GARDEN**
**GOKHAN OZYIGIT**

## 1. ANATOMY

### 1.1. Hypopharynx

- The hypopharynx is the most inferior portion of the pharynx from the level of the hyoid bone, the base of the vallecula and pharyngo epiglottic folds, to the beginning of the esophagus at the plane of the lower border of the cricoid cartilage (Fig. 12-1). It communicates the oropharynx with the esophageal inlet.

- The larynx indents the anterior wall of the hypopharynx to form a horseshoe-shaped hollow cavity. This creates a central aerodigestive passageway and two lateral fossae (i.e., the pyriform sinuses) (Fig. 12-2).

- The hypopharyngeal walls are composed of four layers of tissue: mucosa, fibrous fascia, muscular layer, and areolar coat. The epithelium of the pharyngeal mucous membrane is squamous and continuous with the nasopharyngeal epithelial membrane. There is no visible transitional zone between these two regions. The mucous membrane, lined by ciliated pseudostratified columnar epithelium, is exposed to air. The surfaces that allow the transport of both food and air or food only are lined with stratified squamous epithelium. These differences have importance in the type and differentiation of malignancies occurring in various parts of the pharynx.

- Beneath the mucous membrane of the posterior and lateral walls is the thin muscular layer. The muscular layer of the hypopharynx is composed of two paired constrictor muscles: the middle and the inferior constrictors. These muscles attach anteriorly to the hyoid bone and thyroid cartilage and fuse posteriorly with each other.

- Between the constrictor muscles and the prevertebral fascia that covers the longitudinal spinous muscles is a thin layer of loose areolar tissue called the retropharyngeal space. This is a potential space that may act as a conduit for tumor extension.

- The areaolar layer contains the vessels, nerves, and lymphatics that lie laterally to the pharyngeal walls in a potential parapharyngeal space of loose connective tissue surrounded by the deep cervical and visceral fascia.

- Clinically, the hypopharynx is separated from the other parts of the pharynx by certain anatomic landmarks (Fig. 12-1). The superior border arises anteriorly at the base of the vallecula (inferior border of the hyoid bone) and proceeds laterally to the pharyngoepiglottic folds. The superior border is the plane connecting these points with the posterior pharyngeal wall at the level of the fourth cervical vertebra.

- The posterior and lateral hypopharyngeal walls are continuous with those of the oropharynx without certain anatomic separation. The lateral border of the epiglottis, the aryepiglottic folds, and lateral laryngeal wall composes the medial wall.

- The inferior constrictor muscle has two specialized divisions. The first is the cricopharyngeus muscle, which is composed of the lowermost fibers and the sphincteric guardian of the esophagus. The second part forms the cricothyroid muscle, which is the tensor of the vocal folds. This muscle inserts into the thyroid cartilage. The external branch of the superior laryngeal nerve innervates the cricothyroid muscle.

- The anterior border is the postcricoid region, which extends from the interarytenoid area and cricothyroid muscle. The inferior border is at the inferior edge of the pharyngeal aponeurosis and its cricopharyngeal ligament.

- The hypopharynx is also subdivided into three clinical regions: the pyriform sinus, the posterolateral pharynx, and the postcricoid region. The posterior border of the larynx forms the postcricoid region. The pyriform sinuses lie lateral to the larynx. The medial wall is formed by the aryepiglottic fold and the lateral laryngeal wall (cricothyroid muscle). The anterior and lateral walls are formed by the thyroid ala.

- The posterior wall is open and communicates with the hypopharyngeal lumen. The pyriform sinus apex lies below the level of the vocal cords and occasionally below the cricoid cartilage. The tumors that extend to the pyriform sinus apex or postcricoid area, therefore, are not amenable to voice conservational surgical procedures.

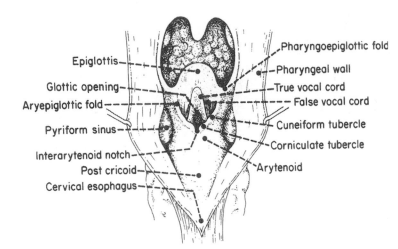

**FIGURE 12-1.** Hypopharynx. Posterior view showing the topography of the pyriform sinus, pharyngeal wall, and postcricoid region (From: Sobotta J. *Atlas of Human Anatomy*, Vol 2. Munich: Urban & Schwarzenberg, 1983.)

- The arterial supply of the hypopharynx is mainly from divisions of the external carotid system: the ascending pharyngeal arteries, superior thyroid arteries, and branches from the lingual artery. A venous plexus drains the pharynx and communicates with the internal jugular vein.
- The lymphatics generally travel in cephalad direction through the thyrohyoid membrane toward the upper deep cervical lymph nodes and then enters the jugulodigastric lymph nodes and the upper and middle jugular chain.
- There is also free communication with the spinal accessory lymph nodes and retropharyngeal lymph nodes; in this group, the highest nodes (Rouviere) are at the skull base. This close proximity of the lymphatics to the mucosa partly explains the high incidence of early metastases.

- The lowest portions of the hypopharynx (the postcricoid region, pyriform apex, and inferior hypopharynx) drains into a lymphatic chain that follows the recurrent laryngeal nerve to the paratracheal, paraesophageal, and supraclavicular nodes.
- The motor neural supply of the hypopharyngeal muscles is from the pharyngeal plexus of nerves, which are motorneural fibers from the glossopharyngeal (IX) and vagus (X) nerves.
- The inferior hypopharynx is innervated by branches from the recurrent laryngeal nerve (X). Efferent pain fibers traveling with the internal branch of the superior laryngeal nerve through the auricular branch of the vagus (nerve of Arnold) to the ipsilateral ear cause a usually ill-defined, dull pain in the superior-posterior wall of the external auditory canal or the posterior skin of the pinna.

## 1.2. Larynx

- The larynx is divided into the supraglottic (epiglottis, false vocal cords, ventricles, aryepiglottic folds, arytenoids), glottic (true vocal cords, anterior commissure), and subglottic (located below the vocal cords) regions[1] (Fig. 12-3).
- The lateral line of demarcation between the glottis and supraglottic larynx clinically is the apex of the ventricle. The demarcation between the glottis and subglottis is ill-defined, but the subglottis is considered to begin 5 mm below the free margin of the vocal cord and to end at the inferior border of the cricoid cartilage and the beginning of the trachea (Fig. 12-4).
- The recurrent laryngeal nerve innervates the intrinsic muscles of the larynx. A branch of the superior laryngeal nerve supplies the cricothyroid muscle, an intrinsic muscle responsible for tensing the vocal cords (Fig. 12-5). Isolated damage to this nerve causes a bowing of the true

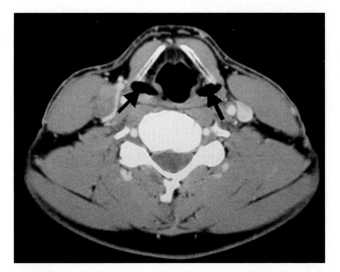

**FIGURE 12-2.** Axial CT section at the level of pyriform sinuses (*arrows*).

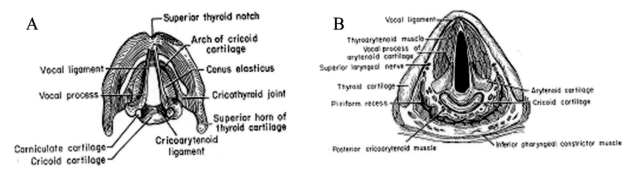

**FIGURE 12-3.** Cross-section of larynx at the level of the vocal cords (**A**). Framework of the larynx (**B**). (From: Sobotta J. In: Clemente CD, ed. *Anatomy: A Regional Atlas of the Human Body.* Philadelphia: Lea & Febiger, 1975; Copyright Munich: Urban & Schwarzenberg, 1975.)

vocal cord, which continues to be mobile, but the voice may become hoarse.

- The supraglottic structures have a rich capillary lymphatic plexus. The trunks pass through the preepiglottic space and thyrohyoid membrane and terminate mainly in the subdigastric lymph nodes; a few drain to the middle internal jugular chain lymph nodes.
- There are essentially no capillary lymphatics of the true vocal cords. Lymphatic spread from glottic cancer oc-

curs only if tumor extends to the supraglottic or subglottic areas.

- The subglottic area has relatively few capillary lymphatics. The lymphatic trunks pass through the cricothyroid membrane to the pretracheal (Delphian) lymph nodes in the region of the thyroid isthmus. The subglottic area also drains posteriorly through the cricotracheal membrane, with some trunks going to the paratracheal lymph nodes and others continuing to the inferior jugular chain.

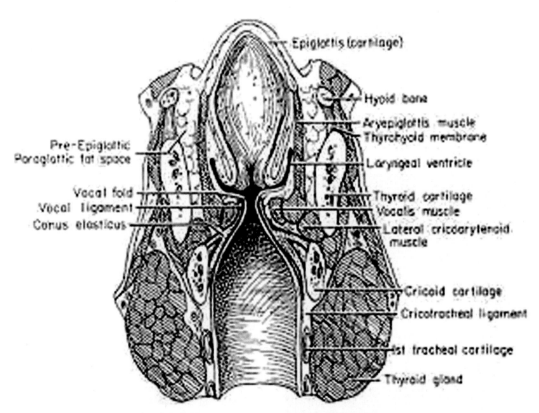

**FIGURE 12-4.** Coronal view of the larynx. (From: Sobotta J. In: Clemente CD, ed. *Anatomy: A Regional Atlas of the Human Body.* Philadelphia: Lea & Febiger, 1975; Copyright Munich: Urban & Schwarzenberg, 1975.)

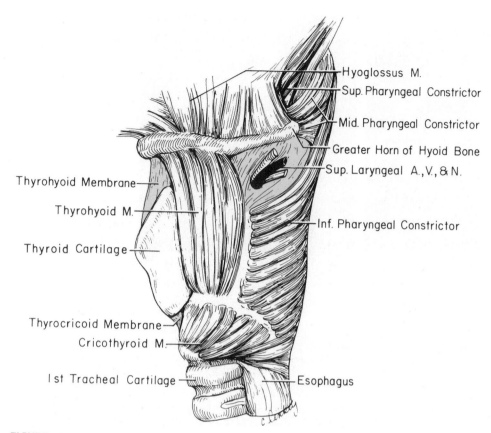

Hyoglossus M.
Sup. Pharyngeal Constrictor
Mid. Pharyngeal Constrictor
Greater Horn of Hyoid Bone
Sup. Laryngeal A.,V.,& N.
Inf. Pharyngeal Constrictor
Thyrohyoid Membrane
Thyrohyoid M.
Thyroid Cartilage
Thyrocricoid Membrane
Cricothyroid M.
1st Tracheal Cartilage
Esophagus

**FIGURE 12-5.** External view of the larynx. (From: Sobotta J. In: Clemente CD, ed. *Anatomy: A Regional Atlas of the Human Body.* Philadelphia: Lea & Febiger, 1975; Copyright Munich: Urban & Schwarzenberg, 1975.)

## 2. NATURAL HISTORY

### 2.1. Hypopharynx

- In the United States, tumors occur in the following decremental frequency: pyriform fossa (>65%), postcricoid (20%), and hypopharyngeal wall (10% to 15%).[2]
- Medial wall pyriform fossa tumors, the most common group, may spread along the mucosal surface to involve the aryepiglottic folds (most common pattern). They sometimes invade medially and deeply into the false vocal folds and larynx via the paraglottic space (Fig. 12-6). Involvement of the paraglottic space allows a lesion to behave as a transglottic carcinoma.[3]
- Cancers of the lateral wall and apex of the pyriform fossa commonly invade the thyroid cartilage and, less frequently, the cricoid cartilage.
- Once they penetrate the constrictor muscle, tumors can spread along the muscle and fascial planes to the base of the skull (the origin and suspension of the constrictor muscles) and along the neurovascular planes following the vagus, glossopharyngeal, and sympathetic nerves.
- Postcricoid area tumors commonly invade the cricoid cartilage, interarytenoid space, and posterior cricohyoid

muscle to produce hoarseness.[4] Because of the tendency for early esophageal spread, some have suggested that these epiesophageal tumors are not hypopharyngeal in origin.[5]

- The abundant lymphatics of the hypopharynx, coupled with extensive primary disease at presentation, account for the high incidence of metastases to the regional lymph nodes (Table 12-1).
- The midcervical lymph nodes are most commonly involved. The incidence of metastases varies according to the site and origin in the hypopharynx (Tables 12-2 and 12-3).[6]
- The contralateral subdigastric nodes are the most common site of harboring metastatic disease.
- Occult disease occurs irrespective of T stage in pyriform fossa tumors, with an incidence of 60% for T1 and T2 and 84% for T3 and T4 disease.[2]
- In 3,419 patients, the most common metastatic site was in level II (69%), and survival decreased as the level of metastases went from level II (39% survival) to the supraclavicular region (level IV, 21% survival).[7]
- Pathologically confirmed node metastases decreased survival by 26% to 28% (N0 vs N+), and size of nodal disease decreased survival by an additional 12% to 18%

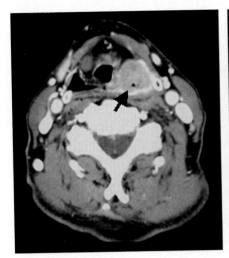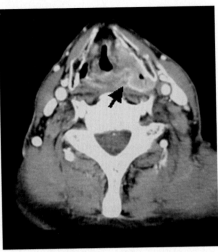

**FIGURE 12-6.** Axial CT sections of a T4N1 squamous cell carcinoma of the pyriform sinus (*arrows*).

## TABLE 12-1. CLINICALLY DETECTED NODAL METASTASES (%) ON ADMISSION BY T STAGE FOR HYPOPHARYNGEAL CARCINOMAS

|  | N0 | N1 | N2–3 |
|---|---|---|---|
| T1 | 37 | 21 | 42 |
| T2 | 30 | 20 | 49 |
| T3 | 21 | 26 | 54 |
| T4 | 26 | 15 | 58 |

Modified from: Lindberg R. Distribution of cervical lymph node metastases from squamous cell carcinoma of the upper respiratory and digestive tracts. *Cancer* 1972;29:1446–1449.

## TABLE 12-2. PERCENTAGE OF NODAL METASTASES (%) AS A FUNCTION OF LOCATION AND TUMOR SIZE

|  | T1 | T2 | T3 | T4 |
|---|---|---|---|---|
| Pyriform sinus | 38%–91% | 67%–83% | 69%–80% | 60%–98% |
| Pharyngeal wall | 33%–70% | 31%–79% | 47%–85% | 70%–82% |
| Postcricoid | 6% | 17% | 38% | 50% |

Modified from: McGavran M, Bauer W, Spjut H, et al. Carcinoma of the pyriform sinus. The results of radical surgery. *Arch Otolaryngol* 1963;78:826–830.

## TABLE 12-3. INCIDENCE AND DISTRIBUTION OF METASTATIC DISEASE IN CLINICALLY NEGATIVE (N–)* AND POSITIVE (N+)† NECK NODES (%)

|  | Radiologically Enlarged Retropharyngeal Nodes | | Pathological Nodal Metastasis | | | | | | | | | |
|---|---|---|---|---|---|---|---|---|---|---|---|---|
|  |  |  | Level I | | Level II | | Level III | | Level IV | | Level V | |
| Clinical presentation | N– | N+ | N– | N+ | N– | N+ | N– | N+ | N– | N+ | N– | N+ |
| Pharyngeal walls | 16 | 21 | 0 | 11 | 9 | 84 | 18 | 72 | 0 | 40 | 0 | 20 |
| Pyriform sinus | 0 | 9 | 0 | 2 | 15 | 77 | 8 | 57 | 0 | 23 | 0 | 22 |
| Supraglottic | 0 | 4 | 6 | 2 | 18 | 70 | 18 | 48 | 9 | 17 | 2 | 16 |
| Glottic | — | — | 0 | 9 | 21 | 42 | 29 | 71 | 7 | 24 | 7 | 2 |

*In patients with hypopharyngeal carcinoma who underwent bilateral neck dissection, 38% to 56% of them were found to have pathological metastasis in both necks.
†Bilateral neck node metastasis was found in 49% of N+ patients at presentation in patients with hypopharyngeal cancer.
Modified from: Chao K, Wippold F, Ozyigit G, et al. Determination and delineation of nodal target volumes for head-and-neck cancer based on patterns of failure in patients receiving definitive and postoperative IMRT. *Int J Radiat Oncol Biol Phys* 2002;53:1174–1184.

(N1 vs N2 and N3).[8,9] There is a decremental survival rate with progressive nodal disease (N0, 57%; N1, 28%; N2, 6%; N3, 0%) and a higher neck recurrence rate with progressively larger neck metastases (N0, 20%; N1, 37%; N2, 48%; N3, 83%).[10]

- Approximately 5% to 15% of presenting cases require an emergent tracheotomy.
- On rare occasions, direct tumor involvement or lymph node extension to the hypoglossal nerve may produce ipsilateral tongue paralysis.

## 2.2. Larynx

- Cancer of the larynx represents about 2% of the total cancer risk and is the most common head and neck cancer (skin excluded).
- The ratio of glottic to supraglottic carcinoma is approximately 3:1.
- Cancer of the larynx is strongly related to cigarette smoking. The risk of tobacco-related cancers of the upper alimentary and respiratory tracts declines among ex-smokers after 5 years and approaches the risk of nonsmokers after 10 years of abstention.[11]

### 2.2.1. Supraglottic Larynx

- Destructive suprahyoid epiglottic lesions tend to invade the vallecula and preepiglottic space, lateral pharyngeal walls, and the remainder of the supraglottic larynx.
- Infrahyoid epiglottic lesions grow circumferentially to involve the false cords, aryepiglottic folds, medial wall of the pyriform sinus, and the pharyngoepiglottic fold. Invasion of the anterior commissure and cords and anterior subglottic extension usually occur only in advanced lesions.
- Extension of false cord tumors to the lower portion of the infrahyoid epiglottis and invasion of the pre-epiglottic space are common.
- It may be difficult to decide whether aryepiglottic fold/arytenoid lesions started on the medial wall of the pyriform sinus or on the aryepiglottic fold. Advanced lesions invade the thyroid, epiglottic, and cricoid cartilages and eventually invade the pyriform sinus and postcricoid area.
- Disease spreads mainly to the subdigastric nodes.
- The incidence of clinically positive nodes is 55% at the time of diagnosis; 16% are bilateral.[12]
- Table 12-4 summarizes the clinically detected nodal metastases (%) on admission by T stage for supraglottic laryngeal carcinoma.
- Elective neck dissection reveals pathologically positive nodes in 16% of cases. Observation of initially node-negative necks eventually identifies the appearance of positive nodes in 33% of cases[13,14] (Table 12-5).

**TABLE 12-4. SUPRAGLOTTIC LARYNX: CLINICALLY DETECTED NODAL METASTASES (%) ON ADMISSION BY T STAGE**

|  | N0 | N1 | N2–3 |
|---|---|---|---|
| T1 | 61 | 10 | 29 |
| T2 | 58 | 16 | 26 |
| T3 | 36 | 25 | 40 |
| T4 | 41 | 18 | 41 |

Compiled from the data of the M. D. Anderson Cancer Center. (From: Lindberg R. Distribution of cervical lymph node metastases from squamous cell carcinoma of the upper respiratory and digestive tracts. *Cancer* 1972;29:1446–1449.)

- Table 12-3 summarizes the incidence and distribution of metastatic disease in clinically negative (N−) and positive (N+) neck nodes for supraglottic laryngeal carcinoma patients.
- The risk of late-appearing contralateral lymph node metastasis is 37% if the ipsilateral neck is pathologically positive (Table 12-6).[15]

### 2.2.2. Glottic Larynx

- At diagnosis, about two-thirds of tumors are confined to the true vocal cords, usually one cord. The anterior portion of the cord is the most common site.
- Subglottic extension may occur by simple mucosal surface growth, but it more commonly occurs by submucosal penetration beneath the conus elasticus. One centimeter of subglottic extension anteriorly or 4 to 5 mm of extension posteriorly brings the border of the tumor to the upper margin of the cricoid, exceeding the anatomic limits for conventional hemilaryngectomy.
- Advanced glottic lesions eventually penetrate through the thyroid cartilage or via the cricothyroid space to enter the neck, where they may invade the thyroid gland.
- In carcinoma of the vocal cord, the incidence of clinically positive lymph nodes at diagnosis approaches zero for T1 lesions and 1.7% for T2 lesions. The incidence of neck metastases increases to 20% to 30% for T3 and T4 lesions.[16]

**TABLE 12-5. ELECTIVE NODAL DISSECTION: INCIDENCE OF NODAL METASTASIS BY T CLASSIFICATION AND SITE IN LARYNX CANCER**

| Primary Site | Tx, T1, T2 | T3, T4 | Total |
|---|---|---|---|
| Supraglottic larynx | 31% | 25% | 26% |
| Glottic larynx | 21% | 14% | 16% |

Modified from: Byers RM, Wolf PF, Ballantyne AJ. Rationale for elective modified neck dissection. *Head Neck Surg* 1988;10:160–167.

**TABLE 12-6. INCIDENCE OF CONTRALATERAL OR BILATERAL NECK NODE METASTASES BY PRIMARY TUMOR SITE (%)**

| Tumor Site | cN+, Bilateral | cN+, Contralateral Only | cN−, pN+ Bilateral |
|---|---|---|---|
| Supraglottis | 39% | 2% | 26% |
| Glottis | — | — | 15% |

c, clinical; p, pathological.
Data compiled from: Northrop M, Fletcher GH, Jesse RH, et al. Evolution of neck disease in patients with primary squamous cell carcinoma of the oral tongue, floor of mouth, and palantine arch, and clinically positive neck nodes neither fixed nor bilateral. *Cancer* 1972;29:23–30
Bataini JP, Bernier J, Brugere J, et al. Natural history of neck disease in patients with squamous cell carcinoma of oropharynx and pharyngo-larynx. *Radiother Oncol* 1985;3:245–255.
Woolger JA. Histological distribution of cervical lymph node metastases from intraoral/oropharyngeal squamous cell carcinomas. *Br J Oral Maxillofac Surg* 1999;37:175–180.
Buckley JG, MacLennan K. Cervical node metastases in laryngeal and hypopharyngeal cancer: a prospective analysis of prevalence and distribution. *Head Neck* 2000;22:380–385.

## 3. DIAGNOSIS AND STAGING SYSTEM

### 3.1. Signs and Symptoms

#### 3.1.1. Hypopharynx

- Early pharyngeal tumors generally produce a mild, non-specific sore throat or vague discomfort on swallowing, which persists for longer than 2 weeks.
- A major neurological finding is referred pain to the ipsilateral ear, which is referred along the internal branch of the superior laryngeal nerve (sensory division to the larynx and hypopharynx) via the vagus nerve (X) to the auricular branch of the vagus nerve (Arnold nerve).
- Dysphagia is produced by bulky tumors, deep constrictor muscle invasion, or prevertebral space invasion of the overlying strap muscles. This finding may be associated with salivary drooling, stiff neck, and a "hot potato" voice. The last finding is especially due to laryngeal, and especially base of tongue, invasion.
- Advanced disease causes significant weight loss.
- Hoarseness by invasion of larynx, blood streaked saliva, airway obstruction, halitosis, and nasal voice are other signs and symptoms that can be seen in hypopharyngeal cancers.

#### 3.1.2. Larynx

- Hoarseness is the initial symptom of carcinomas arising on the true vocal cords. Advanced lesions of vocal cords may cause sore throat, ear pain, pain localized to thyroid cartilage, and airway obstruction.
- Hoarseness is not a prominent sign for supraglottic lesions. Mild odynophagia is the most frequent initial symptom. Pain is referred to the ear by vagus and auricular

nerve of Arnold. Early epiglottic lesions may not present with any signs or symptoms. A mass in the neck may be the first sign of supraglottic lesions. Weight loss, halitosis, dysphagia, and aspiration are late symptoms.

### 3.2. Physical Examination

#### 3.2.1. Hypopharynx

- The initial history and physical examination should include indirect laryngoscopy and a flexible endoscopic examination under topical anesthesia. Posterior pharyngeal wall lesions may be missed during indirect laryngoscopy.

#### 3.2.2. Larynx

- Rigid and flexible fiberoptic endoscopes are routinely used with laryngeal mirrors on examination.
- Determination of the mobility of the vocal cords may require multiple examinations.
- Ulceration of the infrahyoid epiglottis or fullness of the vallecula is an indirect sign of preepiglottic space invasion. Palpation of firm fullness above the thyroid notch with widening of the space between the hyoid and thyroid cartilages also may be a sign of preepiglottic space invasion.
- Tumor may penetrate the thyroid ala and be felt as a subcutaneous mass, suggesting thyroid cartilage invasion.

### 3.3. Imaging

#### 3.3.1. Hypopharynx

- Radiologic evaluation includes chest x-ray and computed tomography (CT) scan with contrast of the head and neck region, which is helpful in delineating cartilage and bone invasion by tumor, as well as extralaryngeal and paraglottic tumor invasion.
- In most cases, delineating the inferior border of the lesion and involvement of the esophageal inlet requires a barium swallow, including a video to evaluate the hypopharynx and cervical esophagus.
- Magnetic resonance imaging (MRI) can clearly distinguish the pharyngeal muscles from the mucosa and the lymphoid tissue lining the inner wall of the hypopharynx.
- The thickness of the posterior and lateral pharyngeal walls seen on MRI is usually less than 3 mm. If it reaches upper limits, it can be a sign of pathologic change.
- The pharyngeal constrictor muscles are relatively easy to distinguish from the mucosal lymphoid tissue on T2-weighted MRI.
- The penetration points of pharyngeal vessels are easily visible on CT and MRI. They are extremely important places, since they may provide early perineural and perivascular spread routes of tumor to the extrapharyngeal soft tissues.

- The constrictor muscle fascia is normally not visible as a separate layer either on CT or MRI, but inflammatory or other invasive changes may cause the fascia to become pathologically visible.
- A small amount of fat is normally seen just lateral to the lateral pharyngeal wall in the deep neck in all patients. Similarly, prevertebral muscles are visible in all patients on axial CT or MRI; however, the prevertebral fascia is not normally visible. The potential retropharyngeal space is located between the constrictor fascia and prevertebral fascia.
- The spaces lateral to the pharynx is referred to as the parapharyngeal space above the level of the hyoid bone.
- The retropharyngeal lymph nodes are located between the posterolateral corners of the pharynx and the carotid artery from the tip of the clivus to the C3 (hyoid) level.
- The degree of distention of the pyriform sinus seen on MRI or CT varies from side to side in any given individual and, more greatly between patients, depends on their anatomy and the study technique. Any thickness on the surface of the pyriform sinus usually represents some type of pathology.
- Imaging can particularly show the deep anatomical relationships of the pyriform sinus apex. The mucosa of the pyriform sinus apex is always seen as a thin line that merges medially with the mucosa in the postcricoid region.
- The postcricoid region is easily visible as the zone posterior to the cricoid cartilage where the constrictor muscle thickens to create the cricopharyngeus muscle. The lumen is not usually distended with air. Since the pharyngeal lumen is typically collapsed, the mucosa on enhanced CT or MRI is normally visible as parallel lines 1 mm or less in thickness, lying along the inner borders of the cricopharyngeus muscle.

### 3.3.2. Larynx

- The neck should be slightly hyperextended and the plane of section for laryngeal studies must be parallel to the true vocal cords with a slice thickness of no more than 3 to 4 mm. Occasionally, 1.5- to 2-mm slice thickness can be used for the false vocal cord, true vocal cord, and subglottic region, where 2- to 3-mm tumor extension might make a difference in treatment approach.
- T1 lesions of the true vocal cord usually require no imaging. Any tumor that is suspicious for deep invasion should be primarily studied with CT. MRI can be better for detection of cartilage invasion. The variation in ossification of the cartilages makes interpretation difficult. In any case, however, both CT and MRI have limited capability in identifying subtle cartilage invasion.
- CT can distinguish extralaryngeal extension of the primary tumor from a lymph node mass and can define extension to the thyroid gland and other adjacent structures.
- CT is the preferred baseline examination for the detection of recurrence in the neck or postirradiation larynx.

## 3.4. Staging

- The American Joint Committee on Cancer (AJCC) staging system for carcinoma of the hypopharynx is shown in Table 12-7.
- The American Joint Committee on Cancer staging system for carcinoma of the larynx is shown in Table 12-8.

## 4. PROGNOSTIC FACTORS

### 4.1. Hypopharynx

- *Age:* Survival progressively declines with increasing age.
- *Gender:* Women have a significantly higher survival rate 3 to 20 years after therapy.
- *Surgical margin:* Pathologic findings in pyriform fossa tumors that adversely affect survival are positive surgical margins or tumor persistence in the irradiation field after initial definitive therapy.
- *Location:* Tumor location influences cure rates. The decremental frequency for survival with hypopharyngeal carcinomas at different sites is pyriform fossa, pharyngeal walls, and postcricoid region.[17] Aryepiglottic fold and medial wall pyriform fossa tumors are usually smaller and more localized, which leads to higher cure rates than with postcricoid and pharyngeal wall tumors. The poorest results are seen with pyriform apex, postcricoid, and two- or three-wall tumors. Furthermore, for mid-cord tumors, anterior commissure involvement is more worrisome for cartilage involvement.
- *Neck metastasis:* In pyriform fossa and aryepiglottic fold tumors, metastases reduce the cure rate by 28% and 26%, respectively (N0 > N+ by 26% to 28%). The presence of extracapsular tumor spread in the cervical lymph nodes and soft tissues of the neck is of paramount importance in survival.[18,19] The presence of neck metastases influences survival.
- *The size and number of neck node metastases:* The size or number of metastases influences survival (higher for N1 than N2 and N3) by an additional 12% to 18%.[8,9]
- *T Stage:* T stage influences survival. Most patients present with large tumors (82% are T3 or T4 pyriform sinus cancers).[20] In pyriform fossa tumors (T1 and T2 exceed T3 and T4 by 28%), there is a significant decrease in cure rates for T3 and T4 disease.[20]

### 4.2. Larynx

- *T Stage:* T stage is the most important prognostic factor determining local control.
- *N Stage:* N stage is an important prognostic factor for predicting distant metastasis and survival.
- *Gender:* Female patients generally have better survival rates than males.

## TABLE 12-7. AMERICAN JOINT COMMITTEE ON CANCER CLASSIFICATION FOR CANCERS OF THE HYPOPHARYNX

**Primary Tumor (T)**

| | |
|---|---|
| TX | Primary tumor cannot be assessed |
| T0 | No evidence of primary tumor |
| Tis | Carcinoma *in situ* |
| T1 | Tumor limited to one subsite of hypopharynx and ≤2 cm in greatest dimension |
| T2 | Tumor involves more than one subsite of hypopharynx or an adjacent site, or measures >2 cm but not >4 cm in greatest dimension without fixation of hemilarynx |
| T3 | Tumor measures >4 cm in greatest dimension or with fixation of hemilarynx |
| T4a | Tumor invades adjacent structures (e.g., thyroid/cricoid cartilage, hyoid bone, thyroid gland, esophagus, or central compartment of soft tissues of neck) |
| T4b | Tumor invades adjacent structures (e.g., prevertebral fascia, encases carotid artery, or involves mediastinal structures) |

**Regional Lymph Nodes (N)**

| | |
|---|---|
| NX | Regional lymph nodes cannot be assessed |
| N0 | No regional lymph node metastasis |
| N1 | Metastasis in a single ipsilateral lymph node, <3 cm in greatest dimension |
| N2 | Metastasis in a single ipsilateral lymph node, >3 cm but not >6 cm in greatest dimension; or in multiple ipsilateral lymph nodes, none > 6 cm in greatest dimension; or in bilateral or contralateral lymph nodes, none >6 cm in greatest dimension |
| N2a | Metastasis in a single ipsilateral lymph node, >3 cm but not >6 cm in greatest dimension |
| N2b | Metastasis in multiple ipsilateral lymph nodes, none >6 cm in greatest dimension |
| N2c | Metastasis in bilateral or contralateral lymph nodes, none >6 cm in greatest dimension |
| N3 | Metastasis in a lymph node >6 cm in greatest dimension |

**Distant Metastasis (M)**

| | |
|---|---|
| MX | Distant metastasis cannot be assessed |
| M0 | No distant metastasis |
| M1 | Distant metastasis |

*Stage Grouping*

| | | | |
|---|---|---|---|
| Stage 0 | Tis | N0 | M0 |
| Stage I | T1 | N0 | M0 |
| Stage II | T2 | N0 | M0 |
| Stage III | T3 | N0 | M0 |
| | T1 | N1 | M0 |
| | T2 | N1 | M0 |
| | T3 | N1 | M0 |
| Stage IVA | T4a | N0, N1, or N2 | M0 |
| | Any T | N2 | M0 |
| Stage IVB | Any T | N3 | M0 |
| | T4b | Any N | M0 |
| Stage IVC | Any T | Any N | M1 |

From: Greene FL, American Joint Committee on Cancer, American Cancer Society. *AJCC Cancer Staging Manual, 6th ed.* New York: Springer; 2002.

## 5. GENERAL MANAGEMENT

### 5.1. Hypopharynx

- The best treatment for hypopharyngeal carcinoma is the one that achieves the highest locoregional control rate with the least functional damage.
- The functions that need to be preserved are respiration, deglutition, and phonation, if possible, with the least risk to the host and without the use of permanent prosthetic devices.
- Most T1N0 and selected T2N0 lesions can be treated equally well with curative irradiation or conservation surgery. Invasion of the larynx by a pyriform fossa tumor with vocal cord fixation predicts a poor outcome to curative irradiation.
- Larger lesions and neck metastases require combined surgical resection and adjuvant radiation therapy.
- Treatment outcomes for hypopharyngeal cancer are summarized in Tables 12-9 through 12-11.

#### 5.1.1. Surgical Management

- Contraindications for conservation surgery include the following: transglottic extension, cartilage inva-

sion, vocal fold paralysis, pyriform apex invasion, postcricoid invasion, and extension beyond the laryngeal framework.

- In all cases, at a minimum, an ipsilateral neck dissection is performed (functional, modified, or radical resection), which is almost always followed by postoperative irradiation.
- Tumors of the aryepiglottic fold are resected with an extended subtotal supraglottic laryngectomy and neck dissection if they fulfill the resection criteria of no extension beyond the larynx, transglottic extension, or vocal cord paralysis.
- Extension into the base of the tongue, epiglottis, and vallecula can be handled by extension of the operative field superiorly to resect these lesions and portions of the base of the tongue.
- Small lesions are amenable to partial laryngopharyngectomy and neck dissection if they are confined to the medial and anterior pyriform fossa walls or aryepiglottic folds, do not extend to the pyriform apex or beyond the larynx, show no postcricoid invasion or vocal cord (paralysis) or contralateral arytenoid involvement, and occur in patients who do not have pulmonary and cardiac disabilities.

**TABLE 12-8. AMERICAN JOINT COMMITTEE ON CANCER CLASSIFICATION FOR CARCINOMA OF THE LARYNX**

**Primary Tumor (T)**

TX    Primary tumor cannot be assessed
T0    No evidence of primary tumor
Tis    Carcinoma *in situ*

*Supraglottis*

T1    Tumor limited to one subsite of supraglottic with normal vocal cord mobility
T2    Tumor invades mucosa of more than one adjacent subsite of supraglottic or glottis or region outside of supraglottis without fixation of the larynx
T3    Tumor limited to larynx with vocal cord fixation and/or invades any of the following: postcricoid area, preepiglottic tissues, paraglottic space, and/or minor thyroid cartilage erosion (e.g., inner cortex)
T4a    Tumor extends through the thyroid cartilage, and/or extends into soft tissues of the neck including deep extrinsic muscle of tongue, strap muscles, thyroid and/or esophagus
T4b    Tumor invades prevertebral space, encases carotid artery, or invades mediastinal structures

*Glottis*

T1    Tumor limited to vocal cords (may involve anterior or posterior commissures) with normal mobility (T1a = limited one vocal cord, T2a = involves both vocal cords)
T2    Tumor extends to supraglottis and/or subglottis, and/or impaired vocal cord mobility
T3    Tumor limited to larynx with vocal cord fixation, and/or invades paraglottic space, and/or minor thyroid cartilage invasion (e.g., inner cortex).
T4a    Tumor extends through the thyroid cartilage, and/or extends into soft tissues of the neck including deep extrinsic muscle of tongue, strap muscles, thyroid and/or esophagus
T4b    Tumor invades prevertebral space, encases carotid artery, or invades mediastinal structures

**Regional Lymph Nodes (N)**

NX    Regional lymph nodes cannot be assessed
N0    No regional lymph node metastasis
N1    Metastasis in a single ipsilateral lymph node, <3 cm in greatest dimension
N2    Metastasis in a single ipsilateral lymph node, >3 cm but not >6 cm in greatest dimension; in multiple ipsilateral lymph nodes, none >6 cm in greatest dimension; or in bilateral or contralateral lymph nodes, none >6 cm in greatest dimension
N2a    Metastasis in a single ipsilateral lymph node >3 cm but not >6 cm in greatest dimension
N2b    Metastasis in multiple ipsilateral lymph nodes, none >6 cm in greatest dimension
N2c    Metastasis in bilateral or contralateral lymph nodes, none >6 cm in greatest dimension
N3    Metastasis in a lymph node >6 cm in greatest dimension

**Distant Metastases (M)**

MX    Presence of distant metastasis cannot be assessed
M0    No distant metastasis
M1    Distant metastasis

*Stage Grouping*

| | | | |
|---|---|---|---|
| Stage 0 | Tis | N0 | M0 |
| Stage I | T1 | N0 | M0 |
| Stage II | T2 | N0 | M0 |
| Stage III | T3 | N0 | M0 |
| | T1 | N1 | M0 |
| | T2 | N1 | M0 |
| | T3 | N1 | M0 |
| Stage IVA | T4a | N0–2 | M0 |
| | Any T | N2 | M0 |
| Stage IVB | Any T | N3 | M0 |
| | T4b | Any N | M0 |
| Stage IVC | Any T | Any N | M1 |

From: Greene FL, American Joint Committee on Cancer, American Cancer Society. *AJCC Cancer Staging Manual*, 6th ed. New York: Springer, 2002.

**TABLE 12-9. PYRIFORM SINUS: LOCAL CONTROL RESULTS CORRELATED WITH T STAGE**

| | No. of Patients | Therapy | Local Tumor Control | | |
|---|---|---|---|---|---|
| | | | T1–T2 | T3–T4 | Overall |
| Bataini et al.[41] | 434 | RT | 67% | 33% | 47% |
| Mendenhall et al.[42] | 50 | RT+ND | 74% | 26% | 49% |
| | 53 | S+RT | 4/6 | 72% | 25% |
| Mendenhall et al.[43] | 30 | RT (qd) | 80% | 20% | — |
| | 8 | RT (bid) | 75% | 25% | — |
| Mendenhall et al.[44] | 53 | RT+ND | 66% | 72% | 100% |
| Dubois et al.[45] | 209 | RT | 73% | 34% | 25% |
| | 154 | S+/−RT | 43% | 33% | 35% |
| Wang et al.[4] | 28 | RT (qd) | 68% | 20% | 44% |
| | 54 | RT (bid) | 82% | 33% | 61% |
| El Badawi et al.[2] | 48 | RT | — | — | 75% |
| | 125 | RT+S | — | — | 89% |
| Vandenbrouck et al.[9] | 152 | RT | 77% | 49% | 45% |
| | 198 | S+RT | | | 80% |
| Marks et al.[46] | 137 | RT+S | — | — | 72% |

RT, radiation therapy; S, surgery; ND, neck dissection; qd, daily; bid, twice daily.

## TABLE 12-10. PHARYNGEAL WALL CANCER: LOCAL CONTROL RESULTS CORRELATED WITH T STAGE

| | No. of Patients | Therapy | Local Tumor Control (%) | | |
| --- | --- | --- | --- | --- | --- |
| | | | T1–T2 | T4–T3 | Overall |
| Meoz-Mendez et al.[47] | 164 | RT | 91–73 | 61–37 | 60 |
| | 25 | S+RT | 5/5 | 75 | 45 |
| Wang et al.[4] | 43 | RT (qd) | 55 | 36 | 47 |
| | 33 | RT (bid) | 74 | 44 | 64 |
| Mendenhall et al.[48] | 49 | RT qd± implant | 10/20 | 9/29 | 39 |
| | 13 | RT (bid) | 5/5 | 5/8 | 77 |
| Chang et al.[49] | 44 | RT (qid) | 3/3–10/18 | 4/19–0/4 | |
| | 13 | RT (bid) | 1/1–1/2 | 5/7–2/3 | |

RT, radiation therapy; S, surgery; qd, daily; bid, twice daily.

- In patients who do not meet the criteria for conservation surgery, either a total laryngopharyngectomy or a total laryngectomy and partial pharyngectomy with reconstruction with neck dissection are performed.

### 5.1.2. Irradiation Alone

- Irradiation alone controls a substantial proportion of small surface lesions in the pyriform sinus. Of 25 T1 and T2 lesions of the pyriform sinus, 16 (64%) were controlled with irradiation alone (65 to 70 Gy in 7 to 8 weeks).[21]

### 5.1.3. Surgery and Irradiation

- Higher doses of adjuvant irradiation (60 to 66 Gy) are better delivered postoperatively than preoperatively because preoperative irradiation (usually 45 to 50 Gy in 4.5 to 5 weeks) retards healing of pharyngeal and cutaneous

suture lines and may cause more complications than postoperative irradiation.[22]

- In pyriform fossa tumors, combined therapy had higher cure rates (71%) than surgery (53%) or irradiation (27%). In aryepiglottic fold tumors, combined therapy (68%) had better disease-free results than surgery (61%) or irradiation (34%) at 5 years.[19]

### 5.1.4. Chemotherapy

- The European Organization for Research and Treatment of Cancer reported results of combined-modality therapy for head and neck cancer: 202 patients with operable, locally advanced squamous cell cancer of the pyriform sinus or the hypopharyngeal aspect of the aryepiglottic fold were randomly assigned to receive treatment with standard surgery and postoperative irradiation or induction chemotherapy (cisplatin and 5-fluorouracil).[23]

## TABLE 12-11. HYPOPHARYNGEAL CANCER: SURVIVAL RESULTS

| | No. of Patients | Therapy | T1 | T2 | T3 | T4 | Overall Survival |
| --- | --- | --- | --- | --- | --- | --- | --- |
| **Pyriform sinus** | | | | | | | |
| Bataini et al.[41]* | 434 | RT | | 26% | | 17% | 19% |
| Mendenhall et al.[32]* | 50 | RT+ND | | 60% | | 23% | 49% |
| | 53 | S+RT | | 43% | | 24% | 25% |
| Dubois et al.[45]* | 209 | RT | | 11% | | 3% | 5% |
| | 154 | S±RT | | 37% | | 30% | 33% |
| Spector et al.[8]† | 128 | RT+S | 9/9(100%) | 19/22(86%) | 50/64(78%) | 20/33(61%) | 98/128 (76.5%) |
| | 49 | S+RT | 5/5(100%) | 7/9(78%) | 13/19(68%) | 7/16(44%) | 32/49 (65.3%) |
| **Pharyngeal wall** | | | | | | | |
| Wang[50]‡ | 43 | RT (qd) | 64% | 29% | 22% | 0% | 30% |

RT, radiation therapy; S, surgery; ND, neck dissection.
*5-year determinate survival.
†5-year overall survival.
5-year disease-free survival.
‡3-year disease-free survival.

- Patients achieving a clinical complete response (CR) at the primary site after two or three cycles of chemotherapy received organ-sparing treatment with definitive irradiation (70 Gy), while those with less than a CR were treated surgically.
- At a median follow-up of 51 months (range, 3 to 106 months), the estimated survival outcomes for patients randomly assigned to receive induction chemotherapy or surgery were 3-year overall survival of 57% versus 43%, 3-year disease-free survival of 43% versus 31%, and median survival of 44 versus 25 months.
- These differences reflected a trend for improved outcome from chemotherapy and meet the statistical criteria for survival equivalence for the two arms. The laryngeal preservation rate was estimated at 42%, considering only deaths from local disease as failure.

## 5.2. Larynx

- Table 12-12 summarizes the results of different treatment strategies used in laryngeal cancer.

### 5.2.1. Vocal Cord Carcinoma

#### Carcinoma In Situ

- Stripping the cord may sometimes control carcinoma in situ; however, it is difficult to exclude the possibility of microinvasion in these specimens.
- Recurrence is frequent, and the cord may become thickened and the voice hoarse with repeated stripping.
- We recommend early radiation therapy because most patients with this diagnosis eventually receive this treatment, and earlier use of irradiation means a better chance of preserving a good voice.

#### Early Vocal Cord Carcinoma

- In most centers, irradiation is the initial treatment for T1 and T2 lesions. Surgery is reserved for salvage after radiation therapy failure.[16,24,25]
- The local control rate with definitive radiation therapy is about 90% for T1 lesions and 70% to 80% for T2 lesions.

## TABLE 12-12. LARNYNGEAL STUDIES WITH SURGERY OR RADIOTHERAPY

| Author | No. of Patients | Site | Stage | Therapy | Outcome |
|---|---|---|---|---|---|
| Mittal et al.[51] | 98 | Glottic | T3–T4 | Surgery alone± adjuvant RT | 75% LC, 50% OS |
| Yuen et al.[52] | 155 | Glottic | T3 | Surgery alone | 82% LC |
| Lundgren et al.[53] | 141 | Glottic | | RT alone | 51% OS |
| Meredith et al.[54] | 68 | Glottic | T3 | RT alone | 64% DSS |
| Razack et al.[55] | 128 | Glottic | T3–T4 | Total laryngectomy | 53% LC, 63% OS |
| Mendenhall et al.[56] | 65 | Glottic | | Surgery alone± adjuvant RT | 75% LC, 71% DSS |
| Simpson et al.[57] | 38 | Glottic | T3N0 | RT alone | 57% OS |
| Simpson et al.[57] | 36 | Glottic | T3N0 | Laryngectomy | 52% OS |
| Foote et al.[58] | 81 | Glottic | T3 | Surgery alone | 74% LC, 78% DSS |
| Kligerman et al.[59] | 76 | Glottic | T3–T4N0 | Surgery alone± adjuvant RT | 72% LC, 52% OS |
| Hao et al.[60] | 114 | Glottic | T3 | Total laryngectomy | 11% 2-year local recurrence rate |
| Bryant et al.[61] | 42 | Glottic | T3N0 | Surgery alone | 69% LC |
| Kowalski et al.[62] | 45 | Glottic | T3N0–1 | RT alone | 59% LC |
| Mendenhall et al.[63] | 75 | Glottic | T3 | RT alone | 63% LC, 78% DSS |
| Nyugen et al.[64] | 116 | Larynx | Stage III | Surgery and adjuvant RT | 76% LC, 68% OS |
| Parsons et al.[65] | 43 | Larynx | T4 | RT alone | 52% LC, 37% OS |
| Mancuso et al.[66] | 63 | Supraglottic | T1–T4 | RT alone | 69% LC |
| MacKenzie et al.[67] | 82 | Larynx | T2N+ | RT alone | 54% OS, 65% ultimate LC (T3–4) |

RT, radiotherapy; LC, local control; OS, overall survival; DSS, disease specific survival.

- Although hemilaryngectomy or cordectomy produces comparable cure rates for selected T1 and T2 vocal cord lesions, irradiation is generally preferred.[26]

## Moderately Advanced Vocal Cord Cancer

- Fixed-cord lesions (T3) can be subdivided into relatively favorable or unfavorable lesions.
- Patients with favorable T3 lesions have disease confined mostly to one side of the larynx, have a good airway, and are reliable for follow-up.
- Patients with unfavorable lesions usually have extensive bilateral disease with a compromised airway and are considered to be in the advanced group.
- Patients with favorable lesions are advised of the alternatives to irradiation with surgical salvage or immediate total laryngectomy.[27] They must be willing to return for follow-up examinations every 4 to 6 weeks for the first year, every 6 to 8 weeks for the second year, every 3 months for the third year, every 6 months for the fourth and fifth years, and annually thereafter.[15]

## Advanced Vocal Cord Carcinoma

- The mainstay of treatment is total laryngectomy, with or without adjuvant irradiation.
- Indications for postoperative irradiation include close or positive margins, significant subglottic extension ($\geq$1 cm), cartilage invasion, perineural invasion, extension of primary tumor into the soft tissues of the neck, multiple positive neck nodes, extracapsular extension, and control of subclinical disease in the opposite neck.[28–30]

## Surgical Treatment

- One entire cord and as much as one-third of the opposite cord is the maximum cordal involvement suitable for hemilaryngectomy in men.
- Women have a smaller larynx, and usually only one vocal cord may be removed without compromising the airway.
- The maximum subglottic extension is 8 to 9 mm anteriorly and 5 mm posteriorly. These limits are necessary to preserve the integrity of the cricoid.
- Tumor extension to the epiglottis, false cord, or both arytenoids is a contraindication to hemilaryngectomy.

## Treatment of Recurrence

- Radiation therapy failures may be salvaged by cordectomy, hemilaryngectomy, or total laryngectomy.
- Biller et al. reported a 78% salvage rate by hemilaryngectomy for eighteen selected patients in whom irradiation failed; total laryngectomy was eventually required in two patients.[31]
- The rate of salvage by irradiation for recurrences or new tumors that appear after initial treatment by hemilaryngectomy is about 50%.

## 5.2.2. Supraglottic Larynx Carcinoma

### Early and Moderately Advanced Supraglottic Lesions

- Treatment of the primary lesion for the early group is by external-beam irradiation or supraglottic laryngectomy, with or without adjuvant irradiation.
- For early-stage primary lesions with advanced neck disease (N2b or N3), combined treatment is frequently necessary to control the neck disease.[30,32] In these cases, the primary lesion is usually treated by irradiation alone, with surgery added to treat the involved neck site(s). If the same patient was treated with supraglottic laryngectomy, neck dissection, and postoperative irradiation, the portals would unnecessarily cover the primary site and the neck.
- If a patient has early, resectable neck disease (N1 or N2a) and surgery is elected for the primary site, postoperative irradiation is added only because of unexpected findings (e.g., positive margins, multiple positive nodes, or extracapsular extension).

### Advanced Supraglottic Lesions

- The surgical alternative for these lesions is total laryngectomy.
- Selected advanced lesions, especially those that are mainly exophytic, may be treated by radiation therapy, with total laryngectomy reserved for irradiation failures.
- Supraglottic laryngectomy is voice-sparing surgery that can be used successfully for selected lesions involving the epiglottis, a single arytenoid, the aryepiglottic fold, or the false vocal cord.
- Extension of tumor to the true vocal cord, anterior commissure, or both arytenoids, fixation of the vocal cord, or thyroid or cricoid cartilage invasion precludes supraglottic laryngectomy.
- Supraglottic laryngectomy may be extended to include the base of the tongue if one lingual artery is preserved.
- All patients have dysphagia with a tendency to aspirate immediately after surgery, but almost all recover within a short time. Motivation and the amount of tissue removed are key factors in regaining swallowing function.
- Preoperatively, adequate pulmonary reserve is evaluated by blood gas determinations, function tests, chest roentgenography, and a work test involving walking a patient up two flights of stairs to determine tolerance to pulmonary stress.

- Voice quality is generally normal after supraglottic laryngectomy.
- Radiation technique and dose are similar to those for glottic tumors; however, because of richer lymphatics in the supraglottic region, regional lymphatics must be treated in tumors greater than T2 size.[15]
- The addition of a neck dissection usually increases the risk of temporary lymphedema; however, it is preferable in terms of tumor control and complications that may arise from higher doses of irradiation required to control large neck nodes.[32]

## Postoperative Treatment

- Irradiation is added for close or positive margins, invasion of soft tissues of the neck, significant subglottic extension ($\geq 1$ cm), thyroid cartilage invasion, multiple positive nodes, and extracapsular extension.
- The postoperative irradiation dose as a function of known residual disease is as follows: negative margins, 60 Gy in 30 fractions; microscopically positive margins, 66 Gy in 33 fractions; and gross residual disease, 70 Gy in 35 fractions.
- If there is subglottic extension, the dose to the stoma is boosted with electrons (typically 10 to 14 MeV) for an additional 10 Gy in 5 fractions.

## Comparison of Surgery and Radiation Therapy

- The 659 patients with stage I (T1N0M0) glottic carcinoma treated with curative intent at Washington University, St. Louis, were subdivided into four groups[28]: 90 patients received low-dose irradiation (mean dose 58 Gy; range 55–65 Gy; daily fractionation 1.5–1.8 Gy)[33]; 104 patients received high-dose irradiation (mean dose 66.5 Gy; range 65–70 Gy; daily fractionation 2–2.25 Gy)[34]; 404 patients underwent conservation surgery; and 61 patients had endoscopic resection.[31] T1A (85%) and T1B (15%) disease was equally distributed among the groups.
- No significant difference in the 5-year cause-specific survival rate was observed among the four therapeutic groups for T1 tumors ($p = 0.68$). Actuarial survival was significantly decreased in the low-dose radiation therapy group as compared with the other three therapeutic groups ($p = 0.04$). Initial local control was poorer for the endoscopic (77%) and low-dose irradiation (78%) groups as compared with the high-dose irradiation (89%) and conservation surgery (92%) groups ($p = 0.02$), but significant differences were not found for ultimate local control following salvage treatment. Unaided laryngeal voice preservation was similar for high-dose radiation therapy (89%), conservation surgery (93%), and endoscopic resection (90%), but significantly poorer for low-dose irradiation (80%; $p = 0.02$).[35]

- Among 134 patients with stage II glottic carcinomas treated with curative intent and function preservation, 47 patients were treated with low-dose radiation therapy (median dose, 58.5 Gy at 1.5- to 1.8-Gy daily fractions), 16 patients with high-dose irradiation (67.5–70 Gy) at higher daily fractionation doses (2–2.25 Gy), and 71 patients underwent conservation surgery. There were no statistical differences in local control, voice preservation, and 5-year actuarial and disease-specific cure rates between conservation surgery and high-dose irradiation ($p = 0.89$). Patients treated with low-dose irradiation had statistically lower local control, 5-year survival, and voice preservation ($p = 0.014$).[36]

## Chemoradiotherapy For Laryngeal Preservation

- The Department of Veterans Laryngeal Cancer Study Group trial first established the use of chemoradiation as an alternative means of preserving the larynx in advanced laryngeal cancer by demonstrating no significant difference in survival between patients receiving induction chemotherapy followed by radiation therapy versus surgery plus adjuvant radiation.[37]
- A meta-analysis including patients with locally advanced laryngeal or hypopharyngeal carcinoma compared radical surgery plus radiation therapy with a neoadjuvant combination of cisplatin and 5-fluorouracil followed by irradiation in responders or radical surgery plus radiation therapy in nonresponders. There were 602 patients identified, with a median follow-up of 5.7 years. The pooled hazard ratio (1.19, 0.97–1.46) showed a nonsignificant trend ($p = 0.1$) in favor of the control group, corresponding to an absolute negative effect in the chemotherapy arm that reduced survival at 5 years by 6% (from 45% to 39%). Adjustment for nodal status (N0, N1–3) or tumor subsite (glottic or subglottic versus supraglottic versus hypopharynx) led to similar results. This meta-analysis suggests that, because of the nonsignificant negative effect of chemotherapy on the organ-preservation strategy, this procedure must remain investigational.[38]
- Recently, the RTOG and Head and Neck Intergroup conducted a multi-institutional randomized trial, RTOG 91-11, for 547 locally advanced laryngeal cancer patients who were randomly assigned to receive induction cisplatin plus fluorouracil followed by radiation, radiation with concurrent cisplatin, or radiation alone. At 2 years, the concurrent regimen preserved the larynx in significantly more patients (88%), which was the primary end point, compared to the induction (75%, $p = 0.05$) or radiation alone (70%, $p < 0.001$) groups. Locoregional control was also significantly better with concurrent chemoradiation ($p = 0.003$), although survival rates were similar in all groups. Moreover, the concurrent group had nearly twice the rate of mucosal toxicity compared to the other two groups. This trial demonstrates

that concurrent chemoradiation with cisplatin plus radiation is the superior modality for preservation of the larynx in advanced laryngeal cancer.[39]

- Table 12-13 summarizes the results of the several randomized larynx preservation trials.

## 6. INTENSITY-MODULATED RADIATION THERAPY IN HYPOPHARYNGEAL AND LARYNGEAL CARCINOMA

### 6.1. Hypopharynx

#### 6.1.1. Target Volume Determination

- If chemotherapy was delivered before radiation, the targets should be outlined on the planning CT according to their prechemotherapy extent.
- Lymph node groups at risk in the hypopharynx include the following:

  a. Submandibular nodes (surgical level I): N2c cases or when level II is involved.
  b. Upper deep jugular (junctional, parapharyngeal) nodes: all cases.
  c. Subdigastric (jugulodigastric) nodes, midjugular, lower neck, and supraclavicular nodes (levels II through IV): all cases, bilaterally.

  d. Posterior cervical nodes (level V): all cases, when jugular node is involved.
  e. Retropharyngeal nodes: all cases, if there is an evidence of jugular nodal metastases.

- The target volume specification for definitive and postoperative IMRT in hypopharynx cancer is summarized in Table 7-5.
- Suggested target volume determination for hypopharynx carcinoma is summarized in Table 12-14.

#### 6.1.2. Target Volume Delineation

- In patients receiving postoperative IMRT, clinical target volume (CTV)1 encompasses residual tumor and the region adjacent to it but not directly involved by the tumor, the surgical bed with soft tissue invasion by the tumor, or extracapsular extension by metastatic neck nodes. CTV2 includes primarily the prophylactically treated neck.
- In patients receiving definitive IMRT, CTV1 encompasses gross tumor (primary and enlarged nodes) and the region adjacent to it but not directly involved. CTV2 includes primarily the prophylactically treated neck.
- CTV1 and CTV2 delineation in a patient with clinically T4N1M0 squamous cell carcinoma of pyriform sinus re-

## TABLE 12-13. RANDOMIZED LARYNX PRESERVATION TRIALS

| Trial | No. of Patients | Site | Stage | Chemotherapy | Local Treatments | Survival | Laryngeal Preservation |
|---|---|---|---|---|---|---|---|
| VALCSG | 332 | Larynx (37% G, 63% SG) | III, IV | Induction: 2–3 CF (98% CR, PR) | RT (if PR) ± salvage surgery | 52% | 31% |
| | | | | | Total laryngectomy+ postop RT | 57% | |
| GETTEC | 68 | Larynx (41% G, 28% TG) | T3 | Induction: 2–3 CF (42% CR, PR) | RT (if PR) ± salvage surgery | 69% | 20% |
| | | | | | Total laryngectomy+ postop RT | 84% | |
| EORTC | 202 | HP/Larynx (78% HP, 22% LE) | II–IV | Induction: 2–3 CF (54% CR, PR) | RT (if PR) ± salvage surgery | 57% | 42% |
| | | | | | Total laryngectomy+ postop RT | 43% | |
| RTOG 91-11 | 547 | Larynx (31% G, 69% SG) | III–IV | Induction: 2–3 CF (85% CR, PR) | RT (if CR or PR) ± salvage surg+ postop RT | 76% | 72% |
| | | | | Concurrent: Cisplatin x 3 | RT | 74% | 84% |
| | | | | | RT alone | 75% | 67% |

VALCSG, Veterans Administration Laryngeal Cancer Study Group; GETTEC, Group d'Études des Tumeurs de la Tête et du Cou; EORTC, European Organization for Research and Treatment of Cancer; G, glottic; SG, supraglottic; TG, transglottic; HP, hypopharynx; CF, cisplatin+5-fluorouracil; CR, complete response; PR, partial response.

**TABLE 12-14. CLINICAL TARGET VOLUME DETERMINATION GUIDELINES FOR HYPOPHARYNGEAL TUMORS**

| Tumor Site | Clinical Presentation | CTV1 | CTV2 | CTV3 |
|---|---|---|---|---|
| **Pyriform Sinus** | Any TN0 | GTVp | Optional@ | IN+CN (II–V, RPLN) |
| **Pharyngeal Wall** | Any TN+ | GTVp+n | IN (adjacent LNs*) | IN+CN+RPLN† (remaining LNs) |

Roman numerals represent neck nodal levels.
CTV, clinical target volume; N0, node negative neck; N+, node positive neck; GTVp, primary gross tumor volume; N, nodal gross tumor volume; IN, ipsilateral nodal levels; CN, contralateral nodal levels; RPLN, retropharyngeal lymph nodes.
*2–3 cm from CTV1 nodal basin.
†Include RPLN for midline and more advanced tumors.
Suggested IMRT dose schedule for chemoradiation: CTV1 = 70 Gy/35 fx or 70 Gy/33 fx; CTV2 = 63 Gy/35 fx or 59.4 Gy/33 fx; CTV3 = 56 Gy/35 fx or 54 Gy/33 fx.
@Optional margins around CTV1.

ceiving definitive IMRT is shown in Figure 12-7. The patient presented with a sore throat and dysphagia. A large mass in the left pyriform sinus extending to the larynx was found. There was also a level III lymph node palpated in the left neck. The patient was treated with concurrent chemotherapy and definitive IMRT.

### 6.1.3. Normal Tissue Delineation

- See Chapter 8 for delineation of normal tissue (Fig. 8-8).

### 6.1.4. Suggested Target and Normal Tissue Doses

- See Chapter 7 for suggested target and normal tissue doses (Table 7-11).

## 6.2. Larynx

### 6.2.1. Target Volume Determination

- If chemotherapy was delivered before radiation, the targets should be outlined on the planning CT according to their prechemotherapy extent.
- Lymph node groups at risk in the larynx include the following:
  a. Submandibular nodes (surgical level I): N2c cases, especially when level II node is involved.
  b. Upper deep jugular (junctional, parapharyngeal) nodes: all cases (at the neck side ipsilateral to the primary tumor).
  c. Subdigastric (jugulodigastric) nodes, midjugular, lower neck, and supraclavicular nodes (levels II through IV): all cases, bilaterally.
  d. Posterior cervical nodes (level V): all cases, at the neck side where there is an evidence of jugular nodal metastases.

  e. Retropharyngeal nodes: if there is an evidence of metastasis.

- The target volume specification for definitive and postoperative IMRT in laryngeal cancer is summarized in Table 7-5.
- Suggested target volume determination for laryngeal carcinoma is summarized in Table 12-15.

### 6.2.2. Target Volume Delineation

- In patients receiving postoperative IMRT, CTV1 encompasses residual tumor and the region adjacent to it but not directly involved by the tumor, the surgical bed with soft tissue invasion by the tumor, or extracapsular extension by metastatic neck nodes. CTV2 includes primarily the prophylactically treated neck.
- In patients receiving definitive IMRT, CTV1 encompasses gross tumor (primary and enlarged nodes) and the region adjacent to it but not directly involved. CTV2 includes primarily the prophylactically treated neck.
- CTV1 and CTV2 delineation in a patient with pathological T3N1M0 squamous cell carcinoma of a supraglottic larynx receiving definitive IMRT is shown in Figure 12-8. The patient presented with hoarseness, a sore throat, and otalgia. Direct laryngoscopy showed a tumor extending mainly in the epiglottic area through the preepiglottic space and left pharyngeal wall and vallecula. There was also a 2.5 cm palpable lymph node in the left level III region. Biopsy taken from this lesion confirmed the diagnosis of squamous cell carcinoma. The patient was treated with concurrent chemoradiation therapy for the preservation of larynx and salivary function.
- CTV1 and CTV2 delineation in a patient with pathological T2N2bM0 squamous cell carcinoma of the supraglottic larynx receiving postoperative IMRT is

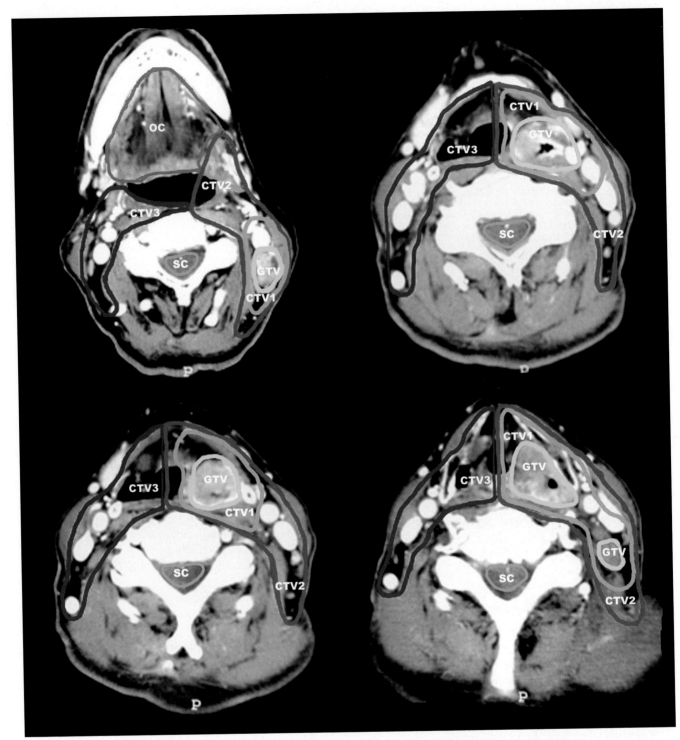

**FIGURE 12-7.** Clinical target volume (CTV) delineation in a patient with a T4N1 pyriform sinus cancer receiving definitive IMRT. Gross tumor volume (GTV), *yellow line;* CTV1, *gold yellow line;* CTV2, *red line;* CTV3 (*dark blue line*); oral cavity (OC), *magenta line;* spinal cord (SC), *green line.*

**TABLE 12-15. CLINICAL TARGET VOLUME DETERMINATION GUIDELINES FOR LARYNGEAL TUMORS**

| Tumor Site | Clinical Presentation | CTV1 | CTV2 | CTV3 |
|---|---|---|---|---|
| **Glottic** | T1–2N0 | GTVp | — | — |
| | T3–4N0 | GTVp | Optional@ | IN+CN (II–V) |
| | Any TN+ | GTVp+n | IN (adjacent LNs*) | IN+CN+RPLN† (remaining LNs) |
| **Supraglottic** | Any TN0 | GTVp | Optional@ | IN+CN (II–V) |
| | Any TN+ | GTVp+n | IN (adjacent LNs*) | IN+CN+RPLN† (remaining LNs) |

CTV, clinical target volume; N0, node negative neck; N+, node positive neck; GTVp, primary gross tumor volume; N, nodal gross tumor volume; IN, ipsilateral nodal levels; CN, contralateral nodal levels; RPLN, retropharyngeal lymph nodes.
Roman numerals represent neck nodal levels.
*2–3 cm from CTV1 nodal basin.
†Include RPLN for midline and more advanced tumors. The chance of RPLN metasis is low.
Suggested IMRT dose schedule for chemoradiation: CTV1 = 70 Gy/35 fx or 70 Gy/33 fx; CTV2 = 63 Gy/35 fx or 59.4 Gy/33 fx; CTV3 = 56 Gy/35 fx or 54 Gy/33 fx.
@Optional margins around CTV1.

shown in Figure 12-9. The patient was presented with hoarseness and a left neck mass. A right-sided supraglottic lesion was seen in direct laryngoscopy. Physical examination revealed two lymph nodes in the right level II neck. A laryngectomy with right modified neck dissection was performed and revealed a surgical staging of T2N2b. Two metastatic lymph nodes were without evidence of extracapsular extension. Postoperative IMRT was given bilaterally to the neck and to the tumor bed.

### 6.2.3. Normal Tissue Delineation

▪ See Chapter 8 for delineation of normal tissue (Fig. 8-8).

### 6.2.4. Suggested Target and Normal Tissue Doses

▪ See Chapter 7 for suggested target and normal tissue doses (Table 7-11).

## 6.3. Intensity-Modulated Radiation Therapy Results

### 6.3.1. Hypopharynx

▪ Following these guidelines, eight patients with hypopharyngeal carcinoma were treated with IMRT between February 1997 and December 2000 at Washington University.[40] Four patients were treated postoperatively while four patients were treated with definitive IMRT. The T stages were one T2, five T3, and two T4. The N stages were four N0, two N1, and two N2 (AJCC staging: one

stage I, three stage III, and four stage IV). Median follow-up time was 21 months (range 11–38 months). We observed two locoregional failures (both in the neck) that were salvaged with surgery. No patients developed distant metastasis. All patients are alive with no evidence of disease, except one who died of intercurrent disease.

▪ G-tube was placed in two patients during the course of IMRT. We observed no grade 3–4 late complications in our patients treated with IMRT. Grade I xerostomia was observed in one patient and trismus developed in another patient as late sequelae.

### 6.3.2. Larynx

▪ Following these guidelines, seven supraglottic larynx carcinoma patients were treated with IMRT between February 1997 and December 2000 at Washington University. All patients were treated with postoperative IMRT. The T stages were two T2, three T3, and two T4. The N stages were three N0, one N1, and three N2 (AJCC staging: two stage III and five stage IV). Median follow-up time was 22 months (range 14–26 months). We observed one locoregional recurrence. This patient subsequently developed distant metastasis and died of disease. We observed no additional distant metastasis. All other patients are alive with no evidence of disease, except one who died of intercurrent disease.

▪ G-tube was placed in three patients during the course of IMRT. We observed no grade 3–4 late complications in our patients treated with IMRT. Grade I xerostomia was observed in three patients and grade II xerostomia in one patient as late sequelae.

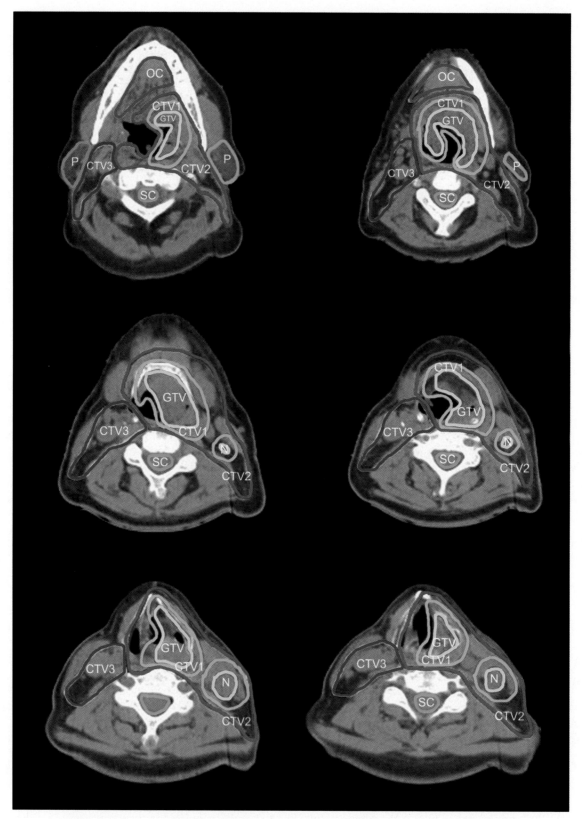

**FIGURE 12-8.** Clinical target volume (CTV) delineation in a patient with a T3N1M0 supraglottic larynx cancer receiving definitive IMRT. Gross tumor volume (GTV), *yellow line*; CTV1, *gold yellow line*; CTV2, *red line*; CTV3 (*dark blue line*); P, parotid gland; right parotid gland, *rust line*; left parotid gland, *aqua line*; oral cavity (OC), *magenta line*; spinal cord (SC), *green line*.

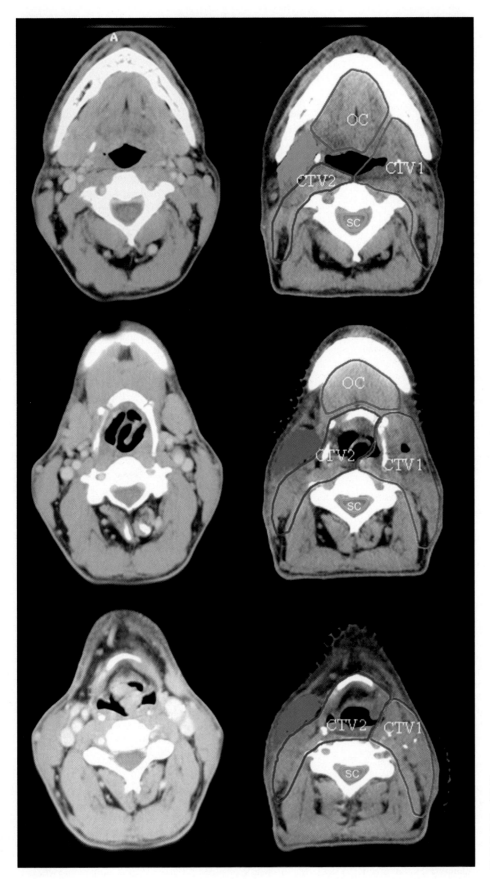

**FIGURE 12-9.** Clinical target volume (CTV) delineation in a patient with a T2N2b supraglottic larynx carcinoma receiving postoperative IMRT. Preoperative CT shown on *left side*, postoperative CT on *right side*. CTV1, *red line*; CTV2, *dark blue line*; oral cavity (OC), *magenta line*.

## REFERENCES

1. Clemente CD. *Anatomy: A Regional Atlas of the Human Body.* Philadelphia: Lea & Febiger, 1975.
2. El Badawi S, Goepfert H, Fletcher G, et al. Squamous cell carcinoma of the pyriform sinus. *Laryngoscope* 1982;92:357–364.
3. Richard J, Sancho-Garnier H, Saravane D, et al. Prognostic factors in cervical lymph node metastasis in upper respiratory and digestive tract carcinomas: study of 1713 cases during a 15-year period. *Laryngoscope* 1987;97:97–101.
4. Wang C, Schulz M, Miller D. Combined radiation therapy and surgery for carcinoma of the supraglottis and pyriform sinus. *Am J Surg* 1972;124:551–554.
5. Marks J, Kurnik B, Powers W, et al. Carcinoma of the pyriform sinus: an analysis of treatment results and patterns of failure. *Cancer* 1978;41:1008–1015.
6. McGavran M, Bauer W, Spjut H, et al. Carcinoma of the pyriform sinus. The results of radical surgery. *Arch Otolaryngol* 1963;78:826–830.
7. Donald P, Hayes R, Dhaliwal R. Combined therapy for pyriform sinus cancer using postoperative irradiation. *Otol Head Neck Surg* 1980;88:738–744.
8. Spector J, Sessions D, Emami B, et al. Squamous cell carcinoma of the pyriform sinus: a nonrandomized comparison of therapeutic modalities and long-term results. *Laryngoscope* 1995;105:397–406.
9. Vandenbrouck C, Eschwege F, De la Rochefordiere A, et al. Squamous cell carcinoma of the pyriform sinus: retrospective study of 351 cases treated at the Institut Gustave-Roussy. *Head Neck Surg* 1987;10:4–13.
10. Lawrence WJ, Terz J, Rogers C, et al. Preoperative irradiation for head and neck cancer: a prospective study. *Cancer* 1974;33:318–323.
11. Wynder EL. The epidemiology of cancers of the upper alimentary and upper respiratory tracts. *Laryngoscope* 1978;88 (Suppl 8):50–51.
12. Lindberg R. Distribution of cervical lymph node metastases from squamous cell carcinoma of the upper respiratory and digestive tracts. *Cancer* 1972;29:1446–1449.
13. Fletcher GH. Elective irradiation of subclinical disease in cancers of the head and neck. *Cancer* 1972;29:1450–1454.
14. Ogura JH, Biller HF, Wette R. Elective neck dissection for pharyngeal and laryngeal cancers: an evaluation. *Ann Otol Rhinol Laryngol* 1971;80:646–651.
15. Mendenhall WM, Parsons JT, Mancuso AA, et al. Larynx. In: Brady LW, ed. *Principles and Practice of Radiation Oncology, 3rd ed.* Philadelphia: Lippincott-Raven;1998:1069–1093.
16. Mendenhall W, Parsons J, Stringer S, et al. T1-T2 vocal cord carcinomas: a basic for comparing the results of the radiotherapy and surgery. *Head Neck Surg.* 1988;10:373–377.
17. Farrington W, Weighill J, Jones P. Postcricoid carcinoma (a 10-year retrospective study). *J Laryngol Otol* 1986;100:79–84.
18. Brugere J, Mosseri V, Mamella G, et al. Nodal failures in patients with N0 N+ oral squamous cell carcinoma without capsular rupture. *Head Neck* 1996;18:133–137.
19. Spector J, Sessions D, Emami B, et al. Squamous cell carcinomas of the aryepiglottic fold: therapeutic results and long-term follow-up. *Laryngoscope* 1995;105:734–746.
20. Emami B, Spector J. Hypopharynx. In: Brady L, ed. *Principles and Practice of Radiation Oncology, 3rd ed.* Philadelphia: Lippincott-Raven;1998:1047–1068.
21. Sasaki T, Baker H, Yeager R. Aggressive surgical management of pyriform sinus carcinoma: a 15-year experience. *Am J Surg* 1986;151:590–592.
22. Cachin Y, Eschwege F. Combination of radiotherapy and surgery in the treatment of head and neck cancers. *Cancer Treat Rev* 1975;2:177–191.
23. McDonald T, DeSanto L, Weiland L. Supraglottic larynx and its pathology as studied by whole laryngeal sections. *Laryngoscope* 1976;86:635–648.
24. Fein DA, Mendenhall WM, Parsons JT, et al. T1-T2 squamous cell carcinoma of the glottic larynx treated with radiotherapy: a multivariate analysis of variables potentially influencing local control. *Int J Radiat Oncol Biol Phys* 1993;25:605–611.
25. Mendenhall WM, Parsons JT, Stringer SP, et al. Management of Tis, T1, and T2 squamous cell carcinoma of the glottic larynx. *Am J Otolaryngol* 1994;15:250–257.
26. O'Sullivan B, Mackillop W, Gilbert R, et al. Controversies in the management of laryngeal cancer: results of an international survey of patterns of care. *Radiother Oncol* 1994;31:23–32.
27. Parsons JT, Mendenhall WM, Mancuso AA, et al. Twice-a-day radiotherapy for T3 squamous cell carcinoma of the glottic larynx. *Head Neck* 1989;11:123–128.
28. Amdur RJ, Parsons JT, Mendenhall WM, et al. Postoperative irradiation for squamous cell carcinoma of the head and neck: an analysis of treatment results and complications. *Int J Radiat Oncol Biol Phys* 1989;16:25–36.
29. Huang DT, Johnson CR, Schmidt-Ullrich R, et al. Postoperative radiotherapy in head and neck carcinoma with extracapsular lymph node extension and/or positive resection margins: a comparative study. *Int J Radiat Oncol Biol Phys* 1992;23:737–742.
30. Mendenhall WM, Parsons JT, Buatti JM, et al. Advances in radiotherapy for head and neck cancer. *Semin Surg Oncol* 1995;11:256–264.
31. Biller HF, Barnhill FR, Jr., Ogura JH, et al. Hemilaryngectomy following radiation failure for carcinoma of the vocal cords. *Laryngoscope* 1968;80:249–253.
32. Mendenhall WM, Parsons JT, Stringer SP, et al. Squamous cell carcinoma of the head and neck treated with irradiation: management of the neck. *Semin Radiat Oncol* 1992;2:163–170.
33. Beahrs OH, Henson DE, Hutter RVP, et al. American Committee on Cancer. *Manual for Staging of Cancer, 4th ed.* Philadelphia: JB Lippincott, 1992.
34. Archer CR, Yeager VL, Herbold DR. Improved diagnostic accuracy in laryngeal cancer using a new classification based on computed tomography. *Cancer* 1984;53:44–57.
35. Spector JG, Sessions DG, Chao KS, et al. Stage I (T1 N0 M0) squamous cell carcinoma of the laryngeal glottis: therapeutic results and voice preservation. *Head Neck* 1999;21:707–717.
36. Spector JG, Sessions DG, Chao KS, et al. Management of stage II (T2N0M0) glottic carcinoma by radiotherapy and conservation surgery. *Head Neck* 1999;21:116–123.
37. Induction chemotherapy plus radiation compared with surgery plus radiation in patients with advanced laryngeal cancer. The Department of Veterans Affairs Laryngeal Cancer Study Group. *N Engl J Med* 1991;324:1685–1690.
38. Pignon J, Bourhis J, Domenge C, et al. Chemotherapy added to locoregional treatment for head and neck squamous-cell carcinoma: three meta-analyses of updated individual data. MACH-NC Collaborative Group. Meta-Analysis of Chemotherapy on Head and Neck Cancer. *Lancet* 2000;18:949–955.
39. Forastiere AA, Goepfert H, Maor M, et al. Concurrent chemotherapy and radiotherapy for organ preservation in advanced laryngeal cancer. *N Engl J Med* 2003;349:2091–2098.
40. Chao K, Wippold F, Ozyigit G, et al. Determination and delineation of nodal target volumes for head-and-neck cancer based on patterns of failure in patients receiving definitive and postoperative IMRT. *Int J Radiat Oncol Biol Phys* 2002;53:1174–1184.
41. Bataini P, Brugere J, Berniere J. Results of radical radiotherapeutic treatment of carcinoma of the pyriform sinus. *Int J Radiat Oncol Biol Phys* 1982;8:1277.
42. Mendenhall W, Parsons J, Cassisi N, et al. Squamous cell carcinoma of the pyriform sinus treated with surgery and/or radiotherapy. *Head Neck Surg* 1987;10:88–92.

43. Mendenhall W, Parsons J, Cassisi N, et al. Squamous cell carcinoma of the pyriform sinus treated with radical radiation therapy. *Radiother Oncol* 1987;9:201–208.

44. Mendenhall W, Parsons J, Stringer S, et al. Radiotherapy alone or combined with neck dissection for T1-T2 carcinoma of the pyriform sinus: an alternative to conservation surgery. *Int J Radiat Oncol Biol Phys* 1993;27:1017–1027.

45. Dubois J, Guerrier B, Di Ruggiero J, et al. Cancer of the pyriform sinus: treatment by radiation therapy alone and after surgery. *Radiology* 1986;160:831–836.

46. Marks J, Sessions D. Hypopharynx. In: Brady L, ed. *Principles and Practice of Radiation Oncology, 2nd ed.* Philadelphia: JB Lippincott, 1992.

47. Meoz-Mendez R, Fletcher G, Guillamondeque O. Analysis of the results of irradiation in the treatment of squamous cell carcinoma of the pharyngeal wall. *Int J Radiat Oncol Biol Phys* 1978;4: 579–585.

48. Mendenhall W, Parsons J, Mancuso A, et al. Squamous cell carcinoma of the pharyngeal wall treated with irradiation. *Radiother Oncol* 1988;11:205–212.

49. Chang L, Stevens K, Moss W, et al. Squamous cell carcinoma of the pharyngeal walls treated with radiotherapy. *Int J Radiat Oncol Biol Phys* 1996;35:477–483.

50. Wang C. *Carcinoma of the Hypopharynx, 2nd ed.* Chicago: Year Book Medical Publishers, 1990.

51. Mittal B, Marks JE, Ogura JH. Transglottic carcinoma. *Cancer* 1984;53:151–161.

52. Yuen A, Medina JE, Goepfert H, et al. Management of stage T3 and T4 glottic carcinomas. *Am J Surg* 1984;148:467–472.

53. Lundgren JA, Gilbert RW, van Nostrand AW, et al. T3N0M0 glottic carcinoma: a failure analysis. *Clin Otolaryngol* 1988;13: 455–465.

54. Meredith AP, Randall CJ, Shaw HJ. Advanced laryngeal cancer: a management perspective. *J Laryngol Otol* 1987;101:1046–1054.

55. Razack MS, Maipang T, Sako K, et al. Management of advanced glottic carcinomas. *Am J Surg* 1989;158:318–320.

56. Mendenhall WM, Parsons JT, Stringer SP, et al. Stage T3 squamous cell carcinoma of the glottic larynx: a comparison of laryn- gectomy and irradiation. *Int J Radiat Oncol Biol Phys* 1992;23: 725–732.

57. Simpson D, Robertson AG, Lamont D. A comparison of radiotherapy and surgery as primary treatment in the management of T3 N0 M0 glottic tumours. *J Laryngol Otol* 1993;107: 912–915.

58. Foote RL, Olsen KD, Buskirk SJ, et al. Laryngectomy alone for T3 glottic cancer. *Head Neck* 1994;16:406–412.

59. Kligerman J, Olivatto LO, Lima RA, et al. Elective neck dissection in the treatment of T3/T4 N0 squamous cell carcinoma of the larynx. *Am J Surg* 1995;170:436–439.

60. Hao SP, Myers EN, Johnson JT. T3 glottic carcinoma revisited. Transglottic vs pure glottic carcinoma. *Arch Otolaryngol Head Neck Surg* 1995;121:166–170.

61. Bryant GP, Poulsen MG, Tripcony L, et al. Treatment decisions in T3N0M0 glottic carcinoma. *Int J Radiat Oncol Biol Phys* 1995;31:285–293.

62. Kowalski LP, Batista MB, Santos CR, et al. Prognostic factors in T3, N0-1 glottic and transglottic carcinoma. A multifactorial study of 221 cases treated by surgery or radiotherapy. *Arch Otolaryngol Head Neck Surg* 1996;122:77–82.

63. Mendenhall WM, Parsons JT, Mancusco AA, et al. Definitive radiotherapy for T3 squamous cell carcinoma of the glottic larynx. *J Clin Oncol* 1997;15:2394–2402.

64. Nguyen TD, Malissard L, Theobald S, et al. Advanced carcinoma of the larynx: results of surgery and radiotherapy without induction chemotherapy (1980–1985): a multivariate analysis. *Int J Radiat Oncol Biol Phys* 1996;36:1013–1018.

65. Parsons JT, Mendenhall WM, Stringer SP, et al. T4 laryngeal carcinoma: radiotherapy alone with surgery reserved for salvage. *Int J Radiat Oncol Biol Phys* 1998;40:549–552.

66. Mancuso AA, Mukherji SK, Schmalfuss I, et al. Preradiotherapy computed tomography as a predictor of local control in supraglottic carcinoma. *J Clin Oncol* 1999;17:631–637.

67. MacKenzie RG, Franssen E, Balogh JM, et al. Comparing treatment outcomes of radiotherapy and surgery in locally advanced carcinoma of the larynx: a comparison limited to patients eligible for surgery. *Int J Radiat Oncol Biol* 2000;47:64–74.

# 13

# THYROID CARCINOMA
## ANESA AHAMAD

## 1. ANATOMY

- The thyroid gland lies in close proximity to the larynx and trachea, cricothyroid ligament, laryngeal nerves (external and recurrent laryngeal) and vagus nerves, common carotid artery and internal jugular vein, hypopharynx, esophagus, strap muscles and prevertebral muscles. These critical structures in the root of the neck and thoracic inlet are at risk for direct invasion by thyroid cancer (Fig. 13-1).
- The gland consists of two lateral lobes and a central isthmus and extends from the level of C5 to T1 vertebra.

### 1.1. Important Anatomical Relations

- As shown in Figure 13-1, the isthmus overlies the second and third tracheal ring and just above it is the arch of the cricoid cartilage and the cricothyroid ligament. The lobes overlie the lateral part of the cricothyroid membrane. The lateral part of this ligament has a free upper margin which is covered in mucous membrane and forms the vocal cord. The lobes surround the upper tracheal rings and esophagus as shown in the same figure.
- The lobes are related antero-laterally laterally to the strap muscles, and just posterior to the lobes are the prevertebral muscles and the inferior constrictor of the pharynx.
- The recurrent laryngeal nerves, which supply all of the intrinsic muscles of the larynx except the cricoarytenoid, may be injured during surgery or by direct tumor infiltration as it enters the larynx under the border of the inferior constrictor behind the cricothyroid joint or in the superior mediastinum.
- The most common site of injury as it crosses the inferior thyroid artery behind the lower part of the lateral lobes is in the region of Berry's ligament.[1] This ligament is the thick part of the pretracheal fascia that suspends the gland from the trachea and cricoid cartilage.
- Important anatomical relations of the normal thyroid gland on CT imaging that are relevant to radiation oncology are shown in Figure 13-2, which shows transverse

sections around the level of the isthmus. Note particularly the spatial relation to the tracheal rings, strap muscles, prevertebral muscles, esophagus, common carotid artery, and the internal jugular vein. Figure 13-3 shows sections more superiorly at the level of the cricoid and thyroid cartilage. Note the position of the thyroid gland to both the cricoid and thyroid cartilage, and that posteriorly the gland abuts the hypopharynx.
- The direct invasion of these local structures is illustrated in Figures 13-4 and 13-5. Figure 13-4 shows CT images of tumor directly invading the trachea, prevertebral muscles, and esophagus. Figure 13-5 shows transverse CT images of tumor directly invading the pyriform sinus, muscles of the hypopharynx, and tracheoesophageal groove.
- Thyroid cancer recurrence postero-laterally in the tracheoesophageal groove is a particularly challenging problem. Figure 13-6 shows examples of the typical location of these recurrences and their threat to the airway, speech, and swallowing. These images may be useful in target volume delineation.

### 1.2. Lymph Nodes

- Regional lymph node spread is common and the distribution of regional nodes is widespread.
- The first station nodes are the level VI nodes: pretracheal, paratracheal, paralaryngeal, and Delphian nodes near the isthmus (Figs. 13-1 and 13-7).[2]
- The secondary nodes are the deep and superficial cervical chains and supraclavicular fossa: nodal levels I through V.
- Inferiorly, the gland drains into level VII, the anterior superior mediastinal nodes.
- Superiorly, it drains as high as the parapharyngeal and retropharyngeal nodes.
- The lymph nodes involved should be described according to the levels of the neck that are involved.[2]
- Nodal metastases from medullary thyroid cancer carry a more ominous prognosis than well-differentiated thyroid cancer.[3]

*Text continues on page 214.*

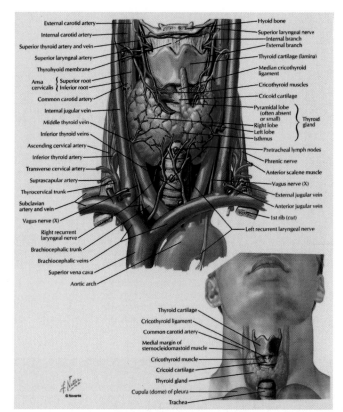

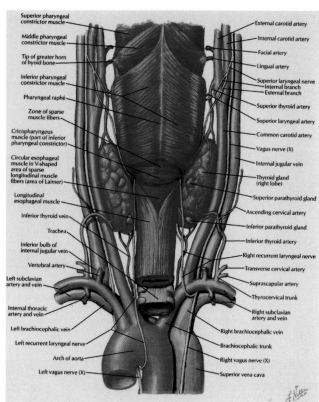

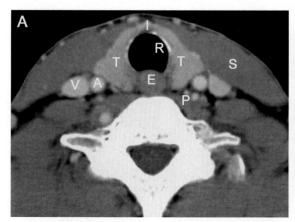

**FIGURE 13-1.** The thyroid gland's close proximity to critical structures in the root of the neck and thoracic inlet. Note its contact with the larynx, trachea, cricothyroid ligament, laryngeal nerves (external and recurrent laryngeal), vagus nerves, common carotid artery and internal jugular vein, hypopharynx, esophagus, strap muscles, and prevertebral muscles. These are at risk for direct invasion by thyroid cancer. (From: Netter FH. *Atlas of human anatomy, 2nd ed.* Teterboro, NJ: Icon Learning Systems; 2003:68–69.)

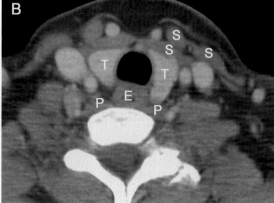

**FIGURE 13-2.** Important anatomical relations of the normal thyroid gland in two separate patients on CT imaging. **A:** Section at the level of the isthmus (*I*). **B:** Section just above the isthmus. Note that the thyroid gland (*T*) overlies the tracheal ring (*R*) and the lobes are in direct contact with the strap muscles (*S*) anteriorly and anterolaterally. The lobes also abut the prevertebral muscles (*P*) posteriorly, the esophagus (*E*) posteromedially, and the common carotid artery (*A*) and the internal jugular vein (*V*) laterally.

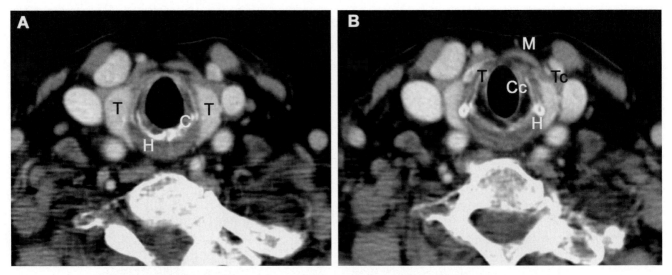

**FIGURE 13-3.** Important anatomical relations of the normal thyroid gland above the isthmus. **A:** Section at the level of the cricoid cartilage (*C*). **B:** Section at the inferior portion of the thyroid cartilage (*Tc*). Note that the thyroid gland (*T*) is closely related to both these intrinsic structures of the larynx, and that posteriorly, it directly abuts the inferior constrictor muscles of the hypopharynx (*H*). Note the position of the cricothyroid ligament (*M*).

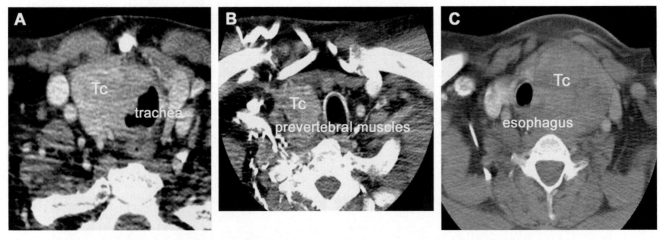

**FIGURE 13-4.** Direct invasion of adjacent structures by thyroid cancer (*Tc*). Invasion of the trachea **(A)**, right prevertebral muscles **(B)**, and esophagus **(C)**.

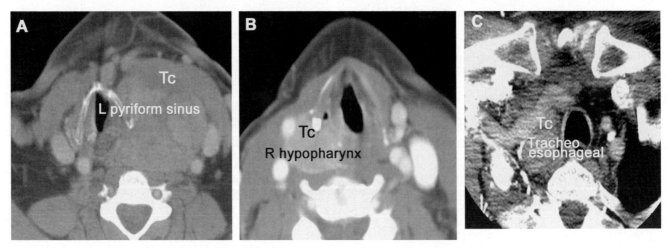

**FIGURE 13-5.** Direct invasion of the adjacent structures by thyroid cancer (Tc). Invasion of the left pyriform sinus **(A)**, right hypopharynx **(B)**, and right tracheoesophageal groove recurrence **(C)**.

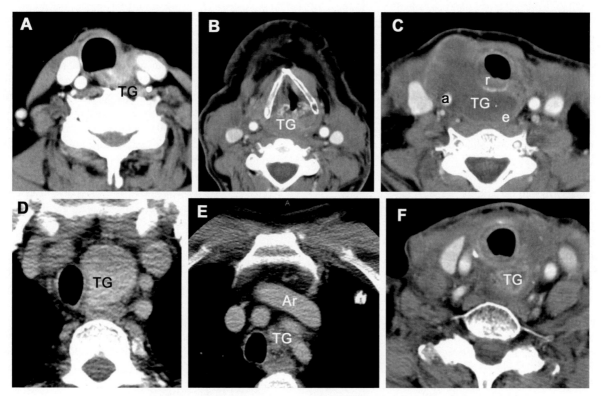

**FIGURE 13-6.** Recurrent tumor in the tracheoesophageal groove (*TG*) after total thyroidectomy. **A:** Small volume recurrence in the left tracheoesophageal groove. Despite aggressive attempt to resect this, there were persistent positive margins. **B:** Recurrence in right tracheoesophageal groove at the level of the vocal cords which threatens the larynx and hypopharynx. **C:** The same patient as in **B** shows tracheoesophageal groove recurrence which involves the tracheal ring (*r*), esophagus (*e*) and encases the common carotid artery (*a*). **D:** Bulky left tracheoesophageal groove recurrence. **E:** Tumor seen in **D** is seen here extending down along the tracheoesophageal groove into the superior mediastinum at the level of the aortic arch (*Ar*). **F:** Recurrence in the left tracheoesophageal groove following radiotherapy with less than 50 Gy given to this region.

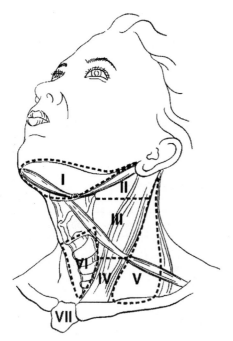

**FIGURE 13-7.** Location of lymph nodes as described in the text and in thyroid staging. (From: Greene FL, et al., eds. *AJCC cancer staging manual*, 6th ed. New York: Springer, 2002.)[2]

## 2. NATURAL HISTORY

### 2.1. Pathology

- Thyroid cancer has a spectrum of histologic types of tumors according to the cells of origin. The main parenchymal cell types are follicular cells and parafollicular neuroendocrine or C cells.
- Follicular cells uptake iodine and produce thyroid hormone. It gives rise to well-differentiated cancers and anaplastic thyroid cancer.
- C cells produce calcitonin and are the cells of origin for medullary thyroid carcinoma (MTC).
- Stromal cells are responsible for sarcoma, and B or T cells give rise to lymphoma.
- The four major histopathologic types of malignant thyroid tumors are: papillary, follicular, medullary, and undifferentiated (anaplastic) carcinoma. The overwhelming majority are favorable well-differentiated tumors (Table 13-1).[4–6]
- More rare tumors include the highly lethal anaplastic or spindle cell thyroid cancer, lymphoma, squamous cell cancer, sarcoma, and metastatic tumors to the thyroid (Table 13-1).[4–6]
- Both papillary and follicular carcinomas have an excellent prognosis if they are confined to the thyroid gland with a well-defined tumor capsule, smaller than 1 cm, or are minimally invasive. Both have adverse outcomes if they are locally invasive or metastatic.[7,8]
- Papillary thyroid carcinoma is the most common histologic type, with a high incidence of multicentricity and lymph node metastasis. Variants of this type, which carry a poorer prognosis, are: tall-cell papillary (25% 10-year mortality), columnar papillary (90% mortality), diffuse sclerosing scirrhous, trabecular and insular variants, and tumor with anaplastic features.[4,9]
- Follicular-variant papillary carcinoma does not have a worse prognosis. Patients with papillary thyroid carcinoma with lymphocytic thyroiditis tend to have more limited disease and better survival.[10]
- Follicular thyroid cancer may be more aggressive than papillary carcinoma with a higher likelihood of hematogeneous spread (30%). It is typically a solitary encapsulated tumor with follicular cell invasion of the capsule or

blood vessels. If capsular penetration is minimal, they are less likely to produce distant metastases or death.[11]
- Nonencapsulated follicular carcinomas, which extensively grow into adjacent tissues and blood vessel, are much less common. Up to 80% of these highly invasive larger cancers will metastasize and 20% of patients will die of their tumor within a few years of diagnosis.[12]
- Hürthle cell tumors are included as a variant of follicular tumors in the WHO classification; however, they are an independent group.
- When oncocytic cells (also know as oxyphil or Askanazy cells) occupy most of the tumor mass, the disease is classified as Hürthle cell carcinoma. They are unpredictable and may be aggressive with a mortality rate as high as 25% in 30 years.[13]
- Anaplastic thyroid cancer contains giant and spindle cells. They rapidly invade local structures and lymph nodes and develop distant metastases. Small cell anaplastic thyroid cancer has a better prognosis.
- Medullary thyroid cancer (MTC) typically presents in the upper pole because the C cells are predominantly located in the upper portion of each lobe of the gland. Approximately half of these patients present with cervical adenopathy.
- Eighty percent of MTCs are sporadic and the typical age of presentation is the fifth or sixth decade. The rest are inherited either as part of a syndrome, such as multiple endocrine neoplasia type 2A (MEN 2A), MEN 2B, or familial medullary thyroid carcinoma (FMTC), and present in the third decade of life.
- Genetic defects have been pinpointed to mutations of the RET proto-oncogene on chromosome 10q11.[14] The RET proto-oncogene codes for a cell membrane-associated tyrosine kinase receptor.

### 2.2. Recurrence Patterns

- Approximately one-third of patients with differentiated thyroid carcinoma have tumor recurrences after several decades.[7]
- Extension into the neck is the first sign of a potentially lethal outcome.[15,16]

### TABLE 13-1. PATHOLOGY OF THYROID CANCER AND ITS ESTIMATED INCIDENCE[4–6]

| Well-Differentiated | Incidence | Other Histology | Incidence |
|---|---|---|---|
| Papillary carcinoma | 78% | Medullary carcinoma | 4% |
| Follicular carcinoma | 13% | Anaplastic carcinoma | 2% |
| Hurthle cell carcinoma | <3% | Lymphoma | <5% |
| | | Squamous cell carcinoma, sarcoma, metastatic tumors | <1% |

- Three-quarters of local recurrences occur in the cervical lymph nodes, and a quarter in the thyroid bed.
- Recurrent disease in the tracheoesophageal groove is particularly challenging to resect and threatens speech, swallowing and airway functions (Fig. 13-6).

## 3. DIAGNOSIS AND STAGING SYSTEMS

### 3.1. Signs and Symptoms

- Differentiated thyroid cancer presents most often as a solitary nodule, similar to the more common benign adenomas and cysts. They grow slowly and therefore, diagnosis is often delayed with approximately 50% of thyroid cancer being discovered during routine examination, imaging, or surgery for presumed benign disease.[7,12]
- Elements of a patient's history which should raise suspicion are

  □ Age: higher in patients less than 15 years and over 60 years.
  □ Symptoms of local invasion such as hoarseness or dysphagia.
  □ Pain.
  □ Rapid growth.
  □ Diarrhea, symptoms of Cushing syndrome, or facial flushing due to the ability of medullary thyroid cancer to secrete hormonally active peptides (adrenocorticotrophic hormone [ACTH], calcitonin-gene related peptide [CGRP]).
  □ Radiation exposure.
  □ Positive family history of thyroid cancer.
  □ Medical history of the diseases associated with

  - MEN 2 syndromes: hyperparathyroidism, pheochromocytoma, a marfanoid habitus, or mucosal neuromas.
  - Familial nonmedullary thyroid carcinoma: Gardner syndrome (a familial adenomatous polyposis with extracolonic manifestations),[17] Carney complex (multiple neoplasia that affects endocrine glands and a lentiginosis syndrome),[18] Cowden syndrome (multiple hamartomas), microscopic familial papillary thyroid carcinoma (more aggressive than the sporadic form)[19] that often metastasizes to lymph nodes and has a high rate of recurrence and distant metastases.[20]

  □ MTC may present with dense calcifications seen on imaging of the anterior neck or metastatic sites.

### 3.2. Physical Examination

- Complete examination of the head and neck is necessary with particular attention to the size, mobility of the mass, attachment to adjacent structures, presence of enlarged lymph nodes, quality of the voice, and presence of stridor.
- Upper airway endoscopy is used to assess vocal cord function.
- Physical findings which raise suspicion of malignancy are

  □ Size: nodules less than 1cm are almost always benign, while nodules over 4 cm have a higher risk of malignancy.[21,22]
  □ Consistency: firm or hard nodules.
  □ Masses fixed to the trachea, larynx, or strap muscles.
  □ Presence of regional lymphadenopathy.
  □ Vocal cord paralysis or paresis due to invasion of the recurrent laryngeal nerve of invasion of muscles and ligaments around the larynx.

### 3.3. Diagnosis and Imaging

#### 3.3.1. Preoperative

- Baseline thyrotropin (TSH) level.
- Fine needle aspiration (FNA) of nodule and enlarged lymph nodes.
- If suspected differentiated thyroid cancer (papillary, follicular, Hürthle cell).

  □ Chest x-ray.
  □ Neck ultrasound.
  □ MRI if suspicious for deep infiltration or extension into the mediastinum. (Iodine contrast with CT is avoided.)

#### 3.3.2. Postoperative

- *Baseline radioactive iodine (RAI) scanning:* thyroid follicular cells physiologically trap and retain iodine. Four to six weeks after thyroidectomy, 3 to 5 mCi of RAI is administered orally and its gamma rays are imaged after 24 hours to produce a whole body map of uptake. This documents any evidence of residual thyroid tissue and enables the calculation of the biological half-life of the isotope, which is useful for deciding doses required for ablation. It may also document metastases, although metastatic lesions which are less avid and may not uptake the presence of a large competing volume of highly avid thyroid tissue.
- *Follow-up—scanning postablation:* remnant thyroid tissue and tumors that uptake iodine are ablated by high dose RAI. Diagnostic scanning is then useful for routine follow-up or diagnosis when there is an elevated thyroglobulin or other signs of recurrence.
- *Thyroglobulin (Tg), Tg antibodies, and TG mRNA:* baseline thyroglobulin and thyroglobulin antibodies are measured postoperatively, post–RAI ablation, or upon suspicion of recurrence. The detection of circulating thyroglobulin mRNA is a more sensitive marker of residual thyroid tissue or cancer than assay for serum thy-

roglobulin, particularly in patients treated with thyroid hormone or patients with circulating antithyroglobulin antibodies; however, this test is not yet standard.[23]

- *Recombinant human thyroid stimulating hormone (rhTSH):* both RAI scanning and measurement of serum Tg during follow-up requires a raised serum TSH concentration sufficient to stimulate thyroid tissue or carcinoma to induce [131]I uptake and Tg release. This can be done by withdrawing thyroid hormone, causing symptomatic hypothyroidism. Alternatively, symptomatic hypothyroidism can be avoided by administering rhTSH intramuscularly while the patient continues thyroid hormone.[24,25]

- *PET scanning in patients with raised TG and negative RAI scans:* fluoro-2-deoxy-d-glucose positron emission tomography (FDG-PET) is a valuable diagnostic tool for localizing residual disease in patients with thyroid cancer who have negative whole-body RAI scans and elevated thyroglobulin. The cancer cells may dedifferentiate and lose the ability to concentrate iodine. FDG-PET is approved for investigation of this group of patients. In one study of patients in this setting, PET localized occult disease in 71% of patients with elevated thyroglobulin levels, and had a positive predictive value of 92%.[26]

- PET scans are clinically indicated in thyroid cancer of follicular call origin for restaging of recurrent or residual thyroid cancers in cases of

  □ Previous treatment by thyroidectomy and RAI ablation.
  □ Serum thyroglobulin of >10 ng/mL.
  □ Negative [131]I whole body scans.

### 3.3.3. Additional Investigations for MTC

- Serum calcitonin, carcinoembryonic antigen (CEA), and calcium.
- Screen for pheochromocytoma (important because this has to be managed prior to thyroid surgery).
- Screen for RET proto-oncogene. Genetic testing for RET proto-oncogene mutations should be offered to all newly diagnosed patients with clinically apparent sporadic MTC since 6% of them carry a germline mutation in RET. Children and adults in known kindreds with inherited forms of MTC should also be screened.
- Neck ultrasound.

## 3.4. Staging

- The American Joint Committee on Cancer staging system for carcinoma of the thyroid is shown in Table 13-2 and Figure 13-7.[2]
- Unlike the TNM staging of other head and neck cancers, it uses *age* and *histology* as criteria.

- The lymph node N classification is unique to this site.
- All papillary and follicular cancers are stage I or II if patients are less than 45 years old.
- Medullary carcinoma staging does not use age as a criterion.
- Note the difference between N1a and N1b in classification of stage III versus IV for patients with medullary cancer or patients older then 45 years with papillary or follicular cancer.
- All anaplastic carcinomas are considered T4.
- This is the most commonly used system. However, the management of a patient with thyroid cancer is dictated by the risk factors, many of which are not included in the TNM staging system.

## 4. PROGNOSTIC FACTORS

### 4.1. Differentiated Thyroid Cancer

- Ten-year relative survival rates for patients with papillary, follicular, Hürthle cell, and undifferentiated/anaplastic carcinomas were 93%, 85%, 76%, and 14%, respectively, according to an analysis of 53,856 thyroid carcinoma cases from the National Cancer Data Base (NCDB: a national electronic registry system which captures approximately 60% of incident cancers in the United States).[6]
- The prognostic factors of a given case are key in determining the treatment plan. Many institutions have collected and analyzed data to assign risk groups which are used to guide extent of surgery, radioactive iodine, and adjuvant radiotherapy.
- The factors which have emerged as important are

  □ Patient-related factors: age, gender.
  □ Tumor-related factors: size, histopathological grade and variant, extra-thyroidal extension in to muscle, larynx, trachea, esophagus, recurrent laryngeal nerve, presence of lymph node or distant metastasis.

- The Mayo Clinic's AGES classification system is based on prognostic factors of age, grade of the tumor, extrathyroidal extension, and size of the tumor.[27]
- The Lahey Clinic's AMES classification system used age, distant metastasis, extra-thyroidal extension, and size.[28,29]
- Both the AGES and AMES systems allow patients to be classified as low risk (long-term mortality less than 2%) or high risk (mortality up to 46%).
- The University of Chicago classification system of four classes

  □ I: disease limited to the thyroid gland.
  □ II: disease involving locoregional lymph nodes.
  □ III: extrathyroid tumor invasion.
  □ IV: distant metastasis.

**TABLE 13-2. AJCC 2002 STAGING FOR THYROID CARCINOMA**

**TNM Definition**

*Primary Tumor (T)*

*Note:* All categories may be subdivided: (a) solitary tumor, (b) multifocal tumor (the largest determines the classification).

| | |
|---|---|
| TX | Primary tumor cannot be assessed. |
| T0 | No evidence of primary tumor. |
| T1 | Tumor ≤2 cm in greatest dimension limited to the thyroid. |
| T2 | Tumor >2 cm but ≤4 cm in greatest dimension limited to the thyroid. |
| T3 | Tumor >4 cm in greatest dimension limited to the thyroid or any tumor with minimal extrathyroid extension (e.g., extension to sternothyroid muscle or perithyroid soft tissues). |
| T4a | Tumor of any size extending beyond the thyroid capsule to invade subcutaneous soft tissues, larynx, trachea, esophagus, or recurrent laryngeal nerve. |
| T4b | Tumor invades prevertebral fascia or encases carotid artery or mediastinal vessels. |

*All anaplastic carcinomas are considered T4 tumors*

| | |
|---|---|
| **T4a** | **Intrathyroidal anaplastic carcinomas–surgically resectable.** |
| **T4b** | **Extrathyroidal anaplastic carcinomas–surgically unresectable.** |

*Regional Lymph Nodes (N)*

Regional lymph nodes are the central compartment, lateral, cervical, and upper mediastinal lymph nodes.

| | |
|---|---|
| NX | Regional lymph nodes cannot be assessed. |
| N0 | No regional lymph node metastasis. |
| N1 | Regional lymph node metastasis. |
| N1a | Metastasis to level VI (pretracheal, paratracheal, and prelaryngeal/Delphian lymph nodes). |
| N1b | Metastasis to unilateral, bilateral, or contralateral cervical or superior mediastinal lymph nodes. |

*Distant Metastasis (M)*

| | |
|---|---|
| MX | Distant metastasis cannot be assessed. |
| M0 | No distant metastasis. |
| M1 | Distant metastasis. |

**Stage Grouping**

*Note:* Separate stage groupings are recommended for papillary or follicular, medullary, and anaplastic (undifferentiated) carcinoma.

| ***Papillary or Follicular*** UNDER 45 YEARS | | | |
|---|---|---|---|
| Stage I | Any T | Any N | M0 |
| Stage II | Any T | Any N | M1 |

| ***Papillary or Follicular*** 45 YEARS AND OLDER | | | |
|---|---|---|---|
| Stage I | T1 | N0 | M0 |
| Stage II | T2 | N0 | M0 |
| Stage III | T3 | N0 | M0 |
| | T1 | N1a | M0 |
| | T2 | N1a | M0 |
| | T3 | N1a | M0 |
| Stage IVA | T4a | N0 | M0 |
| | T4a | N1a | M0 |
| | T1 | N1b | M0 |
| | T2 | N1b | M0 |
| | T3 | N1b | M0 |
| | T4a | N1b | M0 |
| Stage IVB | T4b | Any N | M0 |
| Stage IVC | Any T | Any N | M1 |

| ***Medullary Carcinoma*** | | | |
|---|---|---|---|
| Stage I | T1 | N0 | M0 |
| Stage II | T2 | N0 | M0 |
| Stage III | T3 | N0 | M0 |
| | T1 | N1a | M0 |
| | T2 | N1a | M0 |
| | T3 | N1a | M0 |
| Stage IVA | T4a | N0 | M0 |
| | T4a | N1a | M0 |
| | T1 | N1b | M0 |
| | T2 | N1b | M0 |
| | T3 | N1b | M0 |
| | T4a | N1b | M0 |
| Stage IVB | T4b | Any N | M0 |
| Stage IVC | Any T | Any N | M1 |

| ***Anaplastic Carcinoma*** | | | |
|---|---|---|---|
| All anaplastic carcinomas are considered stage IV. | | | |
| Stage IVA | T4a | Any N | M0 |
| Stage IVB | T4b | Any N | M0 |
| Stage IVC | Any T | Any N | M1 |

From: Greene FL et al., eds. *AJCC cancer staging manual,* 6th ed. New York: Springer, 2002.

- Ohio State University classification system of four stages

  □ 1: primary tumor smaller than 1.5 cm.
  □ 2: primary tumor 1.5 cm to 4.4 cm or presence of cervical lymph node metastases or more than three intrathyroidal foci of tumor.
  □ 3: primary tumor at least 4.5 cm or presence of extrathyroidal invasion.
  □ 4: distant metastases.

- European Organization of Research (EORTC) also uses similar factors in risk stratification.

- While none of these predict the *high risk of recurrences* which occur in patients *less than* 20 years old, the Memorial Sloan-Kettering Cancer Center's GAMES system includes this factor. Their patients were divided into low, intermediate, and high risk groups based on these prognostic factors: grade, age, distant metastasis, extrathyroidal extension, and size of the tumor.[30,31]

  □ Low risk group: below the age of 45 with low risk tumors (99% survival).
  □ Intermediate risk group: young patients with more aggressive tumors and older patients with less aggressive tumors (85% survival).

□ High risk group: patients above the age of 45 with high risk tumors (57% survival).

■ The Mayo Clinic's MACIS system adds a treatment-related factor: completeness of resection along with distant metastasis, age, extra-thyroidal tumor invasion, and size of the tumor. Completeness of resection is a major prognostic factor especially when there is extrathyroidal tumor extension.

## 4.2. Medullary Thyroid Cancer

■ A separate though smaller set of staging approaches exist for MTC. The TNM criteria is given in Table 13-2.

■ Another classification was proposed that characterizes stage III as extrathyroidal or extranodal extension of disease.[32] These patients have significantly worse survival.[33]

■ A third approach is used by the National Thyroid Cancer Treatment Cooperative Study Group to classify tumors into four stages.[34]

□ I: premalignant lesion C-cell hyperplasia.
□ II: primary tumor less than 1 cm without locoregional or distant metastasis.
□ III: tumor greater than 1 cm or locoregional nodal metastasis.
□ IV: distant metastases.

■ Other important poor prognostic factors which must be considered in treatment planning are:

□ Age: patients <40 years old have a 5- and 10-year disease-specific survival rate of about 95% and 75%, respectively, compared with 65% and 50% for those older than age 40 years.[33]
□ MEN 2B: patients with MTC have more locally aggressive disease than those with either MEN 2A or FMTC.[35]
□ Tumors which stain poorly for calcitonin on immunostaining.[36]
□ Rapid rise of serum CEA.[37]
□ Persistent elevated hypercalcitonin.[38]
□ Specific mutations in RET oncogene: exon 16 mutation is associated with more aggressive disease.[39]

## 5. GENERAL MANAGEMENT

■ Multidisciplinary participation is essential in the management of thyroid cancer. While complete surgical removal of the disease is the mainstay of therapy, patients may also require radioactive remnant ablation, adjuvant radioactive iodine therapy, medical suppression of TSH by high dose thyroxine, and/or external beam radiation therapy.

■ A detailed review of the patient and tumor characteristics with respect to the above-mentioned prognostic factors for each histological subtype is necessary is determining the appropriate adjuvant treatment.

## 5.1. Surgery

■ Controversy exists over the extent of initial surgery and neck dissection.[40–43] The extent of surgery depends on the risk of local recurrence based on factors described in the above risk classification systems.

■ The advantages of total thyroidectomy are:

□ Less than 2% risk of permanent hypoparathyroidism or recurrent laryngeal nerve injury.
□ No risk of persistent multifocal cancer in the remnant thyroid tissue.
□ Leaving residual functioning thyroid tissue hampers the detection of metastases or recurrence by radioiodine scanning or serum thyroglobulin.

■ In support of this approach is one study which reported that patients with papillary carcinoma considered to be lowrisk (by age, metastases, extent, and size) had higher rates of local recurrence and nodal metastasis after unilateral lobectomy (14% and 19%, respectively) than after bilateral thyroid lobe resection (2% and 6%, respectively) at 20-years follow-up ($P = 0.0001$). However, there were no significant differences in cancer-specific mortality or distant metastasis rates between the two groups.

■ Advocates of thyroid lobectomy and isthmusectomy or near total thyroidectomy argue

□ There is less risk of injury to the recurrent laryngeal nerve and permanent hypoparathyroidism.
□ Occult residual foci of papillary cancer are rarely of clinical significance.
□ Recurrences after conservative surgery can be managed by re-operation, and therefore, there is no survival advantage of total thyroidectomy over lobectomy for well-differentiated thyroid cancer.

■ While total thyroidectomy allows for radioactive iodine dosimetry and ablation, as well as the use of serum thyroglobulin as a tumor marker in the follow-up of patients, these are generally not necessary in low risk-group patients. Although the incidence of microscopic thyroid cancer in the contralateral lobe ranges between 30% and 80%, the incidence of clinical recurrence in the opposite lobe after ipsilateral lobectomy is only 5% to 7%.[44,45]

■ Lobectomy and isthmusectomy is appropriate for papillary cancers smaller than 1.5 cm.

■ A total or near total thyroidectomy is performed for papillary cancers larger than 1.5 cm, those associated with previous radiation, gross bilateral disease, presence of adverse histopathological features, positive margins, and follicular and Hürthle cell carcinoma.

■ Central compartmental lymph node dissection is recommended. Palpable neck adenopathy or clinical suspicion of nodal metastases requires neck dissection.

■ Total thyroidectomy and bilateral central neck dissection (level VI) is indicated in all patients with MTC, especially when considering the high frequency of bilateral disease in both sporadic and familial disease.[33]

- Modified radical neck dissections (levels II to V) are recommended for all patients with primary tumors larger than 1 cm in diameter (0.5 cm for patients with MEN 2B) or in cases where the tumor is in the central node(s).

- Disfiguring radical node dissections do not improve prognosis and are not indicated. In the presence of grossly invasive disease, more extended procedures with resection of involved neck structures may be appropriate. Function-preserving approaches are preferred.

- Patients with inherited disease are recommended to have total thyroidectomy by age 5 years. Total thyroidectomy is recommended in the first year of life or at diagnosis for MEN 2B patients with specific mutations in (codon 883, 918, or 922 RET mutations). A bilateral central neck dissection (level VI) should be strongly considered for patients with MEN 2B and those identified by genetic testing.[46]

## 5.2. Adjuvant Thyroid Hormone Therapy

- The suppression of endogenous TSH is believed to deprive differentiated thyroid cancer cells of the growth promoting effect of TSH. Supraphysiological oral thyroxine exerts a negative feedback to switch off pituitary production of TSH. Serum TSH concentration is maintained below the lower limit of the normal range ($<0.1$–$0.01$ mU/L). This level is less stringent in patients with low risk disease.

- Postoperative thyroid hormone therapy is indicated in MTC, but TSH suppression is not appropriate because C cells lack TSH receptors.

## 5.3. Radioactive Iodine Remnant Ablation (RRA)

- It is not likely that all thyroid tissue will be removed by routine surgery. It is often necessary to ablate the thyroid remnant with $^{131}$I. This is not the same as RAI therapy, which is the administration of larger doses to destroy neck disease or metastases.

- RRA is the destruction of residual macroscopic thyroid tissue post-thyroidectomy. $^{131}$I is concentrated in thyroid cells and emits short range beta-irradiation, which destroys remnant microscopic tumor cells with a relatively low dose to adjacent organs. This achieves the following:

  □ Thyroid tissue often must be ablated before optimally concentrating in cervical or pulmonary metastatic deposits, which may be less avid than the normal thyroid itself.

  □ Elimination of thyroid remnants allows rendering of a hypothyroid state to achieve a high circulating TSH level necessary for diagnostic RAI scanning.

  □ Viable normal Tg producing thyroid cells are ablated and serum Tg measurement becomes a sensitive test

for follow-up. (Thyroid tissue is the only physiological source of Tg.)

- RRA done after an initial diagnostic RAI scan at four to six weeks. When the amount of tissue is small, 30 mCi is often used. If it demonstrates a significant thyroid remnant or the initial scan shows metastasis tumor, 75 to 150 mCi of RAI is administered to ablate this tissue.

## 5.4. Radioactive Iodine Therapy

- Following remnant ablation, if RAI imaging demonstrates the presence of RAI-avid tumor, RAI therapy is given and repeated at intervals of 6 to 12 months until there is no longer evidence of functioning disease.

- The therapeutic dose of RAI has empirically varied between 100 to 200 mCi, depending upon the extent of local and metastatic disease.

- Complications of RAI include self-limiting thyroiditis and parotitis. Bone marrow depression and pulmonary fibrosis are rare and seen only after very high cumulative doses of RAI.

- Undifferentiated tumors and medullary carcinomas, therefore, are not amenable to RAI therapy. Older patients, those with Hürthle cell or poorly differentiated tumors, and those with bone metastases may also fail to adequately concentrate RAI.

## 5.5. Adjuvant External Beam Radiotherapy

- Aggressive thyroid cancer is frequently treated with adjuvant external beam radiotherapy (EBRT) following thyroidectomy or resection of recurrent disease to reduce the risk of local recurrence, which can threaten the airway, speech, and swallowing.

- Although there is no consensus on what the indications are for EBRT, and no data from randomized trials are available, retrospective analysis suggests that it is effective in reducing local recurrence.

- For example, one review from the Princess Margaret Hospital/University of Toronto studied the impact of EBRT as part of the initial management of differentiated thyroid carcinoma in 382 patients with a median follow-up of 10.8 years. Age older than 60, tumor size larger than 4 cm, multifocality, postoperative residuum, lymph node involvement, less extensive surgery (less than near-total thyroidectomy), and the lack of use of radioiodine were significant with regard to locoregional failure. Although the use of EBRT was associated with more advanced local disease, there were no statistically significant differences in local control between patients who received RT and those who did not, even after adjustment for identified prognostic factors. In the subgroup of 155 patients with papillary histology and microscopic residuum, both 10-year cause-specific survival (100% vs 95%, $P = 0.038$) and local relapse-free rate (93% vs 78%, $P = 0.01$) were higher for patients given RT than for those not given RT. There were 33 patients with macroscopic residual disease who received postoperative RT. Their 5-year local relapse-free rate was 62% and cause-specific survival was 65%.[47]

- Other reports also observed that postoperative EBRT lowers the locoregional recurrence rate of thyroid cancer when used to treat patients who had undergone complete resection but were high risk for local failure.[48–52]
- The favorable effects of RT in advanced patients with medullary thyroid cancer and residual microscopic disease after surgery or those with disease spread to local lymph nodes have also been reported by studies of large thyroid cancer databases in the UK, France, and Canada.[53–56] The present data shows a significantly reduced local relapse in patients with medullary carcinoma on prolonged follow-up.
- The following are some of the indications for EBRT:

  □ Differentiated thyroid cancer.

    • High risk patient with high risk tumor.
    • Extrathyroidal extension and microscopic residual tumor.
    • Gross residual tumor.
    • After resection of recurrent tumor at primary site especially in the tracheoesophageal groove.

- Poorly differentiated thyroid cancer with extensive invasion of central compartment structures, such as muscle, nerve, trachea, esophagus.
- MTC with

  □ Extensive nodal or mediastinal disease.
  □ Persistently elevated calcitonin without distant metastases.
  □ Residual disease.

- Anaplastic thyroid cancer.
- Distant metastasic deposits, such as bone, lung, brain.

# 6. INTENSITY-MODULATED RADIATION THERAPY FOR THYROID CARCINOMA

## 6.1. Rationale

- The thyroid gland itself is closely apposed to the cricoid, larynx, cricothyroid ligament, prevertebral muscles, esophagus and hypopharynx, and common carotid arteries.
- The draining lymph nodes extend from the high cervical level II nodes to central paratracheal level VI nodes and superior mediastinal level VII nodes.
- The target volume therefore extends from the high neck to well below the shoulder. This poses a technical challenge in administering 50–60 Gy to such an extensive concave target, particularly without exceeding the limits of the spinal cord.

- During the early investigation of beam intensity modulation, it was recognized that IMRT could efficiently spare the spinal cord and deliver higher doses than conventional techniques.
- With early clinical experience, it is now evident that IMRT presents significant advantages for this disease: it affords adequate coverage of the high risk volume with sparing of the spinal cord, level II nodes, and parotid glands to avoid significant xerostomia.

## 6.2. Target Volume Determination and Delineation

- The following descriptions are based on the experience at the M. D. Anderson Cancer Center from 1999 to 2004 using IMRT for thyroid carcinoma patients.
- The clinical target volumes (CTVs) can be divided as follows for descriptive purposes: $CTV_{Primary60}$, $CTV_{boost}$, $CTV_{Nodal\ positive}$, $CTV_{Nodal\ negative}$, $CTV_{Mediastinum}$.
- $CTV_{Primary60}$ covers the primary tumor bed, initial thyroid gland volume, central compartment, and immediately adjacent lymph nodes in level VI, and adjacent tissues in the anterior portion of the supraclavicular fossa. The $CTV_{Primary}$ is usually prescribed 60 Gy in 30 fractions. Figures 13-8 and 13-10 to 13-12 show typical examples of $CTV_{Primary60}$.
- The following six sources of information are useful guidelines in determining the $CTV_{Primary60}$:

  (1) **Knowledge of the anatomical location** within the neck at various levels on the transverse CT images. Specifically, the relation of the thyroid gland to normal tissues as illustrated in Figures 13-1 to 13-6.

  (2) **Detailed review of the preoperative physical examination findings.** Ideally, the treating oncologist should examine patients preoperatively in order to establish the extent and location of palpable or visible masses. This is not usually the case because many of the indications for radiotherapy are only discovered intraoperatively or on pathological findings, and the first time the radiation oncologist encounters the patient is following definitive surgery.

  (3) **Review of available preoperative imaging.** Preoperative CT scans are rarely available to aid in localizing the previous thyroid gland and tumor volume, as shown in Figures 13-4 to 13-6. Most patients would not have had CT scans because the administration of iodine contrast interferes with postoperative RAI scans by impairment of the cellular uptake of radioactive iodine. For this reason, MR imaging should be performed if patients are seen preoperatively and it is likely that they will require postoperative radiotherapy.

  (4) **Review of operative notes** with particular attention to these findings

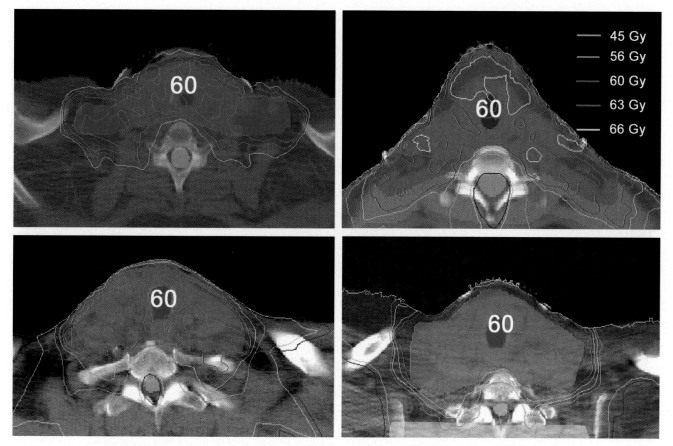

**FIGURE 13-8.** Four examples of typical CTV$_{primary}$, the central compartment CTVs in colorwash prescribed to 60 Gy in 30 fractions. Note that the CTV$_{primary}$ includes the strap muscles, laryngeal nerves, trachea, esophagus, larynx, cricothyroid membrane, vagus nerve and carotid artery, and prevertebral muscles. These patients each had a T4N1M0 papillary cancer with invasion of the trachea, esophagus, and strap muscles. No attempt was made at sparing of the esophagus, trachea, or larynx. In both cases, the level IV and supraclavicular nodal regions are included. The isodoses are shown in the key.

□ The extent of tumor in all directions and planes, the structures invaded such as larynx, trachea, esophagus, strap muscles and prevertebral muscles.

□ The location of adherent tumor which was removed piecemeal or shaved off.

□ The locations where the surgeon felt that residual tumor may have been left in situ.

(5) **Pathology report** with particular attention to location of positive margins, confirmation of structures invaded, and the location of positive nodes.

(6) **Findings on planning CT scan.** Although is this not a diagnostic scan, and contrast is not usually given, gross residual lymphadenopathy may occasionally be seen, and it is useful to review these images with a diagnostic radiologist. In these cases, a boost volume may be customized. An example of gross nodal tumor detected on the CT planning scan is shown in Figure 13-9.

■ CTV$_{boost}$ is a boost subvolume of high priority that covers small regions where a higher dose may be delivered at sites of positive margins, gross macroscopic residual tumor, or in the case of multiply recurrent cancer—the site of the recurrence, such as the tracheoesophageal groove.

■ The goal of this CTV is usually to give 60–66 Gy in 30 fractions. Examples of CTV$_{boost}$ are shown in Figure 13-10 where the boost was taken to 63 Gy and Figure 13-11 where the boost was taken to 66 Gy.

■ CTV$_{Nodal\ positive60}$ is the nodal CTV that covers the regions containing pathologically involved nodes positive plus a margin to include the adjacent nodal levels superiorly and inferiorly. This was usually taken to 60 Gy in 30 fractions.

■ Although this dose is the same goal dose as the as the CTV$_{Primary60}$, it is preferable to delineate it separately for the purpose of prioritizing targets for inverse planning. The CTV$_{Primary60}$ is assigned the highest priority.

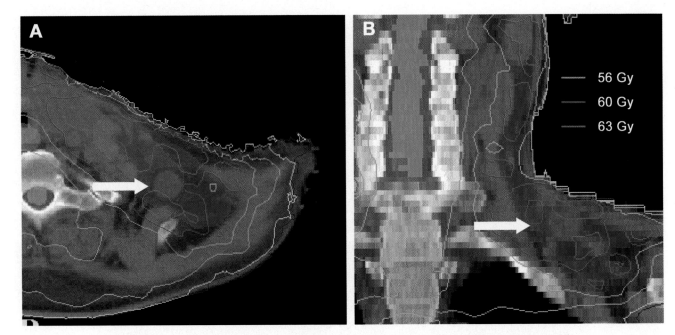

**FIGURE 13-9.** Transverse (**A**) and coronal (**B**) sections of a patient with papillary carcinoma with squamous differentiation who was treated with IMRT following resection of a fungating neck mass. There was a residual left supraclavicular fossa node seen in panels (**A**) and (**B**) contoured in *red colorwash* (*arrows*). This was detected on the simulation scan during radiotherapy planning. The node was boosted to 60 Gy with tentative plan to resect if it was not controlled. The node remained stable, and the rest of the head and neck remained free of disease; however, the patient recurred in the mediastinum.

- Examples of $CTV_{Nodal\ positive60}$ are shown in Figures 13-10 to 13-13. The extent of nodal volumes on either side of the neck varies with the pathological findings, as shown in Figure 13-13 where the nodal volumes were extended up to include the high level II nodes on the left, but just up to level III on the right. This allows better sparing of the parotid gland on the side that receives radiotherapy to level II.

- $CTV_{Nodal\ negative54}$ is the elective nodal volume that covers the nodal levels beyond $CTV_{Nodal\ positive60}$ or the nodal regions of the contralateral neck. This was usually taken to 54–56 Gy in 30 fractions. (The elective dose to undissected elective nodal regions using non–IMRT conventional 3D conformal radiotherapy is 50 Gy is 25 fractions in 5 weeks. The target dose is 54–56 Gy in 30 fractions in 6 weeks to take into account the longer overall treatment time of this region over the 6 weeks with IMRT).

- Examples of $CTV^{Nodal}_{negative\ 54}$ are shown in Figures 13-10 to 13-13.

- At the level of the supraclavicular fossa in patients with positive paratracheal level VI nodes, the posterior supraclavicular fossa nodal regions may be included in the $CTV_{Nodal\ negative54}$. The advantage of this is to avoid irradiating the brachial plexus to >60 Gy, which may occur if hot spots arise in the posterior part of this volume. An example of this is shown is Figure 13-13B,

which shows this sparing in the right supraclavicular fossa.

- In some cases, nodal CTVs may not be necessary. An example of this is shown in Figure 13-14.

- $CTV_{Mediastinum}$ is the superior mediastinal nodal region that is usually taken to a goal dose of 54–56 Gy in 30 fractions.

- For patients with positive mediastinal nodes, the inferior extent of the $CTV_{Mediastinum}$ is taken at the carina.

- For patients without mediastinal nodal involvement, the inferior limit may be considered above this and is usually taken down to the level of the aortic arch. The advantage of a higher inferior limit here is to avoid radiation of the lungs. Examples of $CTV_{Mediastinum}$ are shown in Figures 13-11 and 13-12.

### 6.3. Normal Tissue Delineation

#### 6.3.1. Critical Organs

*The critical avoidance structures which should be outlined are*

- *Spinal Cord.* Traditionally, the dose limit to the spinal cord is set at 45 Gy. Although this is well below tolerance, and since it is being given at 1.5 Gy per fraction (30 fractions), the entire length of the cervical cord and upper

*Text continues on page 227.*

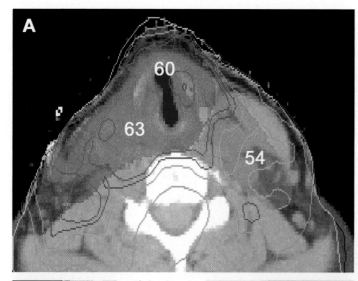

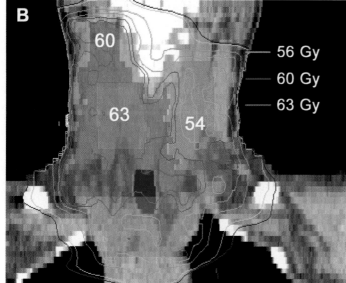

CTV boost63

CTVprimary60 **and** CTVnode positive60

CTVnode negative54 **and** CTVmediastinum54

— 56 Gy
— 60 Gy
— 63 Gy

**FIGURE 13-10.** Transverse (**A**) and coronal (**B**) sections of a patient with papillary carcinoma who was treated with IMRT following resection of a second recurrence involving the right side of the trachea, esophagus, and strap muscles with seven right nodes positive. There was residual microscopic positive margins. The CTV_boost is a smaller subvolume within the primary central compartment CTV_Primary60 outlined in *red colorwash* and represents the region suspicious for microscopic residual disease and is well covered by the corresponding purple 63 Gy isodose. The right neck was prescribed 60 Gy and the left neck and mediastinum (which were node negative) were prescribed 54 Gy. Her tumor was controlled in the head and neck.

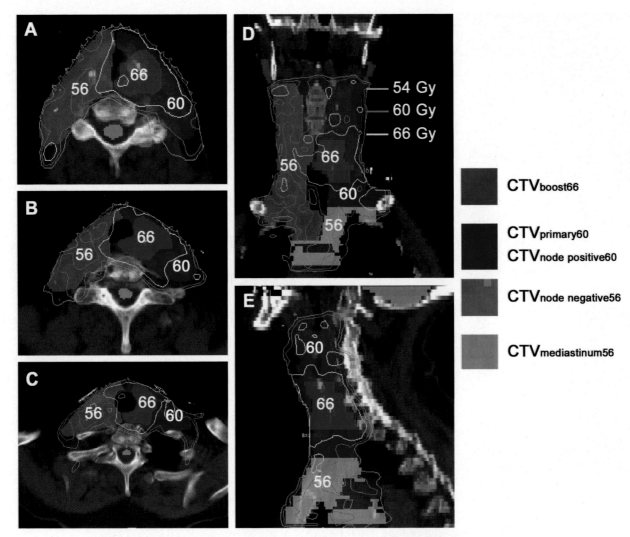

**FIGURE 13-11.** CTV$_{Primary60}$, CTV$_{boost66}$, CTV$_{Nodal\ positive60}$, CTV$_{Nodal\ negative56}$, and CTV$_{Mediastinum56}$ in a patient who was treated with IMRT following resection of left tracheoesophageal recurrence with positive left level III nodes and no nodal disease on the right side. Gross macroscopic residual tumor was left at surgery. **A–C:** Transverse sections through the CTV$_{boost66}$ from the level, subvolumes within the primary CTV$_{Primary60}$ outlined in *red colorwash* and is well covered by the corresponding *yellow* 66 Gy isodose. The ipsilateral neck was prescribed 60 Gy and the contralateral neck and mediastinum was prescribed 56 Gy. Her tumor was controlled in the head and neck.

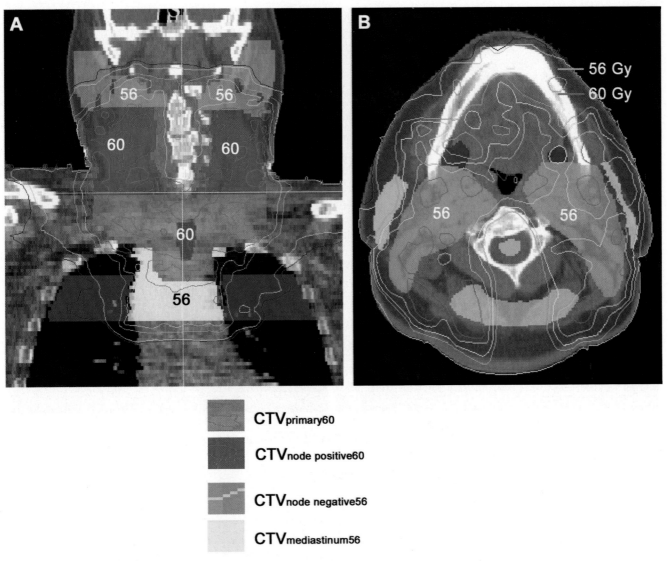

CTVprimary60

CTVnode positive60

CTVnode negative56

CTVmediastinum56

**FIGURE 13-12.** Nodal volume delineation of a patient with recurrent T4N1M0 papillary thyroid cancer. The thyroid bed recurrence measured 6.5 cm. There were multiple nodes positive with extracapsular extension: eight in level VI, eleven on the left from level IV up to level II, and five on the right from level IV up to level II. **A:** Coronal section showing the central CTV in *red color-wash* which includes the CTVprimary60 and CTVnodal positive60. It encompasses the primary tumor bed, adjacent paratracheal nodes (level VI), and the adjacent level IV nodes. **B:** CTVNodal negative56 encompasses the superior part of level II, well above the involved nodes which was contoured as a separate CTV which was prescribed 56 Gy. The superior mediastinum, CTVMediastinum56, in *yellow colorwash*, was also prescribed 56 Gy.

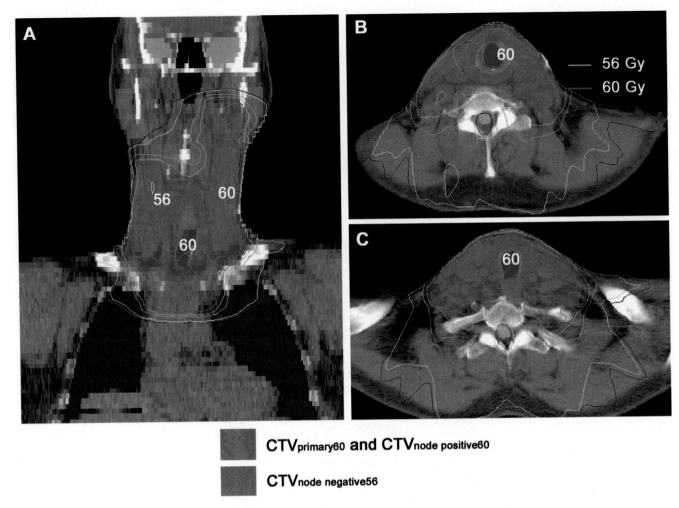

**CTV**primary60 **and CTV**node positive60

**CTV**node negative56

**FIGURE 13-13.** Asymmetrical nodal CTVs in a T4N1M0 multifocal papillary thyroid cancer with squamous differentiation. There were thirteen positive nodes in left level III and IV and seven positive nodes in level VI. The highest involved nodes on the right were level VI (paratracheal). **A:** The CTV prescribed to 60 Gy (in *red colorwash*) includes the primary tumor bed and the nodal volumes on the *left* up to include the superior part of *left* level II (CTVprimary60 and CTVnodal positive60). The nodal CTV on the *right* extends only up to level III only as shown in *purple colorwash*. (CTVNodal negative56). **B:** The central CTV prescribed to 60 Gy (*red colorwash*) includes the paratracheal nodes (level VI), and the adjacent *left* level IV only. The CTVNodal negative56 (*purple colorwash*) at this level is the *right* level III nodes which was prescribed 56 Gy. **C:** CTV at the thoracic inlet was prescribed 60 Gy.

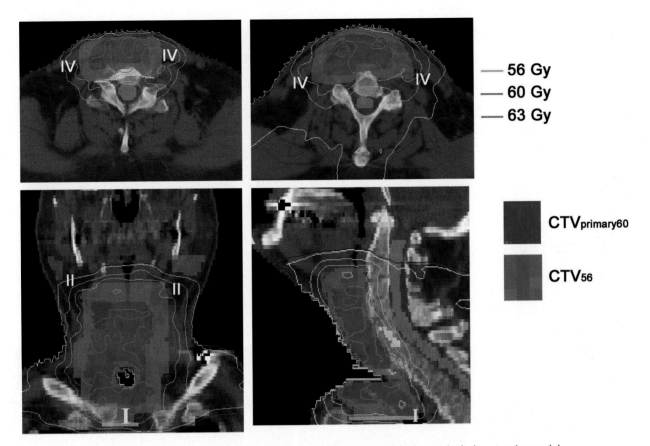

**FIGURE 13-14.** CTV contours for an advanced T4 tumor which do *not include* extensive nodal CTVs in papillary thyroid cancer patient who was found to have tumor extensively invading and destroying the wall of the trachea. There were two small perithyroidal nodes with microscopic tumor deposits. Note that the level II nodes (II) and level IV nodes (IV) are well outside of the CTV. A central (*red*) CTV was prescribed 60 Gy (CTV$_{Primary60}$) and a peripheral expansion of this was prescribed 56 Gy (CTV$_{56}$).

thoracic cord are often adjacent to the target volume and therefore receives a significant dose (Fig. 13-15A). Extra caution is also exercised because thyroid cancer patients have a high likelihood of long-term survival and therefore higher chances of developing complications.

- *Parotid glands.* See Table 7-11.
- *Lungs.* The entire lung should be scanned so that a lung dose volume histogam (DVH) can be generated. Although the lung is not usually outlined in head and neck radiotherapy, this is highly recommended for thyroid cancer where the nodal CTV includes part of the mediastinum. In cases where there are positive nodes in the superior mediastinum, the nodal CTV usually extends to the carina. Failure to generate and inspect the lung DVHs and isodose lines encompassing the lung may easily lead to neglecting that the amount of lung being irradiated is above tolerance. An example of where this may occur if the lung is not specified as an avoidance is shown in Figure 13-15, which compares

plans which were optimized with and without the lungs as avoidance organs. The constraints set should be more stringent than the usual levels used in lung cancer patients ($<40\%$ to $>20$ Gy) because thyroid cancer patients have a high likelihood of long-term survival and therefore a higher chance of manifesting pulmonary dysfunction. They may also develop lung metastases in which they can also survive for a long time, and this may further exacerbate symptomatic pulmonary inadequacy.

- *Submandibular salivary glands.* In many cases, these glands can be spared the high dose volume. They are usually given the same constraints as the parotid glands. An example of sparing is shown in Figure 13-16A–C.
- *Brain and brainstem.* Portions of these structures which lie at the same level of the target volume should be outlined and avoided. The constraint is usually set at around 54 Gy and the dose received is usually well below this, as shown in Figure 13-16D.

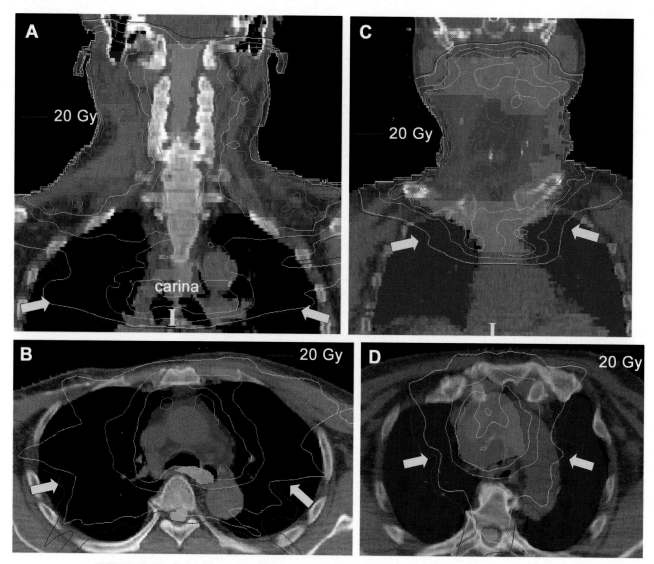

**FIGURE 13-15.** Comparison of resulting dose to the lung if the lung is not scanned and contoured as an avoidance structure. The *dark blue isodose line* is 20 Gy. The lung was not deliberately avoided and the 20 Gy line can be seen encompassing an extensive volume of lung tissue (**A,B**) versus when entire lung was scanned during simulation and strict constraints of >20 Gy to <20% were placed before optimization (**C, D**).

### 6.3.2. Nonspecific Avoidance Regions

- Avoidance structures can be used to assist in optimization. These are not specific organs but regions within tissue that, when specified for avoidance, will generally produce penalties during optimization, facilitating a final plan that gives hot spots well away from the specified region. These are illustrated in Figure 13-16D and include

  □ *Oral cavity avoidance volume* to reduce the dose to the mucosa of the structures of the oral cavity, the mandible, and the lips. Lowering the dose to the mucosa reduces acute mucositis, late xerostomia, and dys-

phasia. Limits of 30–40 Gy can usually be achieved without sacrificing CTV coverage even with high level II nodal CTVs.

  □ *Posterior spinal cord avoidance volume* to aid in reducing the dose to the spinal cord.

  □ *Supraglottic avoidance* includes the suprahyoid epiglottis and aryepiglottic fold. This volume should be kept anteriorly since the lateral lobes of the thyroid gland ascend superiorly along the posterolateral aspect of the thyroid cartilage. It should be well superior to the insertion of the cricothyroid ligament (Fig. 13-1). An example of sparing of some of the supraglottic structures is shown in Figure 13-16D.

☐ *Posterior brachial plexus avoidance volume* in the lower half of neck to reduce the dose to the brachial plexus. This region is at the level of the $CTV_{Primary60}$ where small hot spots within the 60 Gy volume may occur in the brachial plexus. For example, a 10% hot spot would give 66 Gy, which is above the tolerance for this group of patients who are expected to live for a longer period of time. Figure 13-16E gives an example of the hot spots occurring anteriorly within the $CTV_{Primary60}$ **instead** of posteriorly near the brachial plexus.

## 6.4. IMRT Results

■ The efficacy of IMRT and correlative dosimetry with patterns of failure is not yet available because long-term follow-up is needed for this disease with its long natural history.

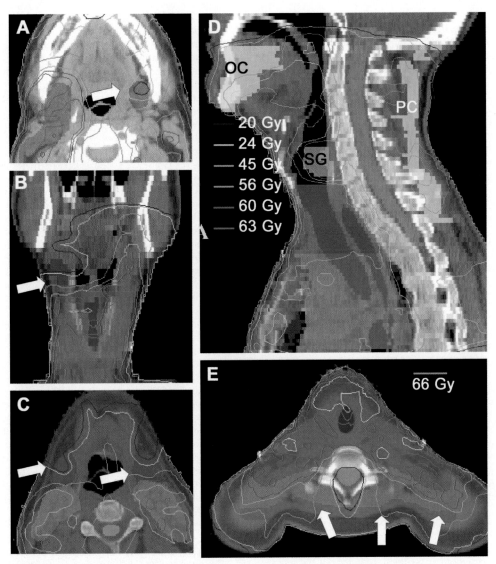

**FIGURE 13-16.** Normal tissue avoidance. **A–C:** The feasibility of avoiding the submandibular gland demonstrated. **D,E:** Illustration of the use of nonspecific avoidance regions which are useful in optimization. These regions within tissue are often specified for avoidance and give penalties during optimization. OC: Oral cavity avoidance volume. Note that much of the mucosa, oral cavity, and lips are well below 45 Gy. PC: Posterior spinal cord avoidance volume. SG: Supraglottic avoidance. This volume should be kept well superior to the insertion of the cricothyroid ligament (See Fig. 13-1). **E:** Posterior brachial plexus avoidance volume (indicated by the *block arrows*). Here, in the lower half of neck, it reduces the dose to the brachial plexus. The *yellow isodose lines* are a 10% hotspot, 66 Gy. This occurs well anterior and off the brachial plexus.

## REFERENCES

1. Cernea CR, Ferraz AR, Nishio S, et al. Surgical anatomy of the external branch of the superior laryngeal nerve. *Head Neck* 1992;14:380–383.
2. Greene FL, American Joint Committee on Cancer, American Cancer Society. *AJCC Cancer Staging Manual, 6th ed.* New York: Springer, 2002.
3. Andersen PE, Kinsella J, Loree TR, et al. Differentiated carcinoma of the thyroid with extrathyroidal extension. *Am J Surg* 1995;170:467–470.
4. Rosai J, Carcangiu M, DeLellis R. *Tumors of the Thyroid Gland, 3rd ed.* Washington, DC: Armed Forces Institute of Pathology, 1996.
5. Hedinger CE. [Problems in the classification of thyroid tumors. Their significance for prognosis and therapy]. *Schweiz Med Wochenschr* 1993;123:1673–1681.
6. Hundahl SA, Fleming ID, Fremgen AM, et al. A National Cancer Data Base report on 53,856 cases of thyroid carcinoma treated in the U.S., 1985–1995 [see comments]. *Cancer* 1998;83: 2638–2648.
7. Mazzaferri EL, Jhiang SM. Long-term impact of initial surgical and medical therapy on papillary and follicular thyroid cancer. *Am J Med* 1994;97:418–428.
8. Brennan MD, Bergstralh EJ, van Heerden JA, et al. Follicular thyroid cancer treated at the Mayo Clinic, 1946 through 1970: initial manifestations, pathologic findings, therapy, and outcome. *Mayo Clin Proc* 1991;66:11–22.
9. LiVolsi V. Unusual variants of papillary thyroid carcinoma. In: Mazzaferri EL, Kreisberg RA, Bar RS, eds. *Advances in Endocrinology and metabolism.* St. Louis: Mosby-Year Book, 1995:39–54.
10. Loh KC, Greenspan FS, Gee L, et al. Pathological tumor-node-metastasis (pTNM) staging for papillary and follicular thyroid carcinomas: a retrospective analysis of 700 patients. *J Clin Endocrinol Metab* 1997;82:3553–3562.
11. LiVolsi VA, Asa SL. The demise of follicular carcinoma of the thyroid gland. *Thyroid* 1994;4:233–236.
12. Mazzaferri EL. Thyroid carcinoma: papillary and follicular. In: Mazzaferri EL, Samaan N, eds. *Endocrine Tumors.* Cambridge: Blackwell Scientific Publications, 1993:278–333.
13. Thompson NW, Dunn EL, Batsakis JG, et al. Hurthle cell lesions of the thyroid gland. *Surg Gynecol Obstet* 1974;139:555–560.
14. Mole SE, Mulligan LM, Healey CS, et al. Localisation of the gene for multiple endocrine neoplasia type 2A to a 480 kb region in chromosome band 10q11.2. *Hum Mol Genet* 1993;2: 247–252.
15. Robie DK, Dinauer CW, Tuttle RM, et al. The impact of initial surgical management on outcome in young patients with differentiated thyroid cancer. *J Pediatr Surg* 1998;33:1134–1138; discussion 1139–1140.
16. Newman KD, Black T, Heller G, et al. Differentiated thyroid cancer: determinants of disease progression in patients <21 years of age at diagnosis: a report from the Surgical Discipline Committee of the Children's Cancer Group. *Ann Surg* 1998;227:533–541.
17. Soravia C, Sugg SL, Berk T, et al. Familial adenomatous polyposis-associated thyroid cancer: a clinical, pathological, and molecular genetics study. *Am J Pathol* 1999;154:127–135.
18. Stratakis CA, Courcoutsakis NA, Abati A, et al. Thyroid gland abnormalities in patients with the syndrome of spotty skin pigmentation, myxomas, endocrine overactivity, and schwannomas (Carney complex). *J Clin Endocrinol Metab* 1997;82:2037–2043.
19. Frankenthaler RA, Sellin RV, Cangir A, et al. Lymph node metastasis from papillary-follicular thyroid carcinoma in young patients. *Am J Surg* 1990;160:341–343.
20. Agostini L, Mazzi P, Cavaliere A. Multiple primary malignant tumours: gemistocytic astrocytoma with leptomeningeal spreading and papillary thyroid carcinoma. A case report. *Acta Neurol (Napoli)* 1990;12:305–310.
21. Tan GH, Gharib H. Thyroid incidentalomas: management approaches to nonpalpable nodules discovered incidentally on thyroid imaging. *Ann Intern Med* 1997;126:226–231.
22. Ezzat S, Sarti DA, Cain DR, et al. Thyroid incidentalomas. Prevalence by palpation and ultrasonography. *Arch Intern Med* 1994;154:1838–1840.
23. Ringel MD, Ladenson PW, Levine MA. Molecular diagnosis of residual and recurrent thyroid cancer by amplification of thyroglobulin messenger ribonucleic acid in peripheral blood. *J Clin Endocrinol Metab* 1998;83:4435–4442.
24. Haugen BR, Pacini F, Reiners C, et al. A comparison of recombinant human thyrotropin and thyroid hormone withdrawal for the detection of thyroid remnant or cancer. *J Clin Endocrinol Metab* 1999;84:3877–3885.
25. Ladenson PW, Braverman LE, Mazzaferri EL, et al. Comparison of administration of recombinant human thyrotropin with withdrawal of thyroid hormone for radioactive iodine scanning in patients with thyroid carcinoma. *N Engl J Med* 1997;337:888–896.
26. Wang W, Macapinlac H, Larson SM, et al. [18F]-2-fluoro-2-deoxy-D-glucose positron emission tomography localizes residual thyroid cancer in patients with negative diagnostic (131)I whole body scans and elevated serum thyroglobulin levels. *J Clin Endocrinol Metab* 1999;84:2291–2302.
27. Hay ID, Grant CS, Taylor WF, et al. Ipsilateral lobectomy versus bilateral lobar resection in papillary thyroid carcinoma: a retrospective analysis of surgical outcome using a novel prognostic scoring system. *Surgery* 1987;102:1088–1095.
28. Cady B, Rossi R. An expanded view of risk-group definition in differentiated thyroid carcinoma. *Surgery* 1988;104:947–953.
29. Cady B, Rossi R, Silverman M, et al. Further evidence of the validity of risk group definition in differentiated thyroid carcinoma. *Surgery* 1985;98:1171–1178.
30. Shah JP, Loree TR, Dharker D, et al. Prognostic factors in differentiated carcinoma of the thyroid gland. *Am J Surg* 1992;164: 658–661.
31. Shaha AR, Loree TR, Shah JP. Intermediate-risk group for differentiated carcinoma of thyroid. *Surgery* 1994;116:1036–1040; discussion 1040–1041.
32. DeGroot LJ. Thyroid carcinoma. *Med Clin North Am* 1975;59: 1233–1246.
33. Saad MF, Ordonez NG, Rashid RK, et al. Medullary carcinoma of the thyroid. A study of the clinical features and prognostic factors in 161 patients. *Medicine (Baltimore)* 1984;63:319–342.
34. Sherman SI, Brierley JD, Sperling M, et al. Prospective multicenter study of thyroid carcinoma treatment: initial analysis of staging and outcome. National Thyroid Cancer Treatment Cooperative Study Registry Group. *Cancer* 1998;83:1012–1021.
35. O'Riordain DS, O'Brien T, Weaver AL, et al. Medullary thyroid carcinoma in multiple endocrine neoplasia types 2A and 2B. *Surgery* 1994;116:1017–1023.
36. Lippman SM, Mendelsohn G, Trump DL, et al. The prognostic and biological significance of cellular heterogeneity in medullary thyroid carcinoma: a study of calcitonin, L-dopa decarboxylase, and histaminase. *J Clin Endocrinol Metab* 1982;54: 233–240.
37. Mendelsohn G, Wells SA, Jr., Baylin SB. Relationship of tissue carcinoembryonic antigen and calcitonin to tumor virulence in medullary thyroid carcinoma. An immunohistochemical study in early, localized, and virulent disseminated stages of disease. *Cancer* 1984;54:657–662.
38. Dottorini ME, Assi A, Sironi M, et al. Multivariate analysis of patients with medullary thyroid carcinoma. Prognostic significance

and impact on treatment of clinical and pathologic variables. *Cancer* 1996;77:1556–1565.

39. Romei C, Elisei R, Pinchera A, et al. Somatic mutations of the ret protooncogene in sporadic medullary thyroid carcinoma are not restricted to exon 16 and are associated with tumor recurrence. *J Clin Endocrinol Metab* 1996;81:1619–1622.

40. Noguchi S, Murakami N, Yamashita H, et al. Papillary thyroid carcinoma: modified radical neck dissection improves prognosis. *Arch Surg* 1998;133:276–280.

41. Samaan NA, Schultz PN, Hickey RC, et al. The results of various modalities of treatment of well differentiated thyroid carcinomas: a retrospective review of 1599 patients. *J Clin Endocrinol Metab* 1992;75:714–720.

42. Hay ID, Grant CS, Bergstralh EJ, et al. Unilateral total lobectomy: is it sufficient surgical treatment for patients with AMES low-risk papillary thyroid carcinoma? *Surgery* 1998;124:958–964; discussion 964–966.

43. Baldet L, Manderscheid JC, Glinoer D, et al. The management of differentiated thyroid cancer in Europe in 1988. Results of an international survey. *Acta Endocrinol (Copenh)* 1989;120: 547–558.

44. Cady B. Hayes Martin Lecture. Our AMES is true: how an old concept still hits the mark: or, risk group assignment points the arrow to rational therapy selection in differentiated thyroid cancer. *Am J Surg* 1997;174:462–468.

45. Shaha AR, Loree TR, Shah JP. Prognostic factors and risk group analysis in follicular carcinoma of the thyroid. *Surgery* 1995;118: 1131–1136; discussion 1136–1138.

46. National Comprehensive Cancer Network Guidelines. CD-ROM; Version 1.2003.

47. Tsang RW, Brierley JD, Simpson WJ, et al. The effects of surgery, radioiodine, and external radiation therapy on the clini-cal outcome of patients with differentiated thyroid carcinoma. *Cancer* 1998;82:375–388.

48. Farahati J, Reiners C, Stuschke M, et al. Differentiated thyroid cancer. Impact of adjuvant external radiotherapy in patients with perithyroidal tumor infiltration (stage pT4). *Cancer* 1996;77: 172–180.

49. Tubiana M, Haddad E, Schlumberger M, et al. External radiotherapy in thyroid cancers. *Cancer* 1985;55:2062–2071.

50. Simpson WJ, Panzarella T, Carruthers JS, et al. Papillary and follicular thyroid cancer: impact of treatment in 1578 patients. *Int J Radiat Oncol Biol Phys* 1988;14:1063–1075.

51. Phlips P, Hanzen C, Andry G, et al. Postoperative irradiation for thyroid cancer. *Eur J Surg Oncol* 1993;19:399–404.

52. Esik O, Nemeth G, Eller J. Prophylactic external irradiation in differentiated thyroid cancer: a retrospective study over a 30-year observation period. *Oncology* 1994;51:372–379.

53. Brierley J, Tsang R, Simpson WJ, et al. Medullary thyroid cancer: analyses of survival and prognostic factors and the role of radiation therapy in local control. *Thyroid* 1996;6: 305–310.

54. Nguyen TD, Chassard JL, Lagarde P, et al. Results of postoperative radiation therapy in medullary carcinoma of the thyroid: a retrospective study by the French Federation of Cancer Institutes—the Radiotherapy Cooperative Group. *Radiother Oncol* 1992;23:1–5.

55. Fife KM, Bower M, Harmer CL. Medullary thyroid cancer: the role of radiotherapy in local control. *Eur J Surg Oncol* 1996;22: 588–591.

56. Hyer SL, Vini L, A'Hern R, et al. Medullary thyroid cancer: multivariate analysis of prognostic factors influencing survival. *Eur J Surg Oncol* 2000;26:686–690.

# 14

# METASTATIC CARCINOMA IN NECK NODE WITH UNKNOWN PRIMARY

GOKHAN OZYIGIT
K. S. CLIFFORD CHAO

## 1. INTRODUCTION

- Neck node metastasis of unknown primary comprises 1% to 2% of head and neck malignancies. Jugulodigastric and midjugular lymph nodes are the most frequent sites.[1]
- The possible site of origin can be estimated from the histology of the neck node, although the biopsy often reveals a poorly differentiated neoplasm. Lymphoma should also be excluded by proper immunohistochemical staining.
- A solitary upper jugular chain is the most common site because most head and neck cancers spread to this area first. This metastasis site is uncommon for tumors below the clavicle.[2]
- A mass between the angle of the mandible and the tip of the mastoid suggests origin in the nasopharynx, oropharynx, parotid, occasionally malignant melanoma, or other skin cancers.
- The oral cavity, larynx, and hypopharynx should be included as likely sites for the mass in the subdigastric region.
- Bilateral upper neck nodes usually originate from the nasopharynx, base of tongue, soft palate, supraglottic larynx, and pyriform sinus.
- A solitary submandibular mass suggests a primary site of origin in the oral cavity, lip, or nasal vestibule, or a primary submandibular salivary gland tumor. A solitary submental node is rare.
- A mass in the mid-neck region suggests a primary site from the larynx or hypopharynx or, less commonly, from the thyroid or cervical esophagus, or a tumor originating below the clavicle.
- A solitary lower neck mass is commonly metastatic from the chest or abdomen. A solitary spinal accessory mass suggests a nasopharyngeal site. Squamous cell carcinoma in the parotid lymph nodes is always from a skin or parotid gland cancer.

## 2. DIAGNOSIS AND STAGING SYSTEM

- Physical examination and assessment under anesthesia conducted by an experienced otolaryngologist can elucidate a primary site in more than 50% of patients with cervical lymph node metastasis.[3,4] In the absence of physical or radiographic suspicion, pan-endoscopy with biopsies yields a 17% detection rate.[5]
- Mendenhall et al.[3] reported that the sites of primary tumor found through this process were at the tonsillar fossa and base of tongue in 82% of patients. Repeat pan-endoscopy did not seem to increase the detection rate.

### 2.1. Imaging

- Repeated examinations and contrast-enhanced computed tomography (CT) or magnetic resonance imaging (MRI) scans are essential for finding primary lesions. CT or MRI to look for a possible primary site follows a diagnosis of squamous cell carcinoma. If the biopsy is not definitive, CT or MRI may redirect the workup.
- The CT or MRI examination should be performed with at least 3-mm sections from the nasopharynx through the entire neck. MRI is used as a supplement for focused evaluation of suspicious regions, but not necessarily when the CT results are positive or normal.
- With negative routine clinical examination and CT, positron emission tomography detects carcinoma in 5% to 25% of patients, whereas ipsilateral tonsillectomy detects carcinoma in approximately 25% of patients.[1] Laser-induced fluorescence imaging with pan-endoscopy and directed biopsies shows encouraging results but requires further investigation. Positron emission tomography has an overall staging accuracy of 69%.[1]

## TABLE 14-1. AMERICAN JOINT COMMITTEE STAGING SYSTEM FOR UNKNOWN PRIMARY CANCERS*

*Primary tumor (T)*
TX     Primary tumor cannot be assessed

*Regional lymph nodes (N)*
NX    Regional lymph nodes cannot be assessed
N0    No regional lymph node metastasis
N1    Metastasis in a single ipsilateral lymph node, 3 cm in greatest dimension
N2    Metastasis in a single ipsilateral lymph node, >3 cm but not >6 cm in greatest dimension; or in multiple ipsilateral lymph nodes, none >6 cm in greatest dimension; or in bilateral or contralateral lymph nodes, none >6 cm in greatest dimension
N2a  Metastasis in a single ipsilateral lymph node, >3 cm but not >6 cm in greatest dimension
N2b  Metastasis in multiple ipsilateral lymph nodes, none >6 cm in greatest dimension
N2c  Metastasis in bilateral or contralateral lymph nodes, none >6 cm in greatest dimension
N3    Metastasis in a lymph node >6 cm in greatest dimension

*Distant metastasis (M)*
MX    Distant metastasis cannot be assessed
M0    No distant metastasis
M1    Distant metastasis

*There is no Roman Numeral Classification of American Joint Committee on Cancer for neck node metastasis of unknown primary cancer. From: Greene FL, American Joint Committee on Cancer, American Cancer Society. *AJCC Cancer Staging Manual, 6th ed.* New York: Springer, 2002.

### 2.2. Staging

- Table 14-1 shows the American Joint Committee on Cancer staging system for carcinoma of the unknown primary.

## 3. GENERAL MANAGEMENT

### 3.1. Surgical Management

- Data from surgery alone series revealed a median nodal recurrence rate of approximately 34% and a 5-year overall survival rate of approximately 66%.[4–7] The crude mucosal carcinoma emergence rate was approximately 25% (30/121 patients).
- Selected patients, especially those with pathologic N1 disease with no extracapsular extension, can be treated adequately with surgery alone.[6]

### 3.2. Irradiation Alone

- Grau et al.[4] reported a group of 213 patients treated with radiation alone. The 5-year actuarial mucosal carcinoma emergence rate was 16%, the nodal relapse rate was 50%, and the survival rate was 37%. It should be noted that se-

ries using radiation alone have more unfavorable prognostic factors.

### 3.3. Surgery and Irradiation

- Colletier et al.[8] reported a series of 136 patients who received radiotherapy after nodal excision or neck dissection. The mucosal carcinoma emergence rate was 10%, the nodal failure rate was 9%, and the 5-year overall survival rate was 60%.

### 3.4. Radiotherapy to Ipsilateral Neck

- Weir et al.[9] compared eighty-five patients who received radiation to the involved nodal region with fifty-nine patients who received radiation to the bilateral neck and putative primary sites. Mucosal primary tumors emerged in 7% of patients who received involved nodal field irradiation compared with 1.7% of patients in the second group. In multivariate analysis, no difference in survival or cause-specific survival was found between these groups.
- Similarly, Marcial-Vega et al.[10] did not show a significant difference of portal volume on mucosal emergence rate and 5-year overall survival in a study of eighty patients.
- In Grau et al.'s series,[4] twenty-six patients received ipsilateral neck radiation. In multivariate analysis, there was no significant difference in the rates of mucosal emergence, nodal failure, disease-specific survival, and overall survival compared with bilateral neck radiation. However, when combining all relapses above the clavicle, unilateral neck radiation showed a relative risk of 1.9 (P = .05) compared with bilateral neck radiation.
- Table 14-2 summarizes the results of comprehensive and limited radiotherapy.

## TABLE 14-2. RESULTS OF COMPREHENSIVE AND LIMITED RADIOTHERAPY*

|  | Unilateral Radiotherapy (Range) | Comprehensive Radiotherapy (Range) |
|---|---|---|
| Medial mucosal emergence rate | 8% (5–44) | 9.5% (2–13) |
| Median neck relapse rate | 51.5% (31–63) | 19% (8–49) |
| Median distant metastasis rate | 38% | 19% (11–23) |
| Median 5-yr overall survival rate | 36.5% (22–41) | 50% (34–63) |

*Comprehensive = irradiation of bilateral neck nodes plus the pharyngeal axis; limited = ipsilateral cervical irradiation.
Modified from: Nieder C, Gregoire V, Ang KK. Cervical lymph node metastases from occult squamous cell carcinoma: cut down a tree to get an apple? *Int Radiat Oncol Biol Phys* 2001;50,731, with permission.

## 3.5. Chemotherapy

- No data have been found to support the benefit of chemotherapy.

## 4. INTENSITY-MODULATED RADIATION THERAPY FOR NECK NODE METASTASIS UNKNOWN PRIMARY CARCINOMA

### 4.1. Target Volume Determination

- Table 7-5 in Chapter 7 summarizes the target volume specification for intensity-modulated radiation therapy (IMRT) in unknown primary carcinoma.
- Table 14-3 summarizes the suggested target volume determination for unknown primary carcinoma.

### 4.2. Target Volume Delineation

- In patients receiving postoperative IMRT, clinical target volume (CTV)1 encompasses the residual tumor and the region adjacent to it but not directly involved by the tumor, the surgical bed with soft tissue invasion by the tumor, or the extracapsular extension by metastatic neck nodes. CTV2 includes primarily the prophylactically treated neck.
- CTV1 and CTV2 delineation in a patient with a clinically TXN2M0 squamous cell carcinoma of unknown primary who received definitive IMRT is shown in Figure 14-1. The patient had multiple level II lymph nodes, and fine-needle biopsy taken from one of the nodes revealed squamous cell carcinoma. The patient underwent examination under anesthesia with biopsies at multiple sites, which were all negative. Both MRI and CT failed to show any primary disease.
- CTV1 and CTV2 delineation in a patient with a clinically TXN2bM0 squamous cell carcinoma of unknown

primary who received postoperative IMRT is shown in Figure 14-2. The patient had multiple right level II lymph nodes and underwent a right supraomohyoid neck dissection. IMRT was given to all mucosal sites and to the involved and uninvolved neck.

### 4.3. Normal Tissue Delineation

- See Chapter 8 for normal tissue delineation (Fig. 8-9).

### 4.4. Suggested Target and Normal Tissue Doses

- See Chapter 7 for suggested target and normal tissue doses (Table 7-11).

### 4.5. Intensity-Modulated Radiation Therapy Results

- Following these guidelines, we treated nine patients with unknown primary carcinoma by using IMRT between February 1997 and December 2000 at Washington University.[11] The N stages were N1 (one patient), N2 (seven patients), and N3 (one patient). The median follow-up time was 34 months (range 10–55 months). We observed one locoregional recurrence, and none of the patients developed lung metastasis. All patients are alive, except 1 who died of recurrent disease.
- A gastrostomy tube was placed in one patient during the course of IMRT. We observed no grade 3 or 4 late complications in our patients who were treated with IMRT. Grade I xerostomia was observed in five patients, and grade II xerostomia developed in one patient as late sequelae.

*Text continues on page 237.*

**TABLE 14-3. TARGET VOLUME DETERMINATION GUIDELINES FOR UNKNOWN PRIMARY CARCINOMA**

| Treatment Type | CTV1 | CTV2 | CTV3 |
|---|---|---|---|
| **Definitive†** | GTVn | Adjacent LNs* | IN+CN+RPLN (remaining LNs) + mucosal area |
| **Postoperative‡** | Surgical bed | IN+CN+RPLN (remaining LNs) + mucosal area | — |

GTVn, nodal gross tumor volume; IN, ipsilateral nodal levels; CN, contralateral nodal levels; RPLN, retropharyngeal lymph node; CTV, clinical target volume.
*Two to 3 cm from CTV1 nodal basin.
†Suggested intensity-modulated radiation therapy (IMRT) dose schedule for chemoradiation: CTV1 = 70 Gy/35 fx or 70 Gy/33 fx; CTV2 = 63 Gy/35 fx or 59.4 Gy/33 fx; CTV3 = 56 Gy/35 fx or 54 Gy/33 fx. When definitive IMRT is used without concomitant chemotherapy, suggested doses are: CTV1 = 66 Gy/30 fx; CTV2 = 60 Gy/30 Gy; CTV3 = 54 Gy/30 fx.
‡Suggested IMRT dose schedule: CTV1 = 60 Gy/30 fx; CTV2 = 54 Gy/30 fx.

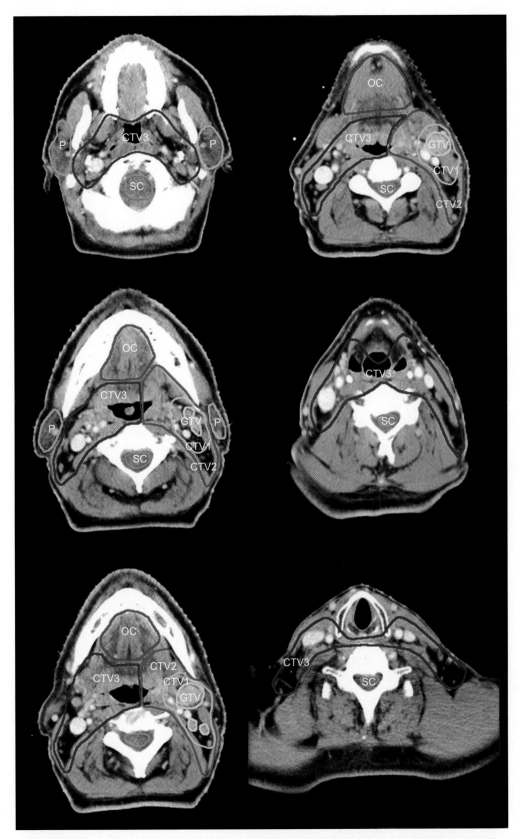

**FIGURE 14-1.** Clinical target volume (CTV) delineation in a patient with TXN2b squamous cell carcinoma of unknown primary who is receiving definitive intensity-modulated radiation therapy (IMRT). CTV1 (*light blue line*); CTV2 (*red line*); CTV3 (*dark blue line*); oral cavity (OC) (*magenta line*); gross tumor volume (GTV) (*yellow line*); left parotid gland (P) (*aqua line*); right parotid gland (P) (*rust line*); spinal cord (SC) (*green line*).

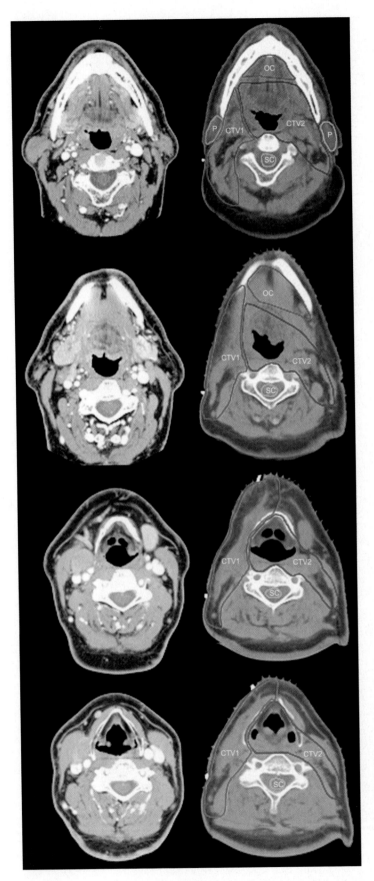

**FIGURE 14-2.** CTV delineation in a patient with TXN2b squamous cell carcinoma of unknown primary who is receiving postoperative IMRT. Preoperative computed tomography (CT) (*left*); postoperative CT (*right*). CTV1 (*red line*); CTV2 (*dark blue line*); oral cavity (OC) (*magenta line*); left parotid gland (P) (*aqua line*); right parotid gland (P) (*rust line*); spinal cord (SC) (*green line*).

# REFERENCES

1. Nieder C, Gregoire V, Ang KK. Cervical lymph node metastases from occult squamous cell carcinoma: cut down a tree to get an apple? *Int J Radiat Oncol Biol Phys* 2001;50:727–733.
2. Jones AS, Cook JA, Phillips DE, et al. Squamous carcinoma presenting as an enlarged cervical lymph node. *Cancer* 1993;72: 1756–1761.
3. Mendenhall WM, Mancuso AA, Parsons JT, et al. Diagnostic evaluation of squamous cell carcinoma metastatic to cervical lymph nodes from an unknown head and neck primary site. *Head Neck* 1998;20:739–744.
4. Grau C, Johansen LV, Jakobsen J, et al. Cervical lymph node metastases from unknown primary tumours. Results from a national survey by the Danish Society for Head and Neck Oncology. *Radiother Oncol* 2000;55:121–129.
5. Coker DD, Casterline PF, Chambers RG, et al. Metastases to lymph nodes of the head and neck from an unknown primary site. *Am J Surg* 1977;134:517–522.
6. Coster JR, Foote RL, Olsen KD, et al. Cervical nodal metastasis of squamous cell carcinoma of unknown origin: indications for withholding radiation therapy. *Int J Radiat Oncol Biol Phys* 1992;23:743–749.
7. Wang RC, Goepfert H, Barber AE, et al. Unknown primary squamous cell carcinoma metastatic to the neck. *Arch Otolaryngol Head Neck Surg* 1990;116:1388–1393.
8. Colletier PJ, Garden AS, Morrison WH, et al. Postoperative radiation for squamous cell carcinoma metastatic to cervical lymph nodes from an unknown primary site: outcomes and patterns of failure. *Head Neck* 1998;20:674–681.
9. Weir L, Keane T, Cummings B, et al. Radiation treatment of cervical lymph node metastases from an unknown primary: an analysis of outcome by treatment volume and other prognostic factors. *Radiother Oncol* 1995;35:206–211.
10. Marcial-Vega VA, Cardenes H, Perez CA, et al. Cervical metastases from unknown primaries: radiotherapeutic management and appearance of subsequent primaries. *Int J Radiat Oncol Biol Phys* 1990;19:919–928.
11. Chao KS, Ozyigit G, Tran BN, et al. Patterns of failure in patients receiving definitive and postoperative IMRT for head-and-neck cancer. *Int J Radiat Oncol Biol Phys* 2003;55: 312–321.

# 15

# BREAST CANCER

## THOMAS A. BUCHHOLZ

## 1. ANATOMY

- The female breast lies on the anterior chest wall superficial to the pectoralis major muscle. The breast can extend mediolaterally from the midline to near the midaxillary line and cranial-caudally from the second anterior rib to the sixth anterior rib.
- The upper-outer quadrant of the breast extends into the region of the low axilla and is frequently referred to as the axillary tail of Spence. This anatomical feature leads the upper-outer-quadrant of the breast to contain a greater percentage of total breast tissue compared to the other quadrants.
- The glandular breast tissue is supported by fibrous septae known as Cooper's ligaments. These septae connect the breast parenchyma to the overlying skin and the pectoralis fascia. These supporting structures can be affected by tumors and lead to skin dimpling.
- The breast parenchyma is composed of lobules and ducts. The function of the lobules is to produce milk and the function of the ducts is to transport lactation products to the nipple. The peripheral ducts converge into major lactiferous ducts, which then communicate with the nipple-areola complex.
- Most breast cancers develop at the interface between the ductal system and the lobules, a region called the terminal ductal lobular unit.
- The breast parenchyma is intermixed with connective tissue, which has a rich vascular and lymphatic network.

### 1.1. Lymphatics

- Figure 15-1 displays a drawing of the breast and regional lymph node anatomy.[1]

### 1.1.1. Axillary Lymph Nodes

- The predominant lymphatic drainage of the breast is to axillary lymph nodes.
- The axilla is commonly described as existing in three levels. The levels of the axillary are based on the relationship of the lymph node regions to the pectoralis minor muscle. The level I axilla is caudal and lateral to the muscle, level II is beneath the muscle, and level III (also known as the infraclavicular region) is cranial and medial to the muscle.
- A standard axillary lymph node dissection resects the tissue and lymph nodes within level I and II. It is very unusual to have involvement of level III of the axilla without disease in level I or II.
- The axillary lymph nodes continue underneath the clavicle to become the supraclavicular lymph nodes, which can be involved in locally advanced breast cancers.

### 1.1.2. Internal Mammary Chain

- Lymphatics can also drain directly into the internal mammary lymph node chain (IMC).
- The internal mammary lymph nodes are intrathoracic structures located in the parasternal space. It is unusual to visualize these lymph nodes with ultrasound or computed tomography (CT), but the anatomical region of the IMC can be determined by the internal mammary artery and vein, which are easily visualized by CT (Fig. 15-2).[2] Most commonly, the IMC lymph nodes are 3 to 4 cm lateral to midline. Figure 15-3 shows the upper one-third of the IMC reconstructed as seen from an anteroposterior projection.[2]
- When breast cancer involves the IMC, the majority of cases will have disease that is limited to lymph nodes in the first three interspaces. It is unusual to have involvement of the lower IMC lymph nodes.
- The use of lymphoscintigraphy as a component of sentinel lymph node imaging has helped to delineate primary lymphatic drainage patterns of breast cancer. Lymphoscintigraphies are performed by injecting technetium-99 radiocolloid into the peritumoral region and followed by scintillation scanning. Figure 15-4 is an example of a lymphoscintigraphy showing drainage of an inner-quadrant breast cancer to both the IMC lymph nodes and axillary lymph nodes.[2]

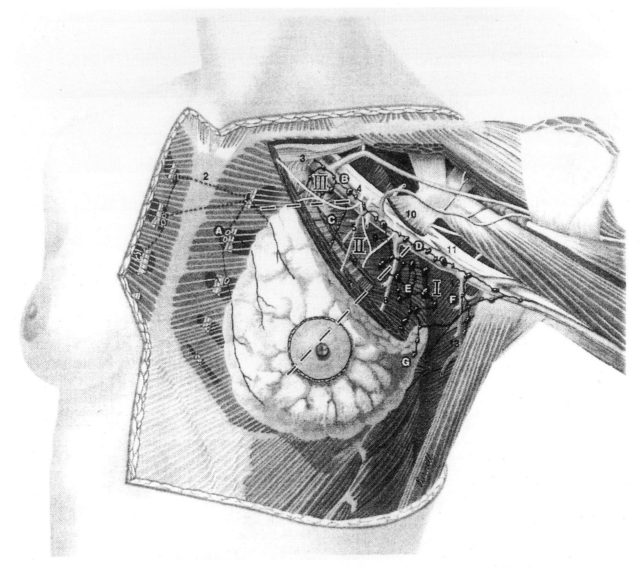

Lymphatic drainage of the breast showing lymph node groups and levels.

1. Internal mammary artery and vein
2. Substernal cross drainage to contralateral internal mammary lymphatic chain
3. Subclavius muscle and Halsted ligament
4. Lateral pectoral nerve (from the lateral cord)
5. Pectoral branch from thoracoacromial vein
6. Pectoralis minor muscle
7. Pectoralis major muscle
8. Lateral thoracic vein
9. Medial pectoral nerve (from the medial cord)
10. Pectoralis minor muscle
11. Median nerve
12. Subscapular vein

13. Thoracodorsal vein
   A. Internal mammary lymph nodes
   B. Apical lymph nodes
   C. Interpectoral (Rotter) lymph nodes
   D. Axillary vein lymph nodes
   E. Central lymph nodes
   F. Scapular lymph nodes
   G. External mammary lymph nodes

Level I lymph nodes: lateral to lateral border of pectoralis minor muscle
Level II lymph nodes: behind pectoralis minor muscle
Level III lymph nodes: medial to medial border of pectoralis minor muscle

**FIGURE 15-1.** Anatomy of the breast and lymphatics.

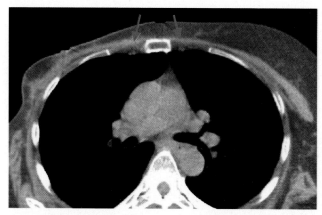

**FIGURE 15-2.** Axial treatment planning CT scan image demonstrating the location and appearance of the internal mammary artery and vein (*arrows*). These vessels can be contoured on sequential slices to show the anatomical region of the internal mammary lymph nodes.

- Breast cancers that develop in the medial, central, or lower breast more commonly drain to the IMC (in addition to the axilla) compared to breast cancer occurring in the lateral and upper quadrants. In our institutional experience using lymphoscintigraphy with sentinel lymph

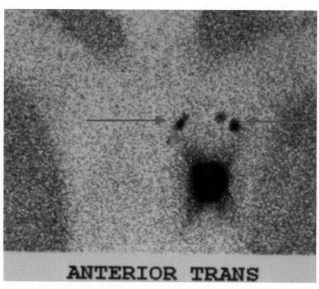

**FIGURE 15-4.** Lymphoscintigraphy from a breast cancer patient with a low central tumor. The scan shows dual drainage to the axilla and internal mammary chain (*arrows*). (From: Buchholz TA, Strom EA, McNeese MD, et al. Radiation therapy as an adjuvant treatment after sentinel lymph node surgery for breast cancer. *Surg Clin N Am* 2003;83:911–930, with permission.)

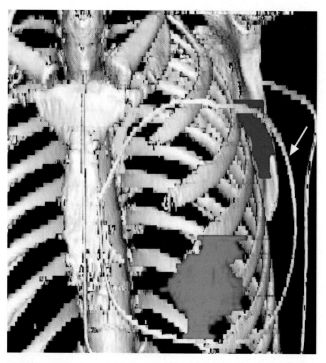

**FIGURE 15-3.** An anterior projection of a digitally reconstructed 6 o'clock tumor bed (*red*), internal mammary chain IMC (*yellow*), and low axilla (*blue*). The contours were reconstructed from volumes outlined on sequential axial slices of a treatment planning CT scan. The circular white volume (*arrow*) is from radiopaque wires placed around the palpable breast tissue at the time of treatment planning simulation. (From: Buchholz TA, Strom EA, McNeese MD, et al. Radiation therapy as an adjuvant treatment after sentinel lymph node surgery for breast cancer. *Surg Clin N Am* 2003;83:911–930, with permission.)

node surgery, drainage to the IMC was 14.1% for upper outer quadrant tumors, 16.7% for upper inner quadrant, 31.6% for lower outer quadrant tumors, 42.9% for lower inner quadrant tumors, and 28.4% for centrally located tumors (N = 88). [3]

## 2. NATURAL HISTORY

### 2.1. Breast Cancer Development

- Breast cancer develops as a consequence of both genetic changes in epithelial cells and complex interactions between cells and the microenvironment. Some, but not all, breast cancers pass through a series of conditions ranging from atypical ductal hyperplasia (ADH), to noninvasive cancer (ductal carcinoma in situ, or DCIS), and finally to invasive breast cancer. It has been estimated that it takes over a decade for most breast cancers to progress through this biological spectrum.
- The progression rate of ductal carcinoma in situ to invasive breast cancer is difficult to estimate and likely dependent on the grade of the lesion. One study found that up to 50% of low grade DCIS progressed to an invasive breast cancer within 20 years. [4] This rate is higher for high grade lesions.
- Many breast cancers develop in the absence of DCIS, suggesting that the ordered progression through the traditional biological spectrum is not required.

- Lobular carcinoma in situ (LCIS) has historically been felt to be more of a marker for breast cancer risk than a true premalignant condition in that the rates of contralateral and ipsilateral breast cancer development for women with LCIS is roughly equivalent.
- The kinetics of breast cancer development is heterogeneous, with some tumors being rather indolent, while others, such as inflammatory breast cancer, are noted for the rapid onset of symptoms and rapid progression.
- Risk factors for the development of breast cancer include

  □ *Genetic:* germline mutations in BRCA1, BRCA2, *p53*, PTEN.
  □ *Family history:* positive family history of breast or ovarian cancer.
  □ *Estrogenic:* nulliparity, late first pregnancy, early menarche, late menopause, postmenopausal estrogen/progesterone replacement.
  □ *Dietary:* moderate or heavy alcohol use.
  □ *Pathology:* personal history of breast cancer, DCIS, LICS, ADH, previous breast biopsies.

## 2.2. Breast Cancer Progression

- Invasive breast cancers can metastasize to lymph nodes or organs at any point in their development history. However, the risk of metastases is low for tumors under 1 cm.
- Risk factors for spread to regional lymph nodes and distant sites include

  □ Primary tumor size.
  □ Grade.
  □ Lymphovascular space invasion.
  □ Non-favorable histology (i.e., not tubular, medullary, or mucinous).
  □ Estrogen-negative disease.

## 3. DIAGNOSIS AND STAGING

### 3.1. Signs and Symptoms

- Most breast cancers present with a palpable mass or as an asymptomatic finding on screening mammogram.
- Signs and symptoms of more advanced disease include: skin retraction, skin edema, skin ulceration, axillary mass, pain, and bleeding.

### 3.2. Physical Examination

- Physical examination of the breast should include: size and location of mass, fixation to chest wall, involvement of skin, skin edema, and skin erythema.
- Physical examination of the axilla and supraclavicular lymph nodes should include: number, size, location of suspicious lymph nodes, and whether the lymph nodes are fixed or matted to one another.

## 3.3. Imaging

- All patients should undergo bilateral diagnostic mammograms, chest x-ray, routine serum chemistries, and blood counts.
- Patients diagnosed with locally advanced breast cancer should undergo a bone scan and imaging of the liver to rule out distant metastases.
- Imaging tools that may benefit selected patients include ultrasound of the breast and regional lymphatics, breast MRI scan, and PET scan.

## 3.4. Staging

- The AJCC implemented a new staging system for breast cancer in 2003.[5] For patients treated with surgery first, the *pathological* staging system should be used. For patients treated with chemotherapy before surgery (neoadjuvant chemotherapy), the *clinical* staging system should be used.
- The 2003 *clinical* staging for breast cancer includes

  □ Primary tumor—Tis: DCIS; T0: no evidence of primary tumor; T1: invasive disease up to 2 cm; T2: 2–5 cm; T3: less than 5 cm; T4: fixation to chest wall (T4a), involvement of skin (T4b), both (T4c), inflammatory breast cancer (T4d).
  □ Lymphatics—N1: suspicious mobile axillary lymph nodes; N2: fixed or matted axillary lymph nodes; N3: infraclavicular or supraclavicular lymph nodes.

- The 2003 *pathological* staging for breast cancer is shown in Table 15-1.

## 4. PROGNOSTIC FACTORS

- Prognostic factors for the development of metastatic disease include: number of positive lymph nodes, location of positive lymph nodes (supraclavicular versus axillary), size of primary tumor, involvement of the skin of the breast, nuclear grade, estrogen and progesterone receptor status, lymphovascular space invasion, and possibly HER2/neu overexpression.
- Prognostic factors for ipsilateral breast tumor recurrence after breast conservation surgery plus radiation include: positive surgical margins, residual diffuse calcifications, lack of systemic therapy, age under 35, germline mutation in BRCA1 or BRCA2, tumor size over 5 cm, and multicentric disease.
- Prognostic factors for locoregional recurrence after mastectomy without radiation include: number of involved lymph nodes, primary tumor size, margin status, and lymphovascular space invasion.

## TABLE 15-1. AJCC BREAST CANCER STAGING 2003 (PATHOLOGIC)[5]

**Primary Tumor (T)**

| | |
|---|---|
| TX | Primary tumor cannot be assessed |
| T0 | No evidence of primary tumor |
| Tis | Carcinoma *in situ:* Intraductal carcinoma, lobular carcinoma *in situ,* or Paget's disease of the nipple with no tumor |
| T1 | Tumor 2 cm or less in greatest dimension* |
| T2 | Tumor more than 2 cm but not more than 5 cm in greatest dimension |
| T3 | Tumor more than 5 cm in greatest dimension |
| T4 | Tumor of any size with direct extension (a) to the chest wall (b) skin, only as described below |
| T4a | Extension to chest wall |
| T4b | Edema or ulceration of the skin of the breast or satellite skin nodules confined to the same breast |
| T4c | (a) and (b) |
| T4d | Inflammatory carcinoma |

**Regional Lymph Nodes (N)**

| | |
|---|---|
| NX | Regional lymph nodes cannot be assessed |
| N0 | No regional lymph node metastasis* |
| N1 | Metastasis in 1 to 3 axillary lymph nodes, and/or in internal mammary nodes with microscopic disease detected by sentinel lymph node dissection but not clinically apparent* |
| N1 | Micrometastasis (>0.2 mm, ≤2.0 mm) |
| N2 | Metastasis in 4 to 9 axillary lymph nodes, or in clinically apparent internal mammary lymph nodes in the absence of axillary lymph node metastasis |
| N3 | Metastasis in 10 or more axillary lymph nodes, or in infraclavicular lymph nodes, or in clinically apparent ipsilateral lymph nodes in the presence of 1 or more axillary lymph nodes; or in more than 3 axillary lymph nodes with clinically negative microscopic metastasis in internal mammary lymph nodes; or in ipsilateral supraclavicular lymph nodes |

**Stage Groupings**

| | | | |
|---|---|---|---|
| Stage 0 | Tis | N0 | M0 |
| Stage I | T1 | N0 | M0 |
| Stage IIa | T0N1M0, T1N1M0, T2N0M0 | | |
| Stage IIb | T2N1M0, T3N0M0 | | |
| Stage IIIa | T0N2M0, T1N2M0, T2N2M0, T3N1M0, T3N2M0 | | |
| Stage IIIb | T4 N0M0, T4N1M0, T4N2M0 | | |
| Stage IIIc | Any T | N3 | |
| Stage IV | Any T | Any N | M1 |

## 5. GENERAL MANAGEMENT

### 5.1. Ductal Carcinoma In Situ

- The majority of patients with DCIS should be managed with a lumpectomy and breast radiation with the consideration of using tamoxifen.
- Three randomized prospective trials have indicated that for DCIS patients, the addition of radiation after lumpectomy reduces ipsilateral breast recurrences (Table 15-2).[6–8]

### 5.2. Early Stage Breast Conservation

- All patients with invasive breast cancer should be managed by a multidisciplinary team including a medical oncologist, surgeon, and radiation oncologist.

- The majority of breast cancer patients should receive systemic therapy (chemotherapy, hormonal therapy, or both). The one category of patients who may not benefit from systemic treatment are those with tumor sizes less than 1 cm who also have negative lymph nodes.
- For patients with clinical T1N0 or T2N0 stages who desire breast preservation, lumpectomy (segmental mastectomy) with a sentinel lymph node dissection or an axillary dissection followed by breast irradiation is the preferred local treatment.
- Sentinel lymph node surgery has less morbidity and allows for a more comprehensive pathological evaluation of the lymph nodes when compared with axillary lymph node dissection.
- An axillary lymph node dissection remains the standard of care for patients with N1 disease.

**TABLE 15-2. RESULTS OF RANDOMIZED PROSPECTIVE TRIALS EVALUATING THE EFFICACY OF RADIATION AFTER BREAST CONSERVATION SURGERY FOR PATIENTS WITH DUCTAL CARCINOMA IN SITU**

| Trial | Follow-up | Event | Ipsilateral Breast Recurrence | | p Value |
|---|---|---|---|---|---|
| | | | No Radiation | Radiation | |
| NSABP B-17[6] | 12 yr | Overall | 31.7% | 5.7% | $p < 0.000005$ |
| | | Invasive | 16.8% | 7.7% | $p = 0.00001$ |
| | | Noninvasive | 14.6% | 8% | $p = 0.001$ |
| EORTC #10853[7] | 4 yr | Overall | 16% | 9% | $p = 0.005$ |
| | | Invasive | 8% | 4% | $p = 0.04$ |
| | | Noninvasive | 8% | 5% | |
| UK/Aus/NZ[8] | 53 mo | Overall | 14% | 6% | $p < 0.0001$ |
| | | Invasive | 6% | 3% | $p = 0.01$ |
| | | Noninvasive | 7% | 3% | $p = 0.0004$ |

- Randomized trials have proven that for patients with early stage breast cancer, a breast conservation approach provides an equivalent outcome as a modified radical mastectomy. The outcome for the largest randomized trial, NSABP B-06, revealed no difference in the 20-year disease-free, distant disease-free, or overall survival between those treated with breast conservation and those treated with mastectomy.[9]
- Radiation is a required component for all cases of invasive breast cancer treated with breast conservation therapy.
- The data from selected trials showing the value of radiation after breast conservation surgery are shown in Table 15-3.[9-14]

## 5.3. Postmastectomy Radiation

- Randomized trials have indicated that radiation can improve the overall survival of patients with a 25% to 30% 10-year risk of locoregional relapse (LRR) treated with mastectomy and systemic treatment.[15-17]

- The data from these trials is shown in Table 15-4.
- A number of studies have evaluated patients treated with mastectomy and chemotherapy without radiation to define pathological factors associated with the risk of LRR. In general, these data indicate that patients with four or more positive lymph nodes, T3 or T4 primary disease, extracapsular extension measuring over 2 mm, or positive surgical margins are at high risk; patients with stage II breast cancer with one to three lymph nodes are at intermediate risk; and patients with small primary and negative lymph nodes are at low risk. These data are summarized in Table 15-5.[18-22]

## 5.4. Chemotherapy

- Adjuvant systemic chemotherapy has been shown to improve survival for both patients with lymph node-negative breast cancer and those with lymph node-positive disease.[23]

**TABLE 15-3. RESULTS OF RANDOMIZED PROSPECTIVE TRIALS EVALUATING THE EFFICACY OF RADIATION AFTER BREAST CONSERVATION SURGERY FOR PATIENTS WITH INVASIVE DISEASE**

| Trial | Follow-up | Eligibility | Ipsilateral Breast Recurrence | | P Value |
|---|---|---|---|---|---|
| | | | No Radiation | Radiation | |
| NSABP B-06[9] | 20 yr | Stage I/II | 39.2% | 14.3% | $P < 0.001$ |
| Milan[10] | 10 yr | <2.5 cm | 23.5% | 5.8% | $P < 0.001$ |
| Finish[11] | 5 yr | Stage I | 14.1% | 6.2% | $P = 0.029$ |
| Scottish[12] | 6 yr | Stage I/II | 24.5% | 5.8% | |
| Swedish[13] | 10 yr | Stage I | 24% | 8.5% | $P = 0.0001$ |
| NSABP B-21[14] | 8 yr | <1.0 cm, N0 | 16.5% | 9.3%/2.8%* | $P = 0.039$ |

*9.3% for those treated with radiation without tamoxifen; 2.8% for those treated with both radiation and tamoxifen.

**TABLE 15-4. RESULTS OF RANDOMIZED PROSPECTIVE TRIALS EVALUATING THE EFFICACY OF RADIATION IN CONJUNCTION WITH MASTECTOMY AND SYSTEMIC THERAPY FOR PATIENTS WITH INVASIVE BREAST CANCER**

| Trial | Follow-up | Eligibility | Locoregional Recurrence | | Overall Survival | |
|---|---|---|---|---|---|---|
| | | | No Radiation | Radiation | No Radiation | Radiation |
| Danish 82b[15] | 10 yr | Premenopausal "high risk" | 32% | 9% | 45% | 54% |
| | | | $p < 0.001$ | | $p < 0.001$ | |
| Danish 82c[16] | 10 yr | Postmenopausal "high risk" | 35% | 8% | 36% | 45% |
| | | | $p < 0.001$ | | $p = 0.03$ | |
| British Columbia[17] | 10 yr | Premenopausal "high risk" | 33% | 13% | 46% | 54% |
| | | | $p < 0.001$ | | $p = 0.07$ | |

- In general, chemotherapy achieves a one-third reduction in the risk of recurrence, with the absolute benefit being largely determined by the de nova risk of recurrence.[23]
- Meta-analysis of the first generation chemotherapy studies suggest that antracyclin-based chemotherapy may offer a modest advantage over non-anthracycline based chemotherapy.[23] These data were generated from studies performed prior to the use of taxanes.
- Emerging evidence suggests that treating with both an anthracycline and a taxane in the adjuvant setting further improves overall survival for women with lymph node-positive breast cancer.[24]
- The optimal systemic treatment for patients with estrogen receptor-positive disease is controversial. Hormonal therapy provides a greater clinical benefit than chemotherapy, but some data suggests that combining chemotherapy and hormonal therapy achieves a greater reduction in risk than either treatment alone.[25]
- Neoadjuvant chemotherapy offers no survival benefit when compared to adjuvant chemotherapy, but can increase the probability of breast conservation for selected patients who would be initially recommended to undergo mastectomy.[26,27]

- Neoadjuvant chemotherapy is the treatment of choice for patients with inoperable locally advanced breast cancer, inflammatory breast cancer, or locally recurrent inoperable breast cancer.

## 6. INTENSITY-MODULATED RADIATION THERAPY FOR BREAST CANCER

- The definition of IMRT has a variety of meanings within breast cancer treatment. The majority of data concerning IMRT refers to use of modulated static tangent fields and the primary goal of IMRT in this setting is to improve dose uniformity with little to no improvement in dose conformality.[28–30]
- IMRT is typically performed through the use of delivery of treatment through sequential open fields and multileaf collimated fields with fixed gantry angles.
- IMRT planning for breast cancer can be implemented both with either forward planning or inverse planning.
- Attempts to improve on conformability of breast cancer treatments with inverse planning IMRT techniques have been limited by trade-offs of increases in doses delivered to the contralateral breast and lung.[31]

**TABLE 15-5. TEN-YEAR LOCAL-REGIONAL RECURRENCE RATES AFTER MASTECTOMY AND SYSTEMIC TREATMENT**

| Investigators | No. of Patients | Systemic Therapy | Local-Regional Recurrence Rate | |
|---|---|---|---|---|
| | | | Patients with 1–3+LN | Patients with <3+LN |
| MDACC[18] | 1,031 | Doxorubicin-based | 10% | 21% |
| ECOG[20] | 2,016 | CMF | 13% | 29% |
| NSABP[21] | 5,758 | Varied | 6%–11%* | 14%–25%* |
| IBCSG[22] | 4,077 | Varied | 14%† | 22%† |

*Range dependent on size of primary tumor.
†Rates based on weighted averages derived from the data presented in the paper.

## 6.1. Target Volume Determination-Breast Conservation

- For patients who undergo lumpectomy for DCIS and who undergo segmental mastectomy with axillary lymph node dissection, the recommended target volume is the ipsilateral breast.
- The patient should be positioned in a reproducible manner with the ipsilateral arm abducted and externally rotated.
- To delineate this target, the external boundaries of the palpable breast tissue and the tumor bed scar should be outlined with radiopaque wire and the entire breast plus a 3 to 5 cm margin should be scanned with a CT-simulator.
- In selected cases, the low axilla may also require treatment and should be considered in the target volume.
- In other cases, the following may be considered at risk and warrant inclusion into the treatment volume:
  □ Low axilla
  □ Entire axilla and supraclavicular (SCV) fossa
  □ Undissected axilla and SVC fossa
  □ IMC

- Table 15-6 provides suggested target volume determination guidelines for certain indications in patients with invasive breast cancer.

## 6.2. Target Volume Delineation

- For breast conservation therapy, the tumor bed and tumor bed scar are contoured in every case. This assists in the arrangements of the primary beams and also is critical for the design of boost fields.
- For patients requiring irradiation to the low axilla or IMC, it is critical that these structures are contoured. This facilitates the design of treatment fields and allows for determination as to whether the target volume can be included in tangent fields or requires matching of a medial electron field with more lateralized tangent fields. Figure 15-5 shows a contoured low axilla and IMC region on a single axilla slice and the structures displayed in a treatment field. Figure 15-6 shows the beam's-eye-view of the treatment field.
- Figure 15-7 delineates the lymph node target volumes for patients requiring comprehensive radiation to the internal mammary lymph nodes, levels I–III of the axilla, and the supraclavicular lymph nodes.

*Text continues on page 248*

**TABLE 15-6. TREATMENT VOLUMES FOR RADIATION FIELDS IN PATIENTS WITH INVASIVE BREAST CANCER**

| Target Volume | Indications | |
| --- | --- | --- |
| Index Breast | When Indicated | All cases treated with breast conservation therapy |
| | When Not Indicated | |
| | Controversial | Whether partial breast treatment will prove to be equally effective |
| Level I/II axilla | When Indicated | Invasive disease without a sentinel lymph node (SLN) or axillary lymph node (ALN) dissection; Positive SLN dissection without an ALN dissection |
| | When Not Indicated | After an adequate negative SLN dissection or an adequate ALN dissection |
| | Controversial | After a negative ALN sampling |
| Level III/SCF | When Indicated | Four or more positive ALNs after an axillary dissection |
| | When Not Indicated | After an adequate negative SLN or ALN dissection |
| | Controversial | One to three positive ALNs after an axillary dissection; Positive SLN without an axillary lymph node dissection |
| Internal Mammary | When Indicated | Positive SLN in axilla with dual drainage to internal mammary chain on esi lymphosintigraphy |
| | When Not Indicated | Negative SLN or ALN dissection with a tumor in the upper outer quadrant |
| | Controversial | Positive SLN or ALN dissection with a tumor in the inner, central or lower quadrant disease with + axilla |

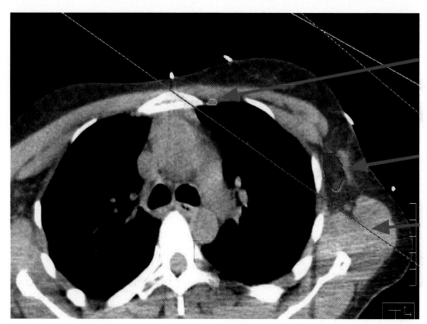

Contoured
IMC Target

Contoured
Axillary Target

Deep Field
Edge

**FIGURE 15-5.** Method of irradiating the upper internal mammary chain (IMC) lymph nodes and low axilla using 3D treatment planning. The IMC lymph nodes (*yellow volume*) and axilla (*blue volume*) are contoured in sequential CT slices, and fields are designed to include these volumes while minimizing the volume of the lung and heart in the field. (From: Buchholz TA, Strom EA, McNeese MD, et al. Radiation therapy as an adjuvant treatment after sentinel lymph node surgery for breast cancer. *Surg Clin N Am* 2003;83:911–930, with permission.)

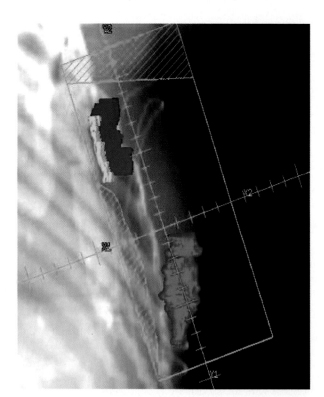

**FIGURE 15-6.** A beam's-eye view of a high tangent radiation treatment field designed to cover the breast, low axilla, and upper internal mammary chain (IMC). The reconstructed contours of a tumor bed (*red*), upper IMC (*yellow*) and the low axilla (*blue*) are shown. In the caudal half of the field, a block is used to minimize the amount of lung and heart that is included in the treatment field. (From: Buchholz TA, Strom EA, McNeese MD, et al. Radiation therapy as an adjuvant treatment after sentinel lymph node surgery for breast cancer. *Surg Clin N Am* 2003;83:911–930, with permission.)

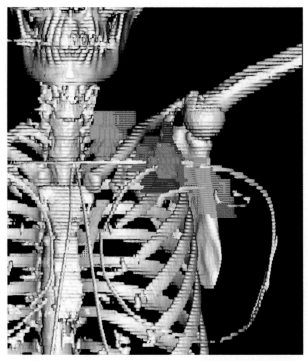

**FIGURE 15-7A.** Coronal image of delineation of lymph nodes regions at risk for a patient requiring comprehensive irradiation of the lymphatics. Displayed are the digitized reconstruction of the internal mammary lymph nodes (*light blue*), the three levels of the axilla (*green, light blue, red*) and their relationship to the pectoralis minor muscle (*dark blue*), and the supraclavicular lymph nodes (*orange*).

.

.

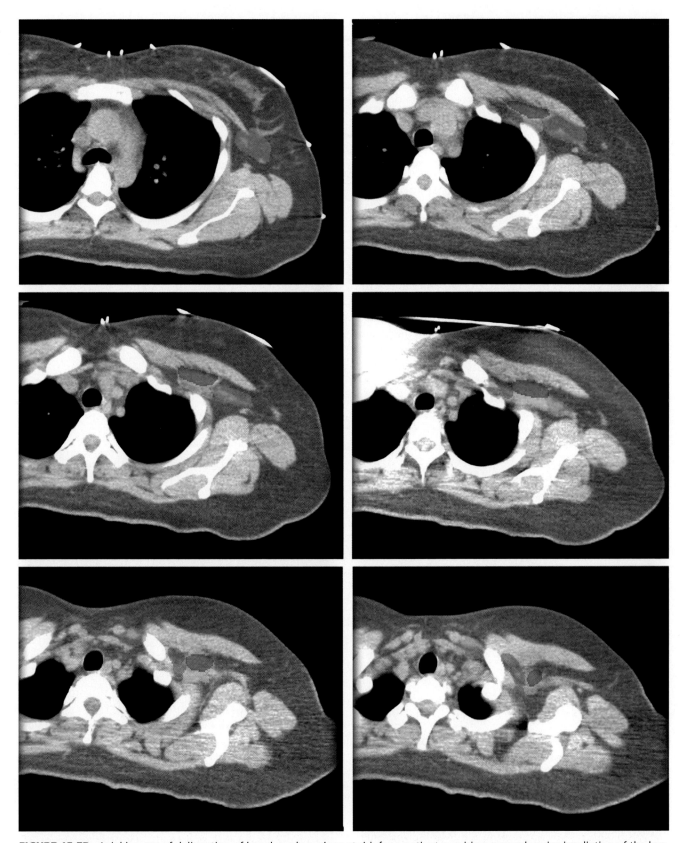

**FIGURE 15-7B.** Axial images of delineation of lymph node regions at risk for a patient requiring comprehensive irradiation of the lymphatics. These images show the anatomical areas displayed in Figure 15-7 in cross-section. Displayed are the internal mammary lymph nodes (*light blue*), the three levels of the axilla (*green, light blue, red*) and their relationship to the pectoralis minor muscle (*dark blue*), and the supraclavicular lymph nodes (*orange*). Note that the three levels of the axilla are determined by their relationship to the pectoralis minor muscle (level I: inferolateral, level II: beneath, level III: superomedial).

## 6.3. Treatment Field Design

- For patients with undissected axillas in whom the entire axilla is to be irradiated, the midaxilla within the supraclavicular field should be contoured to assure adequate lateral coverage and dose are provided to this region.
- Figure 15-8 shows an example of such fields.

## 6.4. IMRT Treatment Planning

- IMRT for breast cancer most commonly attempts to achieve optimal three-dimensional dose distribution within the minimal degree of dose inhomogeneity through forward treatment planning.
- Initially, medial and lateral tangent fields are designed with gantry angles that create a nondivergent posterior field edge and cover the targeted structure while minimizing the volume of normal tissue in the treatment fields.
- The dose distribution of two open fields is examined, with the dose normalized to a point at where the breast and pectoralis major muscle interface at approximately midseparation in the central plane. Adjustments to field weighting are then performed (Fig. 15-9A).
- A dose cloud of the volume included within the 115% isodose curve is generated and projected in the beam's-eye view of the treatment fields. Segments of multileaf collimation are then inserted on the medial tangent field for 15% of the dose.
- A new dose cloud of the volume included within 110% is then generated and the multileaf steps are repeated.
- Typically, four to six fields are needed to optimize the dose distribution (i.e., one open and one collimated medial tangent; one open and two collimated lateral tangents).
- Dose inhomogeneity due to size separation cannot be corrected with collimation; therefore, higher energy photons need to be considered.
- Figure 15-9 shows an example of the IMRT forward planning process and the resulting treatment fields for improving the 3D dose distribution in intact breast irradiation.

## 6.5. IMRT Results

- Three series have indicated that IMRT for breast cancer improves the dose distribution of intact breast treatment compared to conventional wedge planes.[28–30]
- In a study from our institution comparing wedge plans to IMRT in 87 intact breast cancer, IMRT reduced the median maximum dose delivered from 55.5 Gy to 52.8 Gy ($P < 0.0001$).[28] In addition, in the IMRT plans, only 2.2 % of the treated volume received more than 105% of the prescribed dose compared to 19.5 % of the treated volume in the wedge plans ($P < 0.0001$).

*Text continues on page 253*

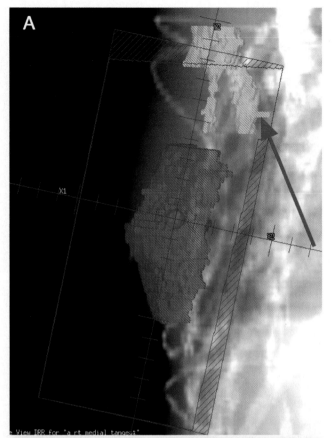
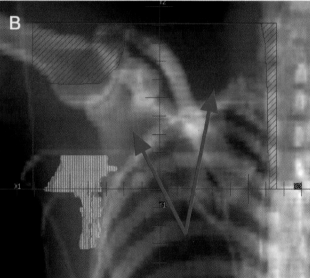

**FIGURE 15-8.** A three-field radiation technique used to comprehensively treat the axilla and supraclavicular fossa (SCF) in addition to the intact breast (**A,B**). The third field is geometrically matched to the cranial edge of the tangent fields and encompasses the high level II and level III axilla (**B**). For this arrangement, the cranial edge of the tangent fields can be lower than when tangent fields are used alone to treat the axilla. The reconstructed contours of a large postoperative tumor bed (*red*) and the low axilla (*yellow*) are shown. A supplemental dose from a posterior field is sometimes required in order to assure that the targeted axillary volume receive the prescribed dose. (From: Buchholz TA, Strom EA, McNeese MD, et al. Radiation therapy as an adjuvant treatment after sentinel lymph node surgery for breast cancer. *Surg Clin N Am* 2003;83:911–930, with permission.)

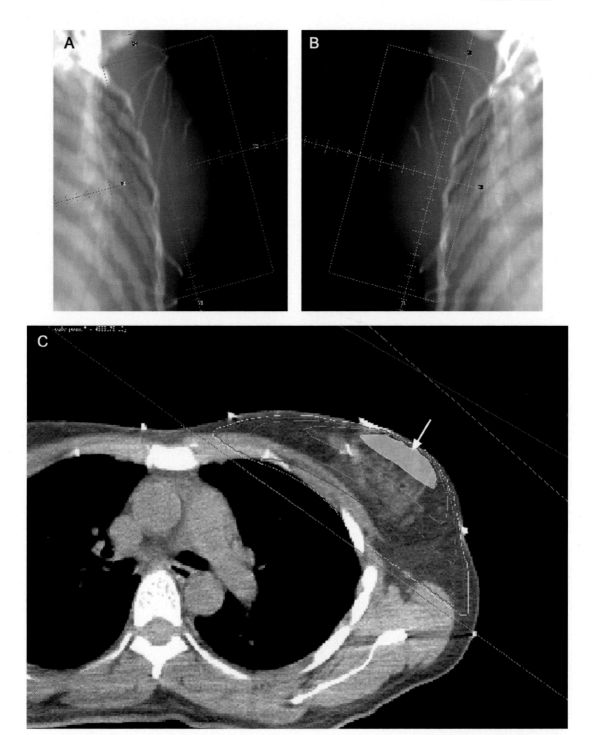

**FIGURE 15-9A.** IMRT planning process and resulting treatment fields. This panel shows beams-eye-view projection of the medial tangent (**A**) and lateral tangent (**B**) and the resulting dose distribution on the central axial CT slice (**C**). As shown, there is a 115% hot spot at the apex of the breast (*arrow*, yellow volume).

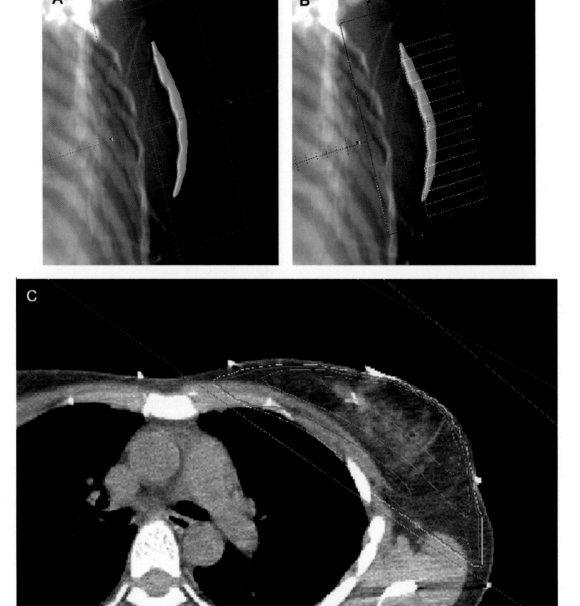

**FIGURE 15-9B.** IMRT planning process and resulting treatment fields. This panel shows the medial tangent (**A**) with the 115% dose cloud (volume in the field that received 115% dose). A collimated field (**B**) that provided 4% of the entire treatment was then designed which eliminated the 115% hot spot (yellow contoured volume in Figure 15-9A) on the axial CT slice.

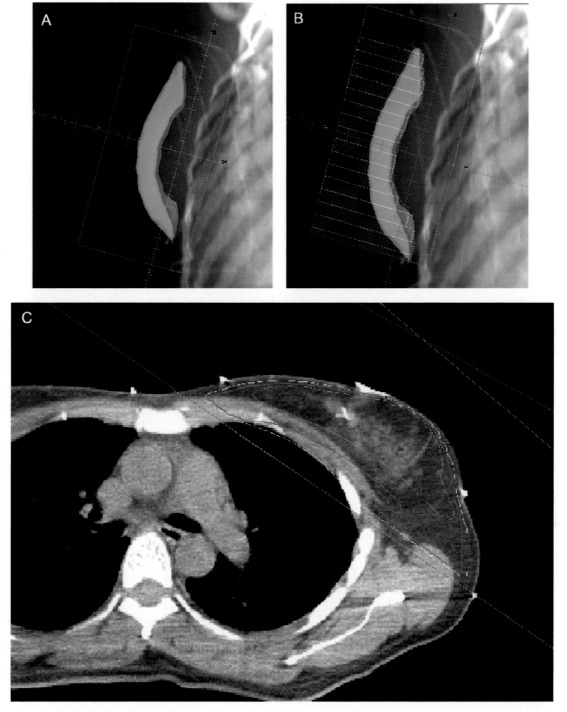

**FIGURE 15-9C.** IMRT planning process and resulting treatment fields. This panel shows the re-peated process used to then eliminate the 110% dose cloud (green isodose line shown in Figure 15-9B). This second collimated field (**B**) provided 5% of the entire treatment.

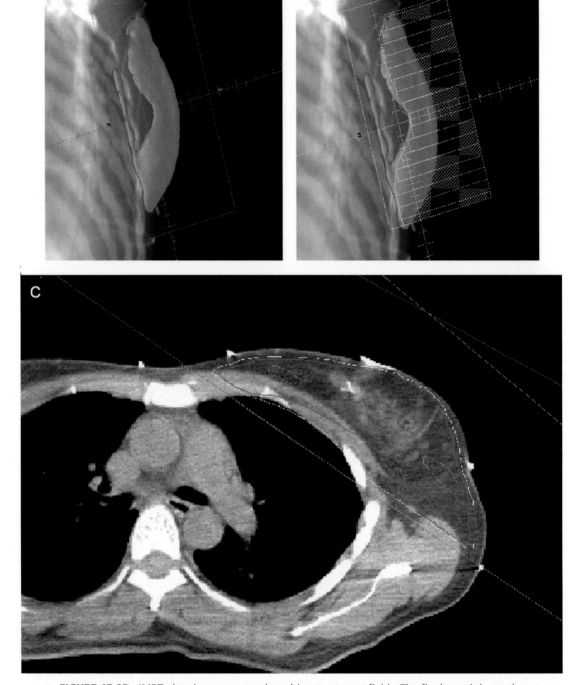

**FIGURE 15-9D.** IMRT planning process and resulting treatment fields. The final panel shows the 105% dose cloud with final collimated field (**B**) that provided 4% of the entire treatment. The final axial isodose CT slice is shown.

## 6.6. Sequela of Treatment

- The acute sequela of breast irradiation is low. Acute effects include fatigue and radiation dermatitis, which can develop into a temporary period of moist desquamation in the minority of the patients. The most common anatomical locations for desquamation are the inframammary sulcus and the axillary region.

- Late sequelae are also unusual. The most common late injury is a change in the aesthetic appearance of the treated breast, but over 80% of women treated with breast, preservation achieve a good or excellent cosmetic outcome. Women with larger breast sizes are more prone to having breast shrinkage, asymmetry, and poor aesthetic outcomes.

- Currently, there are no clinical data to demonstrate that the improved dose distributions achieved with IMRT reduces morbidity from treatment.

- The most significant late sequela of radiation treatment of the axillary and supraclavicular fossa is arm edema.

- Late injuries to the brachial plexus, lung, heart, chest wall, rib cage, skin, or soft tissues are common for patients treated with standard techniques and dosages.

## REFERENCES

1. Osborne MP. Breast development and anatomy. In: Harris JR, Lippman ME, Morrow M, Hellman S, eds. *Diseases of the Breasts.* Philadelphia: Lippincott-Raven, 1996;1–14.
2. Buchholz TA, Strom EA, McNeese MD, et al. Radiation therapy as an adjuvant treatment after sentinel lymph node surgery for breast cancer. *Surg Clin N Am* 2003;83:911–930.
3. Shahar KH, Buchholz TA, Delpassand E, et al. Cancer lower and central tumor location correlates with lymphoscintigraphy: drainage to the internal mammary lymph nodes in breast cancer. *Cancer* 2003;(in press).
4. Page DL, Dupont WD, Rogers LW, et al. Continued local recurrence of carcinoma 15–25 years after a diagnosis of low grade ductal carcinoma in situ of the breast treated only by biopsy. *Cancer* 1995;76:1197–1200.
5. Singletary SE, Allred C, Ashley P, et al. Revision of the American Joint Committee on Cancer staging system for breast cancer. *J Clin Oncol* 2002;20:3628–3636.
6. Fisher B, Land S, Mamounas E, et al. Prevention of invasive breast cancer in women with ductal carcinoma in situ: an update of the national surgical adjuvant breast and bowel project experience. *Semin Oncol* 2001;28:400–418.
7. Julien JP, Bijker N, Fentiman IS, et al. Radiotherapy in breast-conserving treatment for ductal carcinoma in situ: first results of the EORTC randomised phase III trial 10853. EORTC Breast Cancer Cooperative Group and EORTC Radiotherapy Group. *Lancet* 2000;355:528–533.
8. Houghton J, George WD, Cuzick J, et al. Radiotherapy and tamoxifen in women with completely excised ductal carcinoma in situ of the breast in the UK, Australia, and New Zealand: randomised controlled trial. *Lancet* 2003;362:95–102.
9. Fisher B, Anderson S, Bryant J, et al. Twenty-year follow-up of a randomized trial comparing total mastectomy, lumpectomy, and lumpectomy plus irradiation for the treatment of invasive breast cancer. *N Engl J Med* 2002;347:1233–1241.
10. Veronesi U, Marubini E, Mariani L, et al. Radiotherapy after breast-conserving surgery in small breast carcinoma: long-term results of a randomized trial. *Ann Oncol* 2001;12: 997–1003.
11. Holli K, Saaristo R, Isola J, et al. Lumpectomy with or without postoperative radiotherapy for breast cancer with favourable prognostic features: results of a randomized study. *Br J Cancer* 2001;84:164–169.
12. Forrest AP, Stewart HJ, Everington D, et al. Randomised controlled trial of conservation therapy for breast cancer: 6-year analysis of the Scottish trial. Scottish Cancer Trials Breast Group. *Lancet* 1996;348:708–713.
13. Liljegren G, Holmberg L, Bergh J, et al. 10-year results after sector resection with or without postoperative radiotherapy for stage I breast cancer: a randomized trial. *J Clin Oncol* 1999;17: 2326–2333.
14. Fisher B, Bryant J, Dignam J, et al. Tamoxifen, radiation therapy, or both for prevention of ipsilateral breast tumor recurrence after lumpectomy in women with invasive breast cancers of one centimeter or less. *J Clin Oncol* 2002;20:4141–4149.
15. Overgaard M, Hansen PS, Overgaard J, et al. Postoperative radiotherapy in high-risk premenopausal women with breast cancer who receive adjuvant chemotherapy. *N Engl J Med* 1997;337: 949–955.
16. Overgaard M, Jensen MB, Overgaard J, et al. Randomized trial evaluating postoperative radiotherapy in high risk postmenopausal breast cancer patients given adjuvant tamoxifen: results from the DBCG 82c trial. *Lancet* 1999;353:1641–1648.
17. Ragaz J, Jackson SM, Le N, et al. Adjuvant radiotherapy and chemotherapy in node-positive premenopausal women with breast cancer. *N Engl J Med* 1997;337:956–962.
18. Katz A, Strom EA, Buchholz TA, et al. Loco-regional recurrence patterns following mastectomy and doxorubicin-based chemotherapy: implications for postoperative irradiation. *J Clin Oncol* 2000;18:2817–2827.
19. Katz A, Strom EA, Buchholz TA, et al. The influence of pathologic tumor characteristics on locoregional recurrence rates following mastectomy. *Int J Radiat Oncol Biol Phys* 2001;50: 735–742.
20. Recht A, Gray R, Davidson NE, et al. Locoregional failure ten years after mastectomy and adjuvant chemotherapy with or without tamoxifen without irradiation: experience of the Eastern Cooperative Oncology Group. *J Clin Oncol* 1999;17: 1689–1700.
21. Taghian AG, Bryant J, Anderson S, et al. Pattern of loco-regional and distant failure in patients with breast cancer treated with mastectomy and chemotherapy (±tamoxifen) without radiation: results from five NSABP randomized trials. *Int J Radiat Oncol Biol Phys* 2001;51:106–107.
22. Wallgren A, Bonetti M, Gelber RD, et al. Risk factors for locoregional recurrence among breast cancer patients: results from International Breast Cancer Study Group trials I through VII. *J Clin Oncol* 2003;21:1205–1213.
23. Early Breast Cancer Trialists' Collaborative Group. Polychemotherapy for early breast cancer: an overview of the randomised trials. *Lancet* 1998;352:930–942.
24. Henderson IC, Berry DA, Demetri GD, et al. Improved outcomes from adding sequential Paclitaxel but not from escalating Doxorubicin dose in an adjuvant chemotherapy regimen for patients with node-positive primary breast cancer. *J Clin Oncol* 2003;21:976–983.
25. Early Breast Cancer Trialists' Collaborative Group. Tamoxifen for early breast cancer: an overview of the randomised trials. *Lancet* 1998;351:1451–1467.

26. Wolmark N, Wang J, Mamounas E, et al. Preoperative chemotherapy in patients with operable breast cancer: nine-year results from National Su1rgical Adjuvant Breast and Bowel Project B-18. *J Natl Cancer Inst Monogr* 2001;30:96–102.

27. Van der Hage JA, Cornelis JH, van de Velde CJ, et al. Preoperative chemotherapy in primary operable breast cancer: results from the European Organization for Research and Treatment of Cancer trial 10902. *J Clin Oncol* 2001;19:4224–4237.

28. Arzu IY, Perkins GH, Antolak JA, et al. Field-in-field tangent technique improves radiation dose homogeneity in breast conservation. *Proc Am Radium Soc* 2003;61:(#PO41).

29. Vicini FA, Sharpe M, Kestin L, et al. Optimizing breast cancer treatment efficacy with intensity-modulated radiotherapy. *Int J Radiat Oncol Biol Phys* 2002;54:1336–1344.

30. Evans PM, Donovan EM, Partridge M, et al. The delivery of intensity modulated radiotherapy to the breast using multiple static fields. *Radiother Oncol* 2000;57:79–89.

31. Krueger EA, Fraass BA, McShan DL, et al. Potential gains for irradiation of chest wall and regional nodes with intensity modulated radiotherapy. *Int J Rad Oncol Biol Phys* 2003;56:1023–1037.

# 16

# LUNG CANCER

### RITSUKO KOMAKI
### HELEN LIU
### HASAN MURSHED

## 1. ANATOMY

### 1.1. Gross Anatomy

- The right lung has three lobes as a result of a second fissure, the horizontal fissure, which separates the middle lobe from the upper lobe and extends from the anterior margin into the oblique fissure (Fig. 16-1).[1]
- The left lung is composed of two lobes: an upper and lower lobe.[1] The lingular portion of the left upper lobe corresponds to the middle lobe on the right.
- The trachea enters the superior mediastinum and bifurcates approximately at the level of the 5th thoracic vertebra (Fig. 16-2).[2]

### 1.2. Functional Anatomy

- The alveolar epithelium has two types of cells: type I and type II.
- Type I cells are squamous and have little capacity to respond to or repair damage. The type II cells synthesize and secrete surfactant, the lipid-protein complex that prevents alveoli collapse by reducing surface tension at the air-alveolar interface. Type II cells are also the progenitor cells both during normal cell turnover and after damage.
- Other cells that normally present in the lung are pulmonary macrophages and fibroblasts, both of which are critical for pulmonary repair after damage.

### 1.3. Lymphatic Drainage

- Figure 16-3 shows regional nodal stations for lung cancer staging.[3]
- The drainage for each pulmonary lobe is shown in Figure 16-4.[4]
- The lymph from the right upper lobe flows to the tracheobronchial lymph nodes. The lymph from the left upper lobe flows not only to the venous angle of the same side, is but also to the venous angle of the opposite superior mediastinum.

- The right and left lower lobe lymphatics drain into the subcarinal nodes and from there to the right superior mediastinum (the left lower lobe also may drain into the left superior mediastinum) and directly into the inferior mediastinal lymph nodes.
- The intrapulmonary lymph nodes are situated within the lung: the subsegmental nodes, the segmental nodes, and the lobar or interlobar nodes. They are located either at the bifurcation of the bronchi or close to the angle formed by the division of the arteries and veins.
- Hilar nodes are located at the pulmonary hilum outside of the pleural reflection.
- From a radiotherapeutic viewpoint, the bronchopulmonary lymph nodes, situated either along the lower portions of the main bronchi (hilar lymph nodes) or at the bifurcations of the main bronchi into the lobar bronchi (interlobar nodes),[5] are considered hilar nodes.
- The mediastinal lymph nodes are divided into two groups: superior, located above the carina, including the upper paratracheal, pretracheal, retrotracheal, lower paratracheal nodes (azygos nodes), and a group of nodes located in the aortic window; and inferior, situated in the subcarinal region and inferior mediastinum including the subcarinal, paraesophageal, and pulmonary ligament nodes.
- The peritracheobronchial nodes are located around the trachea and the main bronchi.
- In the case of chest wall involvement, there is a risk of spread to the intercostal nodes located close to the intercostal vessels and nerves. Paravertebral nodes situated either lateral to or in front of the vertebral bodies may be located along the pathway of the intercostal lymph collector.

## 2. NATURAL HISTORY

- Lung cancer is the leading cause of cancer death in the United States and the rest of the world.[6] Unfortunately, most patients already have locally advanced lung cancer at the time of diagnosis.

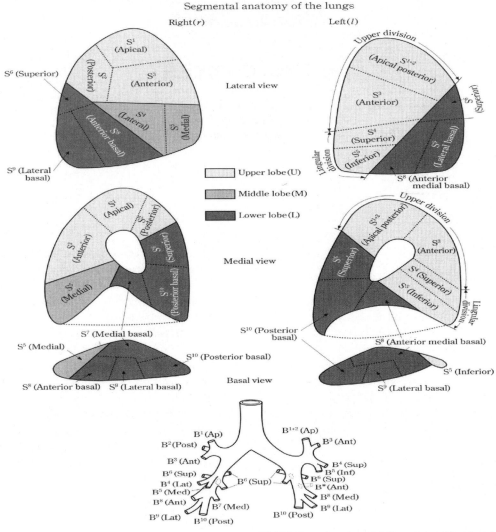

**FIGURE 16-1.** Segmental anatomy of the lungs. (From: The Japan Lung Cancer Society. *Classification of Lung Cancer*, First English ed. Toyko: Kanehara & Co., Ltd., 2000.)

- Squamous cell carcinoma tends to spread more locally or intrathoracically rather than rapid hematogenously, which is the opposite of adenocarcinoma and small cell lung cancer (SCLC).
- Undifferentiated SCLC has more tendencies to spread to lymph nodes and distant sites than does squamous carcinoma.
- Anaplastic or undifferentiated large cell carcinoma and adenocarcinoma spread both locally and distantly, as shown in Table 16-1.

## 3. DIAGNOSIS AND STAGING SYSTEM

### 3.1. Signs and Symptoms

- The majority of patients present with symptomatic disease.

- Cough, hemoptysis, dyspnea, and recurrent pneumonitis are common major symptoms resulting from airway obstruction by central bronchogenic lesions.
- Patients with peripheral tumors are frequently asymptomatic unless there is involvement of the chest wall or intercostal nerves.
- Chest pain is also common when tumors invade the pleura, chest wall, or mediastinal structures.
- Hoarseness may result from recurrent laryngeal nerve involvement by mediastinal metastasis (more common with left lung tumors).
- Compression of the esophagus may cause dysphagia.
- Symptoms from Pancoast syndrome (Horner syndrome, brachial plexus syndrome) or superior sulcus tumor syndrome may result when an apical tumor encroaches on cervical or thoracic nerves.

Segmental anatomy of the tracheobronchial tree

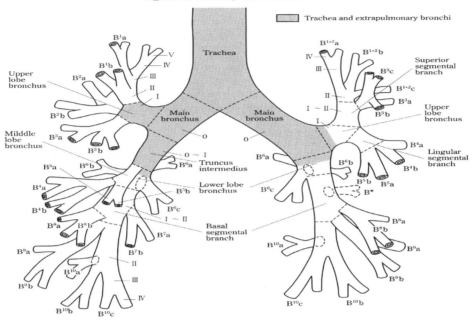

B* : This anomalous bronchial branch is seldom found.

**FIGURE 16-2.** Segmental anatomy of the tracheobronchial tree. The bronchopulmonary tree has sequential divisions down to the alveoli: the trachea (Tr), main bronchus (MB), truncus intermedius (Bint), upper lobe bronchus (Bu), middle lobe bronchus (Bm), lower lobe bronchus (Bl), superior segmental branch, lingular segmental branch, basal segmental branch, and numberous segmental and subsegmental branches. The MR, Bint, Bu, and part of Bl in the right lung, and the MB, and parts of Bu and Bl in the left lung, are defined as extrapulmonary bronchi. All segments are indicated by *S*. (From: The Japan Lung Cancer Society. *Classification of Lung Cancer*, First English Ed. Tokyo: Kanehara & Co., Ltd., 2000.)

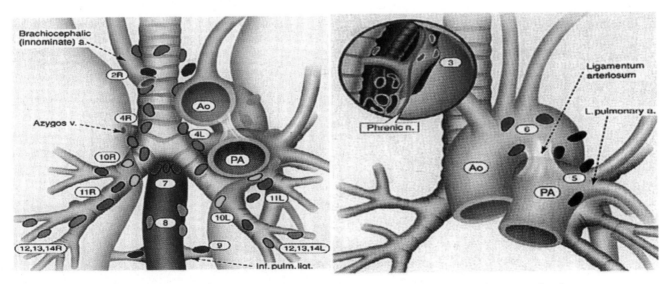

**FIGURE 16-3.** Regional nodal stations for lung cancer. (From: Mountain CF, Dresler CM. Regional lymph node classification for lung cancer staging. *Chest* 1997;111:1718–1723; with permission from the American College of Chest Physicians.)

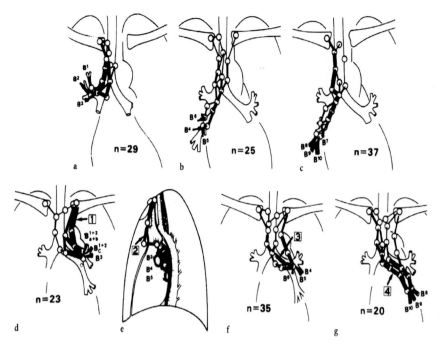

**FIGURE 16-4.** Standard pattern of lymphatic drainage based on 192 lymphoscintigraphies carried out in 179 patients without known nodal dissemination. For the right lobes, most of the lymph flowed into the right scalene nodes through the subcarinal or right tracheobronchial nodes. In contrast, the lymphatic drainage from the left lung was more variable: the lymph flowed both to the left and right scalene lymph nodes, especially in the case of the lower lobe. (From: Hata E, Hayakawa K, Miyamoto H, et al. Rationale for extended lymphadenectomy for lung cancer. *Theor Surg* 1990;5:19–27.)

- Superior vena cava syndrome can arise with right lung tumors or right mediastinal nodal metastasis.
- CNS symptoms are seen with brain metastasis or paraneoplastic disease, such as hyponatremia or hypercalcemia (small cell lung carcinoma).

## 3.2. Physical Examination

- Signs of partial or complete bronchial obstruction, pleural effusion, pneumonia, or atelectasis may be detected by chest examination.

- Inspection of the head and neck may reveal regional lymphatic (N3) spread.
- Metastatic disease can be found by examination of the abdomen (liver metastasis: hepatomegaly) and neuroaxis (cerebral and/or spinal cord metastasis).

## 3.3. Imaging

### 3.3.1. Computed Tomography

- Although the chest x-ray is the principal diagnostic tool for primary lesions, the radiological detection of lymph

**TABLE 16-1. SITE OF METASTASIS CORRELATED WITH HISTOLOGIC TYPE (AT AUTOPSY)**

| Site of Metastasis | Squamous | Small-Cell | Anaplastic | Adenocarcinoma |
|---|---|---|---|---|
| Lymph nodes | 137 (54) | 163 (85) | 134 (76) | 42 (75) |
| Liver | 58 (23) | 122 (64) | 67 (38) | 26 (47) |
| Adrenals | 54 (21) | 84 (44) | 69 (39) | 17 (30) |
| Bones | 59 (23) | 75 (39) | 53 (30) | 23 (41) |
| Brain | 26 (17) | 45 (42) | 30 (24) | 13 (39) |
| Kidney | 39 (15) | 28 (14.5) | 24 (13.5) | 11 (20) |
| Pancreas | 9 (3.5) | 46 (24) | 25 (14) | 3 (5) |
| Lung | 31 (12) | 13 (7) | 15 (8) | 8 (14) |
| Pleura | 18 (7) | 21 (11) | 9 | 3 (5) |
| *Total* | 255 | 191 | 179 | 56 |

Numbers in parentheses indicate percentage.
From: Line DH, Deeley TJ. The necropsy findings in carcinoma of the bronchus. *Br J Dis Chest* 1971;65:238–242.

node metastases is based mainly on findings of nodal enlargement (Fig. 16-5).

- The choice of the upper limit for normal nodal size is a complex issue and varies with nodal position, from 11 mm in the paratracheal region to 3 mm in the hilar region.[7] A convenient and reasonably easy approach is to use a cutoff of 10 mm in the short-axis diameter.[8]
- In a study by McLoud et al., the rate of positive mediastinal lymph node involvement increased from 13% when the node measured less than 1 cm to 62% for nodes of 2 to 2.9 cm.[9]
- CT specificity according to mediastinal nodal site varied from 72% for station 10R (right hilar) to 94% for station 10L (left hilar) when the criteria for positivity were 10 mm or more.[9]

- In the presence of obstructive penumonitis, the rate of false positive lymph node involvement increased to 45%.
- If nodes in the draining territory of the tumor are enlarged (more than 10 mm in the short axis) and at least 5 mm larger than nodes in the nondraining territories, CT specificity improves with a positive predictive value of 95%.[10]

### 3.3.2. Positron-Emission Tomography/Computed Tomography

- Whole body positron-emission tomography (PET) with [18]F-fluorodeoxglucose ([18]F-FDG) is increasingly being used for lung cancer. Mediastinal lymph node metastasis can be accurately detected by PET scan with the sensitivity and specificity of approximately 90%.[11–13]

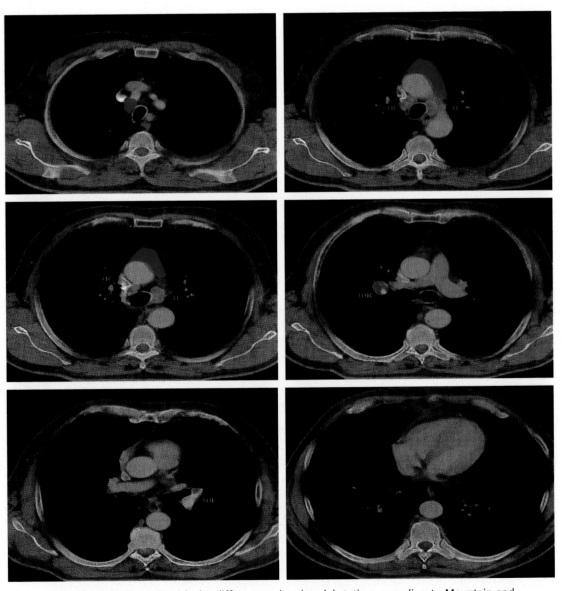

**FIGURE 16-5.** Chest CT with the different regional nodal stations according to Mountain and Dresler[16] (with permission from the American College of Chest Physicians).

- The corresponding values for CT imaging were approximately at 75% and 66%, respectively.
- A disadvantage of PET is its limited anatomical resolution, which has been improved by the fusion of CT and PET (Fig. 16-6).[14]

- A high negative predictive value (~95%) of PET for mediastinal lymph node metastasis implies that invasive procedures are probably not necessary in patients with negative findings of PET in the mediastinum.

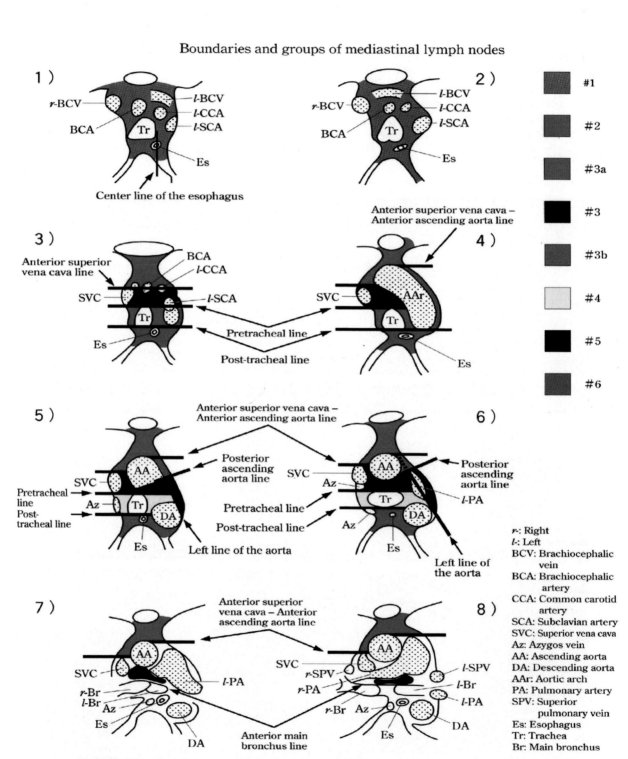

**FIGURE 16-6.** Boundaries and groups of mediastinal lymph nodes. (From: The Japan Lung Cancer Society. Classification of Lung Cancer, 1st English Ed. Tokyo: Kanehara & Co., LTd., 2000; see Appendix for details).

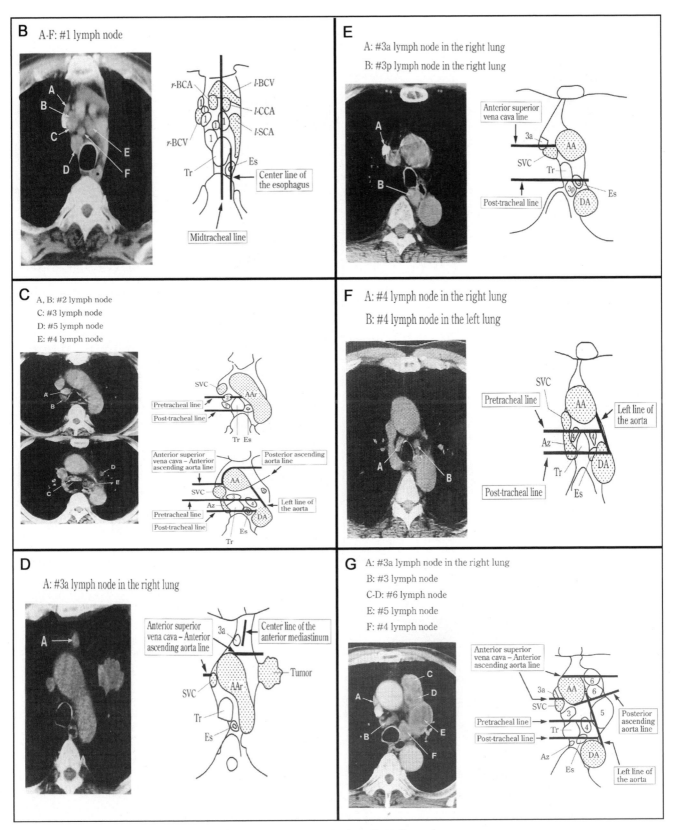

**B** A-F: #1 lymph node

**C** A, B: #2 lymph node
C: #3 lymph node
D: #5 lymph node
E: #4 lymph node

**D** A: #3a lymph node in the right lung

**E** A: #3a lymph node in the right lung
B: #3p lymph node in the right lung

**F** A: #4 lymph node in the right lung
B: #4 lymph node in the left lung

**G** A: #3a lymph node in the right lung
B: #3 lymph node
C-D: #6 lymph node
E: #5 lymph node
F: #4 lymph node

**FIGURE 16-6.** *(continued)*

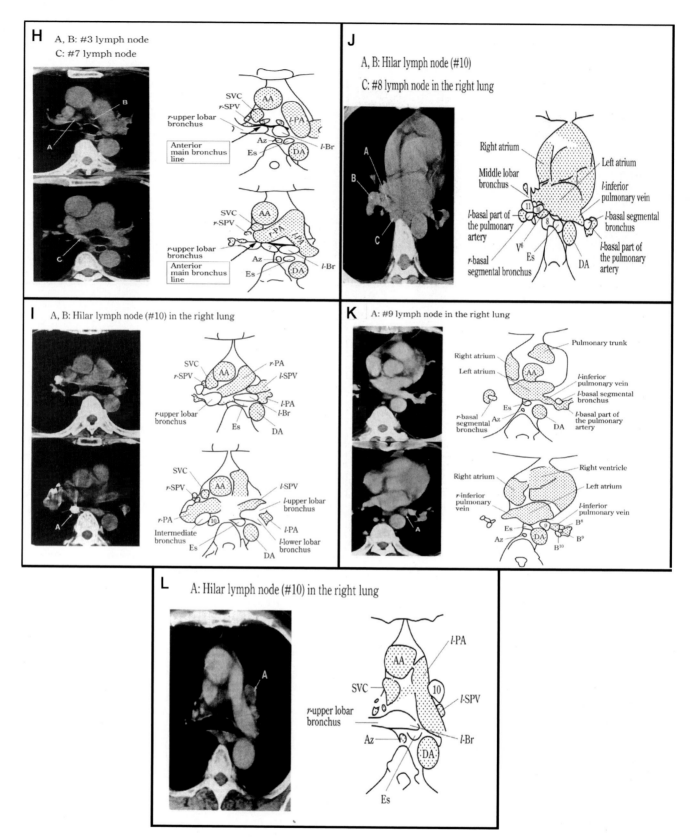

**FIGURE 16-6.** *(continued)*

■ However, 74% positive predictive value means that patients will need cervical mediastinoscopy when a mediastinal hot spot is found on PET.[15]

## 3.4. Staging

■ The American Joint Committee on Cancer (AJCC) staging system for lung cancer is shown in Table 16-2.

■ The location of the lymph nodes within the mediastinum has been described according to the modified 1997 American Thoracic Society's definition (ATS map), which defines the nodal stations in relation to fixed anatomical structures, allowing a correlation between CT and MRI imaging procedures and surgical findings.[16]

■ The anatomical structures concerned are the trachea, bronchi, aortic arch, and other vascular structures (Figure 16-7).

### TABLE 16-2. TNM CLASSIFICATION AND STAGING FOR LUNG CANCER

**Primary Tumor (T)**

| | |
|---|---|
| TX | Primary tumor cannot be assessed, or tumor progression proven by presence of malignant cells in sputum or bronchial washings but not visualized by imaging or bronchoscopy |
| T0 | No evidence of primary tumor |
| Tis | Carcinoma in situ |
| T1 | Tumor ≤3 cm in greatest dimension, surrounded by lung or visceral pleura, without bronchoscopic evidence of invasion more proximal than the lobar bronchus |
| T2 | Tumor with any of the following features of size or extent:<br>>3 cm in greatest dimension<br>Involves main bronchus, ≥2 cm distal to carina<br>Invades visceral pleura<br>Associated with atelectasis or obstructive pneumonitis that extends to hilar region but does not involve entire lung |
| T3 | Tumor of any size that directly invades any of the following: chest wall (including superior sulcus tumors), diaphragm, mediastinal pleura, parietal pericardium; or tumor in the main bronchus <2 cm distal to carina but without involvement of the carina; or associated atelectasis or obstructive pneumonitis of entire lung |
| T4 | Tumor of any size that invades any of the following: mediastinum, heart, great vessels, trachea, esophagus, vertebral body, carina; or separate tumor nodules in the same lobe; or tumor with malignant pleural effusion |

**Regional Lymph Nodes (N)**

| | |
|---|---|
| NX | Regional lymph nodes cannot be assessed |
| N0 | No regional lymph node metastasis |
| N1 | Metastasis to ipsilateral peribronchial and/or ipsilateral hilar lymph nodes, and intrapulmonary nodes including involvement by direct extension of primary tumor |
| N2 | Metastasis to ipsilateral mediastinal and/or subcarinal lymph node(s) |
| N3 | Metastasis to contralateral mediastinal, contralateral hilar, ipsilateral or contralateral scalene, or supraclavicular lymph node(s) |

**Distant Metastasis (M)**

| | |
|---|---|
| MX | Distant metastasis cannot be assessed |
| M0 | No distant metastasis |
| M1 | Distant metastasis present |

**Stage Grouping**

| | | | |
|---|---|---|---|
| Occult Carcinoma | TX | N0 | M0 |
| Stage 0 | Tis | N0 | M0 |
| Stage IA | T1 | N0 | M0 |
| Stage IB | T2 | N0 | M0 |
| Stage IIA | T1 | N1 | M0 |
| Stage IIB | T2 | N1 | M0 |
| | T3 | N0 | M0 |
| Stage IIIA | T1 | N2 | M0 |
| | T2 | N2 | M0 |
| | T3 | N1–2 | M0 |
| Stage IIIB | Any T | N3 | M0 |
| | T4 | Any N | M0 |
| Stage IV | Any T | Any N | M1 |

From: Greene FL, American Joint Committee on Cancer, American Cancer Society. *AJCC Cancer Staging Manual, 6th ed.* New York: Springer; 2002.

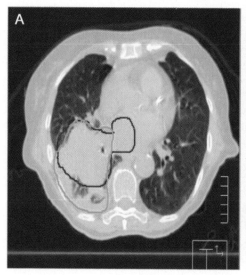
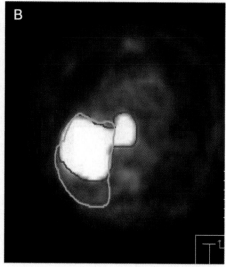

**FIGURE 16-7.** Impact of PET on determination of lung target volumes. GTV was outlined in green on the CT (**A**), which included atelectasis and a small amount of pleural effusion without delineation of the mediastinal node. PET (**B**) showed increased FDG uptake in the mediastinal node outlined in red, which was not delineated on CT. GTV was reduced in the parenchyma excluding atelectasis and post-atelectatic pleural effusion on the PET scan.

## 3.5. Detection of Nodal Metastasis

- Mediastinoscopy is a useful tool for assessing mediastinal lymph node involvement.
- A 4-cm incision is made above the sternal notch. After division of the pretracheal fascia, the trachea is exposed and serves as a guide for further finger dissection and endoscopic exploration.
- The superior mediastinal lymph node (station 2), the upper paratracheal (station 2), the lower paratracheal lymph node (station 4), and the anterior portion of the subcarinal lymph node (station 7) should be identified.
- For left upper lobe lesions, the subaortic and para-aortic mediastinal nodes may require anterior mediastinotomy or an extended cervical mediastinoscopy.
- Video-assisted thoracotomy surgery (VATS) is a minimally invasive technique, but remains investigational for lung cancer.
- Asamura et al. analyzed involvement of the lymph nodes in 337 patients according to tumor size, histologic type, and location (Tables 16-3 to 16-7).[17] Eighty-eight patients (26.1%) had lymph node involvement: 32 (9.5%)

at N1, 55 (16.3%) at N2, and 1 patient at N3 lymph node involvement were found.

- According to this study, complete hilar and mediastinal lymph node dissection should be done routinely because of the relatively high prevalence of the lymph node involvement, especially with adenocarcinoma lesions 2 cm or larger in diameter.
- However, for squamous cell carcinomas, the rate of mediastinal lymph node involvement is very low if the tumor is less than 2 cm in diameter.

## 4. GENERAL MANAGEMENT

- If the disease is not medically operable or surgically resectable, patients are given combined treatment, such as chemotherapy followed by surgery with or without postoperative thoracic radiotherapy (TRT) or chemoradiotherapy.
- Radiation Therapy Oncology Group (RTOG) 73-01 has shown that dose escalation of TRT from 40 Gy in 4 weeks to 60 Gy in 6 weeks has reduced intrathoracic fail-

## TABLE 16-3. LYMPH NODE INVOLVEMENT ACCORDING TO TUMOR DIAMETER

| Tumor Diameter (cm) | Nodal Status | | | | |
|---|---|---|---|---|---|
| | N0 | N1 | N2 | N3 | Total |
| ≤2.0 | 140 (80.5) | 14 (8.0) | 20 (11.5) | 0 (0.0) | 174 (100) |
| >2.0 and ≤3.0 | 10 (66.9) | 18 (11.0) | 35 (21.5) | 1 (0.6) | 164 (100) |
| *Total* | 150 (73.9) | 32 (9.5) | 55 (16.3) | 1 (0.3) | 337 (100) |

Numbers in parentheses indicate percentage.
Statistically significant ($x^2$ test, p+0.028)
From: Asamura H, Nakayama H, Kondo H, et al. Lymph node involvement, recurrence, and prognosis in resected small, peripheral, non-small-cell lung carcinomas: are these carcinomas candidates for video-assisted lobectomy? *J Thorac Cardiovasc Surg* 1996;111:1125–1134.

**TABLE 16-4. LYMPH NODE INVOLVEMENT ACCORDING TO TUMOR HISTOLOGIC TYPE**

| Histologic Type | Nodal Status | | | | Total |
|---|---|---|---|---|---|
| | N0 | N1 | N2 | N3 | |
| Adenocarcinoma | 203 (72.5) | 28 (10.0) | 48 (17.1) | 1 (0.4) | 280 (100) |
| Squamous cell | 38 (86.3) | 1 (2.3) | 5 (11.4) | 0 | 44 (100) |
| Large cell | 7 (70.0) | 1 (10.0) | 2 (20.0) | 0 | 10 (100) |
| Adenosquamous | 1 (33.3) | 2 (66.7) | 0 | 0 | 3 (100) |
| Total | 249 (73.9) | 32 (9.5) | 55 (16.3) | 1 (0.3) | 337 (100) |

Numbers in parentheses indicate percentage.
From: Asamura H, Nakayama H, Kondo H, et al. Lymph node involvement, recurrence, and prognosis in resected small, peripheral, non-small-cell lung carcinomas: are these carcinomas candidates for video-assisted lobectomy? *J Thorac Cardiovasc Surg* 1996;111:1125–1134.

**TABLE 16-5. LYMPH NODE INVOLVEMENT OF 147 PATIENTS WITH TUMORS 2 CM OR LESS IN DIAMETER ACCORDING TO TUMOR HISTOLOGIC TYPE**

| Histologic Type | Nodal Status | | | Total |
|---|---|---|---|---|
| | N0 | N1 | N2 | |
| Adenocarcinoma | 120 (78.9) | 13 (8.6) | 19 (12.5) | 152 (100) |
| Squamous cell | 15 (93.7) | 0 (0.0) | 1 (6.3) | 16 (100) |
| Large cell | 5 (83.3) | 1 (16.7) | 0 (0.0) | 6 (100) |
| Adenosquamous | 0 | 0 | 0 | 3 (100) |
| Total | 140 (80.5) | 14 (8.0) | 20 (11.5) | 174 (100) |

Numbers in parentheses indicate percentage.
From: Asamura H, Nakayama H, Kondo H, et al. Lymph node involvement, recurrence, and prognosis in resected small, peripheral, non-small-cell lung carcinomas: are these carcinomas candidates for video-assisted lobectomy? *J Thorac Cardiovasc Surg* 1996;111:1125–1134.

**TABLE 16-6. LYMPH NODE INVOLVEMENT TO THE MEDIASTINUM ACCORDING TO TUMOR LOCATION**

| Location | Mediastinal Lymph Node Location | | | | | | | | | N2/3 |
|---|---|---|---|---|---|---|---|---|---|---|
| | No.1 | No.2 | No.3 | No.4 | No.5 | No.6 | No.7 | No.8 | No.9 | |
| RUL (122) | 5 (4.1) | 3 (2.5) | 17 (13.9) | 4 (3.3) | | | 2 (1.6) | | | 18 (14.8) |
| RML (31) | 2 (6.5) | 1 (3.2) | 5 (16.1) | | | | 5 (16.1) | | | 7 (22.6) |
| RLL (64) | 3 (4.7) | | 3 (4.7) | | | | 8 (12.5) | | 2 (3.1) | 11 (17.2) |
| LUL (83) | | 3 (3.6) | 2 (2.4) | 6 (7.2) | 5 (6.0) | 6 (7.2) | 4 (4.8) | | | 15 (18.1) |
| LLL (37) | | | | 1 (2.7) | 1 (2.7) | 1 (2.7) | 3 (8.1) | 1 (2.7) | 1 (2.7) | 5 (13.5) |

Numbers in parentheses indicate percentage.
RUL, right upper lobe; RML, right middle lobe; RLL, right lower lobe; LUL, left upper lobe; LLL, left lower lobe.
From: Asamura H, Nakayama H, Kondo H, et al. Lymph node involvement, recurrence, and prognosis in resected small, peripheral, non-small-cell lung carcinomas: are these carcinomas candidates for video-assisted lobectomy? *J Thorac Cardiovasc Surg* 1996;111:1125–1134.

**TABLE 16-7. LYMPH NODE INVOLVEMENT TO HILUM AND LUNG ACCORDING TO TUMOR LOCATION**

| Location | Hilar Intrapulmonary Lymph Node Location | | | | | |
| | No.10 | No.11 | No.12 | No.13 | No.14 | N1* |
| --- | --- | --- | --- | --- | --- | --- |
| RUL (122) | 5 (4.1) | 8 (6.6) | 9 (7.4) | 8 (6.6) | 3 (2.5) | 22 (18.0) |
| RML (31) | 3 (9.7) | 6 (19.4) | 3 (9.7) | 1 (3.2) | 1 (3.2) | 9 (29.0) |
| RLL (64) | 4 (6.3) | 9 (14.1) | 6 (9.4) | 4 (6.3) | 1 (1.6) | 24 (37.5) |
| LUL (83) | 7 (8.4) | 6 (7.2) | 11 (13.3) | 7 (8.4) | 4 (4.8) | 23 (27.7) |
| LLL (37) | 1 (2.7) | 2 (5.4) | 3 (8.1) | 2 (5.4) | 1 (2.7) | 6 (16.2) |

*Patients with both mediastinal and hilar/intrapulmonary metastases were included.
Numbers in parentheses indicate percentage.
RUL, right upper lobe; RML, right middle lobe; RLL, right lower lobe; LUL, left upper lobe; LLL, left lower lobe.
From: Asamura H, Nakayama H, Kondo H, et al. Lymph node involvement, recurrence, and prognosis in resected small, peripheral, non-small-cell lung carcinomas: are these carcinomas candidates for video-assisted lobectomy? *J Thorac Cardiovasc Surg* 1996;111:1125–1134.

ure from 52% to 33%. This intrathoracic improvement was seen in an improvement of the 3-year survival rate from 10% in those who had locally failed to 22% in those who had local control.[18]

- Ninety percent local control of non–small-cell lung cancer (NSCLC) is possible with TRT doses of 80 Gy,[19] provided accurate imaging of nodal metastasis, adequate delineation of the gross tumor volume (GTV), and tumor motion are taken into consideration.[20]

- When TRT is given to the primary tumor and nodal metastasis, toxicities to the surrounding normal tissues including the alveoli, esophagus, heart, and spinal cord, need to be considered.

- Three-dimensional conformal radiation therapy (3-DCRT) has improved the prediction and reduction of normal tissue toxicities in the past several years.[21–24]

- When aggressive hyperfractionated TRT and concurrent cisplatin and etoposide were used for patients with locally advanced NSCLC, the rate of acute grade 3 esophagitis was 60%.[25] The application of 3DCRT reduced this rate to 30%.[26]

## 5. 3D-CONFORMAL RADIATION THERAPY/INTENSITY-MODULATED RADIATION THERAPY FOR LUNG CANCER

### 5.1. Target Volume Determination

- Selection of nodal region(s) to be included in the target volume is determined by the location and presentation of primary tumor (see Section 1.3. Lymphatic Drainage).

- Radiological and anatomical boundaries of each nodal station are detailed below

  1. *Superior mediastinal lymph nodes/highest mediastinal lymph nodes.* Located in the area of the upper one-third of the intrathoracic trachea. The boundary level is from the upper margin of the subclavian artery or the apex to the crossing point of the upper margin of the left brachiocephalic vein and the midline of the trachea.

  2. *Paratracheal lymph nodes.* Located in the area between the superior mediastinal lymph nodes[27] and the tracheobronchial lymph nodes.[28] The paratracheal lymph nodes with primary tumor can be defined as ipsilateral lymph nodes, while paratracheal lymph nodes without primary tumor can be defined as contralateral lymph nodes.

  3. *Pretracheal lymph nodes.* Located in the area anterior to the trachea and inferior to the superior mediastinal lymph nodes.[27] On the right side, the boundary is limited to the posterior wall of the superior vena cava. On the left side, the boundary is limited to the posterior wall of the brachiocephalic vein.

  3a. *Anterior mediastinal lymph nodes.* On the right side, anterior mediastinal lymph nodes are located in the area anterior to the superior vena cava. On the left side, the boundary is limited to the line connecting the left brachiocephalic vein and the ascending aorta.

  3p. *Retrotracheal mediastinal lymph nodes/posterior mediastinal lymph nodes.* Located in the retrotracheal or posterior area of the trachea.

  4. *Tracheobronchial lymph nodes.* Located in the area superior to the carina. On the right side, tracheobronchial lymph nodes are located medial to the azygos vein. On the left side, the lymph nodes are located in the area surrounded by the medial wall of the aortic arch.

  5. *Subaortic lymph nodes/Botallo lymph nodes.* Located in the area adjacent to the ligamentum arteriosum (Botallo ligament). The boundary extends from the aortic arch to the left main-pulmonary artery.

  6. *Para-aortic lymph nodes.* Located along with ascending aorta and in the area of the lateral wall of the aortic arch. The posterior boundary is limited to the site of the vagal nerve.

7. *Subcarinal lymph nodes.* Located in the area below the carina where the trachea bifurcates to the two main bronchi.

8. *Paraesophageal lymph nodes.* Located below the subcarinal lymph nodes, and along the esophagus.

9. *Pulmonary ligament lymph nodes.* Located in the area of the posterior and the lower edge of the inferior pulmonary vein.

10. *Hilar lymph nodes.* Located around the right and left main bronchi.

11. *Interlobar lymph nodes.* Located between the lobar bronchi. On the right side, interlobar lymph nodes are subclassified into two groups.

11s. *Superior interlobar lymph nodes.* Located at the bifurcation of the middle and lower lobar bronchi.

11i. *Inferior interlobar lymph nodes.* Located at the bifurcation of the middle and lower lobar bronchi.

12. *Lobar lymph nodes.* Located in the area around the lobar branches, which are subclassified into three groups.

12u. *Upper lobar lymph nodes.*

12m. *Middle lobar lymph nodes.*

12l. *Lower lobar lymph nodes.*

13. *Segmental lymph nodes.* Located along the segmental branches

14. *Subsegmental lymph nodes.* Located along the subsegmental branches.

## 5.2. Target Volume Delineation

- Parenchymal lesions are better defined in the lung window of a CT image.
- However, in cases in which atelectasis is present, PET helps to delineate the GTV better than CT does alone (Figs. 16-6 and 16-8).

- PET/CT is especially effective in cases of mediastinal nodal metastasis and small parenchymal metastasis, as well as delineation of the GTV (Fig. 16-9).
- Superior sulcus tumors, which are located at the apex of the lung, can be delineated with MRI to define invasion into the neural foramen, brachial plexus, subclavian artery, or vertebral body (Fig. 16-10).
- Addressing the extension of subclinical disease (clinical target volume, or CTV), Giraud and colleagues analyzed microscopic extensions of resected adenocarcinoma and squamous NSCLC. Margins of 8 mm for adenocarcinoma and 6 mm for squamous carcinoma encompassed 95% of microscopic extensions.[29]
- At M. D. Anderson Cancer Center, GTV is defined as any visible gross disease and/or lymph nodes ≥1 cm on CT.
- The CTV is defined as the GTV plus a 6-mm margin for squamous cell carcinoma or an 8-mm margin for adenocarcinoma.
- The PTV is defined as the CTV plus an 8- to 12-mm margin to account for tumor motion and setup uncertainty.
- A 5-mm margin is also added to account for the beam penumbrae if cerrobend blocks are used.
- Because tumors can move up to 8.3 mm, we use a respiration-gating technique for patients who can cooperate and who are receiving treatment with a curative intent.
- Respiration gating (respiration motion effect), accurate setup, and immobilization can reduce the PTV. As Figure 16-11 shows, the tumor moves when the patient breathes. We observed 22 patients who had inoperable lung cancer in various lobes of the lung and had tumors of various sizes. We found no significant differences in the margin of PTV related to tumor size, tumor location, or pulmonary function test results.[30]

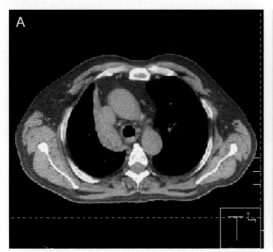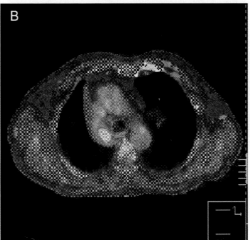

**FIGURE 16-8.** PET assists in differentiation of atelectasis from tumor. A tumor in the right upper bronchus causing collapse of the right upper lobe. CT (**A**) was unable to differentiate the GTV from atelectasis. PET (**B**) shows increased FDG uptake by the tumor. GTV is outlined in *red*, excluding atelectasis.

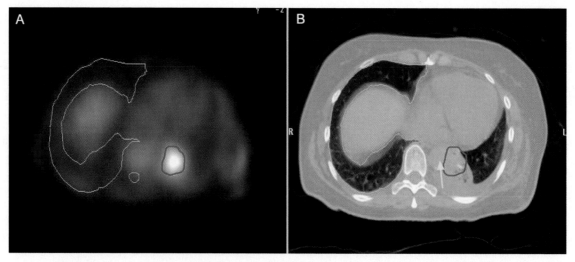

**FIGURE 16-9.** Delineation of GTV by CT vs. PET. **A:** PET shows increased uptake in the CTV outlined in *red*. **B:** CT shows collapse of the left lower lobe (*arrow*) without obvious delineation of the GTV.

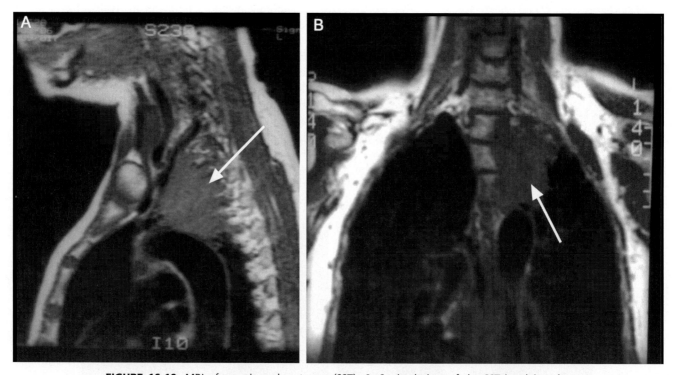

**FIGURE 16-10.** MRI of superior sulcus tumor (SST). **A:** Sagittal view of the SST involving the brachial plexus and vertebral bodies and abutting onto the posterior wall of the subclavian artery and aortic arch. **B:** Coronal view of left SST extending to the vertebral bodies (T1-T4) and aortic arch.

---

*See Chapter 5 for additional discussions on PET for lung cancer.

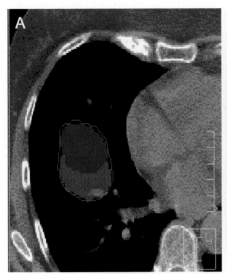
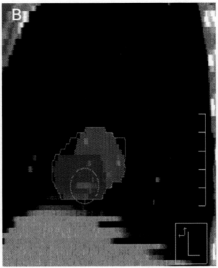
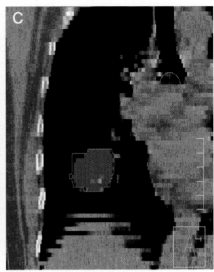

**FIGURE 16-11.** Tumor motion and respiratory gating. **A:** Anterior and posterior tumor (GTV) motion caused by respiration. **B:** Superior and inferior tumor motion with oblique shift caused by respiration. **C:** Elimination of GTV motion with respiratory gating.

## 5.3. Suggested Target and Normal Tissue Doses

- The planning objectives for the IMRT plans reflect the following priorities

  □ Achieve tumor-dose coverage at the prescription dose.
  □ Maintain the maximum dose of the planning spinal cord less than or equal to 45 Gy.
  □ Limit the V20 less than 40% of total lung volume for patients receiving RT alone.
  □ Limit the V20 less than 35% for patients receiving chemoradiation alone.
  □ Limit the V20 less than 20% when chemoradiation followed by surgery is planned. Patients receiving concurrent chemotherapy and radiation therapy followed by surgery had a significantly higher pulmonary complication rate when the total lung volume receiving 10 Gy (V10) exceeded 40%.[31]
  □ Limit the volume of the planning heart receiving 50 Gy (V50) less than 50%.
  □ Limit the length of esophagus to less than 16 cm receiving 60 Gy.

## 5.4. Lung 3DCRT and IMRT Results

- The application of IMRT for lung cancer has been delayed because of the large volume that may be irradiated at lower doses (<V20), potentially causing more profound lung complications.
- Murshed et al. retrospectively analyzed 41 lung cancer cases and found that IMRT may be more suitable than 3D treatment planning for cases of advanced-stage disease with a larger GTV and thus a greater volume of normal lung involvement.[32]
- Using IMRT, the median absolute reduction in the percentage of lung volume irradiated above 10 and 20 Gy was 7% and 10%, respectively. This corresponded with decreases of more than 2 Gy in the mean total lung dose and 10% in the risk of radiation pneumonitis.
- The volumes of the heart and esophagus irradiated above 40–50 Gy and normal thoracic tissue irradiated above 10–40 Gy were reduced using the IMRT plans.
- Significant improvement in the conformity was observed. Both the median value and range of the conformity index (CI) decreased with IMRT, indicating a greater ability to warp high-dose volumes around tumors by introducing intensity modulation within the beams (Table 16-8 and Fig. 16-12).
- To determine whether IMRT could be used to reduce the lung volume treated above low doses (such as 10–20 Gy), various dosimetric and radiobiological indices, including the V5, V10, V20, mean and integral dose, and normal tissue complication probability (NTCP) models were used to compare the isodose distributions of IMRT and 3DCRT plans.
- Figures 16-13 and 16-14 show the advantage of using IMRT to reduce the lung V10 and V20, with a median reduction of 7% and 10%, respectively. When the mean and integral dose delivered to the lung were used for the comparison, we saw a median reduction of 2 Gy and 2.8 J, respectively, for normal lung tissue (Fig. 16-15).
- To comprehend the effect of lung irradiation using IMRT, we must use different sets of NTCP parameters to estimate the risk of radiation pneumonitis (Table 16-9).

**TABLE 16-8. SUMMARY OF THE CI, HI, AND NUMBER OF MUS FOR THE 3DCRT AND IMRT PLANS**

| Parameters | 3DCRT Median (Range) | IMRT Median (Range) | *p* Value |
|---|---|---|---|
| Conformity index | 1.54 (1.26–4.53) | 1.41 (1.06–2.09) | 0.0039 |
| Heterogeneity index | 1.12 (1.06–1.22) | 1.16 (1.06–1.43) | 0.0004 |
| Minimum PTV dose (Gy) | 56.5 (38.4–62.0) | 55.8 (44.4–64.0) | 0.06 |
| Monitor units (sliding window) | 266 (166–991) | 1884 (95–3,838) | <0.0001 |

CI, conformity index; HI, heterogeneity index; MU, monitor unit.
From: Murshed H, Liu HH, Liao Z, et al. Dose and volume reduction for normal lung using intensity-modulated radiotherapy for advanced-stage non-small-cell lung cancer. *Int J Radiat Oncol Biol Phys* 2004;58:1258–1267.

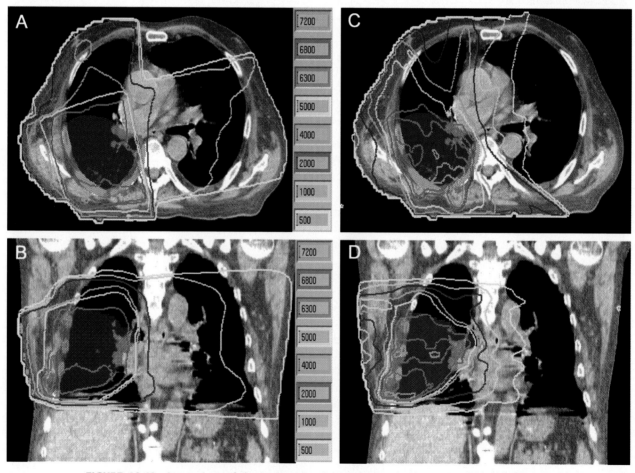

**FIGURE 16-12.** Comparison of the isodose distribution between 3DCRT (*left panel*: **A, B**) and IMRT (*right panel*: **C, D**) in a single case. **A, C:** Axial view. **B, D:** Coronal view. (From: Murshed H, Liu HH, Liao Z, et al. Dose and volume reduction for normal lung using intensity-modulated radiotherapy for advanced-stage non-small-cell lung cancer. *Int J Radiat Oncol Biol Phys* 2004;58:1258–1267.)

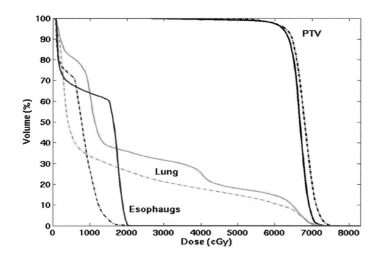

**FIGURE 16-13.** Comparison of DVHs of the PTV, total lung, and esophagus between 3DCRT (*solid lines*) and IMRT (*dashed lines*). (From: Murshed H, Liu HH, Liao Z, et al. Dose and volume reduction for normal lung using intensity-modulated radiotherapy for advanced-stage non-small-cell lung cancer. *Int J Radiat Oncol Biol Phys* 2004;58:1258–1267.)

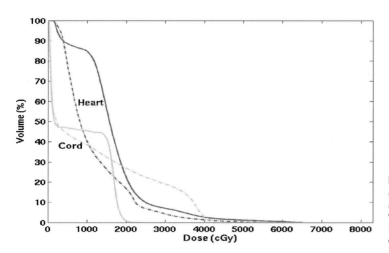

**FIGURE 16-14.** Comparison of DVHs of the spinal cord and heart between 3DCRT (*solid lines*) and IMRT (*dashed lines*). (From: Murshed H, Liu HH, Liao Z, et al. Dose and volume reduction for normal lung using intensity-modulated radiotherapy for advanced-stage non-small-cell lung cancer. *Int J Radiat Oncol Biol Phys* 2004;58:1258–1267.)

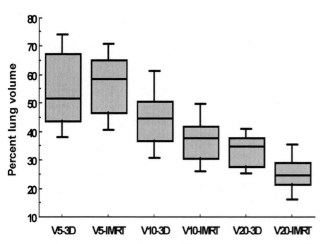

**FIGURE 16-15.** Summary of the total lung V5, V10, and V20 with the 3DCRT and IMRT plans. (From: Murshed H, Liu HH, Liao Z, et al. Dose and volume reduction for normal lung using intensity-modulated radiotherapy for advanced-stage non-small-cell lung cancer. *Int J Radiat Oncol Biol Phys* 2004;58:1258–1267.)

The reduction in the risk of pneumonitis ranged from 3% with Kwa's model[33] to 6% using Hayman's[34] and Yorke's[35] models, and 12% using Graham's model.[22]

- The esophagus and heart volumes above 55 Gy did not increase with the use of IMRT. Because acute esophagitis and long-term cardiac toxicity are limiting factors in the treatment of lung cancer, dose reduction for these structures should benefit this treatment as well (Table 16-10).

- As far as all thoracic tissues are concerned, the V20 and higher dose volumes were all reduced with IMRT. However, the V5 of the thorax increased, possibly because of the MLC leakage with the increased MUs of the IMRT (Tables 16-8 and 16-11).

- Step-and-shoot leaf sequence reduced the monitor units by half compared with the sliding window technique and may help to reduce the lung and normal tissue volumes at very low doses.

### TABLE 16-9. SUMMARY OF THE RISK OF RADIATION PNEUMONITIS AS ESTIMATED BASED ON VARIOUS PARAMETERS

| Parameters | Median RP Risk (Range) 3DCRT | IMRT | *p* Value |
|---|---|---|---|
| V20 (Graham et al.1999[22]) | 20 (2–65) | 6 (1–37) | N/A |
| Total lung mean dose (Yorke et al. 2002[35]) | 22 (4–72) | 16 (4–62) | N/A |
| Total lung mean dose (Kwa et al. 1998[33]) | 12 (1–45) | 9 (1–38) | N/A |
| NTCP (Burman et al. 1991[37]) | 36 (0–90) | 9 (0–82) | <0.0001 |
| NTCP (Emami et al. 1991[38]) | 13 (2–34) | 7 (1–27) | <0.0001 |

RP, radiation pneumonitis; N/A, not performed.
From: Murshed H, Liu HH, Liao Z, et al. Dose and volume reduction for normal lung using intensity-modulated radiotherapy for advanced-stage non-small-cell lung cancer. *Int J Radiat Oncol Biol Phys* 2004;58:1258–1267.

### TABLE 16-10. SUMMARY OF ESOPHAGUS, HEART, AND SPINAL CORD VOLUMES IRRADIATED AT TD 5/5 DOSE LEVELS

| Parameters | Median (Range) 3DCRT | IMRT | *p* Value |
|---|---|---|---|
| Esophagus (% cc at 55 Gy) | 35 (0–72) | 28.82 (0.00–71.00) | <0.0001 |
| Heart (% cc at 40 Gy) | 13 (0–58) | 11 (0–59) | 0.0036 |
| Spinal cord (% cc at 45 Gy) | 0.010 (0.00–33.00) | 0.900 (0.00–31.00) | 0.0261 |
| Spinal cord (% cc at 50 Gy) | 0 (0.00–4.28) | 0 (0.00–9.00) | 0.5228 |
| Spinal cord (maximum dose Gy) | 45.8 (10.6–55.4) | 48.6 (38.6–63.2) | 0.0002 |

From: Murshed H, Liu HH, Liao Z, et al. Dose and volume reduction for normal lung using intensity-modulated radiotherapy for advanced-stage non-small-cell lung cancer. *Int J Radiat Oncol Biol Phys* 2004;58:1258–1267.

### TABLE 16-11. SUMMARY OF NORMAL THORACIC TISSUE V5, V10, V20, V30, V40, AND INTEGRAL DOSE

| Parameters | Median (Range) 3DCRT | IMRT | *p* Value |
|---|---|---|---|
| V5 (cc) | 5,658 (3,040.3–11,596.0) | 6,929 (2,759–10,788) | 0.0064 |
| V10 (cc) | 4,905 (2,550–8,751) | 4,931 (2,066–8,722) | 0.6362 |
| V20 (cc) | 3,919 (1,919–6,776) | 3,398 (1,509–6,535) | 0.0014 |
| V30 (cc) | 3,212 (1,560–5,489) | 2,673 (1,242–5,402) | <0.0001 |
| V40 (cc) | 3,213 (1,560–5,489) | 2,673 (1,242–5,402) | <0.0001 |
| Integral dose | 180.46 (87.97–311.92) | 185.71 (72.32–13,511.00) | 0.7805 |

From: Murshed H, Liu HH, Liao Z, et al. Dose and volume reduction for normal lung using intensity-modulated radiotherapy for advanced-stage non-small-cell lung cancer. *Int J Radiat Oncol Biol Phys* 2004;58:1258–1267.

- We are now investigating IMRT applications for lung cancer patients to reduce the volume of V20, V15 and V10 with adequate immobilization techniques that could make IMRT more applicable to patients with compromised lung function.
- Our current results are limited to the treatment planning study without fully accounting for the tumor motion and its effect on the accuracy of the IMRT dosimetry.
- For IMRT to be feasible and more effective in treating the NSCLC, motion reduction techniques should be explored further, such as those relying on respiratory gating, breath holding, and tumor tracking.

## REFERENCES

1. Boyden EA. *Segmental anatomy of the lungs: a study of the patterns of the segmental bronchi and related pulmonary vessels.* New York: McGraw-Hill, 1955.
2. Gray H. *Gray's Anatomy: the Anatomical Basis of Medicine and Surgery, 38th ed.* New York: Churchill Livingstone, 1995.
3. Greene FL, American Joint Committee on Cancer, American Cancer Society. *AJCC Cancer Staging Manual, 6th ed.* Philadelphia: Lippincott-Raven-1997.
4. Nagaishi C. *Functional Anatomy and Histology of the Lung.* Baltimore: University Park Press, 1972.
5. Borri J. Primary carcinoma of the bronchus: prognoses following surgical resection (Hunterian lecture). *Ann Royal Coll Surg Engl* 1952;10:165–186.
6. Jemal A, Tiwari RC, Murray T, et al. Cancer statistics, 2004. *CA Cancer J Clin* 2004;54:8–29.
7. Hanson J, Armstrong P. Radiological evaluation of intrathoracic extension and respectibility of non-small cell lung cancer. In: Van Houtte P, Klastersky J, Rocmans P, eds. *Progress and Perspectives in Lung Cancer.* Berlin Heidelberg; New York: Springer, 1999: 23–38.
8. Glazer GM, Gross BH, Quint LE, et al. Normal mediastinal lymph nodes: number and size according to American Thoracic Society mapping. *AJR Am J Roentgenol* 1985;144:261–265.
9. McLoud TC, Bourgouin PM, Greenberg RW, et al. Bronchogenic carcinoma: analysis of staging in the mediastinum with CT by correlative lymph node mapping and sampling. *Radiology* 1992;182:319–323.
10. Buy JN, Ghossain MA, Poirson F, et al. Computed tomography of mediastinal lymph nodes in nonsmall cell lung cancer. A new approach based on the lymphatic pathway of tumor spread. *J Comput Assist Tomogr* 1988;12:545–552.
11. Vansteenkiste JF, Stroobants SG, De Leyn PR, et al. Lymph node staging in non-small-cell lung cancer with FDG-PET scan: a prospective study on 690 lymph node stations from 68 patients. *J Clin Oncol* 1998;16:2142–2149.
12. Steinert HC, Hauser M, Allemann F, et al. Non-small cell lung cancer: nodal staging with FDG PET versus CT with correlative lymph node mapping and sampling. *Radiology* 1997;202:441–446.
13. Chin R, Jr., Ward R, Keyes JW, et al. Mediastinal staging of non-small-cell lung cancer with positron emission tomography. *Am J Respir Crit Care Med* 1995;152:2090–2096.
14. Vansteenkiste JF, Stroobants SG, Dupont PJ, et al. FDG-PET scan in potentially operable non-small cell lung cancer: do anatometabolic PET-CT fusion images improve the localisation of regional lymph node metastases? The Leuven Lung Cancer Group. *Eur J Nucl Med* 1998;25:1495–1501.
15. Lewis PJ, Salama A. Uptake of fluorine-18-fluorodeoxyglucose in sarcoidosis. *J Nucl Med* 1994;35:1647–1649.
16. Mountain CF, Dresler CM. Regional lymph node classification for lung cancer staging. *Chest* 1997;111:1718–1723.
17. Asamura H, Nakayama H, Kondo H, et al. Lymph node involvement, recurrence, and prognosis in resected small, peripheral, non-small-cell lung carcinoma: are these carcinomas candidates for video-assisted lobectomy? *J Thorac Cardiovasc Surg* 1996;111:1125–1134.
18. Perez CA, Bauer M, Edelstein S, et al. Impact of tumor control on survival in carcinoma of the lung treated with irradiation. *Int J Radiat Oncol Biol Phys* 1986;12:539–547.
19. Vijayakumar S, Myrianthopoulos LC, Rosenberg I, et al. Optimization of radical radiotherapy with beam's eye view techniques for non-small cell lung cancer. *Int J Radiat Oncol Biol Phys* 1991;21:779–788.
20. Komaki R, Liao Z, Forster K, et al. Target definition and contouring in carcinoma of the lung and esophagus. *Rays* 2003;28: 225–236.
21. Socinski MA, Rosenman JG, Halle J, et al. Dose-escalating conformal thoracic radiation therapy with induction and concurrent carboplatin/paclitaxel in unresectable stage IIIA/B nonsmall cell lung carcinoma: a modified phase I/II trial. *Cancer* 2001;92: 1213–1223.
22. Graham MV, Purdy JA, Emami B, et al. Clinical dose-volume histogram analysis for pneumonitis after 3D treatment for non-small cell lung cancer (NSCLC). *Int J Radiat Oncol Biol Phys* 1999;45:323–329.
23. Sibley GS, Mundt AJ, Shapiro C, et al. The treatment of stage III nonsmall cell lung cancer using high dose conformal radiotherapy. *Int J Radiat Oncol Biol Phys* 1995;33:1001–1007.
24. Armstrong J, Raben A, Zelefsky M, et al. Promising survival with three-dimensional conformal radiation therapy for non-small cell lung cancer. *Radiother Oncol* 1997;44:17–22.
25. Komaki R, Lee JS, Kaplan B, et al. Randomized phase III study of chemoradiation with or without amifostine for patients with favorable performance status inoperable stage II–III non-small cell lung cancer: preliminary results. *Semin Radiat Oncol* 2002;12:46–49.
26. Komaki R, Lee J, Milas L, et al. Effects of amifostine on acute toxicity from concurrent chemotherapy and radiation therapy for inoperable non-small cell lung cancer: report of a randomized comparative trial. *Int J Radiat Oncol Biol Phys* 2004;58: 1369–1377.
27. VanHoutte P, Mornex F, Rocmans P, et al. Lung cancer. In: *Clinical Target Volumes in conformal and Intensity Modulated Radiation Therapy: A clinical guide to cancer treatment* Gregoire V. Scalliet P, Ang KK, etds., Berlin Springer-Verlag; 2002;91–106.
28. Hata E. Hayakawa K, Miyamoto H, et al. Rationale for extended lymphadenectomy for lung cancer. *Theor Surg* 1990;5:19–27.
29. Giraud P, Antoine M, Larrouy A, et al. Evaluation of microscopic tumor extension in non-small-cell lung cancer for three-dimensional conformal radiotherapy planning. *Int J Radiat Oncol Biol Phys* 2000;48:1015–1024.
30. Stevens CW, Munden RF, Forster KM, et al. Respiratory-driven lung tumor motion is independent of tumor size, tumor location, and pulmonary function. *Int J Radiat Oncol Biol Phys* 2001;51: 62–68.
31. Lee HK, Vaporciyan AA, Cox JD, et al. Postoperative pulmonary complications after preoperative chemoradiation for esophageal carcinoma: correlation with pulmonary dose-volume histogram parameters. *Int J Radiat Oncol Biol Phys* 2003;57: 1317–1322.
32. Murshed H, Liu HH, Liao Z, et al. Dose and volume reduction for normal lung using intensity-modulated radiotherapy for advanced-stage non-small-cell lung cancer. *Int J Radiat Oncol Biol Phys* 2004;58:1258–1267.

33. Kwa SL, Lebesque JV, Theuws JC, et al. Radiation pneumonitis as a function of mean lung dose: an analysis of pooled data of 540 patients. *Int J Radiat Oncol Biol Phys* 1998;42:1–9.
34. Hayman JA, Martel MK, Ten Haken RK, et al. Dose escalation in non-small-cell lung cancer using three-dimensional conformal radiation therapy: update of a phase I trial. *J Clin Oncol* 2001;19:127–136.
35. Yorke ED, Jackson A, Rosenzweig KE, et al. Dose-volume factors contributing to the incidence of radiation pneumonitis in non-small-cell lung cancer patients treated with three-dimensional conformal radiation therapy. *Int J Radiat Oncol Biol Phys* 2002;54:329–339.
36. Line DH, Deeley TJ. The necropsy findings in carcinoma of the bronchus. *Br J Dis Chest* 1971;65:238–242.
37. Burman C, Kutcher GJ, Emami B, et al. Fitting of normal tissue tolerance data to an analytic function. *Int J Radiat Oncol Biol Phys* 1991;21:123–135.
38. Emami B, Lyman J, Brown A, et al. Tolerance of normal tissue to therapeutic irradiation. *Int J Radiat Oncol Biol Phys* 1991;21:109–122.
39. Hata E, Hayakawa K, Miyamoto H, et al. Rationale for extended lymphadenectomy for lung cancer. *Theor Surg* 1990;5:19–27.

## APPENDIX

## Boundaries and Groups of Mediastinal Lymph Nodes

1. *Superior (highest) lymph nodes in the upper mediastinum.* Lymph nodes from the apex of the lung to the level of the intersection of the left brachiocephalic vein and midtracheal line including the slice containing the intersection (Figs. 16-7A, B).
2. *Paratracheal lymph nodes.* Lymph nodes caudal to 1 and cephalad to the azygos arch with the center of the node located between the pretracheal line and the retrotracheal line, excluding the slice containing the intersection of the left brachiocephalic vein, midtracheal line, and the azygos arch (Figs. 16-7A, C).
3. *Anterior mediastinal lymph nodes.* Lymph nodes caudal to 1 with the center of the node located anterior to the line from the superior vena cava to the anterior wall of the ascending aorta (Figs. 16-7A, D, E, and G).
3a. *Paratracheal lymph nodes.* Lymph nodes caudal to 1 and cephalad to the right main pulmonary artery with the center of the node located anterior to the paratracheal line or posterior to the line of the anterior wall of the superior vena cava and to the right of the left margin of the aorta (Figs. 16-7A, C, G, and H). Lymph nodes located superior to the aortic arch and on the left of the left subclavian artery and left common carotid artery should be classified as 6, if these nodes are contiguous to 6.
3b. *Retrotracheal lymph nodes.* Lymph nodes caudal to 1 and cephalad to the carina with the center of the node located posterior to the retrotracheal line, excluding the nodes on the slice showing bilateral main stem bronchi (Figs. 16-7A, E).
4. *Tracheobronchial lymph nodes.* Lymph nodes caudal to the azygos vein including the slice level showing the azygos vein. The center of the node is located between pretracheal and retrotracheal lines. Lymph nodes are located on the right of the left margin line of the aorta and in contact with the trachea on the left of the azygos arch (Figs. 16-7A, C, F, and G). The center of the node is located in the region of the left 4, but the nodes that clearly separate from the trachea should be classified as 5.
5. *Subaortic lymph nodes.* Lymph nodes between the aortic arch and the left main pulmonary artery. The center of the node is located on the left of the left margin of aorta and posterior to the posterior wall of the ascending aorta (Figs. 16-7A, C, and G).
6. *Paraortic lymph nodes.* Lymph nodes located on the left of the ascending aorta and aortic arch. The center of the node is posterior to the anterior wall line of the ascending aorta. In the region where the posterior wall of the ascending aorta is illustrated, lymph nodes are located anterior to the posterior wall line of the ascending aorta (Figs. 16-7A, G).
7. *Subcarinal lymph nodes.* Lymph nodes in contact with the subcarina. The center of the node is located posterior to the anterior wall line of the main stem bronchi (Figs. 16-7A, H). Lymph nodes in contact with the mediastinal side of the bilateral main stem bronchi or truncus intermedius, and the nodes which are not contiguous to the subcarina are classified as 10.
8. *Paraesophageal lymph nodes.* Lymph nodes caudal to the carina (on the slice showing bilateral main stem bronchi separately) in contact with the esophagus, but apart from the bronchi (Figs. 16-7A, J).
9. *Pulmonary ligament lymph nodes.* Lymph nodes located caudal to the interior pulmonary veins (Figs. 16-7A, K).

Note 1: If it is difficult to determine the station number of the mediastinal lymph nodes on CT images, the smaller number should be recorded.

Note 2: The border of the right and left sides should be determined according to the following line.

　1: SNL Midtracheal line.

　3a: SNL Center line of the anterior mediastinum.

　3 and 8: SNL Center line of the esophagus.

Note 3: The lymph node group close to the left side of the left main pulmonary artery should be recorded as 10(*l*).

# 17

# MESOTHELIOMA

**CRAIG W. STEVENS**
**KENNETH M. FORSTER**
**W. ROY SMYTHE**

## 1. ANATOMY

- Mesothelioma arises from the mesothelial lining of the pleural cavity. It can arise either from the visceral or parietal pleura.
- The pleural space is bounded anteriorly, posteriorly, laterally, and superiorly by the ribs/chest wall, medially by the mediastinum and heart, and inferiorly by the diaphragm.
- The inferior portion of the parietal pleura is intimately associated with the central tendon of the diaphragm.
- The pleural space extends into the intrapulmonary fissures.
- The pleural space extends into the costodiaphragmatic sulcus, which can extend posteriorly to the level of L4.
- The pleural space can also cross midline in the costomediastinal recess.
- The pleura is only a few cells thick at most, though much of the parietal mesothelium is adjacent to the endothoracic fascia. This structure can be a barrier to tumor invasion of the chest wall.
- Tumors of the pleural space can dramatically influence normal pleural anatomy. Occasionally, accumulation of pleural fluid can exert a positive pressure on the mediastinum and shift it towards the contralateral side. Other times, a thick rind of mesothelioma can encase the lung, resulting in volume loss and a mediastinal shift towards the involved side.

## 2. DIAGNOSIS AND STAGING SYSTEM

### 2.1. Signs and Symptoms

- Dyspnea, chest pain, cough, and weight loss are all common symptoms of malignant pleural mesothelioma (MPM).
- All patients should be queried about their history of asbestos exposure. This could include exposure during childhood by a parent that was an asbestos worker or environmental exposure. Even a history of living near asbestos-using businesses, such as automotive shops (from break linings) or cement manufacturers (which may have added asbestos), can increase the risk of mesothelioma.
- Tobacco use does not increase the risk of mesothelioma, although asbestos exposure can increase the risk of lung cancer.

### 2.2. Physical Examination

- All sites of previous instrumentation should be identified and examined for evidence of tumor seeding. This may manifest as pain, a nodule, or an ulcer.
- The axillary and supraclavicular lymph nodes should be palpated for possible involvement.
- Occasionally, new scoliosis can occur because of ipsilateral lung volume loss.

### 2.3. Imaging

#### 2.3.1. Chest x-ray

- Pleural effusion
- Irregular nodularity
- Lung volume loss
- Scoliosis

#### 2.3.2. Computed Tomography of the Chest

- Irregular pleural masses, particularly near the diaphragm
- Invasion of adjacent structures, such as the chest wall, mediastinum, great vessels, vertebral body, or heart
- Pleural effusions
- Nodularity within the fissures
- Mediastinal or hilar adenopathy
- Pericardial effusion
- The anterior-medial extent of tumor. In particular, extension across the midline needs to be determined before surgery. This can be quite problematic because surgery will obliterate the costomediastinal space, so it is not easily detected on postoperative studies
- Ascites, a poor prognostic sign

### 2.3.3. Magnetic Resonance Imaging

- The utility of MRI in the staging of mesothelioma is controversial.
- The extent of invasion can be better identified by MRI. This should not necessarily preclude surgery, as long as the region of invasion can be removed with a limited chest wall resection.
- Invasion of the diaphragm can be better appreciated on MRI because the scan time is much shorter than CT; however, invasion to the peritoneal surface of the diaphragm cannot always be appreciated without invasive staging.

### 2.3.4. $^{18}$FDG-PET

- Mesotheliomas tend to be quite FDG avid. Results can guide mediastinoscopy or identify extrathoracic sites of metastases. However, reimbursement may limit availability.

### 2.3.5. Invasive Staging

- *Mediastinoscopy:* at our institution, contralateral mediastinoscopy is only performed because we have achieved 100% local control even with pathologically involved ipsilateral mediastinal lymph nodes. At other institutions, ipsilateral mediastinal metastases preclude potentially curative surgery.

- *Laparoscopy:* all patients at our institution undergo laparoscopy at the time of mediastinoscopy. This study is positive in about 10% of patients that were otherwise negative for metastases, even by FDG-PET.

## 2.4. Staging

- The American Joint Committee on Cancer staging system for mesothelioma is shown in Table 17-1 and is based on the International Mesothelioma Interest Group (IMIG) staging system.[1]

## 3. PROGNOSTIC FACTORS

- *Performance status:* patients with minimal symptoms tend to do better than those with pronounced dyspnea, pain, or weight loss.
- *Stage:* primary tumor stage and involvement of hilar or mediastinal lymph nodes have a significant correlation with survival. Note that T3 includes any "technically resectable" tumors, which may vary somewhat between institutions.
- *Histology:* epithelioid histology has been shown to have a better outcome than sarcomatoid or mixed histology.
- *Thrombocytosis:* several studies have demonstrated that thrombocytosis predicts a poor outcome. This is con-

### TABLE 17-1. TNM CLASSIFICATION FOR MESOTHELIOMA

**Primary Tumor (T)**

| | |
|---|---|
| TX | Primary tumor cannot be assessed |
| T0 | No evidence of primary tumor |
| T1 | Tumor involves ipsilateral parietal pleura, with or without local involvement of visceral pleura |
| T1a | Tumor involves ipsilateral parietal (mediastinal, diaphragmatic) pleura. No involvement of the visceral pleura |
| T1b | Tumor involves ipsilateral parietal (mediastinal, diaphragmatic) pleura with focal involvement of the visceral pleura. |
| T2 | Tumor involves any of the ipsilateral pleural surfaces with at least one of the following:<br>-confluent visceral pleural tumor (including fissure)<br>-invasion of diaphragmatic muscle<br>-invasion of lung parenchyma |
| T3* | Tumor involves any of the ipsilateral pleural surfaces, with at least one of the following:<br>-invasion of the endothoracic fascia<br>-invasion into mediastinal fat<br>-solitary focus of tumor invading the soft tissues of the chest wall<br>-non-transmural involvement of the pericardium |
| T4† | Tumor involves any of the ipsilateral pleural surfaces, with at least one of the following:<br>-diffuse or multifocal invasion of soft tissues of the chest wall |

-any involvement of rib
-invasion through the diaphragm to the peritoneum
-invasion of any mediastinal organ(s)
-direct extension to the contralateral pleura
-invasion into the spine
-extension to the internal surface of the pericardium
-pericardial effusion with positive cytology
-invasion of the myocardium
-invasion of the brachial plexus

**Regional Lymph Nodes (N)**

| | |
|---|---|
| NX | Regional lymph nodes cannot be assessed |
| N0 | No regional lymph node metastases |
| N1 | Metastases in the ipsilateral bronchopulmonary and/or hilar lymph node(s) |
| N2 | Metastases in the subcarinal lymph node(s) and/or the ipsilateral internal mammary or mediastinal lymph node(s) |
| N3 | Metastases in the contralateral mediastinal, internal mammary, or hilar lymph node(s) and/or the ipsilateral or contralateral supraclavicular or scalene lymph node(s) |

**Distant Metastasis (M)**

| | |
|---|---|
| MX | Distant metastasis cannot be assessed |
| M0 | No distant metastasis |
| M1 | Distant metastasis |

*Describes locally advanced, but potentially resectable tumor.
†Describes locally advanced, technically unresectable tumor.
From: Rusch VW. A proposed new international TNM staging system for malignant pleural mesothelioma. From the International Mesothelioma Interest Group. *Chest* 1995;108:1122–1128.

**TABLE 17-2. RESULTS OF LARGE STUDIES COMBINING SURGERY WITH POSTOPERATIVE RADIOTHERAPY FOR MESOTHELIOMA**

| Study | Surgery | Number of Patients | RT Dose | Local Failure | Survival |
|---|---|---|---|---|---|
| Maasilta[16] | P | 34 | 55–70 Gy | 33% progression, remainder "stable" | Median 12 mo |
| Hilaris et al.[17] | P | 41 | 45 Gy + implant | 29/41 (71%) | Median 12.6 mo |
| Lee et al.[18] | P | 24 | Median 41.4 Gy 5–15 Gy IORT | "Most" | Median 18 mo |
| Baldini et al.[19] | EPP | 49 | 30.6 Gy ~ 20 Gy boost | 21/49 (43%) | 22 mo |
| Rusch et al.[20] | EPP | 55 | 54 Gy | 7/55 (13%) | Stage I-II:34 mo Stage III-IV: 10 mo |
| Ahamad et al.[11] | EPP | 28 | 45–50 Gy | 0 2 marginal misses | Not yet reached (2 yr–OS 62%) |
| Yajnik et al.[4] | EPP | 35 | 54 Gy | 13/35 (37%) | Not reported |

RT, radiation therapy; P, pleurectomy; EPP, extrapleural pneumonectomy; IORT, intra-operative radiation therapy.

sistent with the observation that MPMs, which produce platelet-derived growth factor, also have a poor prognosis.

- *Treatment related factors:* the completeness of surgical resection has been shown to predict survival.

## 4. GENERAL MANAGEMENT

- "Standard" therapy for MPM is quite varied and ranges from best supportive care to trimodality therapy with surgery, radiation, and chemotherapy.
- There have been no prospective randomized trials that demonstrate the superiority of one approach over another. There is a current registration trial in the UK to compare surgery/radiation with best supportive care.
- There have been problems with the reporting of locoregional failure, such that the true failure rate within the presurgical thoracic space (from the insertion of the diaphragm/crus to the thoracic inlet, and from the surgically violated chest wall to the anterior-medial pleural reflection) has not been described in great detail.
- We have noted that the insertion of the neodiaphragm at EPP averages 16.5 cm above the lowest surgical clips. This essentially "abdominalizes" a large portion of what was intrathoracic prior to EPP. Not irradiating this region will result in true local failure, which may be reported as an abdominal failure.

### 4.1. Surgery

- A biopsy is often required for diagnosis, particularly if pleural cytology is negative. Any site of thoracic instrumentation can potentially spread tumor. Surgical entry points and chest tube sites should be irradiated.

- Surgery alone has a very high incidence of locoregional thoracic failure, which has been reported as high as 80% in some series.
- In pleurectomy/decortication, the visceral and parietal pleura are removed. In some institutions, parts of the diaphragm and/or pericardium may be removed. Generally, gross involvement of the intrapleural fissures contraindicates pleurectomy except for symptom control. Pleurectomy/decortication followed by radiation also has a high incidence of local failure (Table 17-2), but it is much less than 80%.
- *Extrapleural pneumonectomy (EPP):* attempts to remove the entire pleural space intact, including the lung. The diaphragm and pericardium are also removed.
- *Potential problems:* surgery can often remove all visible disease; however, this is not usually sufficient for cure of MPM. The pleural space containing mesothelioma is only a few cells away from the endothoracic fascia adjacent to the parietal pleura. Thus, surgery alone is rarely curative, except in the rare circumstance of a well-circumscribed small tumor.

### 4.2. Chemotherapy

- The role of chemotherapy in MPM is not well defined. Active regimens include cisplatin/gemcitabine and cisplatin/pemetrexed. This latter combination has been shown to improve survival in unresected patients in a prospective randomized trial.
- The pattern of failure after EPP/irradiation is no longer primarily locoregional. This suggests that systemic treatment needs to be integrated into a combined approach. The regimen and timing are currently under investigation.
- Because of the high rates of locoregional control with EPP followed by radiation, concurrent chemoradiation will probably not be required.

- A recent prospective randomized trial suggested that pemetrexed-cisplatin chemotherapy can slightly improve survival compared with cisplatin monotherapy ($p = 0.02$).[2] This suggests that pemetrexed should be a component of future MPM trials.

## 4.3. Radiation Therapy

- MPMs are nearly impossible to cure with radiotherapy as a single modality. Because they are large tumors, large radiation doses and extensive target volume coverage are required. The target volumes should extend from the thoracic inlet to the insertion of the diaphragm and include the intrapulmonary fissures. These target volumes are very close to radiosensitive structures such as the lung, kidney, liver, esophagus, and heart. Thus, radiation therapy alone should be considered only for palliative treatment.

- Because surgical margins are rarely generous, some form of additional therapy is necessary to eliminate microscopic residual disease. Since mesothelioma cells are not particularly radioresistant, radiotherapy should be an effective adjuvant to surgery.

- EPP followed by radiation therapy has the best locoregional control, although it results in the greatest toxicity.

## 4.4. Conformal Radiotherapy (After Extrapleural Pneumonectomy)

- The 3D-conformal radiotherapy (3DCRT) approach has been described best in two reports from the Memorial Sloan-Kettering Cancer Center.[3,4] The technique applies AP/PA beam geometry to the hemithorax using roughly the volumes described above as CTV.

- For right-sided cases, an abdominal block is present throughout treatment to shield the liver, and the region is boosted with electrons (1.53 Gy per day, which accounts for scatter under the block).

- For left-sided cases, the kidney and heart are blocked. The kidney block is present throughout treatment, and the heart block is added after 19.8 Gy. The spinal cord is shielded after 41.4 Gy in all cases. The goal dose to the target volume was 54 Gy in 30 fractions, with the dose calculated at the mid-plane with equally weighted beams. Patients are treated with arms akimbo without other immobilization.

- Treatment by this simple approach results in good coverage of the vast majority of the volumes at risk to the target dose of 54 Gy. Doses seem very homogeneous within the regions at risk, although some regions such as the crus, the pericardium, and the neodiaphragm may be difficult to treat. The radiosensitive structures such as the liver and heart can be spared quite well. Protection of the ipsilateral kidney is clearly better than with IMRT (see below).

## 4.5. Palliation

- A radiation dose-response has been demonstrated in 29 courses of palliative external beam radiotherapy delivered to 17 patients with MPM.[5] Four of six patients treated with more than 40 Gy achieved significant relief of symptoms. Thoracic pain was better controlled than symptoms of superior vena cava (SVC) syndrome and dyspnea.

- In another study, 26 radiotherapy courses were reviewed for any symptomatic improvement.[6] Pain improved in 13 of 18 cases, but was similar irrespective of dose/fractionation (20 Gy/5 fx or 30 Gy/10 fx). Palliative treatment was also delivered for "mass", Pancoast complex, and SVC syndrome. Palliation was achieved approximately half the time in this heterogeneous patient group.

- At our institution, patients with good performance status receive palliative radiotherapy with 45 Gy in 15 fractions. This combines the benefit of a dose above 40 Gy with a relatively short treatment course. Although an outcome analysis of these patients has not yet been completed, anecdotal evidence suggests that the response may be similar to that achieved in non–small-cell lung cancer with this regimen.[7]

## 4.6. Prophylaxis

- Unlike most malignancies, MPM has a tendency to recur along tracks of previous chest wall instrumentation.[8]

- Boutin et al. randomized 40 consecutive patients with pathologically proven MPM to immediate prophylactic radiotherapy to each site of instrumentation or to observation.[9] Prophylactic treatment was given in three 7 Gy fractions for a total of 21 Gy. Treatment geometry was simple and generally used *en face* electron fields. Tissue equivalent bolus material overlaid each target to improve dose delivery to the skin. After a median follow-up of 6 months, there was no subcutaneous MPM progression in the irradiated patients, while such nodules developed in 8 of 20 (40%) of the untreated patients. In the unirradiated group, subcutaneous recurrence did not correlate with positive cytology, histologic type, disease stage, subsequent chemotherapy, or the size of the tracts. The authors concluded that since such recurrences are typically painful, short course prophylactic irradiation was an effective means of maintaining patient quality of life.

## 5. INTENSITY-MODULATED RADIATION THERAPY FOR MESOTHELIOMA

## 5.1. Target Volume Determination and Delineation (After Extrapleural Pneumonectomy)

- There is general consensus among authors that the ipsilateral mediastinum should be included in the target volume because of the high incidence of mediastinal involvement.[10–13] The superior border should be the thoracic inlet. The medial border should include the ipsilateral nodal regions, trachea and subcarinal regions, or should extend to the edge of the vertebral body.[4,10,11] While there may be paraesophageal lymph nodes posterior to the heart, our institution has not included this region in the target volume and has had no retrocardiac failures.

- All authors also include all sites of skin instrumentation, as has been previously described. These should be contoured to the skin, as should any regions of subcutaneous tissue disruption.[14] Typically, the skin incision does not directly overlie the regions where the ribs are entered. Since there is tunneling under the subcutaneous fat, the entire disturbed region should be irradiated; this often includes the subscapular tissues.

- Potential problem areas in the delineation of target volumes for MPM include

  □ *The anterior-medial pleural reflection:* the costomediastinal recess can be quite variable, and can even cross the midline. This anatomic relationship can be lost after surgery. When possible, this region is best identified by the placement of radiopaque clips intraoperatively. The medial extent of the pleura should be identified on preoperative CT scans, and this extent is estimated on the treatment planning CT. Failure to ac-

count for this variability led to one of the two marginal misses in our study.[11]

  □ *Variable inferior extent of the diaphragm:* the insertion of the diaphragm is quite variable, ranging from L1 to L4. Using a population-based estimate of the point of diaphragm insertion will result in the clinical target volume (CTV) being too large for some patients and too small for others. Because of this variability, the diaphragm insertion should ideally be marked either by intraoperative placement of radiopaque clips or by suturing the neodiaphragm at the point of insertion.[4,10,14] When the border of the intrathoracic and abdominal contents are well marked, the radiotherapy margins can be individualized and maximally reduced. Figure 17-1 shows two cases in which the lowest clips are at the bottom of L2 (note proximity of the rib, Fig. 17-1A) or at the bottom of L3 (no ribs, Fig. 17-1B). Note how the change in chest shape and the point of diaphragm reconstruction (higher in Fig. 17-1A) significantly affect the proximity of the target volumes to organs at risk. Use of a radiopaque neodiaphragm helps to differentiate thoracic fluid from liver (Fig. 17-2).

  □ *Medial extent of the crus of the diaphragm:* especially at its most inferior extent (Fig. 17-3). The ipsilateral crus can be difficult to identify without clips. Compare the remnants of the crus on the right (*black arrow*) with the contralateral crus (*white arrow*). The best way to

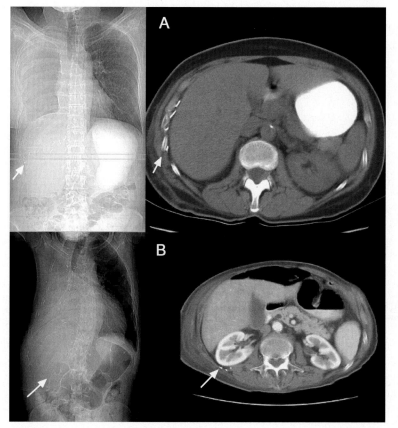

**FIGURE 17-1.** The diaphragmatic insertion is variable. The lowest point of the diaphragm is identified in two cases in which radiopaque clips were placed at the time of EPP. The lowest insertion point in patient (**A**) was above the ribs (*arrow*), while in the other case (**B**) it was well below the ribs. Note also that the neodiaphragm was reconstructed much lower in patient (**A**) than (**B**), which helped to keep the ipsilateral kidney far from the CTV.

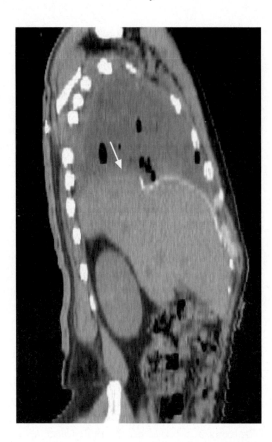

**FIGURE 17-2.** A radiopaque neodiaphragm makes contouring easier. This example demonstrates a case in which the posterior insertion of the neodiaphragm has dehisced. Regions bounded by the Gortex neodiaphragm are easily identified, while the extent of the liver is more difficult to identify. In such cases, more generous margins have been used to ensure that the regions at risk are within the CTV. This approach tends to irradiate more liver than would be necessary if the interface is more clearly seen.

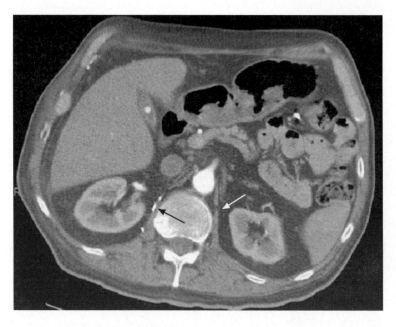

**FIGURE 17-3.** The crus can be difficult to identify without clips. The crus (inferior-medial extent of the diaphragm) is resected as low as possible and clips placed (*black arrow*). This region is much more difficult to identify than the unresected crus (*white arrow*). The medial extent of the resection can also be difficult to determine postoperatively.

individualize the inferior edge of the target volume is with extensive intraoperative placement of radiopaque clips with particular attention to the crus.

- When the entire resection margin is extensively clipped, a pattern such as that seen in Figure 17-4 emerges. Regions of potential pitfall are highlighted. These include the anterior medial reflection (*1*), the crus of the diaphragm (*2*), and the insertion of the diaphragm (*3*).
- Our institution has found it helpful to have the surgeon, radiation oncologist, and radiation physicist discuss the target volumes at the planning workstation.[14] This allows for unambiguous target volume identification and helps the radiation oncologist to better understand the anatomy and extent of disease. It helps the surgeons to better understand the limits of target volume identification/clipping. It also helps the physicist to understand which regions of this very large CTV are critical and gives the physicist more insight into the planning constraints for each case.

## 5.2. Normal Tissue Delineation

- Delineation of normal tissues can be done by experienced well-trained dosimetrists or planning therapists. However, they must be checked by the treating physician.

- As shown in Figure 17-5, we routinely contour the spinal cord, esophagus, lung, heart, and liver. Each kidney is contoured separately.
- We now also contour the small bowel/stomach as avoidance structures (not shown). Limiting the dose to these structures reduces nausea/vomiting during treatment.
- The most difficult structure to contour is the heart, which should be done with reference to an anatomy atlas.

## 5.3. Suggested Target and Normal Tissue Doses

- The doses prescribed for the target volumes and the dose–volume limits for the critical structures are listed in Table 17-3. Treatment typically is delivered with 16–24 intensity-modulated fields using 8–10 gantry angles, typically with 100 segments per intensity-modulated field.[14]
- Lung dose should be kept as low as possible, since only one lung remains.
- The contralateral kidney dose should also be kept as low as possible, since the ipsilateral kidney typically cannot be spared.
- The dose limits for critical structures were the standard values used in clinical practice at the M. D. Anderson Cancer Center, with the exception of the contralateral lung dose. Because patients have only one lung after EPP,

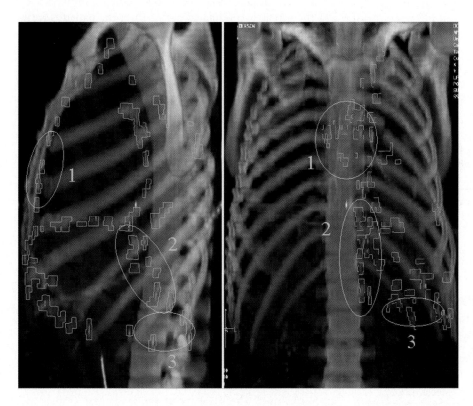

**FIGURE 17-4.** Regions of challenge. Three parts of the CTV are potentially difficult to appreciate without great care. These are: *(1)* the anterior-medial pleural reflection of the sterno-pericardial recess; *(2)* the inferior and medial extents of the crus of the diaphragm; and *(3)* the inferior insertion of the diaphragm.

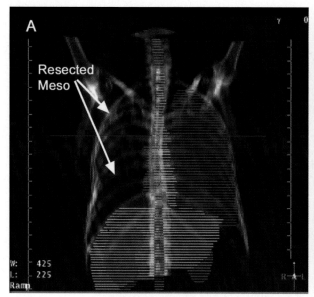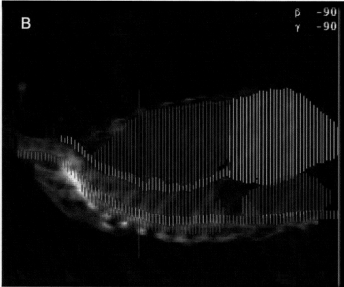

**FIGURE 17-5.** Normal tissue delineation for mesotheliomas. The extent of normal tissue contouring is shown from anterior-posterior (**A**) and lateral (**B**) perspective. The CT scan was so long that the inferior extent is not seen on these windows, since the patient is routinely scanned at least to the anterior-superior iliac spines. Spinal cord, red; esophagus, *green*; left lung, *dark purple*, heart; *light blue*; liver, *yellow*; right kidney, *dark blue* (green when superimposed on liver); left kidney, *light purple*.

it was decided to limit the volumes of contralateral lung irradiated such that the mean lung dose was less than 9.5 Gy. This is consistent with results of whole lung irradiation.[15] Patient setup and treatment were within a 45-minute period.

### 5.4. Verification Process

- Four components comprise the verification process: delivered dose, relative dose distributions, leaf sequences, and patient position. Measurements to verify all four components are acquired for each patient using a variety of standard techniques customized for these unusual cases.

- Ion chamber measurements are used to verify the absolute dose for each patient. Before making these measurements, the dose distribution that results from delivering the intensity-modulated beams from the patient's treatment plan to a phantom should calculated. Initially, three ion chamber measurements should be made: one point near the apex of the field, one near the center, and one corresponding to a point roughly at the center of the liver. The measurement points were selected in regions of relatively uniform doses. The phantom, ion chamber, and electrometer should be appropriately calibrated for each set of measurements.[14]

- On the first day of treatment, a dry run should be performed in which AP and lateral isocenter verification films are acquired. The isocenter verification films should be compared with the AP and lateral digitally reconstructed radiographs generated from the treatment plan. During the first week of treatment, two sets of isocenter verification films are also acquired. Weekly isocenter verification films should be obtained thereafter.

- Clearly, IMRT is more complicated to deliver than 3DCRT. However, very good coverage of the target can be achieved. As shown in Figure 17-6, the 50 Gy isodose line encompasses the CTV quite well. The dose volume histograms confirm that target volume coverage is adequate and normal tissue tolerances are preserved (Fig. 17-7). The liver and contralateral lung are spared with this technique. The majority of the ipsilateral kidney will

**TABLE 17-3. TARGET DOSES AND DOSE-VOLUME CONSTRAINTS OF ORGANS AT RISK IN MESOTHELIOMA**

| Target or Organ | Goal Dose or Constraint Dose |
| --- | --- |
| Clinical target volume (CTV) | 50 Gy in 25 fractions |
| bCTV | 60 Gy in 25 fractions |
| Lung | <20% to receive >20 Gy and mean less than 9.5 Gy |
| Liver | <33% to receive >30 Gy |
| Contralateral kidney | <20% to receive >15 Gy |
| Heart | <50% to receive >45 Gy |
| Spinal cord | <10% to receive >45 Gy  No portion to receive >50 Gy |
| Esophagus | <30% to receive >55 Gy |

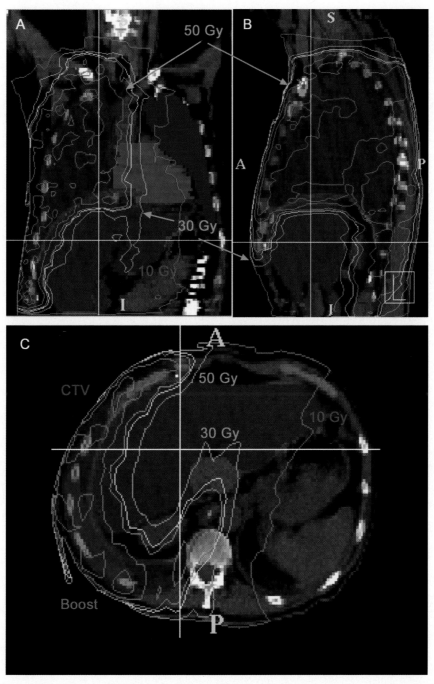

**FIGURE 17-6.** IMRT dose distributions. The dose distribution demonstrates good coverage of the CTV and the high dose gradients achievable with this technique. The goal was 50 Gy to the CTV, and a boost to close margin of 60 Gy (panel **C**). Note the clips visible at the inferior extent of panels **A** and **B**, and the medial CTV extent in panel **C**.

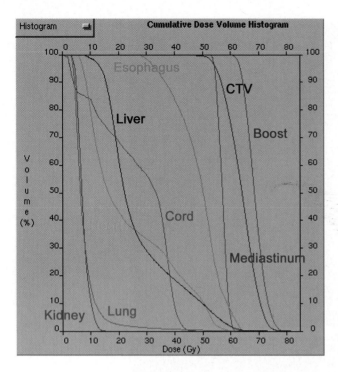

**FIGURE 17-7.** IMRT dose-volume histogram (DVH) from the case in Figure 17-6. Coverage of the target volumes is quite good. There is substantial inhomogeneity within the CTV and the boost volume. Both the liver and ipsilateral kidney (not shown) receive more dose than with the traditional approach. The mean lung dose was about 8.5 Gy.

likely be destroyed by this treatment. Adequate contralateral renal function is assured by pretreatment renal ultrasounds. For left-sided lesions, the spleen is also likely to receive a high radiation dose. Therefore, pneumococcal prophylaxis is recommended.

## 5.5. IMRT Results

■ Ahamad et al. demonstrated 100% in-field local control in the first 45 patients treated with IMRT.[11] There were

two marginal misses: one in the anterior-medial pleural reflection, and one at the ipsilateral crus. Both of these occurred before these regions were adequately clipped.
■ Major toxicities have been tabulated for the first 28 patients (Table 17-4). Most significant among these are nausea/vomiting, fatigue, and anorexia. The grade 3 pulmonary toxicities were residual dyspnea from surgery ($O_2$ requirements) which resolved before radiotherapy. Of the 17 subsequent patients, one died of probable radiation pneumonitis several weeks after treatment.

## TABLE 17-4. ACUTE TOXIC EFFECTS OF IMRT POST-EPP FOR MESOTHELIOMA*

| Symptom | Grade: [Incidence (%)] | | | | Overall Incidence (%) | Modal Grade (min–max) |
|---|---|---|---|---|---|---|
| | Grade 0 | Grade 1 | Grade 2 | Grade 3 | | |
| Fatigue | 20 | 17 | 38 | 24 | 80 | 2 (0–3) |
| Dehydration/anorexia | 72 | 0 | 17 | 10 | 27 | 0 (0–3) |
| Dysphagia/esophagitis | 59 | 14 | 21 | 7 | 41 | 0 (0–3) |
| Nausea/vomiting | 21 | 14 | 55 | 10 | 89 | 2 (0–3) |
| Weight loss | 69 | 31 | 0 | 0 | 0 | 0 (0–1) |
| Cough | 62 | 31 | 7 | 0 | 0 | 0 (0–2) |
| Dyspnea | 52 | 10 | 21 | 17 | 48 | 0 (0–3) |
| Depression/anxiety | 45 | 21 | 27 | 7 | 55 | 0 (0–3) |
| Skin changes | 28 | 45 | 21 | 6 | 72 | 1 (0–3) |

*According to Revised Common Toxicity Criteria.
From: Ahamad A, Stevens CW, Smythe WR, et al. Promising early local control of malignant pleural mesothelioma following postoperative intensity-modulated radiotherapy (IMRT) to the chest. *Cancer J* 2003;9:476–484.

# REFERENCES

1. Rusch VW. A proposed new international TNM staging system for malignant pleural mesothelioma. From the International Mesothelioma Interest Group. *Chest* 1995;108:1122–1128.

2. Vogelzang NJ, Rusthoven JJ, Symanowski J, et al. Phase III study of pemetrexed in combination with cisplatin versus cisplatin alone in patients with malignant pleural mesothelioma. *J Clin Oncol* 2003;21:2636–2644.

3. Kutcher GJ, Kestler C, Greenblatt D, et al. Technique for external beam treatment for mesothelioma. *Int J Radiat Oncol Biol Phys* 1987;13:1747–1752.

4. Yajnik S, Rosenzweig KE, Mychalczak B, et al. Hemithoracic radiation after extrapleural pneumonectomy for malignant pleural mesothelioma. *Int J Radiat Oncol Biol Phys* 2003;56:1319–1326.

5. Gordon W, Jr., Antman KH, Greenberger JS, et al. Radiation therapy in the management of patients with mesothelioma. *Int J Radiat Oncol Biol Phys* 1982;8:19–25.

6. Ball DL, Cruickshank DG. The treatment of malignant mesothelioma of the pleura: review of a 5-year experience, with special reference to radiotherapy. *Am J Clin Oncol* 1990;13:4–9.

7. Nguyen LN, Komaki R, Allen P, et al. Effectiveness of accelerated radiotherapy for patients with inoperable non-small cell lung cancer (NSCLC) and borderline prognostic factors without distant metastasis: a retrospective review. *Int J Radiat Oncol Biol Phys* 1999;44:1053–1056.

8. van Ooijen B, Eggermont AM, Wiggers T. Subcutaneous tumor growth complicating the positioning of Denver shunt and intrapleural port-a-cath in mesothelioma patients. *Eur J Surg Oncol* 1992;18:638–640.

9. Boutin C, Rey F, Viallat JR. Prevention of malignant seeding after invasive diagnostic procedures in patients with pleural mesothelioma. A randomized trial of local radiotherapy. *Chest* 1995;108:754–758.

10. Ahamad A, Stevens CW, Smythe WR, et al. Intensity-modulated radiation therapy: a novel approach to the management of malignant pleural mesothelioma. *Int J Radiat Oncol Biol Phys* 2003;55:768–775.

11. Ahamad A, Stevens CW, Smythe WR, et al. Promising early local control of malignant pleural mesothelioma following postoperative intensity-modulated radiotherapy (IMRT) to the chest. *Cancer J* 2003;9:476–484.

12. Rusch VW. Surgical techniques for pulmonary metastasectomy. *Semin Thorac Cardiovasc Surg* 2002;14:4–9.

13. Sugarbaker DJ, Flores RM, Jaklitsch MT, et al. Resection margins, extrapleural nodal status, and cell type determine postoperative long-term survival in trimodality therapy of malignant pleural mesothelioma: results in 183 patients. *J Thorac Cardiovasc Surg* 1999;117:54–63; discussion 63–65.

14. Forster KM, Smythe WR, Starkschall G, et al. Intensity-modulated radiotherapy following extrapleural pneumonectomy for the treatment of malignant mesothelioma: clinical implementation. *Int J Radiat Oncol Biol Phys* 2003;55:606–616.

15. Della Volpe A, Ferreri AJ, Annaloro C, et al. Lethal pulmonary complications significantly correlate with individually assessed mean lung dose in patients with hematologic malignancies treated with total body irradiation. *Int J Radiat Oncol Biol Phys* 2002;52:483–488.

16. Maasilta P. Deterioration in lung function following hemithorax irradiation for pleural mesothelioma. *Int J Radiat Oncol Biol Phys* 1991;20:433–438.

17. Hilaris BS, Nori D, Kwong E, et al. Pleurectomy and intraoperative brachytherapy and postoperative radiation in the treatment of malignant pleural mesothelioma. *Int J Radiat Oncol Biol Phys* 1984;10:325–331.

18. Lee TT, Everett DL, Shu HK, et al. Radical pleurectomy/decortication and intraoperative radiotherapy followed by conformal radiation with or without chemotherapy for malignant pleural mesothelioma. *J Thorac Cardiovasc Surg* 2002;124:1183–1189.

19. Baldini EH, Recht A, Strauss GM, et al. Patterns of failure after trimodality therapy for malignant pleural mesothelioma. *Ann Thorac Surg* 1997;63:334–338.

20. Rusch VW, Rosenzweig K, Venkatraman E, et al. A phase II trial of surgical resection and adjuvant high-dose hemithoracic radiation for malignant pleural mesothelioma. *J Thorac Cardiovasc Surg* 2001;122:788–795.

# 18

# ESOPHAGUS

## ZHONGXING LIAO

## 1. ANATOMY

### 1.1. Anatomical Course

- The esophagus begins in the neck at the cricoid cartilage at the level of vertebra C7, passes through the thorax in the posterior mediastinum, and extends for several centimeters past the diaphragm to its junction with the stomach, which is near the lower border of vertebra T11. The endoscopic distance of the esophagus is approximately 40 to 43 cm from the upper incisor teeth.
- The cervical esophagus is posterior to the trachea and bounded on both sides by the recurrent laryngeal nerve and the carotid sheath. The thoracic esophagus continues posterior to the trachea to the level of bifurcation, then courses posteriorly to the left atrium, with the azygous veins ascending on either side of the thoracic segment.

### 1.2. Classification

- For the purpose of classification, staging, and reporting of an esophageal malignancy, the American Joint Committee on Cancer[1] has recommended dividing the esophagus into four regions

  □ *Cervical esophagus*: extends from the lower edge of the cricoid cartilage to the thoracic inlet, approximately 18 cm from the incisors.
  □ *Upper thoracic esophagus*: part of the intrathoracic and abdominal esophagus, which extends from the thoracic inlet to the tracheal bifurcation, approximately 24 cm from the incisor teeth.
  □ *Middle thoracic esophagus*: also part of the intrathoracic and abdominal esophagus, which extends from the tracheal bifurcation to the level of the distal esophagus just above the esophagogastric junction, 32 cm from the incisor teeth.
  □ *Lower thoracic and abdominal esophagus*: includes the lower thoracic esophagus, approximately 3 cm distal to the esophagus, and the intra-abdominal portion and

the esophagogastric junction, 40 to 43 cm from the incisors.

### 1.3. Layers

- The esophagus has four layers: the mucosa, submucosa, muscularis propria, and serosa. Figure 18-1 shows the layers and lymphatic anatomy of the esophagus.
- The mucosa consists of a nonkeratinizing, stratified, squamous epithelium, the lamina propria, and the muscularis mucosa.
- The submucosa comprises the loose connective tissue containing vessels, nerve fibers, lymphatics, and submucosal glands.
- The muscularis propria is composed of the inner, circular and outer, longitudinal layers.
- The serosa lines the short segment of the thoracic and intra-abdominal esophagus and is absent in other esophageal regions.[2]

### 1.4. Blood Supply

- The cervical esophagus is supplied mainly by branches of the inferior thyroid artery. Branches of the bronchial arteries, intercostal arteries, and aorta supply the thoracic segment, and branches of the left gastric and inferior phrenic artery supply the abdominal segment. Branches from these arteries run within the muscularis propria and give rise to branches that course within the submucosa with extensive anastomosis.
- The venous system of the esophagus consists of four layers. The radially arranged epithelial layer channels communicate with the superficial venous plexus in the upper submucosa, the latter of which communicates with the deep intrinsic veins in the lower submucosa. From here, perforating veins pierce the muscularis propria and connect with the adventitial veins on the esophageal surface. Branches from the upper two-thirds of the esophagus lead into the inferior thyroidal vein and the azygous system, eventually to the superior vena cava. The lower seg-

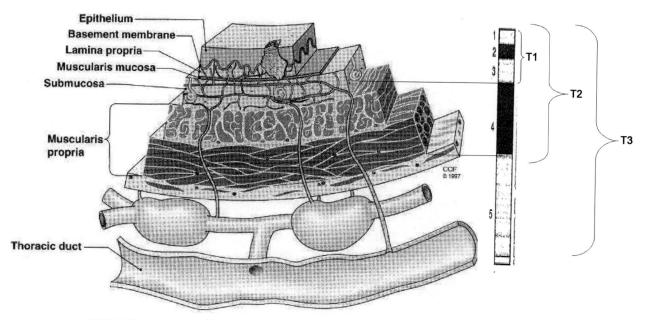

**FIGURE 18-1.** Layers and lymphatic anatomy of the esophagus. The *black and white bar* indicates the ultrasound presentation of the layers. (Modified from: Rice TW, Zuccaro G Jr, Adelstein DJ, et al. Esophageal carcinoma: depth of tumor invasion is predictive of regional lymph node status. *Ann Thorac Surg* 1998;65:787–792.)

ment drains into the systemic vasculature through the branches of the azygous and left gastric veins and into the splenic vein through the short gastric veins. The caval and portal systems communicate through the veins within the submucosa.[2]

## 1.5. Lymphatics

- A rich network of lymphatics in the lamina propria and submucosa connects with the lymphatics in the muscularis propria and adventitia.
- The lymphatics in the esophagus are oriented primarily in a longitudinal direction. Because of this arrangement, extensive intramucosal and submucosal spread beyond a grossly visible tumor is common. This feature becomes an important consideration in the delineation of the clinical target volume (CTV) in esophageal cancer.
- The lymphatic network of the esophagus drains into three areas: the upper, middle, and lower lymphatic trunks. All three groups of lymphatics drain into the paraesophageal lymph nodes located immediately adjacent to the esophagus. The cervical esophagus drains into the internal jugular and upper tracheal lymph node groups. The thoracic esophagus drains into the superior, middle, and lower mediastinal lymph node groups. The abdominal segment drains into the superior gastric artery, celiac axis, common hepatic artery, and splenic artery lymph nodes. However, extensive communication among the lymphatics results in a varied and unpredictable nodal involvement pattern.[2]

- Figures 18-2A, B demonstrate the lymph nodal regions of the esophagus according to Akiyama (1990).[3]

## 2. NATURAL HISTORY

### 2.1. EPIDEMIOLOGY

- In 2003, the incidence of esophageal carcinoma in the United States was 13,900 with approximately 13,000 deaths per year.
- The highest incidence is found in western Turkey, northern and eastern China, and Zimbabwe.
- In the past 20 years, there has been a dramatic change in the epidemiology in North America and most western countries characterized by a very rapid rise in the incidence at a rate of 5% to 10% increase per year, and a shift of histology from squamous cell carcinoma occurring mostly in the middle and lower esophagus to adenocarcinoma arising at the distal esophagus and gastroesophageal (GE) junction.[4]
- Predisposing factors for squamous cell carcinoma include high alcohol intake, heavy smoking, and nutritional deficiencies of minerals and vitamins.
- Predisposing factors for adenocarcinoma are acid reflux and Barrett's esophagus.

### 2.2. Histopathologic Features

- Esophageal cancer, regardless of its histopathology features, may extend over wide areas of the mucosal surface.
- Squamous cell carcinoma often arises as multifocal tumors, presumably as a result of field cancerization.

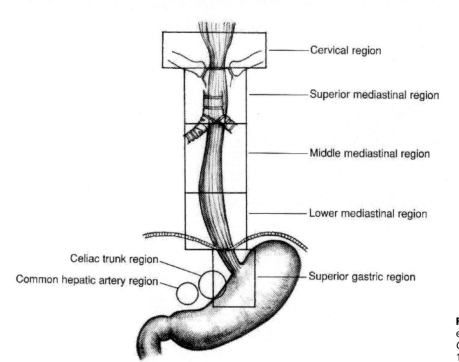

**FIGURE 18-2A.** Lymph node regions of the esophagus. (From: Akiyama H. *Surgery for Cancer of the Esophagus*. Baltimore; 1990: 19–131.)

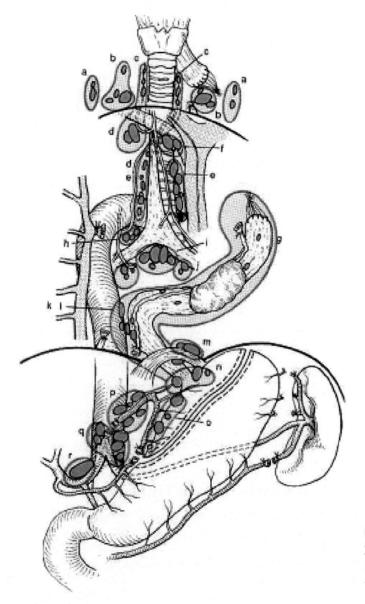

**FIGURE 18-2B.** Classification of lymph nodes according to Akiyama (1990) in "3 field nodal dissection," in which more than 100 lymph nodes were completely dissected from the lower neck, mediastinum, and upper abdomen. (From: Akiyama H. *Surgery for Cancer of the Esophagus*. Baltimore; 1990:19–131.)

**TABLE 18-1. RELATIONSHIP BETWEEN DEPTH OF TUMOR INFILTRATION AND INCIDENCE OF LYMPH NODE METASASES IN ESOPHAGEAL CANCER**

| Depth of Infiltration | % of N+ | (N+/Total) |
|---|---|---|
| M1 | 0 | (0/199) |
| M2 | 3.3 | (5/153) |
| M3 | 12.2 | (28/230) |
| Sm1 | 26.5 | (58/219) |
| Sm2 | 26.5 | (133/372) |
| Sm3 | 45.9 | (260/567) |

Both mucosal and submucosal layers are divided into 3 sublayers. N+, positive lymph nodes; M, mucosa; Sm, submucosa. From: Kodama M, Kakegawa T. Treatment of superficial cancer of the esophagus: a summary of responses to a questionnaire on superficial cancer of the esophagus in Japan. *Surgery* 1998;123:432–439.

- Adenocarcinomas may have varying lengths of mucosal and submucosal disease, particularly in patients with the long segment of Barrett's esophagus.

## 2.3. Patterns of Lymph Node Metastasis

- Lymph node metastasis occurs both upwards and downwards at a very early stage (Fig. 18–3). The incidence of lymph nodes metastasis is directly correlated with the depth of tumor invasion (Table 18-1).[5]
- Furthermore, larger tumors are more likely to present with locoregional nodal metastasis (Table 18-2).

## 3. DIAGNOSIS AND STAGING SYSTEM
## 3.1. Signs and Symptoms

- Early symptoms include those related to acid reflux and Barrett's esophagus.
- Odynophagia as a result of esophageal ulceration.

- Progressive dysphagia is the most common clinical symptom for all lesions as a result of tumor obstruction of the esophageal lumen and deep invasion of the esophageal wall. Both are indications of locally advanced disease.
- Complete medical evaluation with focus on history of alcohol consumption, cigarette smoking, acid reflux, history of Barrett's, dysphagia, odynophagia, weight loss, and other constitutional symptoms.

## 3.2. Imaging

- Pretreatment evaluation of esophageal cancer typically includes a combination of esophagogram, endoscopic examination with biopsy, endoscopic ultrasound examination, computed tomography (CT) of the chest, MRI, and PET.
- The accuracy of staging by esophagography, esophagoscopy, endoscopic ultrasonography, and CT scan for T staging was 80% and for N staging, 72% with a sensitivity of 78%, specificity of 60% and positive predictive value of 78%. The overall accuracy of stage group was 56%.[6]

### 3.2.1. Esophagogram

- Esophagograms provide good assessment of the structure of the esophageal lumen and mucosal surface. Mucosal irregularity, an intraluminal filling defect, and stricture seen on a barium esophagogram are suggestive of an esophageal malignancy (Fig. 18-4A).
- Although the length of a tumor can be estimated from a barium esophagogram, a noticeable discrepancy exists when it is compared with the length measured from CT and histopathology.[7]

### 3.2.2. Esophagastroduodenoscopic Examination

- Esophagastroduodenoscopic (EGD) examination with biopsy is the procedure of choice for diagnosing esophageal cancer (Fig. 18-5). The lesion seen at the

**TABLE 18-2. PROBABILITY OF POSITIVE LOCOREGIONAL NODES ACCORDING TO STAGE IN ESOPHAGEAL CANCER**

| Stage | % Possibility of Positive Locoregional Node | Reference |
|---|---|---|
| T1 (intra-epithelial) | 0 | Nishimaki 1993[39] |
| T1b | 31–56 | Nishimaki 1994[40] |
| T2 | 58–78 | Akiyama 1990[3]; Altorki 2002[23] |
| T3 | 74–81 | Lerut 1999[41]; Natsugoe 1995[42]; Nishimaki 1993[39], 1994[40], 1999[6]; Altorki 2002[23] |
| T4 | 83–100 | Lerut 1999[41]; Natsugoe 1995[42]; Nishimaki 1993[39], 1994[40], 1999[6] |

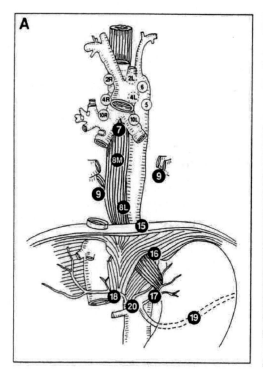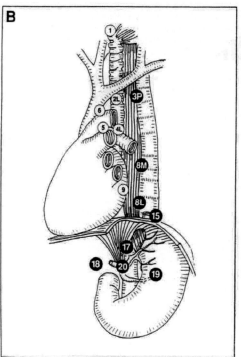

**FIGURE 18-3.** Regional lymph nodes stations for staging esophageal cancer. **A:** front side and **B:** back side. (From: Korst RJ, Rusch VW, Venkatraman E, et al. Proposed revision of the staging classification for esophageal cancer. *J Thorac Cardiovasc Surg* 1998;115:660–669; discussion 669–670.)

endoscope examination must be brushed and then biopsied. The accuracy of brushing cytology plus biopsy is 98.8% compared to 93.9% with biopsy alone and 87.9% with brushing cytology alone.

- Although both procedures allow for an excellent structural examination of the esophageal lumen, neither a barium swallow procedure nor an EGD plus biopsy can assess the extraluminal extension of the disease for nodal status.

### 3.2.3. Endoscopic Ultrasonography

- Endoscopic ultrasonography (EUS) is an ideal modality for determining clinical tumor and nodal stage according to the TNM staging system. Because it can distinguish wall layers of the esophagus, EUS provides a more accurate determination of the depth of tumor invasion, which is the basis of tumor staging, than a CT scan.

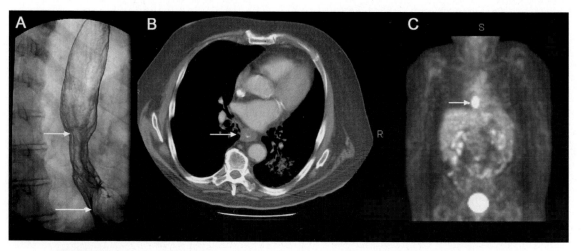

**FIGURE 18-4. A:** Esophagogram showing a distal stricture characteristic of esophageal cancer. **B:** Chest CT scan of the same lesion. **C:** PET scan showing hypermetabolism in the distal esophagus. *Arrows* indicate the lesion.

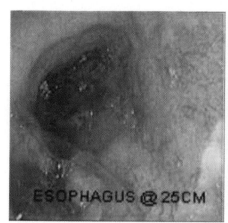
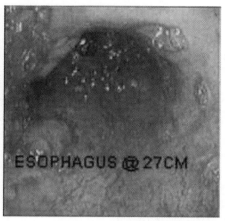

**FIGURE 18-5.** EGD shows multicentric lesions in a patient with a midthoracic esophageal tumor.

- The reported accuracy of EUS in tumor staging ranges from 75% to 90% compared with pathological examination of the resected specimen.[8–11] The accuracy of EUS in measuring tumor invasion ranges from 76% to 89%, compared with 49% to 59% for CT.[9–12] EUS is also more accurate than CT in staging regional nodal metastasis. The accuracy of EUS ranges from 70% to 90%,[13–16] compared with 46% to 58% for CT scan.[9,12]
- Although EUS is the most powerful procedure for accurately staging tumors of the esophagus, its role in target delineation is limited by the fact that EUS defines no spatial relationship between the tumor and adjacent structure and that the examination sometimes cannot be completed because of severe stricture. In addition, EUS does not provide information on the status of distant metastases.

- derestimate tumor length up to 3 cm, compared with a barium swallow test.[18]
- Regional lymph nodes are readily visualized in paraesophageal and retroperitoneal fat. Enlarged lymph nodes or clusters of multiple lymph nodes are abnormal. A short axis that is longer than 1 cm in the intrathoracic and intra-abdominal region is enlarged. Supraclavicular lymph nodes with a short axis longer than 0.5 cm and retrocrural lymph nodes longer than 0.6 cm are pathologic.[17]
- Normal-sized nodes may contain metastatic deposits, and not all the enlarged lymph nodes may be malignant. Accuracy of 61% to 90%, sensitivity of 8% to 75%, and specificity of 60% to 98% were reported for cervical, mediastinal, and abdominal nodes.[17,18]

### 3.2.4. CT Scan

- For preclinical evaluation and target delineation of esophageal cancer, CT is the most used diagnostic modality.
- The normal esophageal wall thickness seen on a CT scan is 3 mm or less; a wall thickness of more than 5 mm is considered abnormal.[17] Evident thickening of the esophageal wall and proximal lumen dilatation caused by obstruction characterize an esophageal malignancy. An asymmetric thickening of the esophageal wall is the principal, but nonspecific CT finding of an esophageal carcinoma.
- Although CT does not define the layers of the esophagus, the lack of a fat plane between a tumor mass and an adjacent structure seen on CT scan indicates a stage IV tumor.
- The cephalad extent of the tumor often can be identified by its interface with a dilated air- or fluid-filled proximal esophageal lumen; whereas, the caudal tumor margin may be difficult to delineate using CT. CT scan can un-

### 3.2.5. PET Scan

- PET scan can detect hypermetabolism in 92% to 100% of esophageal cancers.[19,20]
- The specificity for regional and distant lymph nodes is 98% with a sensitivity of 43% compared to the combined use of EUS and CT scan (Fig. 18-6).[21]
- FDG-PET relies on the size of the metastatic deposit and on the intensity of the FDG uptake and decay, thereby making the identification of microscopic disease possible. Through tomographic imaging, whole-body PET scanning can provide detailed images that can be superimposed on conventional CT scans, enabling the areas of hypermetabolism to be correlated with anatomic sites of disease.[17]
- Although FDG-PET has no value in determining the tumor stage because it provides no definition of the esophageal wall, it can nevertheless be a powerful complementary tool to CT for delineating the target volume in esophageal cancer treatment planning (Figs. 18-4C and 18-6).

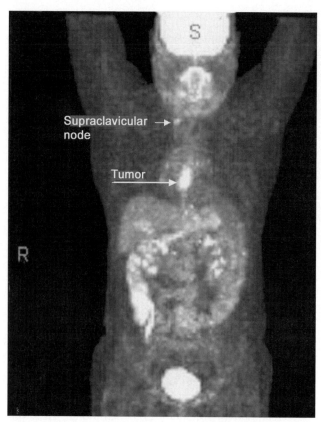

**FIGURE 18-6.** PET scan of a distal esophageal cancer (*arrow*) patient with supraclavicular lymph node metastasis (*arrow*).

### 3.3. Staging System

- The current staging system for esophageal cancer is limited by the fact that only the depth of invasion into the esophageal wall and nodal status are considered in staging. The length of the primary tumor, which is a critical factor in target delineation during treatment planning and a factor in the 1983 staging system, is not included in the current staging manual.
- The 2002 AJCC staging system is shown in Table 18-3.[1]
- Figure 18-3 demonstrates the regional lymph node stations for staging esophageal cancer in the 2002 AJCC staging system.[1]

### 4. PROGNOSTIC FACTORS

- Depth of invasion (T).
- Presence of nodal disease.
- Distant organ metastasis is associated with a worse prognosis compared to extensive nonregional nodal metastases.
- R0 resection is a strong indication for better outcome in patients treated with surgical resection.
- Complete pathological response after neoadjuvant chemoradiation is a strong indication of better overall survival.

### TABLE 18-3. AJCC 2002 STAGING SYSTEM

**Primary Tumor (T)**
| | |
|---|---|
| TX | Primary tumor cannot be assessed |
| T0 | No evidence of primary tumor |
| Tis | Carcinoma in situ |
| T1 | Tumor invades lamina propria or submucosa |
| T2 | Tumor invades muscularis propria |
| T3 | Tumor invades adventitia |
| T4 | Tumor invades adjacent structures |

**Regional Lymph Nodes (N)**
| | |
|---|---|
| NX | Regional lymph nodes cannot be assessed |
| N0 | No regional lymph node metastasis |
| N1 | Regional lymph node metastasis |

**Distant Metastasis (M)**
| | |
|---|---|
| MX | Distant metastasis cannot be assessed |
| M0 | No distant metastasis |
| M1 | Distant metastasis |

Tumors of the lower thoracic esophagus:
| | |
|---|---|
| M1a | Metastasis in celiac lymph nodes |
| M1b | Other distant metastasis |

Tumors of the midthoracic esophagus
| | |
|---|---|
| M1a | Not applicable |
| M1b | Nonregional lymph nodes and/or other distant metastasis |

Tumors of the upper thoracic esophagus:
| | |
|---|---|
| M1a | Metastasis in cervical nodes |
| M1b | Other distant metastasis |

**Stage Grouping**
| | | | |
|---|---|---|---|
| Stage 0 | Tis | N0 | M0 |
| Stage I | T1 | N0 | M0 |
| Stage IIA | T2 | N0 | M0 |
| | T3 | N0 | M0 |
| Stage IIB | T1 | N1 | M0 |
| | T2 | N1 | M0 |
| Stage III | T3 | N1 | M0 |
| | T4 | Any N | M0 |
| Stage IV | Any T | Any N | M1 |
| Stage IVA | Any T | Any N | M1a |
| Stage IVB | Any T | Any N | M1b |

From: Greene FL, American Joint Committee on Cancer, American Cancer Society. *AJCC cancer staging manual, 6th ed.* New York: Springer, 2002.

# 5. GENERAL MANAGEMENT

## 5.1. Surgical Approach

### 5.1.1. Surgery Alone

- Esophagectomy continues to be the treatment of choice for patients with resectable tumors.
- Esophageal cancer is characterized by its ability to spread intramurally to distant locations from the primary lesion, resulting in multicentric lesions. Therefore, the whole esophagus is considered at risk for disease involvement.
- The entire esophagus or at least 5 cm surgical margins has been the principle of esophagectomy.
- Regional lymph nodes should be dissected during esophagectomy. For thoracic esophageal cancer, a 3-field lymphadenectomy (3-FD) technique has been advocated by Udagawa and Akiyama.[22] More than 100 lymph nodes from the lower neck, mediastinum, and upper abdomen are removed during this procedure. In a retrospective report including more than 700 patients, the 5-year survival rates of patients with curative surgical resection were 53.8% overall, 77.4%, 49%, 44%, and 28% for patients with T1, T2, T3, and T4 lesions.
- The pattern of lymph node metastases in 519 patients who underwent 3-FD resection is shown in Figure 18-7A and B.[22]
- In a prospective observational study of 80 patients, Altorki et al. reported 69% (55 of 80) overall nodal metastases.[23] Twenty patients had nodal disease in only 1-field, 17 had 2-field, and 18 had 3-field nodal involvement. Unsuspected cervicothoracic nodal involvement was found in 36% of the entire whole group, 32% of patients with lower-third tumors, and 60% of patients with middle-third tumors (Table 18-4). The prevalence of nodal disease increased with advancing T-stage and exceeded 80% for T2 and T3 lesions. The overall 5-year survival rate was 88% and 33% for node negative and positive patients, respectively. There was no difference in the prevalence of nodal metastasis between different cell types. The overall survival was not influenced by cell type: 46% for adenocarcinoma and 65% for squamous cell carcinoma.
- Locoregional recurrence after surgery ranges from 21% to 39%.[16,24–26] Anastomotic recurrence is reported at 3% to 7% after 3-FD resection compared to 77% after transhiatal esophagectomy.[3,27]

### 5.1.2. Neoadjuvant Therapy

- Neoadjuvant chemotherapy before surgery has not shown to improve outcomes measured by resectability, local regional control, and overall survival (Fig. 18-8).[28]
- Results of neoadjuvant chemoradiation are shown in Table 18-5.
- A phase II study using chemotherapy, chemoradiation, and surgery for locally advanced esophageal cancer was

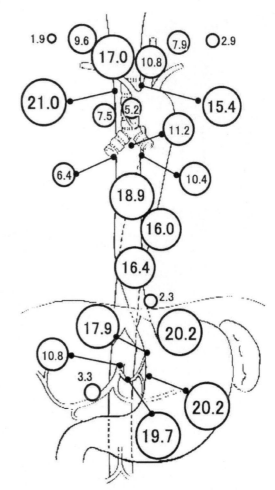

**FIGURE 18-7A.** The pattern of lymph node metastasis in 519 patients who underwent 3-FD resection. Note the extensive and almost homogeneous distribution of the lymph node metastasis. (From: Udagawa H, Akiyama H. Surgical treatment of esophageal cancer: Tokyo experience of the three-field technique. *Dis Esophagus* 2001;14:110–114.)

reported by Swisher et al. Of the 38 patients enrolled in the protocol, 35 had surgery. The complete pathological response or microscopic residual carcinoma (<10% viable) was found in 71% with an associated disease-free survival rate of 72% at 3 years and 51% at 5 years. The

**TABLE 18-4. PREVALENCE OF CERVICOTHORACIC NODES IN ESOPHAGEAL CANCER BY CELL TYPE AND TUMOR SITE**

| | |
|---|---|
| Adenocarcinoma | 37.42% (18/48) |
| Squamous carcinoma | 34.3% (11/32) |
| Lower-third | 32.73% (18/55) |
| Middle-third | 58.82% (10/17) |
| Upper-third | 12.5% (1/8) |

Modified from: Altorki N, Kent M, Ferrara C, et al. Three-field lymph node dissection for squamous cell and adenocarcinoma of the esophagus. *Ann Surg* 2002;236:177–183.

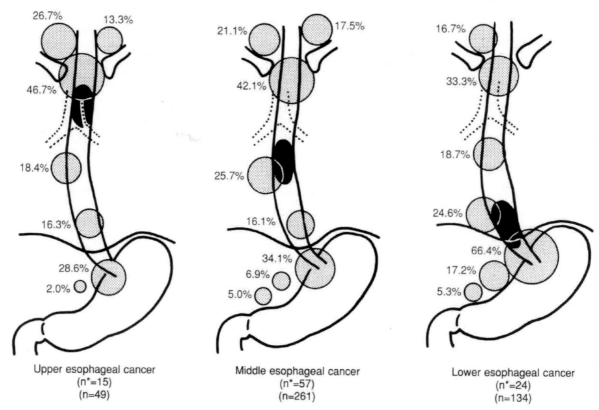

Upper esophageal cancer
(n*=15)
(n=49)

Middle esophageal cancer
(n*=57)
(n=261)

Lower esophageal cancer
(n*=24)
(n=134)

**FIGURE 18-7B.** The pattern of lymph node metastases according to Akiyama. (From: Akiyama H. *Surgery for Cancer of the Esophagus.* Baltimore: Williams & Wilkins; 1990:19–131.)

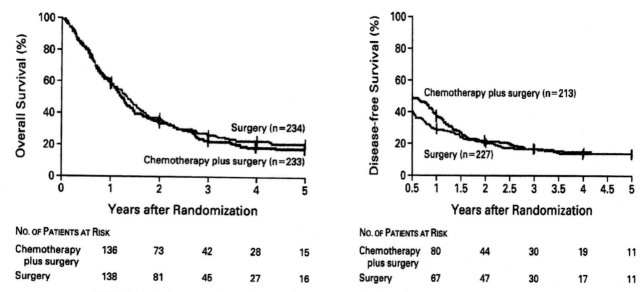

NO. OF PATIENTS AT RISK

| | | | | | |
|---|---|---|---|---|---|
| Chemotherapy plus surgery | 136 | 73 | 42 | 28 | 15 |
| Surgery | 138 | 81 | 45 | 27 | 16 |

NO. OF PATIENTS AT RISK

| | | | | | |
|---|---|---|---|---|---|
| Chemotherapy plus surgery | 80 | 44 | 30 | 19 | 11 |
| Surgery | 67 | 47 | 30 | 17 | 11 |

**FIGURE 18-8.** Outcome of neoadjuvant chemotherapy for esophageal cancer. (From: Kelsen DP, Ginsberg R, Pajak TF, et al. Chemotherapy followed by surgery compared with surgery alone for localized esophageal cancer. *N Engl J Med* 1998;339:1979–1984.).

**TABLE 18-5. RESULTS OF RANDOMIZED TRIALS USING NEOADJUVANT CHEMORADIATION FOLLOWED BY SURGICAL RESECTION FOR ESOPHAGEAL CANCER**

| Study | No. Pt. | Histology | Treatment | PCR | 3-yr OS |
|---|---|---|---|---|---|
| Urba 2001[43] | 100 | ADC 75% SCC 25% | Surgery only<br>5-FU/CDDP + 45 Gy/30 fx, 1.5 Gy bid | —<br>28% | 15%<br>32% |
| Bosset 1997[44] | 282 | SCC | Surgery only<br>5-FU/CDDP + 370 cGy x 5, followed by 2 weeks break, then 370 cGy x 5 | —<br>26% | 36%<br>36% |
| Walsh 1996[45] | 113 | ADC | Surgery only<br>5-FU + 40 Gy/15 Fx | —<br>25% | 6%<br>32% |
| Le Prise 1994[46] | 86 | SCC | Surgery only<br>5-FU/CDDP + RT 2.67 Gy x 10 fx | — | 14%<br>19% |
| Nygaard 1992[47] | 103 | SCC | Surgery only<br>CDDP/Bleo + 35 Gy/20 fx | | 9%<br>17% |

PCR, pathological complete response; OS, overall survival; ADC, adenocarcinoma; SCC, squamous cell carcinoma; 5-FU, 5-fluorouracil; CDDP, cisplatin; Bleo, bleomycin.

overall survival rates for all 38 patients were 63% and 39% at 3- and 5-years, respectively. This strategy is under further investigation at the University of Texas M. D. Anderson Cancer Center.

- Adjuvant chemotherapy or radiation therapy alone has not shown to improve patient outcome after surgery.

## 5.2. Nonsurgical Approach

### 5.2.1. Radiation Therapy Alone

- No patients treated with radiation alone in the RTOG 85-01 trial survived at 3 years.[29]

- Radiation therapy alone as a single modality is reserved for palliation and for patients who are not candidates for chemotherapy.

### 5.2.2. Concurrent Chemoradiation

- Concurrent chemoradiation is the treatment of choice for patients who are not surgical candidates.
- Table 18-6 demonstrates the outcomes of randomized studies comparing radiation alone with concurrent chemoradiation. The long-term overall survival after chemoradiation is similar to that of surgery.

**TABLE 18-6. OUTCOMES OF RANDOMIZED TRIALS COMPARING RADIATION ALONE VERSUS CHEMORADIATION**

| Study | Rx | No. Pts | LRF (%) | 5-yr OS (%) |
|---|---|---|---|---|
| Cooper 1998 | RT<br>CT/RT<br>CT/RT | 62<br>61<br>69 | 68<br>45<br>54 | 0<br>27<br>30 (3 yr) |
| NCI Brazil | RT<br>CT/RT | 31<br>28 | 84<br>61 | 6<br>16 |
| EORTC | RT<br>CT/RT | 69<br>75 | 12 | 6 (3 yr) |
| Scandinavia | RT<br>CT/RT 46 | 51<br>96 | | 6 (3 yr) |
| Pretoria | RT<br>CT/RT | 36<br>34 | | 5 mo (MST)<br>6 mo (MST) |
| ECOG | RT | 60 | | 7 |
| EST 1282 | CT/RT 59 | | | 9 |

LRF, locoregional failure; OS, overall survival; RT, radiation therapy; CT, chemotherapy.

- An intergroup study (RTOG 94-05, INT 0123) compared different doses of concurrent chemotherapy: 50.4 Gy vs 64.8 Gy.[30] The higher radiation dose did not lead to improved survival or locoregional control. It is believed that the failure to find a dose-response may be due to geographic underdosage to subclinical disease from inadequate treatment field size; the treatment fields were only extended to 5 cm from the primary tumor.[31]

## 6. INTENSITY-MODULATED RADIATION THERAPY IN ESOPHAGEAL CANCER

### 6.1. Gross Tumor Volume Determination

- Gross tumor volume (GTV) includes the primary tumor mass and enlarged lymph nodes determined by the combination of all available pretreatment evaluation modalities. Information from barium swallow, endoscopic examination, and PET scan should be reviewed and incorporated in GTV contouring (Fig. 18-9).

- If chemotherapy was delivered before radiation, the pre-chemotherapy target volume should be outlined on the planning CT or PET/CT.

- An esophageal wall thickness of more than 0.5 cm on CT scan is usually considered abnormal and should be included in the GTV. A barium swallow procedure that images the treatment area may be helpful in delineating the length of a primary tumor.

- PET/CT simulation, which is becoming readily available and popular in the clinical setting, is highly recommended for target delineation and treatment planning (Fig. 18-10).

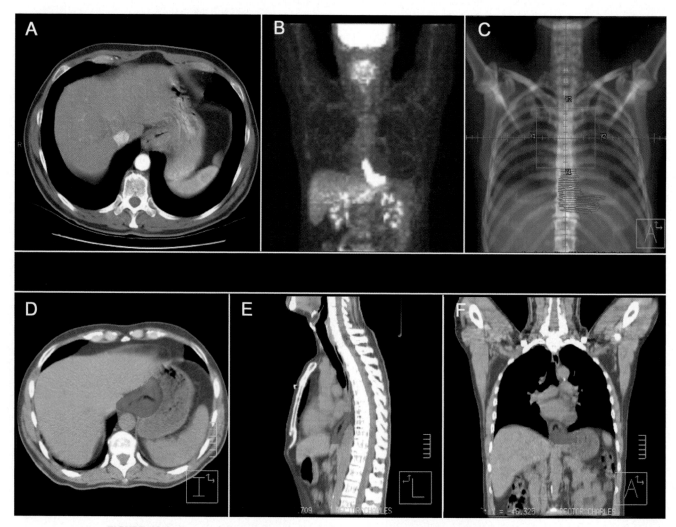

**FIGURE 18-9.** Target delineation using planning CT (**A, C–F**) and diagnostic PET (**B**) for a distal esophageal cancer (delineated in *red*).

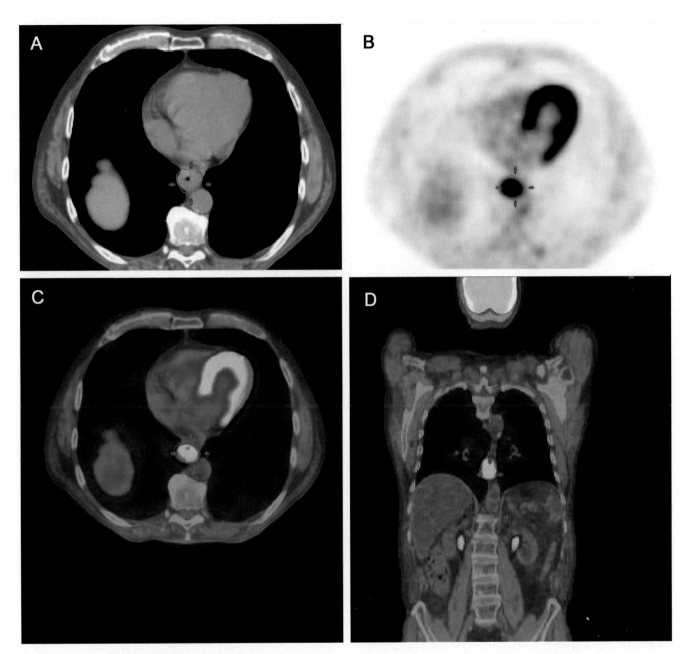

**FIGURE 18-10.** Target delineation using PET/CT scanner. A distal esophageal tumor is delineated in red on CT (**A**) and PET (**B**), and treatment is subsequently planned on PET/CT fusion in axial (**C**) and coronal views (**D**).

## 6.2. Clinical Target Volume Delineation

- Esophageal cancer may be associated with multicentric disease or submucosal "skip" metastasis sometimes found at a considerable distance from the primary tumor.[32] This tendency supports the use of generous proximal and distal margins for treating the primary tumor.

- Analyses of the patterns of failure after radiation therapy showed that marginal failure or failure outside the radiation field in the esophagus occurred when 5-cm longitudinal margins were used[33,34]; hence, these investigators have advocated that the entire esophagus be included in an initial treatment.[35] The Radiation Therapy Oncology Group (RTOG) 85-01 included the entire esophagus in the radiation portals. However, toxicity was severe, especially when concurrent chemotherapy was administered. Therefore, in the follow-up RTOG 94-05 study, 5-cm proximal and distal margins and a 2-cm lateral margin from the lateral border of the GTV were recommended.

- Esophageal cancer is characterized by a high rate of nodal involvement; thus, uninvolved regional lymph nodes should also be included in the CTV. If the primary tumor is above the carina (proximal esophagus), the supraclavicular nodes should be included in the CTV. For tumors of the lower two-thirds of the esophagus, treatment of the celiac nodes warrants consideration.

- For cervical esophageal cancer, the treatment fields usually extend from the laryngopharynx to the upper two-thirds of the esophagus and encompass the lower cervical, supraclavicular, and superior mediastinal nodes. Inclusion of the nodal basin of the upper jugular, subgastric region in the treatment field is still debated. The routine inclusion of these nodes in the CTV of oral pharyngeal or hypopharyngeal cancer treatment supports the inclusion of these nodes when treating cervical esophageal cancer.

- Another critical consideration in determining target volume and treatment planning for esophageal cancer is tumor motion caused by respiration and peristalsis, especially in cases of esophagogastric junction tumors. Unfortunately, motion of esophageal cancer is severely understudied, although longitudinal respiratory motion of 2 to 3 cm has been reported.[36]

## 6.3. Intensity-Modulated Radiation Therapy Results

- IMRT for esophageal cancer is advantageous in reducing total lung volume and dose that exceeds the tolerance of the normal lung tissue.

- Lee et al. reported higher rates of postoperative pulmonary complications of pneumonia and acute respiratory distress syndrome (ARDS) when higher volumes of lung received low doses of lung radiation in the preoperative setting.[37] Specifically, when the volume of lung receiving ≥10 Gy (V10) was ≥40% vs. <40%, the rates of pulmonary complication were 35% vs 8% (Table 18-7).

- In a study by Chandra et al., ten patients with cancer of the distal esophagus and gastro-esophageal junction were gathered for a treatment planning study.[38] Three sets of IMRT plans each using 4, 7, and 9 fields, were developed for each patient and compared to the 4-field 3DCRT plan used clinically. All IMRT plans significantly ($p < 0.05$) decreased the total lung V10, V20, Veff at 30 Gy, mean lung dose, and lung integral dose compared to the 3DCRT plans. For the total lung V10, V20, and mean lung dose parameters, the median absolute improvement of IMRT over 3DCRT plans was approximately 10%, 5% and 2.5 Gy, respectively. The authors concluded that a clinical trial is warranted to further investigate the potential of lung toxicity reduction using IMRT for esophageal cancer (Figures 18-11 and 18-12).[38]

- At the M. D. Anderson Cancer Center, IMRT is used routinely for cervical esophageal tumors.

- The challenge of using IMRT in treating tumors located at the lower esophagus and GE junction is accurate target delineation, especially the distal extension of the tumor, and respiratory motion. The tumor could move 1.5 to 2 cm longitudinally.[36] A clinical trial using PET/CT and a new technique using Feed-Back Guided Breath Hold has been developed at our institution to address these two questions.

## TABLE 18-7. CORRELATION OF PULMONARY COMPLICATIONS AFTER PREOPERATIVE CHEMORADIATION FOR ESOPHAGEAL CARCINOMA WITH

|  | No. Experiencing Pulmonary Complications (%) | P Value |
|---|---|---|
| V10 |  |  |
| ≥40% | 8/23 (35) | 0.014 |
| <40% | 3/38 (8) |  |
| V15 |  |  |
| ≥30% | 7/21 (33) | 0.036 |
| <30% | 4/40 (10) |  |
| V20 |  |  |
| ≥20% | 7/22 (32) | 0.079 |
| <20% | 4/39 (10) |  |

V10, percentage of lung receiving ≥10 Gy; V15, percentage of lung receiving ≥15 Gy; V20, percentage of lung receiving ≥20 Gy: From: Lee H, Vaporciyan A, Cox J, et al. Postoperative pulmonary complications following preoperative chemoradiation for esophageal carcinoma: correlation with pulmonary dose-volume histogram. *Int J Radiat Oncol Biol Phys* 2003;57:1317–1322.

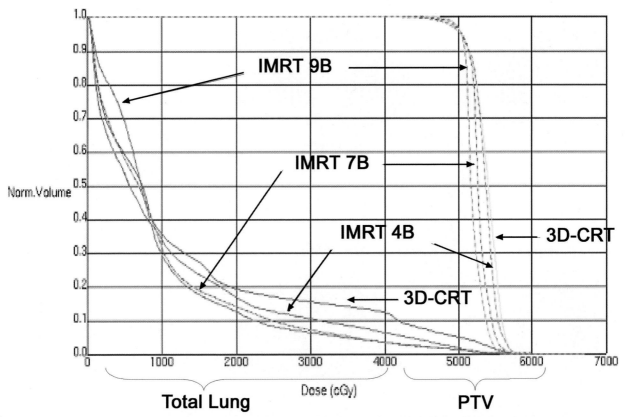

**FIGURE 18-11.** A sample dose volume histogram (DVH) showing the DVH for 3DCRT and IMRT plans for PTV and total lung structures. The PTV is normalized to 95% coverage at prescription dose (50.4 Gy). The three IMRT plans show reduced total lung V10 and V20 compared to 3DCRT ($P < 0.05$ by Wilcoxon matched pairs signed-rank test). The V5 for 9-field IMRT plans appeared to be increased compared to 3DCRT, but did not reach statistical significance ($P = 0.139$).

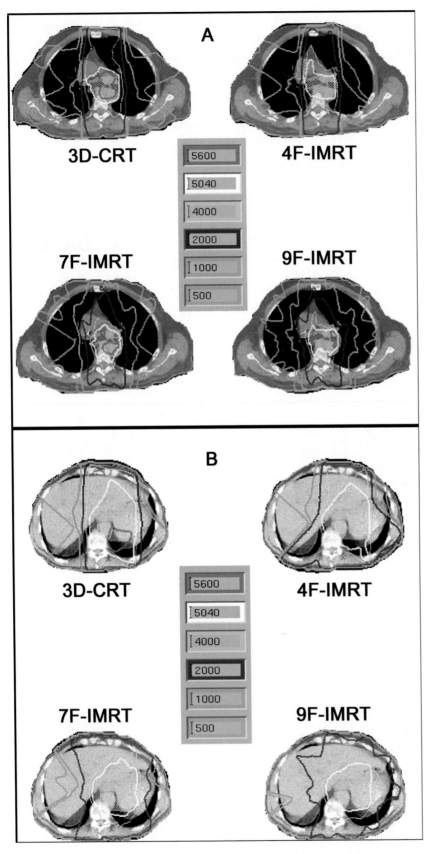

**FIGURE 18-12.** A sample transverse image showing the sample IMRT isodose distributions in axial images at the level of the thorax (**A**) and gastroesophageal junction (**B**). Comparison of 3DCRT and 4-field, 7-field, and 9-field IMRT is shown.

# REFERENCES

1. Greene FL, American Joint Committee on Cancer, American Cancer Society. *AJCC Cancer Staging Manual, 6th ed.* New York: Springer, 2002.
2. DeNardi FG, Riddell RH. The normal esophagus. *Am J Surg Pathol* 1991;15:296–309.
3. Akiyama H. *Surgery for cancer of the esophagus.* Baltimore: Lippincott Williams & Wilkins, 1990.
4. Devesa S, Blot W, Fraumeni JF. Changing patterns in the incidence of esophageal and gastric carcinoma in the United States. *Cancer* 1998;83:2049–2053.
5. Kodama M, Kakegawa T. Treatment of superficial cancer of the esophagus: a summary of responses to a questionnaire on superficial cancer of the esophagus in Japan. *Surgery* 1998;123:432–439.
6. Nishimaki T, Suzuki T, Kanda T, et al. Extended radical esophagectomy for superficially invasive carcinoma of the esophagus. *Surgery* 1999;125:142–147.
7. Drudi FM, Trippa F, Cascone F, et al. Esophagogram and CT vs endoscopic and surgical specimens in the diagnosis of esophageal carcinoma. *Radiol Med* 2002;103:344–352.
8. Grimm H, Binmoeller KF, Hamper K, et al. Accuracy of endoscopic ultrasound (EUS) in preoperative staging of esophageal carcinoma [abstract]. *Endoscopy* 1992;24:652.
9. Hordijk ML, Zander H, van Blankenstein M, et al. Influence of tumor stenosis on the accuracy of endosonography in preoperative T staging of esophageal cancer. *Endoscopy* 1993;25:171–175.
10. Kallimanis GE, Gupta PK, al-Kawas FH, et al. Endoscopic ultrasound for staging esophageal cancer, with or without dilation, is clinically important and safe. *Gastrointest Endosc* 1995;41:540–546.
11. Rosch T, Lorenz R, Zenker K, et al. Local staging and assessment of resectability in carcinoma of the esophagus, stomach, and duodenum by endoscopic ultrasonography. *Gastrointest Endosc* 1992;38:460–467.
12. Tio TL, Cohen P, Coene PP, et al. Endosonography and computed tomography of esophageal carcinoma. Preoperative classification compared to the new (1987) TNM system. *Gastroenterology* 1989;96:1478–1486.
13. Rosch T. Endosonographic staging of esophageal cancer: a review of literature results. *Gastrointest Edosc Clin N Am* 1995;5:537–547.
14. Lightdale C. Practice guidelines: esophageal cancer. *Am J Gastroenterol* 1999;94:20–29.
15. Yoshikane H, Tsukamoto Y, Niwa Y, et al. Superficial esophageal carcinoma: evaluation by endoscopic ultrasonography. *Am J Gastroenterol* 1994;89:702–707.
16. Fok M, Sham J, Choy D, et al. Postoperative radiotherapy for carcinoma of the esophagus: a prospective, randomized controlled study. *Surgery* 1993;113:138–147.
17. Rice T. Clinical Staging of esophageal carcinoma CT, EUS, and PET. *Chest Surg Clin N Am* 2000;10:471–485.
18. Saunders HS, Wolfman NT, Ott DJ. Esophageal cancer. Radiologic staging. *Radiol Clin North Am* 1997;35:281–294.
19. Flanagan FL, Dehdashti F, Siegel BA, et al. Staging of esophageal cancer with 18F-fluorodeoxyglucose positron emission tomography. *Am J Roentgenol* 1997;168:417.
20. Rankin SC, Taylor H, Cook GJ, et al. Computed tomography and positron emission tomography in the pre-operative staging of oesophageal carcinoma. *Clin Radiol* 1998;53:659–665.
21. Mallery S, Van Dam J. Increased rate of complete EUS staging of patients with esophageal cancer using the nonoptical, wire-guided echoendoscope. *Gastrointest Endosc* 1999;50:53–57.
22. Udagawa H, Akiyama H. Surgical treatment of esophageal cancer: Tokyo experience of the three-field technique. *Dis Esophagus* 2001;14:110–114.
23. Altorki N, Kent M, Ferrara C, et al. Three-field lymph node dissection for squamous cell and adenocarcinoma of the esophagus. *Ann Surg* 2002;236:177–183.
24. Bhansali M, Fujita H, Kakegawa T, et al. Pattern of recurrence after extended radical esophagectomy with three-field lymph node dissection for squamous cell carcinoma in the thoracic esophagus. *World J Surg* 1997;21:275–281.
25. Law S, Fok M, Wong J. Pattern of recurrence after oesophageal resection for cancer: clinical implications. *Br J Surg* 1996;83:107–111.
26. Altorki N, Skinner D. Should en bloc esophagectomy be the standard of care for esophageal carcinoma? *Ann Surg* 2001;234:581–587.
27. Law S, Fok M, Cheng S, et al. A comparison of outcome after resection for squamous cell carcinomas and adenocarcinomas of the esophagus and cardia. *Surg Gynecol Obstet* 1992;125:107–112.
28. Kelsen D, Ginsberg R, Pajak T, et al. Chemotherapy followed by surgery compared with surgery alone for localized esophageal cancer. *N Engl J Med* 1998;339:1979–1984.
29. Cooper J, Guo M, Herskovic A, et al. Chemoradiotherapy of locally advanced esophageal cancer: long-term follow-up of a prospective randomized trial (RTOG 85-01). Radiation Therapy Oncology Group. *JAMA* 1999;281:1623–1627.
30. Minsky B, Pajak T, Ginsberg R, et al. INT 0123 (Radiation Therapy Oncology Group 94-05) phase III trial of combined-modality therapy for esophageal cancer: high-dose versus standard-dose radiation therapy. *J Clin Oncol* 2002;20:1167–1174.
31. Haustermans K, Lerut A. Esophageal tumors. In: Brady L, Heilmann H, Molls M, eds. *Clinical target volumes in conformal and intensity modulated radiation therapy: a clinical guide to cancer treatment.* New York: Springer; 2003:107–119.
32. Mauer AM, Weichselbaum RR. Multimodality therapy for carcinoma of the esophagus. In: Steele GD, Phillips TL, Chabner BA, eds. *American Cancer Society atlas of clinical oncology cancer of the upper gastrointestinal tract.* Chicago: BC Decker Inc.; 2002.
33. Miller C. Carcinoma of the esophagus and gasric cardia. *Br J Surg* 1962;49:507–522.
34. Elkon D, Lee MS, Hendrickson FR. Carcinoma of the esophagus: sites of recurrence and palliative benefits after definitive radiotherapy. *Int J Radiat Oncol Biol Phys* 1978;4:615–620.
35. Herskovic A, Martz K, al-Sarraf M, et al. Combined chemotherapy and radiotherapy compared with radiotherapy alone in patients with cancer of the esophagus. *N Engl J Med* 1992;326:1593–1598.
36. Konski A, Chen L, Doss M, et al. Preliminary analysis of incorporating PET and MRI scans into the treatment planning process for esophageal carcinoma. American Radium Society, 85th Annual Meeting. Houston, TX; 2003.
37. Lee H, Vaporciyan A, Cox J, et al. Postoperative pulmonary complications following preoperative chemoradiation for esophageal carcinoma: correlation with pulmonary dose-volume histogram. *Int J Radiat Oncol Biol Phys* 2003;57:1317–1322.
38. Chandra A, Guerrero T, Liu H, et al. IMRT reduces lung irradiation in distal esophageal cancer over 3D CRT. *Int J Radiat Oncol Biol Phys* 2003;57(Suppl 2):S384–385.
39. Nishimaki T, Tanaka O, Suzuki T, et al. Tumor spread in superficial esophageal cancer: histopathologic basis for rational surgical treatment. *World J Surg* 1993;17:766–771; discussion 771–772.
40. Nishimaki T, Tanaka O, Suzuki T, et al. Patterns of lymphatic spread in thoracic esophageal cancer. *Cancer* 1994;74:4–11.

41. Lerut T, Coosemans W, De Leyn P, et al. Is there a role for radical esophagectomy? *Eur J Cardiothorac Surg* 1999;16:s44–s47.

42. Natsugoe S, Aikou T, Yoshinaka H, et al. Lymph node metastasis of early stage carcinoma of the esophagus and of the stomach. *J Clin Gastroenterol* 1995;20:325–328.

43. Urba S, Orringer M, Turrisi A, et al. Randomized trial of preoperative chemoradiation versus surgery alone in patients with locoregional esophageal carcinoma. *J Clin Oncol* 2001;19: 305–313.

44. Bosset J, Gignoux M, Triboulet J, et al. Chemoradiotherapy followed by surgery compared with surgery alone in squamous-cell cancer of the esophagus. *N Engl J Med* 1997;337: 161–167.

45. Walsh T, Noonan N, Hollywood D, et al. A comparison of multimodal therapy and surgery for esophageal adenocarcinoma. *N Engl J Med* 1996;335:462–467.

46. Le Prise E, Etienne PL, Meunier B, et al. A randomized study of chemotherapy, radiation therapy, and surgery versus surgery for localized squamous cell carcinoma of the esophagus. *Cancer* 1994;73:1779–1784.

47. Nygaard K, Hagen S, Hansen H, et al. Pre-operative radiotherapy prolongs survival in operable esophageal carcinoma: a randomized, multicenter study of pre-operative radiotherapy and chemotherapy. The second Scandinavian trial in esophageal cancer. *World J Surg* 1992;16:1104–1110.

# 19

# PELVIC AND PARA-AORTIC NODAL TARGET DELINEATION

## K. S. CLIFFORD CHAO

## 1. INTRODUCTION

- Definitive or adjuvant radiotherapy (RT) has contributed significantly to the successful management of gynecologic malignancies. Conventional RT is performed through either AP parallel-opposed fields or a 4-field technique consisting of an anterior, a posterior, and two lateral portals. However, the use of conventional portals has been reported to result in incomplete coverage of the intended target volume.[1] Bonin et al. and Pendelbury et al. reported inadequate coverage of the external iliac lymph nodes using standard irradiation fields in 45% and 62% of patients.[2,3]

- The lack of conformality via conventional techniques is also associated with normal tissue complications. According to various criteria to classify the severity of the radiation side effects, severe complications may develop in 8% to 10% of patients treated with a conventional beam arrangement. The incidence of complications requiring surgical management is approximately 5%.[4]

- As chemoradiotherapy has become the integral therapeutic measure in either the definitive or postoperative setting, gastrointestinal complications have been the most significant concern other than hematologic side effects.

- The results from the Radiation Therapy Oncology Group (RTOG) study 79-20 suggest that in a select group of patients, the use of extended fields covering the para-aortic lymph nodes is associated with better disease-free and overall survival compared with pelvic RT alone.[5] However, when the lymph nodes are grossly enlarged, para-aortic lymph node RT combined with chemotherapy proved to be highly toxic in the RTOG 92-10 study.[6] Although the acute hematologic toxicity was higher in patients receiving chemoradiotherapy than in those receiving RT alone, RTOG 92-10 clearly showed that 50% (15 of 30 patients) experienced grade 4 nonhematologic toxicity after therapy, and all 15 of those toxicities were bowel related. The cumulative in-

cidence of late Grade 3 and 4 toxicity was 34% at 36 months.[6]

- Techniques such as IMRT, which allows adequate target coverage in the pelvic and para-aortic lymph nodes while keeping the dose delivered to the critical organs such as the small bowel to a minimum, would be of tremendous interest and may permit combining high-dose RT and chemotherapy without prohibitive gastrointestinal complications. Minimizing the volume of the gastrointestinal tract inside the radiation field is pivotal to the potential improvement of the therapeutic ratio by IMRT.

- Portelance et al. demonstrated that IMRT for cervical cancer yields similar tumor coverage with superior normal tissue sparing compared with conventional beam arrangements.[7] Similar findings were also reported in a study from the University of Chicago.[8]

- The dosimetric advantage of IMRT may potentially improve the therapeutic outcome in patients with locally advanced cervical cancer, especially when the pelvic/para-aortic lymph nodes are grossly enlarged and a higher radiation dose is required.

- Patient- and tumor-related issues have hindered the acceptance of IMRT for patients with gynecologic malignancies.

  □ The first is related to the organ motion of the pelvic structures; for example, the uterus and cervix may shift as much as 4 to 5 cm on AP projection, depending on whether the bladder and rectum are empty or full.[1]

  □ The second concern that hinders the widespread use of IMRT for gynecologic cancer is the lack of an objective description of pertinent lymph node locations in a 3-dimensional (3D) projection. However, because the lymph node status is extremely important in determining the prognosis of patients with gynecologic malignancies, IMRT plans must provide adequate coverage of the pelvic, para-aortic, and inguinal draining nodes when these are at risk.

## 2. IMAGING FOR PARA-AORTIC, PELVIC, AND INGUINAL LYMPH NODES

- CT and MRI may be equally effective as lymphangiography (LAG) in detecting enlarged lymph nodes; however, small lymph nodes containing microscopic disease (clinical target volume [CTV]) are often difficult to identify using CT and MRI on the basis of size.

- Most institutions use CT to gather imaging data for IMRT treatment planning. Inconsistencies in visualizing unenlarged lymph nodes on pelvic and abdominal CT imaging could impose significant variations in target delineation among different physicians.

- Bipedal LAG has been shown to be an accurate method of assessing the nodal status and location in patients with cervical cancer. Performing routine LAG on each patient would greatly aid in determining the target volumes; however, only a few institutions still perform these technically difficult, uncomfortable, and time-consuming studies.

- LAG was considered the best option for detecting para-aortic nodal metastasis in an early Gynecologic Oncology Group study. The Gynecologic Oncology Group studied the clinical-pathologic correlation of para-aortic lymph node involvement by CT, LAG, and ultrasonography in patients with Stage IIB, III, and IVA cervical carcinoma. Of 264 patients evaluated, the LAG sensitivity was 79%, with a specificity of 73%. The sensitivity of CT and ultrasonography was 34% and 19%, with a specificity of 96% and 99%, respectively.[9] However, LAG was also associated with some shortcomings in detecting metastatic internal iliac and presacral nodes, which are only occasionally seen.

- In a more recent meta-analysis, Scheidler et al. concluded that LAG, CT, and MRI perform equivalently in the detection of grossly enlarged metastatic pelvic lymph nodes from cervical cancer.[10]

- We demonstrated that the nodal CTV can be better delineated by LAG-aided CT imaging.[11] The combination of LAG to demonstrate nodal texture and CT for spatial orientation has provided a better tool to delineate the CTV for the para-aortic, pelvic, and inguinal lymph nodes than relying solely on CT or MRI.

## 3. PARA-AORTIC, PELVIC, AND INGUINAL NODAL TARGET VOLUME DELINEATION

- The lymph node locations are described relative to the aorta, inferior vena cava, common iliac, external iliac, and femoral vessels. Lymph nodes lying adjacent to the aorta and inferior vena cava from T12 to the aortic bifurcation are designated as para-aortic.

- Nodes adjacent to the common iliac vessels (from the aortic bifurcation to the branching of the internal iliac artery) are designated as common iliac.

- Nodes adjacent to the external iliac vessels and extending anteriorly above the iliopsoas muscle and posteriorly, including the obturator group, are deemed the external iliac group.

- Nodes located adjacent to the femoral vessels to the level of the inner edge of the ischial tuberosities are designated as inguinal nodes.

- When the distance from the vessel wall to the furthest lymph node are measured in each nodal region, of all the lymph node areas, the lymph nodes on the left side of the para-aortic region are located the greatest distance from the corresponding vessel, at an average of 22.2 ± 12.2 mm from the aorta (range 10.3–44.5). In contrast, the right-side para-aortic nodes are located within an average of 9.1 ± 3.3 mm from the inferior vena cava (range 5.9–14.9). Very few lymph nodes are found ventral to the aorta, with an average distance of 1.8 mm (range 0–5.6). Figure 19-1 depicts a measurement example, and Table 19-1 details the results.

- Because lymph nodes generally follow the path of the major blood vessels, contouring vessels followed by radial expansion may be a practical method to define the nodal CTV. However, we showed that vessel contour expansion alone was not sufficient to cover the nodal areas fully and reasonably exclude normal tissue.[11] Expanding the vessel contours (aorta plus 20 mm, inferior vena cava plus 10 mm, common iliac plus 15 mm, external iliac plus 20 mm, and femoral plus 20 mm) could still miss 17.7% of LAG-avid nodal volume. This approach, although simple, not only led to inadequate CTV coverage, but also resulted in the inclusion of a substantial amount of normal tissue inside the CTV.

- In the second approach, we added a 15 mm strip medial to the iliacus muscle to cover the lateral external iliac nodes and a 17-mm strip medial to the pelvic sidewall to cover the obturator nodes. In addition, we truncated the volume 5 mm anterior to the walls of the aorta and common iliac arteries to minimize the amount of normal tissue encompassed within the CTV. When including grossly enlarged nodes greater than or equal to 2 cm, this modification provided complete coverage of the LAG-avid nodal regions and included less than 7% of the small bowel and less than 5% of the large bowel, bladder, and rectum.

- The modification is made to cover the lateral external iliac nodes by defining a volume that encompassed the region less than or equal to 15 mm medial to the iliacus muscle beginning at the S2-S3 interspace and continuing inferiorly until it fuses with the vessel expansion volumes.

- To cover the obturator nodes, a volume should be added 17 mm medial to the pelvic sidewall, beginning 1 cm superior to the S2-S3 interspace and continuing inferiorly to the beginning of the inguinal nodes.

- Additionally, the preliminary CTV should be focally expanded to fully encompass grossly enlarged nodes greater than or equal to 2 cm. With these three additions, the CTV definition yielded 100% coverage of LAG-avid lymph nodes in every patient.

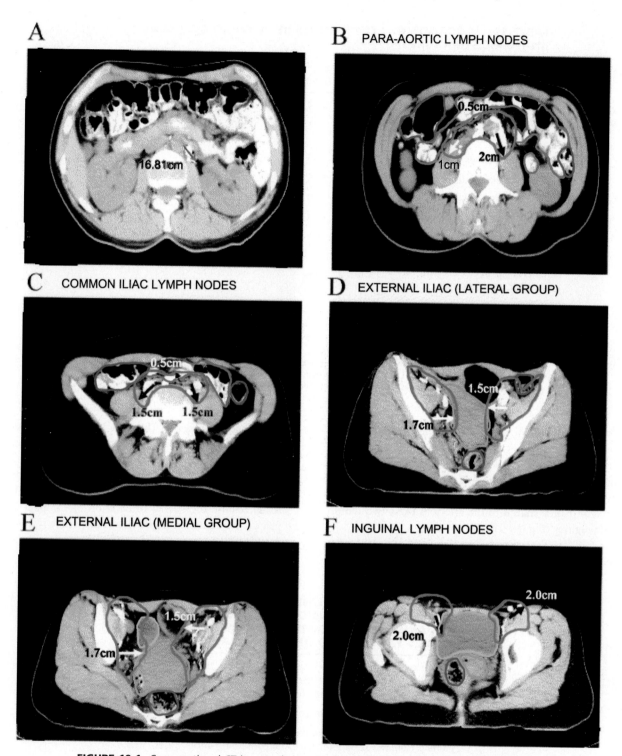

**FIGURE 19-1.** Cross-sectional CT images demonstrating technique to measure distance of LAG-avid lymph nodes to adjacent vessel and nodal CTV delineation at various anatomic levels. **A:** Furthest distance from lymph node to vessel wall determined on a Voxel-Q computer (Marconi, Cleveland, OH). **B:** Para-aortic lymph node CTV. **C:** Common iliac lymph node CTV. **D:** External iliac CTV, including lateral group. **E:** External iliac CTV, including medial (obturator) group. **F:** Inguinal lymph node CTV. CTV depicted by thick orange line. Small bowel demarcated by thin magenta, large bowel by thin blue, rectum by thin dark purple, bladder by thin turquoise, and uterus by thin yellow-green line. (From: Chao KS, Lin M. Lymphangiogram-assisted lymph node target delineation for patients with gynecological malignancies. *Int J Radiat Oncol Biol Phys* 2002;54: 1147–1152).

**TABLE 19-1. LOCATION OF LYMPH NODES RELATIVE TO ADJACENT ANATOMIC STRUCTURES**

| | Average Distance (mm) | Range (mm) | Standard Deviation (mm) |
|---|---|---|---|
| Para-aortic nodes left to aorta | 22.1 | 10.3–44.5 | 12.2 |
| Para-aortic nodes right to inferior vena cava | 9.1 | 5.9–14.9 | 3.3 |
| Para-aortic nodes ventral to aorta | 1.8 | 0–5.8 | 2.4 |
| Common iliac nodes, right | 11.9 | 5.3–15.8 | 3.9 |
| Common iliac nodes, left | 15.6 | 6.2–22.5 | 6.3 |
| Common iliac nodes, ventral | 0.3 | 0–1.8 | 0.7 |
| External iliac nodes relative to pelvic side wall, right | 16.2 | 11.1–22.2 | 4.2 |
| External iliac nodes relative to pelvic side wall, left | 13.8 | 7.4–16.7 | 3.5 |
| Inguinal nodes relative to femoral artery, right | 16.8 | 6.6–27.7 | 7.4 |
| Inguinal nodes relative to femoral artery, left | 15.3 | 7.5–23.3 | 6.5 |

Modified from Chao KS, Lin M. Lymphangiogram-assisted lymph node target delineation for patients with gynecological malignancies. *Int J Radiat Oncol Biol Phys* 2002;54:1147–1152.

- To refine the CTV definition further and maximally spare normal tissue, particular attention should be focused on the nodes most ventral to the aorta and common iliac arteries. Because they lay no more than 5 mm away from the vessel wall, the vessel expansions are truncated at 5 mm ventral to the artery in these two lymph node regions (Fig. 19-1B).
- The CTV is also truncated of bone and air. When the nodal CTV intersected bowel or bladder, it is truncated after 5 mm of overlap (Fig. 19-1D–F). We chose this value to offset nodal tissue that may have been omitted during CT image processing of these 5-mm sections.
- To assist radiation oncologists in correctly delineating the nodal target volume, we previously reported our guidelines to determine the spatial orientation of the para-aortic, pelvic, and inguinal nodes on the basis of the relationship of the nodal groups to nearby anatomic structures with the aid of bipedal LAG on CT images (Table 19-2).[11]

**TABLE 19-2. THE GUIDELINES FOR DELINEATING THE PARA-AORTIC, COMMON ILIAC, EXTERNAL ILIAC, AND INGUINAL LYMPH NODE TARGET VOLUMES WITH THE AID OF BIPEDAL LAG**

- Aorta plus 2 cm, inferior vena cava plus 1 cm (Fig. 19-1B), common iliac artery plus 1.5 cm (Fig. 19-1C), external iliac artery plus 2 cm, and femoral artery plus 2 cm (Fig. 19-1F)

- Focally expand to encompass lymph nodes ≥2 cm fully

- Add volume 15 mm medial to iliopsoas muscle (Fig. 19-1D) beginning from the S2-S3 interspace and continuing until it fuses with the vessel expansion volumes to cover the lateral external iliac nodes

- Add volume 17 mm medial to the pelvic sidewall (Fig. 19-1D and E), beginning 1 cm superior to S2-S3 interspace and continuing inferiorly to the inguinal nodes to cover the obturator (or medial external iliac) nodes

- Truncate out bone and air

- Truncate 5 mm into bowel or bladder (Fig. 19-1D–F) and 5 mm ventral to the aorta and common iliac arteries (Fig.19-1B and C)

- The information derived from these guidelines could result in the avoidance of performing invasive and uncomfortable LAG on every patient receiving IMRT. Furthermore, we also determined the volume of normal tissue encompassed by the CTV and the CTV with a 1- or 2-cm margin.

## REFERENCES

1. Greer BE, Koh WJ, Figge DC, et al. Gynecologic radiotherapy fields defined by intraoperative measurements. *Gynecol Oncol* 1990;38:421–424.
2. Bonin SR, Lanciano RM, Corn BW, et al. Bony landmarks are not an adequate substitute for lymphangiography in defining pelvic lymph node location for the treatment of cervical cancer with radiotherapy. *Int J Radiat Oncol Biol Phys* 1996;34:167–172.
3. Pendlebury SC, Cahill S, Crandon AJ, et al. Role of bipedal lymphangiogram in radiation treatment planning for cervix cancer. *Int J Radiat Oncol Biol Phys* 1993;27:959–962.
4. Perez CA, Brady LW. *Principles and Practice of Radiation Oncology*. Philadelphia: Lippincott-Raven, 1998.
5. Rotman M, Pajak TF, Choi K, et al. Prophylactic extended-field irradiation of para-aortic lymph nodes in stages IIB and bulky IB and IIA cervical carcinomas. Ten-year treatment results of RTOG 79-20. *JAMA* 1995;274:387–393.
6. Grigsby PW, Heydon K, Mutch DG, et al. Long-term follow-up of RTOG 92-10: cervical cancer with positive para-aortic lymph nodes. *Int J Radiat Oncol Biol Phys* 2001;51:982–987.
7. Portelance L, Chao KS, Grigsby PW, et al. Intensity-modulated radiation therapy (IMRT) reduces small bowel, rectum, and bladder doses in patients with cervical cancer receiving pelvic and para-aortic irradiation. *Int J Radiat Oncol Biol Phys* 2001;51:261–266.
8. Roeske JC, Lujan A, Rotmensch J, et al. Intensity-modulated whole pelvic radiation therapy in patients with gynecologic malignancies. *Int J Radiat Oncol Biol Phys* 2000;48:1613–1621.
9. Heller PB, Maletano JH, Bundy BN, et al. Clinical-pathologic study of stage IIB, III, and IVA carcinoma of the cervix: extended diagnostic evaluation for paraaortic node metastasis—a Gynecologic Oncology Group study. *Gynecol Oncol* 1990;38:425–430.
10. Scheidler J, Hricak H, Yu KK, et al. Radiological evaluation of lymph node metastases in patients with cervical cancer. A meta-analysis. *JAMA* 1997;278:1096–1101.
11. Chao KS, Lin M. Lymphangiogram-assisted lymph node target delineation for patients with gynecologic malignancies. *Int J Radiat Oncol Biol Phys* 2002;54:1147–1152.

# 20

# PROSTATE

## STEVEN J. FEIGENBERG
## ALAN POLLACK
## ROBERT A. PRICE
## SHAWN W. MCNEELEY
## ERIC M. HORWITZ

## 1. ANATOMY

- The prostate is bounded superiorly by the bladder, inferiorly by the urogenital diaphragm, anteriorly by the pubic symphysis, and posteriorly by Denonvilliers' prostatic fascia and the rectum.
- The urethra courses from the bladder neck superiorly to the prostatic urethra and through the urogenital diaphragm, bulbous urethra and penile urethra anteroinferiorly.
- A sagittal view of the prostate is shown in Figure 20-1.
- The prostate is triangular in shape, with the base situated superiorly and the apex inferiorly.
- A capsule encases the prostate except at the apex of the gland, where the prostate blends into the urogenital diaphragm.

## 1.1. Zonal Anatomy

- The prostate is divided into anatomical zones (Fig. 20-2).[1] The peripheral zone, located posteriorly, is the largest, comprising 70% of the glandular tissue. About 75% of prostatic malignancies occur in the peripheral zone.
- The transition zone surrounds the urethra in the midprostate and tends to enlarge with age as a consequence of benign prostatic hypertrophy (BPH), causing urinary obstructive symptoms. The transition zone comprises 5% to 10% of the glandular tissue and 20% of malignancies.
- The central zone, located superiorly, contains about 20% of the glandular tissue, but only 5% of the prostatic malignancies. The ejaculatory ducts pass through the central zone and empty into the urethra at the verumontanum.
- The anterior fibromuscular stroma has very little glandular tissue and malignancies rarely originate in this region.

## 1.2. Erectile Tissues

- Erectile function is controlled mainly by the neurovascular bundles, which are located posterolaterally to the prostate.[2–4]
- Radiation dose to be penile bulb and corporal bodies has been implicated as a determinant of erectile function.[5,6]

## 1.3. Seminal Vesicles

- The seminal vesicles are located superior and posterior to the base of the prostate.
- Invasion of the seminal vesicles is a relatively common pattern of spread for intermediate and high risk prostate cancer.[7]

## 2. NATURAL HISTORY

## 2.1. Lymphatics

- Lymphatic spread has been related to pretreatment PSA, Gleason score, and stage.[8–13]
- The most common sites of involvement are the obturator, external iliac, and internal iliac lymph nodes. The presacral lymph nodes are also at risk.[14, 15]
- Lymph node dissection prior to radical prostatectomy involves an en bloc resection of the fatty tissue from the external iliac vein medially to the obturator vessels and nerve, extending inferiorly from the inguinal ligament to the bifurcation of the common iliac vessels superiorly.

## 2.2. Metastasis

- Lymph node metastasis is typically less than 15% in the absence of T3 disease[12]; however, high rates may be seen

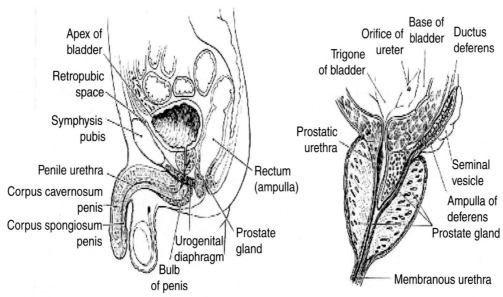

**FIGURE 20-1.** Sagittal section through the pelvis. **A:** The relationship of the prostate to the surrounding pelvic structures. **B:** An enlargement at the region of the prostate and bladder neck. (Reprinted from: Pollack A. *Radiation Oncology: Rationale, Technique and Results, 8th ed.* St. Louis: Mosby, 2003, with permission.)

in T1/T2 tumors when the Gleason score is 8–10 and/or the PSA is >20 ng/mL.[10] The Roach formula has been used to estimate lymph node risk in patients with T1/T2 disease utilizing only two variables, the pretreatment PSA, and the Gleason score.[16,17]

- Hematogenous metastases are typically to the axial skeleton (vertebral bodies and ribs).
- Soft tissue metastases, such as to the liver, lung or brain, can rarely occur late in the disease course.

## 3. DIAGNOSIS AND STAGING SYSTEM

### 3.1. Signs and Symptoms

- Many patients with prostate cancer present with urinary obstructive symptoms. In most cases, this is due to BPH, which is common in elderly men.
- An assessment of urinary function using the International Prostate Symptom Score (IPSS) questionnaire is a useful tool for determining whether patients will have

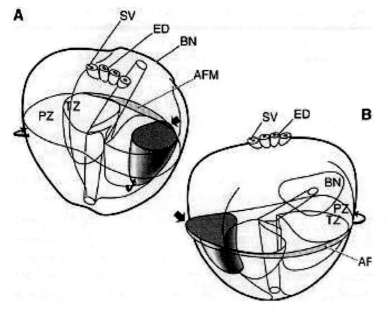

**FIGURE 20-2.** Transparent 3-D images of the prostate showing two zones of origin. A representative cancer in each zone is related to a transverse section through the midprostate (*curved arrows*). **A:** Transition zone cancer on left is viewed from the rectal surface and base. Cancer conforms to Z boundary but invades anteriorly into anterior fibromuscular stroma (*arrow*). **B:** Nontransition zone cancer on right is viewed from the anterior surface. Cancer conforms to TZ boundary but invades posterolaterally through the capsule (*arrow*) in the region where nerve penetration of capsule is common. TZ, transition zone; PZ, peripheral zone; AFM, anterior fibromuscular stroma; BN, bladder neck; ED, ejaculatory duct; SV, seminal vesicle. (Redrawn from: McNeal JE, Villers AA, Redwine EA, et al. Capsular penetration in prostate cancer. Significance for natural history and treatment. *Am J Surg Pathol* 1990;14:240–247, with permission.)

significantly more acute urinary morbidity with a seed implant compared with external beam radiotherapy (IPSS >8–10) or whether they should be considered for a transurethral resection of the prostate (TURP) prior to EBRT (IPSS >20).[18–22]

- Diagnosis is usually made by ultrasound-guided prostate biopsies provoked by either a change in the rate of increase in PSA (velocity >0.75 ng/mL per year), a high absolute PSA (>4.0 ng/mL) and/or a low free to total PSA (<25% when the absolute PSA is greater than 4.0–10 ng/mL).[23–25]
- When high risk features are present (a positive family history or African American descent),[26, 27] biopsies may be recommended at lower absolute PSAs (>2.5 ng/mL).[28–31]
- Bone pain is a sign of metastatic disease.

## 3.2. Physical Examination

- Digital rectal exam (DRE) is fundamental to the staging of prostate cancer.

## 3.3. Imaging

- Bone scan and CT scan of the pelvis are recommended when high risk features are present (palpable T3 disease, Gleason score of 8–10, or a pretreatment PSA >20 ng/mL).[32,33] Although the yield is low, some advocate a bone scan if the PSA is greater than 10 ng/mL.[33]
- Endorectal coil MRI has been advocated as a routine test for identifying extraprostatic extension.[34–37] We have used it when DRE reveals bulky disease suspicious for extraprostatic extension. If obvious extraprostatic extension

is identified in this setting, androgen deprivation would then be recommended for the patient. We have also used it for patients with limited intermediate risk features who are adamant about undergoing a seed implant.

- Because the consistency of the Prostascint scan has been criticized, it is not routinely used to evaluate for metastatic disease.[38,39]
- PET scanning has not been proven to contribute to prostate cancer staging.[38,40]

## 3.4. Staging

- The American Joint Committee on Cancer (AJCC) staging system for adenocarcinoma of the prostate is shown in Table 20-1.
- The current T-staging system is primarily based on the findings of the DRE.
- Although imaging studies, such as ultrasound and MRI, and laterality findings at biopsy are allowed in staging, this information has not been consistently applied.[41] The inclusion of imaging and biopsy results have resulted in stage migration and have not adequately been documented to predict for outcome independently of the DRE. A T2a on DRE may be upstaged to a T2b or T2c based on ultrasound or biopsy findings.
- As mentioned above, endorectal MRI has proven to be promising in the categorization of extraprostatic extension and has promise for supplementing the digital rectal exam.[34,35,42] However, it has not been routinely used.
- If imaging is included in the staging, it should be documented.

## TABLE 20-1. TNM CLASSIFICATION FOR CARCINOMA OF THE PROSTATE

**Primary Tumor (T)**

| | |
|---|---|
| TX | Primary tumor cannot be assessed |
| T0 | No evidence of primary tumor |
| T1 | Clinically inapparent tumor neither palpable nor visible by imaging |
| T1a | Tumor incidental histologic finding in 5% or less of resected tissue |
| T1b | Tumor incidental histologic finding in more than 5% of resected tissue |
| T1c | Tumor identified by needle biopsy (i.e., elevated PSA) |
| T2 | Tumor confined within prostate |
| T2a | Tumor involves one half of one lobe or less |
| T2b | Tumor involves more than one-half of one lobe but not both lobes |
| T2c | Tumor involves both lobes |
| T3 | Tumor extends through the prostate capsule |
| T3a | Extracapsular extension |
| T3b | Tumor invades seminal vesicle(s) |
| T4a | Tumor stris fixed or invades adjacent structures other than seminal vesicles: bladder neck, external sphincter, rectum, levator muscles, and/or pelvic wall |

**Regional Lymph Nodes (N)**

| | |
|---|---|
| NX | Regional lymph nodes cannot be assessed |
| N0 | No regional lymph node metastasis |
| N1 | Metastasis in regional lymph nodes |

**Distant Metastases (M)**

| | |
|---|---|
| MX | Presence of distant metastasis cannot be assessed |
| M0 | No distant metastasis |
| M1 | Distant metastasis |
| M1a | Non-regional lymph nodes |
| M1b | Bone(s) |
| M1c | Other site(s) with or without bone disease |

**Stage Grouping**

| | | | | |
|---|---|---|---|---|
| Stage I | T1a | N0 | M0 | G1 |
| Stage II | T1a | N0 | M0 | G2,3-4 |
| | T1b | N0 | M0 | Any G |
| | T1c | N0 | M0 | Any G |
| | T2 | N0 | M0 | Any G |
| Stage III | T3 | N0 | M0 | Any G |
| Stage IV | T4 | N0 | M0 | Any G |
| | Any T | N1 | M0 | Any G |
| | Any T | Any N | M1 | Any G |

From: Greene FL, American Joint Committee on Cancer, American Cancer Society. *AJCC Cancer Staging Manual, 6th ed.* New York: Springer, 2002.

# 4. ENDPOINTS

- Perhaps the most significant endpoint used is freedom from a rising PSA or freedom from biochemical failure. The rising PSA profile has been defined by an ASTRO consensus conference as three consecutive rises at follow-up visits measured at 3- to 6-month intervals with back-dating of the failure to the midpoint between the nadir and the first rise in PSA.[43] Backdating distorts the shape of the Kaplan-Meier curves, causing a flattening at the end of the curves, thereby resulting in falsely high estimates of biochemical-free survival exacerbated with short follow-up.[44–47]

- Biochemical failure is strongly related to local failure as well as distant metastasis and cause-specific death.[48–57] The relationship of biochemical failure to overall mortality is still not well defined.[50]

- When androgen deprivation is used, the ASTRO consensus definition is not accurate, with as many as 20% to 30% of patients being misclassified as a failure.[58] Several definitions have been proposed,[45,59–61] with the Houston definition[62] (rise of PSA of 2 over the last nadir) emerging as a promising alternative.

# 5. PROGNOSTIC FACTORS

## 5.1. T-Stage

- When patients with distant metastasis and lymph node involvement are excluded, T-stage is a significant predictor of biochemical, local, and distant failure.[63–65]

## 5.2. Prostate Specific Antigen

- Pretreatment PSA is the strongest predictor of biochemical failure and is also significantly associated with local and distant failure, cause specific death, and overall mortality.[48,56,64,65]

## 5.3. Gleason Score

- Adenocarcinoma is the most common histology and is seen in over 95% of cases of prostate cancer.

- The Gleason scoring system is the most frequently used grading system. A major and minor pattern, ranging from 1 to 5, are assigned based on the glandular pattern. The total score is the sum of the major and minor glandular patterns, which ranges from 2 to 10. The higher scores predict for more aggressive disease.[66]

- The Gleason score is a strong predictor of distant metastasis and survival.[64–66]

## 5.4. Percentage of Positive Biopsies

- The percentage of positive biopsies in the surgical literature has been found to be predictive of tumor volume, extracapsular extension, seminal vesicle invasion, lymph node involvement, and pathologic upgrading of Gleason score.[67–71]

- When the percentage of cores involved with cancer is greater than 50%, overall survival and cancer specific survival for patients with intermediate risk disease treated with radical prostatectomy or external beam radiotherapy (EBRT) is significantly worse, and becomes similar to the high-risk group.[64,65,72–78]

# 6. GENERAL MANAGEMENT

- Expectant management (i.e., watchful waiting) is a treatment option for elderly patients with a low likelihood of living 10 to 15 more years due to comorbid conditions. Patients who underwent expectant management died of prostate cancer in 18% to 30%, 42% to 70%, and 60% to 87% of cases when their Gleason score was 6, 7, or 8 to 10, respectively.[79–81]

- When undergoing curative therapy, patients at Fox Chase Cancer Center are stratified into risk groups based on the T stage, pretreatment PSA, and Gleason score (Table 20-2).

## TABLE 20-2. THE SINGLE AND DOUBLE HIGH RISK FACTOR MODELS

|  | Single Factor | Double Factor |
|---|---|---|
| **Low Risk** | PSA ≤10<br>GS 2–6<br>T1–T2c* | PSA <10<br>GS 2–6<br>T1–T2c |
| **Intermediate Risk** | Presence of 1 or more<br>PSA 10–20<br>GS 7<br>T1-T2c | Presence of 1<br>PSA >10<br>GS 7<br>T3 |
| **High Risk** | Presence of 1 or more<br>PSA >20<br>GS 8–10<br>T3 | Presence of 2 or 3<br>PSA >10<br>GS 7<br>T3 |

The single and double factor high risk models are patterned after that described by D'Amico et al.[142] and Zelefsky et al.[125]
*T2b has sometimes been considered intermediate risk and T2c has sometimes been considered intermediate or high risk.[123,142] In the Fox Chase Cancer Center database, these patients have about the same prognosis as patients with T2a disease in univariate and multivariate analysis, and so have been grouped in a favorable category here.
From: Chism DB, Hanlon AL, Horwitz EM, et al. A comparison of the single vs. double high-risk factor stratification systems for prostate cancer treated radiotherapy without androgen deprivation. *Int J Radiat Oncol Biol Phys* 2003;57:S270, with permission.

- Radical prostatectomy and radiotherapy offer comparable control rates for patients with favorable risk features (PSA <10 ng/mL, Gleason score <7 and T1/T2 disease), and for most patients with intermediate risk features (PSA 10–20 ng/mL or Gleason score 7 in the absence of high risk features).[82] However, there are no contemporary randomized studies to support this assumption.

- When intermediate features are present, low dose rate brachytherapy as monotherapy may have inferior results compared to external beam radiotherapy or surgery.[83,84]

- When high risk features are present (T3/T4 disease, PSA >20 or Gleason score 8–10), EBRT is typically recommended due to the high likelihood of positive surgical margins, extracapsular disease, seminal vesicle invasion and/or lymph node involvement, which would necessitate postoperative radiotherapy.[85]

- Long-term (2 to 3 years) androgen deprivation is combined with EBRT when any high risk feature is present.[66,86–89]

## 7. INTENSITY-MODULATED RADIATION THERAPY FOR PROSTATE CANCER

### 7.1. Target Volume Determination

- Gross tumor volume (GTV) for adenocarcinoma of the prostate is not visualized well and therefore is not contoured separately. Some investigators use functional imaging to distinguish a GTV for dose escalation with MR spectroscopy[90–92] or Prostascint scans,[93] but these are clearly investigational.

- The clinical target volume (CTV) is determined by the patient's respective risk group (low, intermediate, or high), which includes the prostate with or without the seminal vesicles and periprostatic lymph nodes (Tables 20-2 and 20-3).

- The CTV for low risk disease includes the prostate ± the proximal seminal vesicles.[94,95] The CTV for high risk disease covers the prostate, seminal vesicles, and periprostatic lymph nodes as outlined in Table 20-3.

- The coverage of lymph nodes outside the periprostatic and periseminal vesical nodal stations should be considered in the CTV for high risk patients based on the recent publication of RTOG 94-13.[96] The target volume specification for definitive IMRT in low, intermediate, and high risk prostate cancer is summarized in Table 20-3.

### 7.2. Target Volume Delineation

- At Fox Chase Cancer Center, the prostate, seminal vesicles, and periprostatic lymph node volumes are contoured on an MRI (0.23 Tesla open MRI simulator, Philips Panorama, Philips Medical Systems, Highland Heights, OH), which is coregistered to the simulation CT (Fig. 20-3).[97–100] The two scans are obtained within 1 hour of each other. Using CT simulation alone, the volume of the prostate may be overestimated by 30% to 40% due to difficulty in precisely determining the apex, base, and radial borders of the prostate (Fig. 20-4).[98,101]

- The seminal vesicles are contoured as described in Table 20-3 and shown in Figure 20-5.

- The peri-prostatic lymph nodes are contoured in patients with high risk features (Fig. 20-5).

### 7.3. Planning Target Volume Determination

- The planning target volume (PTV) is the added margin, which takes into account all the uncertainties in target position, including daily patient setup and positional changes due to rectal filling, bladder filling, and respiration during treatment.[102–106]

- Interfractional motion requires an additional 1.1 cm margin to ensure that the CTV is within the PTV 95% of the time.[105] In order to reduce this uncertainty, the prostate must be immobilized[107,108] (i.e., daily rectal balloon) or localized every day (i.e., using implantable fiducial with portal imaging,[109–112] daily transabdominal ultrasounds[113] or daily CT scans in

**TABLE 20-3. TARGET VOLUME AND DOSE SPECIFICATION FOR DEFINITIVE IMRT IN PROSTATE CANCER**

| Target | Low Risk Disease (Dose) | Intermediate Risk Disease (Dose) | High Risk Disease (Dose) |
|---|---|---|---|
| CTV 1 | Prostate +/− proximal seminal vesicles (74 Gy) | Prostate and proximal seminal vesicles (76–78 Gy) | Prostate, gross extracapsular disease and proximal seminal vesicles† (76–78 Gy) |
| CTV 2 | N/A* | Distal seminal vesicles (56 Gy) | Distal seminal vesicles and periprostatic lymph nodes (56 Gy) |

CTV, clinical target volume.
*Not applicable.
†For T3b disease: most, if not all, of the seminal vesicles are treated to the full dose.

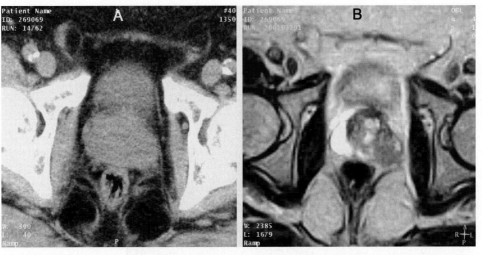

**FIGURE 20-3.** Axial images from CT and MR are coregistered for treatment planning. The MR image (**B**) demonstrates obvious extracapsular disease, which is not appreciated on the the CT scan (**A**).

the treatment room[114]). Displacement of the prostate during radiotherapy (intrafraction motion) is minimal,[111,115,116] although it can be increased in the prone position.[103,109,117]

- The absolute PTV margin used at Fox Chase Cancer Center is 5 mm posteriorly and 8 mm in all other dimensions. These tight margins can be used since the patients undergo daily imaging using the Nomos BAT ultrasound system (Nomos Corporation, Sewickey, PA) to correct for interfractional motion.[118–120]

### 7.4. Dose Specification

- There are several sequential dose escalation trials in the PSA era that have demonstrated a dose response for patients treated with 3D conformal radiotherapy (3DCRT).[121–126] The benefit seems to be most pronounced in patients with intermediate risk disease.

- These findings are echoed by the prospective randomized trial published by the M. D. Anderson Cancer Center, which demonstrated a significant benefit in freedom from failure for patients with a pretreatment PSA greater than 10 treated when treated to 78 Gy as compared to 70 Gy (Fig. 20-6).[121,127] In this trial, the dose was prescribed to the isocenter.

- The dose specifications used for definitive IMRT for prostate cancer at Fox Chase Cancer Center is dependent on the patient's risk stratification (Table 20-3). The prescription ensures that at least 95% of the PTV (D95) receives the prescription dose.

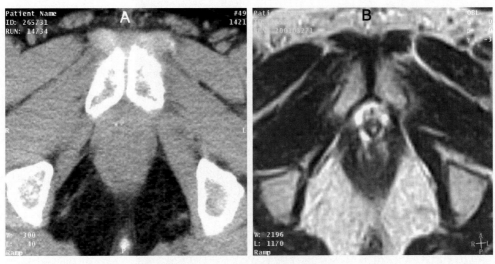

**FIGURE 20-4.** Corresponding axial CT (**A**) and MR (**B**) images of the prostate apex demonstrate a clear benefit at delineating the apex and the rectal/prostate interface.

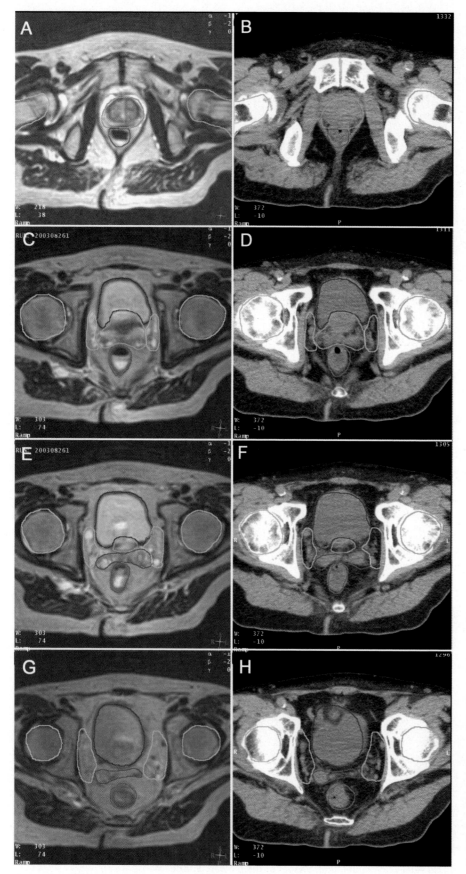

**FIGURE 20–5.** Delineation of the clinical target volume (CTV) in a prostate cancer patient with high risk disease through MR (*left column*) and CT (*right column*) axial images. The normal structures, including the rectum, bladder, and femoral necks are also delineated. At the mid-prostate, the prostate is contoured on the MR (**A, B**). Nearing the base, the prostate and proximal (1 cm) seminal vesicles are contoured (**C, D**) corresponding to the high risk CTV (*orange*). The periprostatic lymph nodes are contoured separately (*green*). At the base, the prostate (*orange*) alone makes up the high risk CTV, while the distal seminal vesicles (*blue*) and periprostatic lymph nodes (*green*) make up the low risk CTV (**E, F**). More superiorly, only the distal seminal vesicles (*blue*) and periprostatic lymph nodes (*green*) are contoured and make up the low risk CTV (**G, H**).

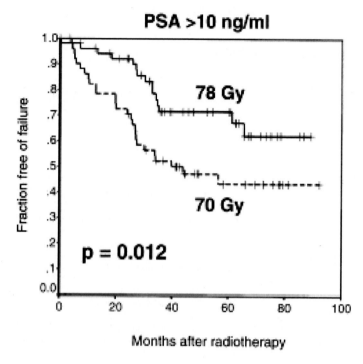

**FIGURE 20-6.** The Kaplan-Meier freedom from failure (FFF), which includes biochemical and clinical failures, curves are displayed for patients in the M. D. Anderson Cancer Center randomized trial who had a pretreatment PSA >10 ng/mL and were treated to 70 or 78 Gy. (Reprinted from: Pollack A, Zagars GK, Starkschall G, et al. Prostate cancer radiation dose response: results of the M. D. Anderson phase III randomized trial. *Int J Radiat Oncol Biol Phys* 2002;53:1097–1105, with permission)

## 7.5. Normal Tissue Delineation

- The entire circumference of the rectum is outlined from the ischial tuberosities to the sigmoid flexure with the rectum empty (Fig. 20-5). The patients are given an enema prior to simulation, which gives a worse case scenario in regards to planning and evaluating the dose volume histogram (DVH) of the rectum.

- At Fox Chase Cancer Center, patients are treated with a half-full bladder, since daily localization is performed with an abdominal ultrasound. The half-full bladder also minimizes the volume of bladder receiving a significant dose of radiation during treatment. The entire circumference of the bladder is contoured.

- Currently, no effort is made to contour the urethra, neurovascular bundle, or penile bulb.

## 7.6. Suggested Normal Tissue Dose Constraints

- The relationship between normal tissue complication risk in the management of prostate and radiation dose and volume for grade 2 and 3 late rectal bleeding has been well-established.[125,128–136] In contrast, predictors of late bladder injuries are more elusive due to the longer onset of injury and the more severe volume changes during therapy.

- DVH analysis from the M. D. Anderson Cancer Center randomized dose finding study demonstrated higher rectal complications (≥grade 2) when more than 25% of the rectal volume received at least 70 Gy (Fig. 20-7).[137,138] The volume of rectum was outlined completely from the ischial tuberosities to 11 cm superiorly.

- Other significant published DVH criteria demonstrating increased rectal bleeding are greater than 15 cc (absolute volume) of rectum receiving the prescription dose and enclosure of the entire rectum by the 50% isodose line at the isocenter.[134,136,139]

- Several investigators have determined that the rectal volume that receives an intermediate dose (40–60 Gy) is also a significant predictor of rectal morbidity.[131,134]

- The constraints for the rectum used at Fox Chase Cancer Center are to keep the volume of rectum that receives greater than or equal to 65 Gy at less than or equal to 17%. A second constraint is to keep the volume of rectum that receives greater than or equal to 40 Gy at less than or equal to 35%.

- The constraints for the bladder are more arbitrary, limiting the volume of bladder receiving greater than or equal to 65 Gy and greater than or equal to 40 Gy to less than or equal to 25% and less than or equal to 50%, respectively.

- The constraint for the right and left femoral head is to limit the volume receiving 50 Gy below 10%.

- In addition to DVH analyses, a slice-by-slice (axial and sagittal) analysis of the isodose lines is essential to ensure that the 90% isodose line falls within the half-width margin of the rectum and the 50% isodose line falls within the full-width of the rectum on all axial slices (Fig. 20-8A–C).

*Text continues on page 320.*

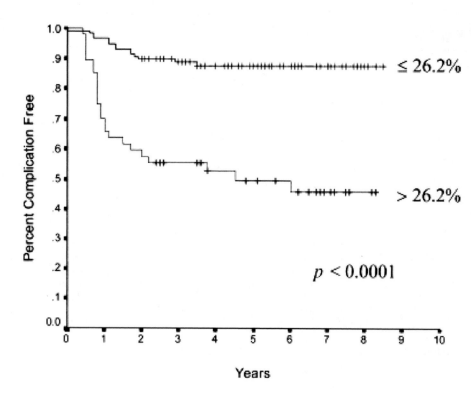

**FIGURE 20-7.** The Kaplan-Meier freedom from a grade 2 or higher rectal complication curves are for patients treated with conformal radiotherapy boost technique in the M. D. Anderson Cancer Center randomized trial. The patients are subdivided through DVH analysis by whether ≤26.2% vs >26.2% of the rectal volume received ≥70 Gy. (Reprinted from: Huang EH, Pollack A, Levy L, et al. Late rectal toxicity: dose-volume effects of conformal radiotherapy for prostate cancer. *Int J Radiat Oncol Biol Phys* 2002;54:1314–1321, with permission.)

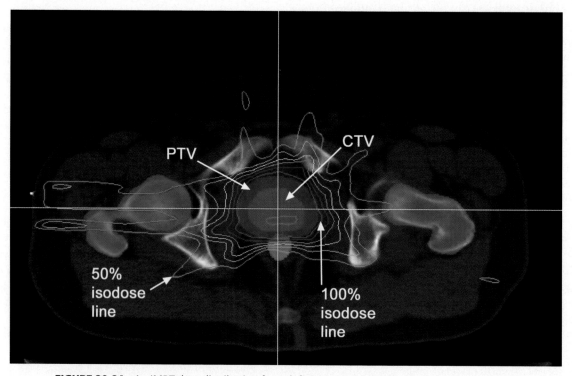

**FIGURE 20-8A.** An IMRT dose distribution for a definitive treatment for prostate cancer. The axial isodose distribution from the 50% (*dark green*) to 100% (*magenta*) are illustrated in 10% increments. This plan demonstrates the 100% isodose line to conform to the PTV (*outer red colorwash*) with a rapid fall-off in the dose posteriorly. CTV, *inner red colorwash*; rectum, green colorwash; femoral heads, *purple and orange colorwash.*

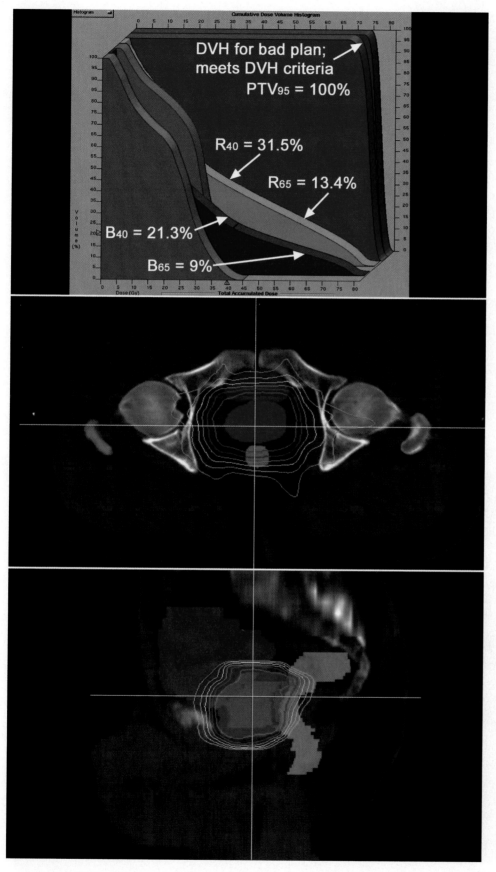

**FIGURE 20-8B.** An IMRT dose distribution for a definitive treatment for prostate cancer. The DVH criteria were met with this IMRT plan, although the corresponding axial and sagittal isodose distributions are poor with the entire circumference of the rectum receiving >50% of the dose. CTV, *inner red colorwash*; bladder, *dark purple colorwash*; rectum, *green colorwash*; femoral heads, *purple and orange colorwash*.

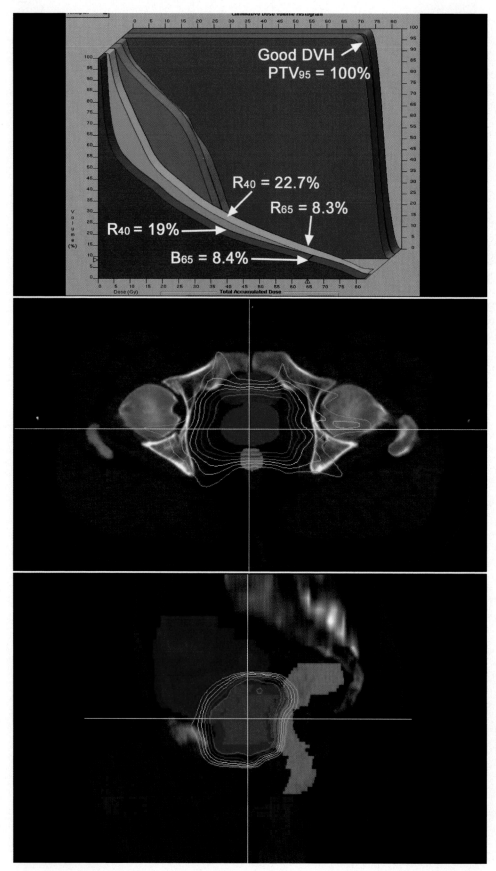

**FIGURE 20-8C.** An IMRT dose distribution for a definitive treatment for prostate cancer. The same patient with an improved plan demonstrates a similar DVH meeting the criteria for PTV coverage and normal tissue contraints, although the corresponding axial and sagittal isodose distributions are much better with a much more rapid falloff in the dose posteriorly. CTV, *inner red colorwash*; bladder, *dark purple colorwash*; rectum, *green colorwash*; femoral heads, *purple and orange colorwash*.

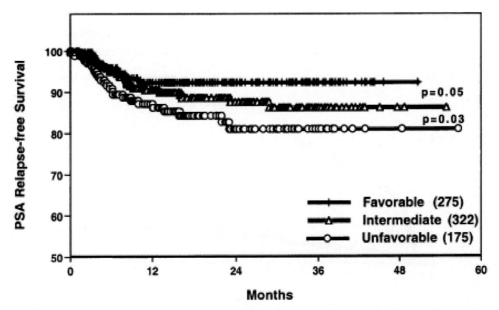

**FIGURE 20-9.** The Kaplan-Meier freedom from PSA relapse curves for favorable, intermediate, and high risk patients treated with IMRT at Memorial Sloan-Kettering Cancer Center. (Reprinted from: Zelefsky MJ, Fuks Z, Hunt M, et al. High-dose intensity modulated radiation therapy for prostate cancer: early toxicity and biochemical outcome in 772 patients. *Int J Radiat Oncol Biol Phys* 2002;53:1111–1116, with permission.)

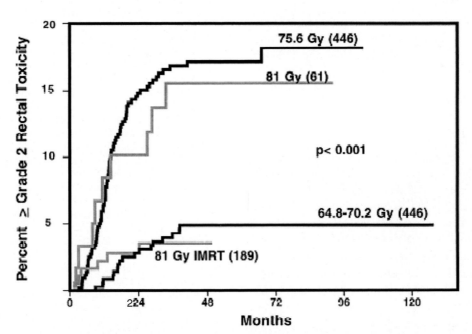

**FIGURE 20-10.** The Kaplan-Meier freedom from a grade 2 or higher rectal complication curves are displayed for patients treated with 3D-conformal and IMRT at Memorial Sloan-Kettering Cancer Center. (Reprinted from: Zelefsky MJ, Fuks Z, Happersett L, et al. Clinical experience with intensity modulated radiation therapy (IMRT) in prostate cancer. *Radiother Oncol* 2000;55:241–249, with permission.)

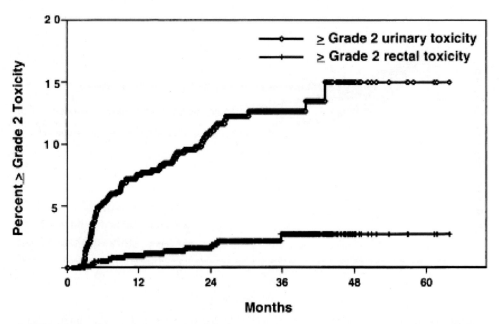

**FIGURE 20-11.** The Kaplan-Meier freedom from a grade 2 or higher late rectal and urinary toxicity curves for IMRT to 81 Gy and 86.4 Gy at Memorial Sloan-Kettering Cancer Center. (Reprinted from: Zelefsky MJ, Fuks Z, Hunt M, et al. High-dose intensity modulated radiation therapy for prostate cancer: early toxicity and biochemical outcome in 772 patients. *Int J Radiat Oncol Biol Phys* 2002;53:1111–1116, with permission.)

## 7.7. IMRT Results

■ The 3-year actuarial PSA relapse-free survival for 772 patients treated with IMRT at Memorial Sloan-Kettering Cancer Center (MSKCC) was 92%, 86%, and 81% for patients with low risk, intermediate risk, and high risk, respectively (Fig. 20-9).[140] The risk groups used at MSKCC were defined by the double factor system.

## 7.8. IMRT Morbidity

■ Zelefsky et al. from MSKCC, who have the most experience with IMRT for prostate cancer, has demonstrated a significant decrease in grade 2 and higher rectal complications with the use of IMRT as compared to 3DCRT (Fig. 20-10).[141] The complication risk with IMRT at 81 Gy was equivalent to 3DCRT at doses 10 to 15 Gy and lower.

■ A more recent update continues to show low rectal toxicities, but no significant decrease in acute or chronic urinary morbidity (Fig. 20-11) with peripheral doses of 81 and 86.4 Gy.[140] This lack of clinical benefit with IMRT has been attributed to the inability to minimize the dose to the prostatic urethra, but could also be related to the use of an empty bladder during treatment.

## REFERENCES

1. McNeal JE, Redwine EA, Freiha FS, et al. Zonal distribution of prostatic adenocarcinoma. Correlation with histologic pattern and direction of spread. *Am J Surg Pathol* 1988;12:897–906.

2. Carrier S, Hricak H, Lee SS, et al. Radiation-induced decrease in nitric oxide synthase—containing nerves in the rat penis. *Radiology* 1995;195:95–99.

3. Goldstein I, Feldman MI, Deckers PJ, et al. Radiation-associated impotence. A clinical study of its mechanism. *JAMA* 1984;251:903–910.

4. Merrick GS, Butler WM, Dorsey AT, et al. A comparison of radiation dose to the neurovascular bundles in men with and without prostate brachytherapy-induced erectile dysfunction. *Int J Radiat Oncol Biol Phys* 2000;48:1069–1074.

5. Fisch BM, Pickett B, Weinberg V, et al. Dose of radiation received by the bulb of the penis correlates with risk of impotence after three-dimensional conformal radiotherapy for prostate cancer. *Urology* 2001;57:955–959.

6. Merrick GS, Butler WM, Wallner KE, et al. The importance of radiation doses to the penile bulb vs. crura in the development of postbrachytherapy erectile dysfunction. *Int J Radiat Oncol Biol Phys* 2002;54:1055–1062.

7. Diaz A, Roach M, 3rd, Marquez C, et al. Indications for and the significance of seminal vesicle irradiation during 3D conformal radiotherapy for localized prostate cancer. *Int J Radiat Oncol Biol Phys* 1994;30:323–329.

8. Partin AW, Yoo J, Carter HB, et al. The use of prostate specific antigen, clinical stage and Gleason score to predict pathological stage in men with localized prostate cancer. *J Urol* 1993;150:110–114.

9. Khan MA, Partin AW, Mangold LA, et al. Probability of biochemical recurrence by analysis of pathologic stage, Gleason score, and margin status for localized prostate cancer. *Urology* 2003;62:866–871.

10. Partin AW, Kattan MW, Subong EN, et al. Combination of prostate-specific antigen, clinical stage, and Gleason score to predict pathological stage of localized prostate cancer. A multi-institutional update. *JAMA* 1997;277:1445–1451.

11. Polascik TJ, Pearson JD, Partin AW. Multivariate models as predictors of pathological stage using Gleason score, clinical stage, and serum prostate-specific antigen. *Semin Urol Oncol* 1998;16:160–171.

12. Khan MA, Partin AW. Partin tables: past and present. *BJU Int* 2003;92:7–11.

13. Blute ML, Bergstralh EJ, Partin AW, et al. Validation of Partin tables for predicting pathological stage of clinically localized prostate cancer. *J Urol* 2000;164:1591–1595.

14. Heidenreich A, Varga Z, Von Knobloch R. Extended pelvic lymphadenectomy in patients undergoing radical prostatectomy: high incidence of lymph node metastasis. *J Urol* 2002; 167:1681–1686.

15. Clark T, Parekh DJ, Cookson MS, et al. Randomized prospective evaluation of extended versus limited lymph node dissection in patients with clinically localized prostate cancer. *J Urol* 2003;169:145–147; discussion 147–148.

16. Roach M, 3rd, Marquez C, Yuo HS, et al. Predicting the risk of lymph node involvement using the pre-treatment prostate specific antigen and Gleason score in men with clinically localized prostate cancer. *Int J Radiat Oncol Biol Phys* 1994;28:33–37.

17. Woo S, Kaplan I, Roach M, et al. Formula to estimate risk of pelvic lymph node metastasis from the total Gleason score for prostate cancer. *J Urol* 1988;140:387.

18. Locke J, Ellis W, Wallner K, et al. Risk factors for acute urinary retention requiring temporary intermittent catheterization after prostate brachytherapy: a prospective study. *Int J Radiat Oncol Biol Phys* 2002;52:712–719.

19. Gelblum DY, Potters L, Ashley R, et al. Urinary morbidity following ultrasound-guided transperineal prostate seed implantation. *Int J Radiat Oncol Biol Phys* 1999;45:59–67.

20. Terk MD, Stock RG, Stone NN. Identification of patients at increased risk for prolonged urinary retention following radioactive seed implantation of the prostate. *J Urol* 1998;160: 1379–1382.

21. Lee N, Wuu CS, Brody R, et al. Factors for predicting postimplantation urinary retention after permanent prostate brachytherapy. *Int J Radiat Oncol Biol Phys* 2000;48:1457–1460.

22. Crook J, McLean M, Catton C, et al. Factors influencing risk of acute urinary retention after TRUS-guided permanent prostate seed implantation. *Int J Radiat Oncol Biol Phys* 2002;52: 453–460.

23. Catalona WJ, Southwick PC, Slawin KM, et al. Comparison of percent free PSA, PSA density, and age-specific PSA cutoffs for prostate cancer detection and staging. *Urology* 2000;56: 255–260.

24. Partin AW, Oesterling JE. The clinical usefulness of percent free-PSA. *Urology* 1996;48:1–3.

25. Partin AW, Catalona WJ, Southwick PC, et al. Analysis of percent free prostate-specific antigen (PSA) for prostate cancer detection: influence of total PSA, prostate volume, and age. *Urology* 1996;48:55–61.

26. Roach M, 3rd, Lu J, Pilepich MV, et al. Race and survival of men treated for prostate cancer on radiation therapy oncology group phase III randomized trials. *J Urol* 2003;169: 245–250.

27. Catalona WJ, Partin AW, Slawin KM, et al. Percentage of free PSA in black versus white men for detection and staging of prostate cancer: a prospective multicenter clinical trial. *Urology* 2000;55:372–376.

28. Uzzo RG, Pinover WH, Horwitz EM, et al. Free prostate-specific antigen improves prostate cancer detection in a high-risk population of men with a normal total PSA and digital rectal examination. *Urology* 2003;61:754–759.

29. Catalona WJ, Partin AW, Finlay JA, et al. Use of percentage of free prostate-specific antigen to identify men at high risk of prostate cancer when PSA levels are 2.51 to 4 ng/mL and digital rectal examination is not suspicious for prostate cancer: an alternative model. *Urology* 1999;54:220–224.

30. Carlson GD, Calvanese CB, Partin AW. An algorithm combining age, total prostate-specific antigen (PSA), and percent free PSA to predict prostate cancer: results on 4298 cases. *Urology* 1998;52:455–461.

31. Walsh PC, Partin AW. Family history facilitates the early diagnosis of prostate carcinoma. *Cancer* 1997;80:1871–1874.

32. Engeler CE, Wasserman NF, Zhang G. Preoperative assessment of prostatic carcinoma by computerized tomography. Weaknesses and new perspectives. *Urology* 1992;40:346–350.

33. Oesterling JE, Martin SK, Bergstralh EJ, et al. The use of prostate-specific antigen in staging patients with newly diagnosed prostate cancer. *JAMA* 1993;269:57–60.

34. D'Amico AV, Schnall M, Whittington R, et al. Endorectal coil magnetic resonance imaging identifies locally advanced prostate cancer in select patients with clinically localized disease. *Urology* 1998;51:449–454.

35. D'Amico AV, Whittington R, Schnall M, et al. The impact of the inclusion of endorectal coil magnetic resonance imaging in a multivariate analysis to predict clinically unsuspected extraprostatic cancer. *Cancer* 1995;75:2368–2372.

36. Tempany CM, Zhou X, Zerhouni EA, et al. Staging of prostate cancer: results of Radiology Diagnostic Oncology Group project comparison of three MR imaging techniques. *Radiology* 1994;192:47–54.

37. Perrotti M, Kaufman RP, Jr, Jennings TA, et al. Endo-rectal coil magnetic resonance imaging in clinically localized prostate cancer: is it accurate? *J Urol* 1996;156:106–109.

38. Yu KK, Hricak H. Imaging prostate cancer. *Radiol Clin North Am* 2000;38:59–85, viii.

39. Elgamal AA, Troychak MJ, Murphy GP. ProstaScint scan may enhance identification of prostate cancer recurrences after prostatectomy, radiation, or hormone therapy: analysis of 136 scans of 100 patients. *Prostate* 1998;37:261–269.

40. Hofer C, Laubenbacher C, Block T, et al. Fluorine-18-fluorodeoxyglucose positron emission tomography is useless for the detection of local recurrence after radical prostatectomy. *Eur Urol* 1999;36:31–35.

41. Buyyounouski MK, Horwitz EM, Hanlon AL, et al. Positive prostate biopsy laterality and implications for staging. *Urology* 2003;62:298–303.

42. D'Amico AV, Whittington R, Malkowicz SB, et al. Role of percent positive biopsies and endorectal coil MRI in predicting prognosis in intermediate-risk prostate cancer patients. *Cancer J Sci Am* 1996;2:343.

43. Cox JD, Gallagher MJ, Hammond EH, et al. Consensus statements on radiation therapy of prostate cancer: guidelines for prostate re-biopsy after radiation and for radiation therapy with rising prostate-specific antigen levels after radical prostatectomy. American Society for Therapeutic Radiology and Oncology Consensus Panel. *J Clin Oncol* 1999;17:1155.

44. Horwitz EM, Thames HD, Kuban DA, et al. Definitions of biochemical failure that best predict clinical failure in prostate cancer patients treated with external beam radiation alone—a multi-institutional pooled analysis. *Int J Radiat Oncol Biol Phys* 2003;57:S147.

45. Kestin LL, Vicini FA, Ziaja EL, et al. Defining biochemical cure for prostate carcinoma patients treated with external beam radiation therapy. *Cancer* 1999;86:1557–1566.

46. Vicini FA, Kestin LL, Martinez AA. The importance of adequate follow-up in defining treatment success after external beam irradiation for prostate cancer. *Int J Radiat Oncol Biol Phys* 1999;45:553–561.

47. Horwitz EM, Uzzo RG, Hanlon AL, et al. Modifying the American Society for Therapeutic Radiology and Oncology definition of biochemical failure to minimize the influence of backdating in patients with prostate cancer treated with 3-dimensional conformal radiation therapy alone. *J Urol* 2003;169: 2153–2157; discussion 2157–2159.

48. Zagars GK, Kavadi VS, Pollack A, et al. The source of pretreatment serum prostate-specific antigen in clinically localized prostate cancer--T, N, or M? *Int J Radiat Oncol Biol Phys* 1995;32:21–32.

49. Zagars GK, Pollack A. Kinetics of serum prostate-specific antigen after external beam radiation for clinically localized prostate cancer. *Radiother Oncol* 1997;44:213–221.

50. Pollack A, Hanlon AL, Movsas B, et al. Biochemical failure as a determinant of distant metastasis and death in prostate cancer treated with radiotherapy. *Int J Radiat Oncol Biol Phys* 2003;57:19–23.

51. Zagars GK, Pollack A. The fall and rise of prostate-specific antigen. Kinetics of serum prostate-specific antigen levels after radiation therapy for prostate cancer. *Cancer* 1993;72:832–842.

52. Pollack A, Zagars GK, Kavadi VS. Prostate specific antigen doubling time and disease relapse after radiotherapy for prostate cancer. *Cancer* 1994;74:670–678.

53. Hanks GE, Hanlon AL, Pinover WH, et al. Survival advantage for prostate cancer patients treated with high-dose three-dimensional conformal radiotherapy. *Cancer J Sci Am* 1999;5:152–158.

54. Sandler HM, Dunn RL, McLaughlin PW, et al. Overall survival after prostate-specific-antigen-detected recurrence following conformal radiation therapy. *Int J Radiat Oncol Biol Phys* 2000;48:629–633.

55. Valicenti R, Lu J, Pilepich M, et al. Survival advantage from higher-dose radiation therapy for clinically localized prostate cancer treated on the Radiation Therapy Oncology Group trials. *J Clin Oncol* 2000;18:2740–2746.

56. Zagars GK, Pollack A. Radiation therapy for T1 and T2 prostate cancer: prostate-specific antigen and disease outcome. *Urology* 1995;45:476–483.

57. Kupelian PA, Buchsbaum JC, Patel C, et al. Impact of biochemical failure on overall survival after radiation therapy for localized prostate cancer in the PSA era. *Int J Radiat Oncol Biol Phys* 2002;52:704–711.

58. Buyyounouski MK, Hanlon AL, Pollack A. The temporal kinetics of PSA after 3D-conformal radiotherapy with androgen deprivation. *Int J Radiat Oncol Biol Phys* 2003;57:S147–S148.

59. Sandler HM, DeSilvio ML. Surrogate end points for prostate cancer: what is prostate-specific antigen telling us? *J Natl Cancer Inst* 2003;95:1352–1353.

60. Kuban DA, Thames HD, Levy LB, et al. Long-term multi-institutional analysis of stage T1-T2 prostate cancer treated with radiotherapy in the PSA era. *Int J Radiat Oncol Biol Phys* 2003;57:915–928.

61. Thames H, Kuban D, Levy L, et al. Comparison of alternative biochemical failure definitions based on clinical outcome in 4839 prostate cancer patients treated by external beam radiotherapy between 1986 and 1995. *Int J Radiat Oncol Biol Phys* 2003;57:929–943.

62. Pickles T, Kim-Sing C, Morris WJ, et al. Evaluation of the Houston biochemical relapse definition in men treated with prolonged neoadjuvant and adjuvant androgen ablation and assessment of follow-up lead-time bias. *Int J Radiat Oncol Biol Phys* 2003;57:11–18.

63. Zagars GK, Geara FB, Pollack A, et al. The T classification of clinically localized prostate cancer. An appraisal based on disease outcome after radiation therapy. *Cancer* 1994;73:1904–1912.

64. D'Amico AV, Cote K, Loffredo M, et al. Pretreatment predictors of time to cancer specific death after prostate specific antigen failure. *J Urol* 2003;169:1320–1324.

65. D'Amico AV, Cote K, Loffredo M, et al. Determinants of prostate cancer specific survival following radiation therapy during the prostate specific antigen era. *J Urol* 2003;170:S42–S46; discussion S46–S47.

66. Hanks GE, Pajak TF, Porter A, et al. Phase III trial of long-term adjuvant androgen deprivation after neoadjuvant hormonal cytoreduction and radiotherapy in locally advanced carcinoma of the prostate: the Radiation Therapy Oncology Group Protocol 92-02. *J Clin Oncol* 2003;21:3972–3978.

67. D'Amico AV, Whittington R, Malkowicz SB, et al. Combination of the preoperative PSA level, biopsy gleason score, percentage of positive biopsies, and MRI T-stage to predict early PSA failure in men with clinically localized prostate cancer. *Urology* 2000;55:572–577.

68. Cheng L, Slezak J, Bergstralh EJ, et al. Preoperative prediction of surgical margin status in patients with prostate cancer treated by radical prostatectomy. *J Clin Oncol* 2000;18:2862–2868.

69. Veltri RW, Miller MC, Partin AW, et al. Prediction of prostate carcinoma stage by quantitative biopsy pathology. *Cancer* 2001;91:2322–2328.

70. Lewis JS, Jr., Vollmer RT, Humphrey PA. Carcinoma extent in prostate needle biopsy tissue in the prediction of whole gland tumor volume in a screening population. *Am J Clin Pathol* 2002;118:442–450.

71. Graefen M, Ohori M, Karakiewicz PI, et al. Assessment of the enhancement in predictive accuracy provided by systematic biopsy in predicting outcome for clinically localized prostate cancer. *J Urol* 2004;171:200–203.

72. D'Amico AV, Whittington R, Malkowicz SB, et al. Clinical utility of the percentage of positive prostate biopsies in defining biochemical outcome after radical prostatectomy for patients with clinically localized prostate cancer. *J Clin Oncol* 2000;18:1164–1172.

73. D'Amico AV, Whittington R, Malkowicz SB, et al. Clinical utility of percent-positive prostate biopsies in predicting biochemical outcome after radical prostatectomy or external-beam radiation therapy for patients with clinically localized prostate cancer. *Mol Urol* 2000;4:171–175;discussion 177.

74. D'Amico AV, Schultz D, Silver B, et al. The clinical utility of the percent of positive prostate biopsies in predicting biochemical outcome following external-beam radiation therapy for patients with clinically localized prostate cancer. *Int J Radiat Oncol Biol Phys* 2001;49:679–684.

75. D'Amico AV, Keshaviah A, Manola J, et al. Clinical utility of the percentage of positive prostate biopsies in predicting prostate cancer-specific and overall survival after radiotherapy for patients with localized prostate cancer. *Int J Radiat Oncol Biol Phys* 2002;53:581–587.

76. Lieberfarb ME, Schultz D, Whittington R, et al. Using PSA, biopsy Gleason score, clinical stage, and the percentage of positive biopsies to identify optimal candidates for prostate-only radiation therapy. *Int J Radiat Oncol Biol Phys* 2002;53:898–903.

77. Yoon JH, Chen MH, Renshaw AA, et al. Predictive factor analysis as the basis for the clinical utility of percent positive prostate biopsies in patients with intermediate-risk prostate cancer. *Urology* 2002;60:454–457.

78. D'Amico AV, Whittington R, Malkowicz SB, et al. Investigating the clinical utility of the percent of positive prostate biopsies in predicting PSA outcome following local therapy for patients with clinically localized prostate cancer. *Prostate Cancer Prostatic Dis* 2000;3:259–264.

79. Albertsen PC, Hanley JA, Gleason DF, et al. Competing risk analysis of men aged 55 to 74 years at diagnosis managed conservatively for clinically localized prostate cancer. *JAMA* 1998;280:975–980.

80. Johansson JE, Holmberg L, Johansson S, et al. Fifteen-year survival in prostate cancer. A prospective, population-based study in Sweden. *JAMA* 1997;277:467–471.

81. Chodak GW, Thisted RA, Gerber GS, et al. Results of conservative management of clinically localized prostate cancer. *N Engl J Med* 1994;330:242–248.

82. Vicini FA, Martinez A, Hanks G, et al. An interinstitutional and interspecialty comparison of treatment outcome data for patients with prostate carcinoma based on predefined prognostic categories and minimum follow-up. *Cancer* 2002;95:2126–2135.

83. D'Amico AV, Whittington R, Malkowicz SB, et al. Biochemical outcome after radical prostatectomy, external beam radiation therapy, or interstitial radiation therapy for clinically localized prostate cancer. *JAMA* 1998;280:969–974.

84. Brachman DG, Thomas T, Hilbe J, et al. Failure-free survival following brachytherapy alone or external beam irradiation alone for T1-2 prostate tumors in 2222 patients: results from a single practice. *Int J Radiat Oncol Biol Phys* 2000;48:111–117.

85. Pound CR, Partin AW, Eisenberger MA, et al. Natural history of progression after PSA elevation following radical prostatectomy. *JAMA* 1999;281:1591–1597.

86. Bolla M, Collette L, Blank L, et al. Long-term results with immediate androgen suppression and external irradiation in patients with locally advanced prostate cancer (an EORTC study): a phase III randomised trial. *Lancet* 2002;360:103–106.

87. Bolla M, Gonzalez D, Warde P, et al. Improved survival in patients with locally advanced prostate cancer treated with radiotherapy and goserelin. *N Engl J Med* 1997;337:295–300.

88. Lawton CA, Winter K, Murray K, et al. Updated results of the phase III Radiation Therapy Oncology Group (RTOG) trial 85-31 evaluating the potential benefit of androgen suppression following standard radiation therapy for unfavorable prognosis carcinoma of the prostate. *Int J Radiat Oncol Biol Phys* 2001;49:937–946.

89. Pilepich MV, Caplan R, Byhardt RW, et al. Phase III trial of androgen suppression using goserelin in unfavorable-prognosis carcinoma of the prostate treated with definitive radiotherapy: report of Radiation Therapy Oncology Group Protocol 85-31. *J Clin Oncol* 1997;15:1013–1021.

90. Roach M, 3rd, Kurhanewicz J, Carroll P. Spectroscopy in prostate cancer: hope or hype? *Oncology (Huntingt)* 2001;15:1399–1410; discussion 1415–1416, 1418.

91. Xia P, Pickett B, Vigneault E, et al. Forward or inversely planned segmental multileaf collimator IMRT and sequential tomotherapy to treat multiple dominant intraprostatic lesions of prostate cancer to 90 Gy. *Int J Radiat Oncol Biol Phys* 2001;51:244–254.

92. Pickett B, Vigneault E, Kurhanewicz J, et al. Static field intensity modulation to treat a dominant intra-prostatic lesion to 90 Gy compared to seven field 3-dimensional radiotherapy. *Int J Radiat Oncol Biol Phys* 1999;44:921–929.

93. Ellis RJ, Vertocnik A, Kim E, et al. Four-year biochemical outcome after radioimmunoguided transperineal brachytherapy for patients with prostate adenocarcinoma. *Int J Radiat Oncol Biol Phys* 2003;57:362–370.

94. Sohayda C, Kupelian PA, Levin HS, et al. Extent of extracapsular extension in localized prostate cancer. *Urology* 2000;55:382–386.

95. Teh BS, Bastasch MD, Wheeler TM, et al. IMRT for prostate cancer: defining target volume based on correlated pathologic volume of disease. *Int J Radiat Oncol Biol Phys* 2003;56:184–191.

96. Roach M, 3rd, DeSilvio M, Lawton C, et al. Phase III trial comparing whole-pelvic versus prostate-only radiotherapy and neoadjuvant versus adjuvant combined androgen suppression: Radiation Therapy Oncology Group 9413. *J Clin Oncol* 2003;21:1904–1911.

97. Schubert K, Wenz F, Krempien R, et al. [Possibilities of an open magnetic resonance scanner integration in therapy simulation and three-dimensional radiotherapy planning]. *Strahlenther Onkol* 1999;175:225–231.

98. Krempien RC, Schubert K, Zierhut D, et al. Open low-field magnetic resonance imaging in radiation therapy treatment planning. *Int J Radiat Oncol Biol Phys* 2002;53:1350–1360.

99. Kagawa K, Lee WR, Schultheiss TE, et al. Initial clinical assessment of CT-MRI image fusion software in localization of the prostate for 3D conformal radiation therapy. *Int J Radiat Oncol Biol Phys* 1997;38:319–325.

100. Mah D, Steckner M, Hanlon A, et al. MRI simulation: effect of gradient distortions on three-dimensional prostate cancer plans. *Int J Radiat Oncol Biol Phys* 2002;53:757–765.

101. Rasch C, Barillot I, Remeijer P, et al. Definition of the prostate in CT and MRI: a multi-observer study. *Int J Radiat Oncol Biol Phys* 1999;43:57–66.

102. Schild SE, Casale HE, Bellefontaine LP. Movements of the prostate due to rectal and bladder distension: implications for radiotherapy. *Med Dosim* 1993;18:13–15.

103. Crook JM, Raymond Y, Salhani D, et al. Prostate motion during standard radiotherapy as assessed by fiducial markers. *Radiother Oncol* 1995;37:35–42.

104. Beard CJ, Kijewski P, Bussiere M, et al. Analysis of prostate and seminal vesicle motion: implications for treatment planning. *Int J Radiat Oncol Biol Phys* 1996;34:451–458.

105. Antolak JA, Rosen II, Childress CH, et al. Prostate target volume variations during a course of radiotherapy. *Int J Radiat Oncol Biol Phys* 1998;42:661–672.

106. Mageras GS, Fuks Z, Leibel SA, et al. Computerized design of target margins for treatment uncertainties in conformal radiotherapy. *Int J Radiat Oncol Biol Phys* 1999;43:437–445.

107. McGary JE, Teh BS, Butler EB, et al. Prostate immobilization using a rectal balloon. *J Appl Clin Med Phys* 2002;3:6–11.

108. Teh BS, McGary JE, Dong L, et al. The use of rectal balloon during the delivery of intensity modulated radiotherapy (IMRT) for prostate cancer: more than just a prostate gland immobilization device? *Cancer J* 2002;8:476–483.

109. Kitamura K, Shirato H, Shimizu S, et al. Registration accuracy and possible migration of internal fiducial gold marker implanted in prostate and liver treated with real-time tumor-tracking radiation therapy (RTRT). *Radiother Oncol* 2002;62:275–281.

110. Wu J, Haycocks T, Alasti H, et al. Positioning errors and prostate motion during conformal prostate radiotherapy using on-line isocentre set-up verification and implanted prostate markers. *Radiother Oncol* 2001;61:127–133.

111. Malone S, Crook JM, Kendal WS, et al. Respiratory-induced prostate motion: quantification and characterization. *Int J Radiat Oncol Biol Phys* 2000;48:105–109.

112. Pouliot J, Aubin M, Langen KM, et al. (Non)-migration of radiopaque markers used for on-line localization of the prostate with an electronic portal imaging device. *Int J Radiat Oncol Biol Phys* 2003;56:862–866.

113. Chandra A, Dong L, Huang E, et al. Experience of ultrasound-based daily prostate localization. *Int J Radiat Oncol Biol Phys* 2003;56:436–447.

114. Hua C, Lovelock DM, Mageras GS, et al. Development of a semi-automatic alignment tool for accelerated localization of the prostate. *Int J Radiat Oncol Biol Phys* 2003;55:811–824.

115. Huang E, Dong L, Chandra A, et al. Intrafraction prostate motion during IMRT for prostate cancer. *Int J Radiat Oncol Biol Phys* 2002;53:261–268.

116. Mah D, Freedman G, Milestone B, et al. Measurement of intrafractional prostate motion using magnetic resonance imaging. *Int J Radiat Oncol Biol Phys* 2002;54:568–575.

117. McLaughlin PW, Wygoda A, Sahijdak W, et al. The effect of patient position and treatment technique in conformal treatment of prostate cancer. *Int J Radiat Oncol Biol Phys* 1999;45:407–413.

118. Lattanzi J, McNeeley S, Donnelly S, et al. Ultrasound-based stereotactic guidance in prostate cancer—quantification of organ motion and set-up errors in external beam radiation therapy. *Comput Aided Surg* 2000;5:289–295.

119. Lattanzi J, McNeeley S, Hanlon A, et al. Ultrasound-based stereotactic guidance of precision conformal external beam radiation therapy in clinically localized prostate cancer. *Urology* 2000;55:73–78.

120. Lattanzi J, McNeeley S, Pinover W, et al. A comparison of daily CT localization to a daily ultrasound-based system in prostate cancer. *Int J Radiat Oncol Biol Phys* 1999;43:719–725.

121. Pollack A, Zagars GK, Starkschall G, et al. Prostate cancer radiation dose response: results of the M. D. Anderson phase III randomized trial. *Int J Radiat Oncol Biol Phys* 2002;53:1097–1105.

122. Pollack A, Smith LG, von Eschenbach AC. External beam radiotherapy dose response characteristics of 1127 men with prostate cancer treated in the PSA era. *Int J Radiat Oncol Biol Phys* 2000;48:507–512.

123. Lyons JA, Kupelian PA, Mohan DS, et al. Importance of high radiation doses (72 Gy or greater) in the treatment of stage T1-T3 adenocarcinoma of the prostate. *Urology* 2000;55:85–90.

124. Kupelian PA, Kuban D, Thames H, et al. Improved biochemical relapse-free survival with increased external radiation doses in patients with localized prostate cancer: the combined experience of nine institutions in patients treated in 1994 and 1995. *Int J Radiat Oncol Biol Phys* 2003;57:S271–S272.

125. Zelefsky MJ, Leibel SA, Gaudin PB, et al. Dose escalation with three-dimensional conformal radiation therapy affects the outcome in prostate cancer. *Int J Radiat Oncol Biol Phys* 1998;41:491–500.

126. Hanks GE, Hanlon AL, Epstein B, et al. Dose response in prostate cancer with 8–12 years' follow-up. *Int J Radiat Oncol Biol Phys* 2002;54:427–435.

127. Pollack A, Zagars GK, Smith LG, et al. Preliminary results of a randomized radiotherapy dose-escalation study comparing 70 Gy with 78 Gy for prostate cancer. *J Clin Oncol* 2000;18:3904–3911.

128. Shipley WU, Verhey LJ, Munzenrider JE, et al. Advanced prostate cancer: the results of a randomized comparative trial of high dose irradiation boosting with conformal protons compared with conventional dose irradiation using photons alone. *Int J Radiat Oncol Biol Phys* 1995;32:3–12.

129. Lee WR, Hanks GE, Hanlon AL, et al. Lateral rectal shielding reduces late rectal morbidity following high dose three-dimensional conformal radiation therapy for clinically localized prostate cancer: further evidence for a significant dose effect. *Int J Radiat Oncol Biol Phys* 1996;35:251–257.

130. Ryu JK, Winter K, Michalski JM, et al. Interim report of toxicity from 3D conformal radiation therapy (3DCRT) for prostate cancer on 3DOG/RTOG 9406, level III (79.2 Gy). *Int J Radiat Oncol Biol Phys* 2002;54:1036–1046.

131. Benk VA, Adams JA, Shipley WU, et al. Late rectal bleeding following combined X-ray and proton high dose irradiation for patients with stages T3-T4 prostate carcinoma. *Int J Radiat Oncol Biol Phys* 1993;26:551–557.

132. Boersma LJ, van den Brink M, Bruce AM, et al. Estimation of the incidence of late bladder and rectum complications after high-dose (70–78 GY) conformal radiotherapy for prostate cancer, using dose-volume histograms. *Int J Radiat Oncol Biol Phys* 1998;41:83–92.

133. Wachter S, Gerstner N, Goldner G, et al. Rectal sequelae after conformal radiotherapy of prostate cancer: dose-volume histograms as predictive factors. *Radiother Oncol* 2001;59:65–70.

134. Jackson A, Skwarchuk MW, Zelefsky MJ, et al. Late rectal bleeding after conformal radiotherapy of prostate cancer. II. Volume effects and dose-volume histograms. *Int J Radiat Oncol Biol Phys* 2001;49:685–698.

135. Fiorino C, Cozzarini C, Vavassori V, et al. Relationships between DVHs and late rectal bleeding after radiotherapy for prostate cancer: analysis of a large group of patients pooled from three institutions. *Radiother Oncol* 2002;64:1–12.

136. Kupelian PA, Reddy CA, Carlson TP, et al. Dose/volume relationship of late rectal bleeding after external beam radiotherapy for localized prostate cancer: absolute or relative rectal volume? *Cancer J* 2002;8:62–66.

137. Storey MR, Pollack A, Zagars G, et al. Complications from radiotherapy dose escalation in prostate cancer: preliminary results of a randomized trial. *Int J Radiat Oncol Biol Phys* 2000;48:635–642.

138. Huang EH, Pollack A, Levy L, et al. Late rectal toxicity: dose-volume effects of conformal radiotherapy for prostate cancer. *Int J Radiat Oncol Biol Phys* 2002;54:1314–1321.

139. Skwarchuk MW, Jackson A, Zelefsky MJ, et al. Late rectal toxicity after conformal radiotherapy of prostate cancer (I): multivariate analysis and dose-response. *Int J Radiat Oncol Biol Phys* 2000;47:103–113.

140. Zelefsky MJ, Fuks Z, Hunt M, et al. High-dose intensity modulated radiation therapy for prostate cancer: early toxicity and biochemical outcome in 772 patients. *Int J Radiat Oncol Biol Phys* 2002;53:1111–1116.

141. Zelefsky MJ, Fuks Z, Happersett L, et al. Clinical experience with intensity modulated radiation therapy (IMRT) in prostate cancer. *Radiother Oncol* 2000;55:241–249.

142. D'Amico AV, Desjardin A, Chung A, et al. Assessment of outcome prediction models for localized prostate cancer in patients managed with external beam radiation therapy. *Semin Urol Oncol* 1998;16:153–159.

143. Chism DB, Hanlon AL, Horwitz EM, et al. A comparison of the single vs. double high-risk factor stratification systems for prostate cancer treated radiotherapy without androgen deprivation. *Int J Radiat Oncol Biol Phys* 2003;57:S270.

144. Pollack A. *Radiation Oncology: Rationale, Technique and Results*, 8th ed. St. Louis: Mosby; 2003.

145. McNeal JE, Villers AA, Redwine EA, et al. Capsular penetration in prostate cancer. Significance for natural history and treatment. *Am J Surg Pathol* 1990;14:240–247.

# 21

# GYNECOLOGIC CANCERS

## ANUJA JHINGRAN

## 1. ANATOMY

- Gynecologic cancers can be subdivided into five major groups: endometrial, cervical, vulvar, vaginal, and ovarian/fallopian tube carcinomas. This chapter will discuss only carcinomas of the vulva, vagina, endometrium, and cervix, as these are the ones most commonly treated by radiation therapy.

### 1.1. Vulva

- The vulva comprises the mons pubis, clitoris, labia majora and minora, vestibule (containing the urethral meatus and hymenal remnant), perineal body, associated erectile tissues and muscles, and supporting subcutaneous tissues. Figure 21-1 shows the sections of the vulva.
- The vulva is bound by the anterior abdominal wall superiorly, the labial-crural folds laterally, and the anus posteriorly. It is perforated by the distal vagina, the urethra, and the greater vestibular glands.
- In women, the mons pubis is a hair-bearing, mounded fat pad that overlies the pubic symphysis.
- The clitoris is situated at the inferior aspect of the mons pubis, and the labia majora, which consist of elongated bands of skin, connective tissue, and subcutaneous fat that bridge the vulva and come together at the posterior labial commissure.
- Immediately medial to the labia majora are the labia minora, which are thin, pigmented structures comprising mostly of skin and fibrous tissue with little fat. At the junction of the labia minora and the vaginal vestibule is the duct opening for the greater vestibular (Bartholin's) gland.
- In addition to the clitoris, the midline vulvar structures below the mons pubis are the urethral meatus, the vaginal opening, and the perineal body.
- Lymphatic drainage of the vulva and lower portion of the vagina is primarily via the inguinal nodes (Fig. 21-2). These nodes are situated in the subcutaneous tissue overlying the femoral triangle and are bounded by the inguinal ligament in the cephalad direction, the sartorius muscle inferiorly and laterally, and the adductor longus

medially. Anatomically, this nodal group is divided into superficial and deep nodes on the basis of their location in reference to the fascia lata, the cribriform fascia over the fossa ovalis, and the femoral vessels.
- The ipsilateral flow from the vulva to the lymph nodes for the most part does not cross the labial crural fold laterally; in general, only midline structures (e.g., the clitoris and perineum) have bilateral drainage. Direct drainage from the clitoris to the pelvic nodes, bypassing the inguinal nodes, has been reported but is rare. The drainage from the vulva usually proceeds in an orderly fashion from the inguinal nodes to the external iliac and pelvic nodal chains.

### 1.2. Vagina

- The vagina is a hollow, pliable viscous structure that opens onto the vulva caudally and attaches to the cephalad uterine cervix.
- The vagina is richly supplied with mucosal and submucosal lymph nodes. The specific nodes at risk for metastasis depend on the primary tumor location. The drainage of the apical vagina is similar to that in the cervix, with initial spread to the obturator and hypogastric nodes. The lymph nodes of the posterior wall of the vagina anastomose with those of the anterior rectal wall, draining to the superior and inferior gluteal nodes. Tumors involving the lower third of the vagina drain either to the pelvic nodes or to the inguinofemoral lymph nodes by way of the vulvar lymph nodes (Fig. 21-3).

### 1.3. Endometrium and Cervix

- The uterus is a flattened, muscular, thick-walled, hollow structure that lies in the true pelvis between the bladder and the rectum and sigmoid colon. The uterus is divided by the internal os into two regions: the corpus (or body) and the cervix (Fig. 21-4).
- Uterine cancer that occurs in the uterine corpus is known as endometrial cancer. The endometrium is the mucous membrane of the uterus.

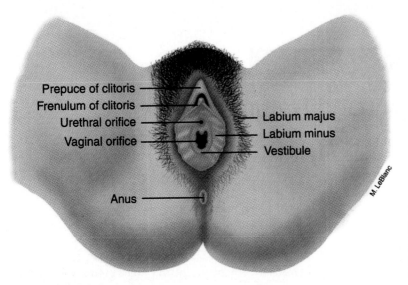

**FIGURE 21-1.** Anatomy of the external female genitalia. The major anatomic landmarks are labeled. (Adapted from: Eifel PJ, Levenback C. Cancer of the female lower genital tract. In: *ACS atlas of oncology: cervix, vulva, and vagina*. Ontario: B.C. Decker, Inc.; 2001:48.)

In the figure the following labels are shown:
- Prepuce of clitoris
- Frenulum of clitoris
- Urethral orifice
- Vaginal orifice
- Labium majus
- Labium minus
- Vestibule
- Anus

M. LeBlanc

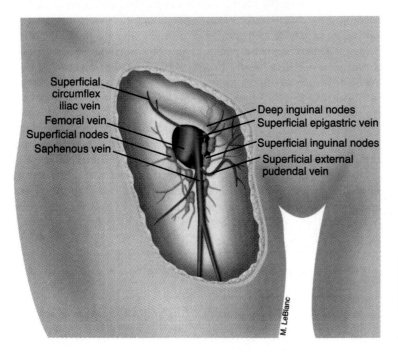

**FIGURE 21-2.** The anatomic relationship of the groin nodes to the femoral vasculature. The superficial nodal group contains approximately 7 to 10 nodes; the deep group contains approximately 3 to 5 nodes. (Adapted from: Eifel PJ, Levenback C. Cancer of the female lower genital tract. In: *ACS atlas of oncology: cervix, vulva, and vagina*. Ontario: B.C. Decker, Inc.; 2001:49.)

In the figure the following labels are shown:
- Superficial circumflex iliac vein
- Femoral vein
- Superficial nodes
- Saphenous vein
- Deep inguinal nodes
- Superficial epigastric vein
- Superficial inguinal nodes
- Superficial external pudendal vein

M. LeBlanc

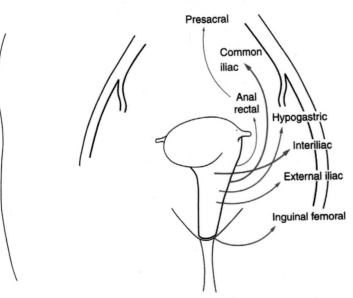

**FIGURE 21-3.** Lymphatic drainage of the vagina. (From: Jhingran A, Eifel PJ, Wharton JT, et al. Neoplasms of the cervix. In: Holland J.F. and Frei E., eds. *Cancer medicine 6*, Vol. 2. Ontario: B.C. Decker, Inc.; 2003:1779–1808.)

In the figure the following labels are shown:
- Presacral
- Common iliac
- Anal rectal
- Hypogastric
- Interiliac
- External iliac
- Inguinal femoral

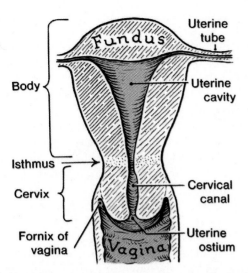

**FIGURE 21-4.** Diagram of the uterus and vagina illustrating the parts of the uterus and the relationship of its cervix to the superior end of the vagina. (From: Moore KL. *Clinically oriented anatomy.* Baltimore: Williams & Wilkins Co.; 1980:383.)

- The cervix is normally approximately 2.5 cm long, but the length can vary depending on the age of the patient and other cervical or uterine factors. The cervix is divided into two parts, the upper or supravaginal cervix and the lower or vaginal cervix, which is also known as the portio vaginalis cervicis. The external os is visible as a depression on the vaginal cervix.
- The cervical lymph nodes merge and form three dominant trunks: the lateral, posterior, and anterior trunks.
- The lateral trunk is the most dominant and exits laterally from the uterine isthmus in three groups: the upper branch follows the uterine artery and terminates in the uppermost hypogastric nodes; the middle branch drains to the deeper hypogastric (i.e., obturator) nodes; and the lowest branch courses posteriorly to the inferior and superior gluteal, common iliac, and presacral nodes.
- The posterior trunk drains to the superior rectal nodes or passes through the retrorectal space to the subaortic nodes, which lie at the level of the sacral promontory.
- The anterior trunk drains into the distal external iliac nodes. It is important to remember, however, that in cervical cancer, the pelvic lymph nodes are involved first almost all of the time (Fig. 21-5).
- The uterus also has a very rich supply of lymph nodes and differs from the cervix in that it can drain directly into the para-aortic nodes without involving the pelvic nodes. The lymphatic system of the uterus is composed of four lymphatic trunks that emerge from the lateral border of the corpus.
- The more superior lymphatic trunks pass through the broad ligament and drain to the external iliac nodes near the ovary and then to the para-aortic nodes.
- The inferior branch passes through the broad ligament to the common iliac nodes.

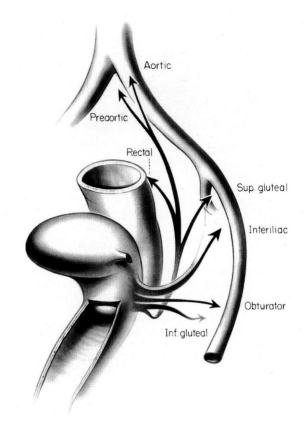

**FIGURE 21-5.** Diagram of the major lymphatic trunks leaving the cervix. There are three dominant trunks (anterior, lateral, and posterior). (From: Plentl AA, Friedman EA. *Lymphatic system of the female genitalia.* Philadelphia: W.B. Saunders Co.; 1971:83.)

- Subserosal lymph nodes near the junction of the fallopian tubes and the uterine body anastomose with lymph nodes of the fallopian tube to drain directly to the para-aortic lymph nodes.
- Lymph nodes also pass from the corpus by way of the ovarian pedicle to anastomose with lymph nodes of the fallopian tube and then empty into the femoral lymph nodes (Fig. 21-6).

## 2. NATURAL HISTORY

### 2.1. Vulva

- More than 85% of invasive vulvar carcinomas are epidermoid carcinomas. Two variants of these cancers, verrucous carcinoma and the so-called spray-pattern carcinoma, have distinctive histopathologic features and characteristic clinical behaviors.
- Verrucous carcinomas tend to be locally destructive, but rarely metastasize to the regional lymph nodes or distant sites.
- The spray-pattern variant is associated with a high probability of marginal recurrence (or "skip" lesions) after surgery, despite surgical margins that are free of disease, and so usually requires postoperative radiotherapy (RT).

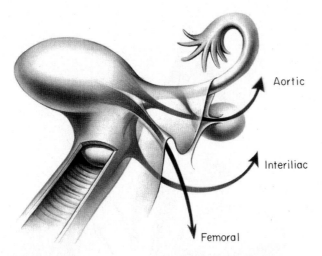

**FIGURE 21-6.** Diagram of the major lymphatic trunks leaving the uterus. There are three dominant trunks, one leaving the broad ligament and joining the lymphatics of the ovary and terminated directly to the para-aortic nodes. A smaller trunk follows the round ligament toward the inguinal regions, and a larger one arises from the subserosal network on the lateral aspect of the uterus and joins the uppermost branches of the cervix towards the interiliac nodes. (From: Plentl AA, Friedman EA. *Lymphatic system of the female genitalia.* Philadelphia: W.B. Saunders Co.; 1971:122.)

- Two-thirds of vulvar squamous carcinomas involve the labia majora or minora. A smaller percentage arise in the clitoris or gynecologic perineum.
- Carcinomas of the vulva can extend from the site of origin to invade the vagina, urethra, or anus; advanced vulvar carcinoma can invade adjacent pelvic bones, particularly the pubis.
- Approximately 20% of patients with clinically uninvolved groin nodes will have histologic evidence of groin metastasis if the nodes are radically dissected.[1,2] Conversely, approximately 22% of patients with clinically suspicious groin nodes will show no histologic evidence of nodal spread if the groin nodes are dissected and studied pathologically.[1,2]
- The vulva is richly supplied with lymphatic vessels that often cross the midline. As a result, lymph node metastasis is quite common, with an incidence of 3.1% in patients with lesions less than 1 mm thick and 31% in patients with lesions that are 4 mm or greater in thickness.
- The primary site of drainage from the vulva is the superficial inguinal nodes. Although carcinomas of the clitoris and Bartholin's gland occasionally spread directly to the deep femoral and even obturator lymph nodes, these nodal groups are rarely involved without evidence of superficial inguinal metastases.
- The most common site of hematogenous metastasis from vulvar cancer is the lung; however, advanced cancer can also spread to the liver, bone, and other sites.

## 2.2. Vagina

- Squamous cell carcinoma comprises approximately 90% of all vaginal cancers; most cases occur in the upper third of the vagina. Sixty percent of the primary apical lesions are diagnosed in women who have undergone hysterectomy.
- Vaginal cancer spreads laterally to involve the paravaginal tissues and may become fixed to pelvic wall structures. Fewer than 10% of cases involve the mucosa of adjacent structures, such as the urethra, the bladder, or the rectum.
- The location of the tumor determines the areas of lymphatic spread. The drainage pattern of apical lesions is similar to that of cervical lesions, with initial spread primarily to the obturator and hypogastric nodes, whereas lesions involving the lower third of the vagina drain similarly to vulvar carcinomas, with initial spread primarily to the inguinofemoral lymph nodes.
- Although few data exist on the risk for regional spread of vaginal cancer, available studies suggest that at least 25% of patients with FIGO (International Federation of Gynecology and Obstetrics) stage II vaginal cancer have pelvic node metastases.[3,4]
- The most common site of distant metastasis is the lung.

## 2.3. Cervix

- Invasive tumors of the cervix may develop as exophytic growths protruding from the cervix into the vagina or as endocervical lesions that can cause massive expansion of the cervix, despite a relatively normal-appearing cervical portio.
- From the cervix, a tumor may extend superiorly to the lower uterine segment, inferiorly to the vagina, or into the paracervical spaces by way of the broad or uterosacral ligaments.
- The tumor may become fixed to the pelvic wall by direct extension or by coalescence of the central tumor with regional adenopathy.
- The tumor may also extend anteriorly to involve the bladder or posteriorly to involve the rectum, although rectal mucosal involvement is a rare finding at initial presentation.
- Cervical cancer usually follows a relatively orderly pattern of metastatic progression, spreading first to the primary echelon nodes in the pelvis then to the para-aortic nodes, and then to distant sites.
- Table 21-1 summarizes the reported incidences of pelvic and para-aortic node involvement for patients who underwent lymphadenectomy as part of their primary surgical treatment or before RT for cervical carcinoma.
- The most frequent sites of distant metastasis are the lung, extrapelvic nodes, liver, and bone.

**TABLE 21-1. THE INCIDENCE OF PELVIC AND PARA-AORTIC LYMPH NODE METASTASIS IN PATIENTS WITH CERVICAL CARCINOMAS**

| Study | Primary Treatment | IB | | | IIA | | | IIB | | | III | | |
|---|---|---|---|---|---|---|---|---|---|---|---|---|---|
| | | No. Patients | Pelvic Nodes | PA Nodes | No. Patients | Pelvic Nodes | PA Nodes | No. Patients | Pelvic Nodes | PA Nodes | No. Patients | Pelvic Nodes | PA Nodes |
| Girardi and Haas[106] | RH | 163 | 31% | | 8 | 0% | | 249 | 45% | | | | |
| Averette et al.[107] | RH | 866 | 14% | 5% | 95 | 21% | 8% | | | | | | |
| Kamura et al.[26] | RH | 211 | 12% | | 48 | 17% | | 86 | 34% | | | | |
| Alvarez et al.[19] | RH | 401 | 12% | 1% | | | | | | | | | |
| Delgado et al.[81] | RH | 645 | 16% | | | | | | | | | | |
| Lee et al.[108] | RH | 596 | 13% | | 250 | 27% | | 108 | 35% | | | | |
| Fuller et al.[109] | RH | 285 | 15% | | 133 | 22% | | | | | | | |
| Barber[110] | RH/EX | 273 | 14% | | | | | 283* | 28% | | 67 | 42% | |
| Creasman et al.[111] | RH | 258 | 14% | | 10 | 10% | | | | | | | |
| Sudarsanam et al.[112] | RH/RT | 155 | | 7% | 21 | | 14% | 22 | | 18% | 19 | | 19% |
| Stehman et al.[113] | RT | | | | | | | 321 | 18% | | 188 | 23%† | |
| LaPolla et al.[114] | RT | 8 | 75% | 50% | 8 | 38% | 0% | 39 | 33% | 15% | 38 | 55% | 37% |
| Berman et al.[115] | RT | 158 | | 5% | 25 | 12% | | 240 | | 17% | 180 | | 25% |
| Ballon et al.[116] | RT | 22 | 27% | 23% | 16 | 38% | 19% | 32 | 16% | 19% | 24 | 38% | 17% |
| Lagasse et al.[117] | RT | 143 | | 6% | 22 | | 18% | 58 | | 33% | 64 | | 30% |
| Wharton et al.[33] | RT | 21 | 38% | 0% | | | | 67* | 35% | 18% | 42 | 29%† | 33% |
| Nelson et al.[118] | RT | | | | 16 | 13% | | 47 | | 15% | 39 | | 38% |

FIGO, International Federation of Gynecology and Obstetrics; RH, radical hysterectomy; RT, radiation treatment; EX, RT, radiation therapy.
\* Stage IIA and IIB combined.
† Patients with positive para aortic excluded.
Adapted from: Eifel PJ, Berek JS, Thigpen JT. Gynecologic Cancer. In: DeVita VT, Hellman S, Rosenberg SA, eds. *Cancer principles and practice of oncology*. Philadelphia: Lippincott Williams & Wilkins; 2001.

## 2.4. Endometrium

- Endometrial carcinoma is a disease that affects mostly postmenopausal women, with an average age at diagnosis of 60 years.
- The initial neoplasm forms a polypoid mass within the uterine lining, resulting in bleeding and an early diagnosis in most cases.
- Ninety percent of endometrial tumors present with the disease confined to the uterus, and 90% of these tumors are typical endometrial adenocarcinomas.
- With further growth, however, the primary tumor may extend to involve a greater proportion of the endometrial surface and ultimately extend to the lower uterine segment and cervix.
- Tumors that penetrate the uterine serosa may directly invade adjacent tissues, such as the bladder, colon, or adnexa(e), or they may exfoliate into the abdominal cavity to form implant metastases.
- The largest prospective study of surgical staging conducted by the Gynecologic Oncology Group (GOG) provides some of the best data available about the relationship between hysterectomy findings, nodal involvement, and outcome (Tables 21-2 and 21-3).[5] In this series, lymph node metastases were reported in 70 of 621 evaluable patients (11%). Approximately half of the patients with documented nodal involvement had positive para-aortic nodes; 32% of those with pelvic node metastases also had positive para-aortic nodes, and 12 of the 70 patients with regional metastases had only para-aortic node involvement.
- Although hematogenous dissemination is uncommon, the sites of distant spread include the lung, liver, bone, and brain.

## 3. DIAGNOSIS AND STAGING

### 3.1. Signs and Symptoms

#### 3.1.1. Vulva

- Burning, pruritus, and a mass are the most common presenting symptoms of vulvar cancer.
- Pain is associated with locally advanced disease.
- Vulvar carcinomas can be mistaken for a number of other entities, and benign entities such as flat condylomas and various forms of chronic inflammatory changes may be mistaken for carcinomas.

**TABLE 21-2. ASSOCIATION BETWEEN DEPTH OF MYOMETRIAL INVASION, TUMOR GRADE, AND PELVIC NODE INVOLVEMENT IN PATIENTS WITH ENDOMETRIAL CARCINOMA**

| Depth of Invasion | No. (%) Patients with Pelvic Node Involvement | | |
| --- | --- | --- | --- |
| | Grade 1 (n = 180) | Grade 2 (n = 288) | Grade 3 (n = 153) |
| Endometrium (n = 86) | 0 (0) | 1 (3) | 0 (0) |
| Inner third (n = 281) | 3 (3) | 7 (5) | 5 (9) |
| Middle third (n = 115) | 0 (0) | 6 (9) | 1 (4) |
| Outer third (n = 139) | 2 (11) | 11 (19) | 22 (34) |

From: Creasman W, Morrow C, Bundy B, et al. Surgical pathologic spread patterns of endometrial cancer. A Gynecologic Oncology Group Study. *Cancer* 1987;60:2035–2041.

### 3.1.2. Vagina

- Abnormal bleeding is the most common symptom of vaginal cancer.
- Pain (including dyspareunia), discharge, and a mass are other symptoms that patients can have on initial presentation.

### 3.1.3. Cervix

- The most common symptoms of cervical cancer are abnormal vaginal bleeding, discharge, and pain.
- The triad of back pain, leg edema, and a nonfunctioning kidney is evidence of an advanced carcinoma with extensive pelvic wall involvement.
- Hematuria and incontinence suggest possible involvement of the bladder.
- Severe back pain, especially in the para-aortic area, may be a manifestation of nodal disease.

### 3.1.4. Endometrium

- The most common symptom of endometrial cancer is abnormal postmenopausal vaginal bleeding.

## 3.2. Physical Examination

### 3.2.1. Vulva

- In addition to a complete history and physical examination, a complete examination of the pelvic and groin area is mandatory for diagnosing vulvar cancer.
- A careful examination of the vulva is required, with special care taken to determine the dimensions of the lesion and its distance from the major midline structures, including the clitoris, urethral meatus, and anus.
- A digital rectal examination is also mandatory to accurately assess the extent of the primary tumor and rule out a rare coexisting squamous carcinoma of the anus.
- The groin areas similarly need to be carefully examined, with the patient in a supine position.

### 3.2.2. Vagina

- In addition to a complete history and physical examination, a complete examination of the pelvis is mandatory for diagnosing vaginal cancer.
- Cystoscopy and proctoscopy should be performed on patients with symptoms or clinical findings suspicious for bladder or rectal infiltration, respectively.

**TABLE 21-3. ASSOCIATION BETWEEN DEPTH OF MYOMETRIAL INVASION, TUMOR GRADE, AND PARA-AORTIC NODE INVOLVEMENT**

| Depth of Invasion | No. (%) Patients with Para-aortic Node Involvement | | |
| --- | --- | --- | --- |
| | Grade 1 (n = 180) | Grade 2 (n = 288) | Grade 3 (n = 153) |
| Endometrium (n = 86) | 0 (0) | 1 (3) | 0 (0) |
| Inner third (n = 281) | 1 (1) | 5 (4) | 2 (4) |
| Middle third (n = 115) | 1 (5) | 0 (0) | 0 (0) |
| Outer third (n = 139) | 1 (6) | 8 (14) | 15 (23) |

From: Creasman W, Morrow C, Bundy B, et al. Surgical pathologic spread patterns of endometrial cancer. A Gynecologic Oncology Group Study. *Cancer* 1987;60:2035–2041.

- Careful evaluation of the vaginal lesion should be performed, with attention paid to its location and the presence of any paravaginal or sidewall extension.

### 3.2.3. Cervix/Endometrium

- Careful inspection of the external genitalia, vagina, and cervix should be performed for diagnosing cervical or endometrial cancer, with particular care taken to examine all the mucosal surfaces of the vagina.
- A digital vaginal examination should be performed to evaluate any irregularities of the vaginal mucosa. The size and configuration of the exophytic cervical lesions should be noted.
- A careful bimanual examination should also be performed. The size and shape of the uterus should be assessed by balloting it between the vagina and suprapubis. The position (anteverted, axial, or retroverted), flexion (anteflexed or retroflexed), size, and mobility of the uterus should be noted, as should any nodularity.
- The adnexa should be carefully examined for any masses or tenderness. Tenderness may indicate the presence of pelvic inflammatory disease.
- A rectovaginal examination should always be performed, with particular attention paid to the parametrium and pelvic wall. Paracervical nodularity, fixation, and distortion of the normal anatomy should be noted. The size of the cervix should also be noted.
- Cystoscopy and proctoscopy should be performed on patients with symptoms or clinical findings suspicious for bladder or rectal infiltration, respectively.

## 3.3. Imaging of the Pelvis

- Intravenous pyelography and radiography of the chest and bones are the only radiographic examinations to determine a patient's cancer stage according to the FIGO staging system.
- Recently, imaging techniques such as lymphangiography, intravenous pyelography, and barium enema have been replaced by computed tomography (CT) and magnetic resonance imaging (MRI) to help diagnose gynecologic cancer.
- CT and MRI are equally effective in detecting positive nodes, with an accuracy of approximately 72% to 93%. However, the accuracy of both of these imaging modalities is compromised by their inability to detect small metastases. Moreover, many enlarged nodes are caused not by metastases but by inflammation associated with advanced disease.
- Compared with MRI, CT has the advantage of wider availability and quick imaging time. It is most useful for staging more advanced disease and detecting (and guiding biopsies of) suspicious lymph nodes and suspected metastases.
- MRI is superior to CT, physical examination, and ultrasonography in the evaluation of the tumor location and size, the depth of stromal invasion, and the vaginal or parametrial extension of most gynecologic cancers (Fig. 21-7).[6,7]
- Positron emission tomography (PET) is a new and rapidly expanding modality that may be useful in the diagnosis of gynecologic cancer (Fig. 21-8).

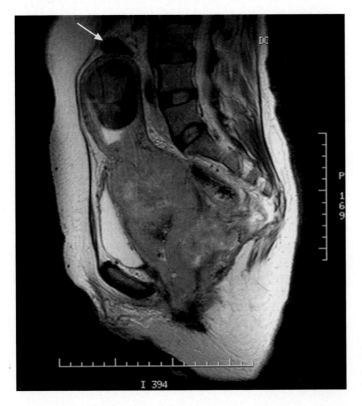

**FIGURE 21-7.** MRI scan of a patient with a large cervical tumor. The mass at the fundus, however, is a large fibroid and not a tumor. An air cavity inside the large intestine is shown above the mass (*arrow*).

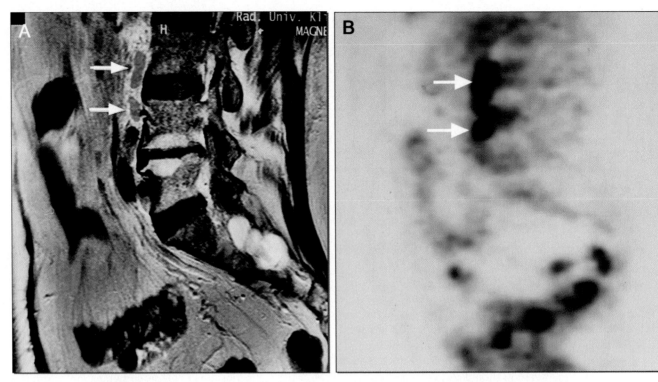

**FIGURE 21-8.** Positive para-aortic nodes (*arrows*) are contoured on sagittal MRI (**A**) and PET (**B**) scans.

- In a study of 101 patients with carcinoma of the cervix, Grigsby and colleagues reported that with CT, enlarged pelvic lymph nodes were detected in 20% of patients and enlarged para-aortic lymph nodes in 7%; whereas with PET, abnormal fluorodeoxyglucose uptake was detected in 67% of pelvic lymph nodes, 21% of para-aortic nodes, and 8% of supraclavicular nodes.[8]

### 3.4. Staging

- The FIGO staging systems for carcinoma of the vulva, vagina, cervix, and endometrium are shown in Tables 21-4 to 21-7.

## 4. PROGNOSTIC FACTORS

### 4.1. Vulva

- *Lymph node status:* the presence or absence of inguinal lymph node involvement is considered one of the strongest predictors of prognosis in cases of vulvar cancer (Table 21-8).[9]
- *Predictors for nodal metastasis:* tumor size, depth of invasion, tumor thickness, and the presence or absence of lymphovascular space invasion.[10]
- *Margin status:* an association between the margin status in excised vulvar specimens and the incidence of local failure has been noted, especially if the margin is smaller than 8 mm.[11]

### 4.2. Vagina

- *Stage:* the disease stage is probably the most important prognostic factor in terms of ultimate outcome in cases of vaginal carcinoma.[12–15]
- *Size:* tumor size (measured in centimeters or as the percentage of the vaginal wall involved) has been found by several investigators to be correlated with local control.[12,13]
- *Age:* several investigators have found age to be prognostic (i.e., women younger than 60 years had a better outcome), whereas others have not.[13,17]

### 4.3. Cervix

- *Tumor size and local extent:* large tumor size has been consistently shown to be one of the most important predictors of local recurrence of and death from cervical cancer, whether patients were treated with hysterectomy[18,19] or RT.[20–22]
- *Lymph node involvement:* an important predictor of outcome; the location, size, and number of affected lymph nodes all correlate with survival.[19,23–25]
- *Lymphovascular space invasion:* associated with an increased risk for recurrence independently from lymph node involvement.[26,27]
- *Tumor grade and histologic type:* the prognostic importance of the histologic grade of squamous cell carcinomas is unclear. However, the degree of differentiation

**TABLE 21-4. INTERNATIONAL FEDERATION OF GYNECOLOGY AND OBSTETRICS CLINICAL STAGING SYSTEM FOR CARCINOMA OF THE CERVIX (1994)**

| Stage | Tumor Description |
|---|---|
| 0 | Carcinoma in situ, intraepithelial carcinoma; *cases of stage 0 should not be included in any therapeutic statistics for invasive carcinoma.* |
| I | The carcinoma is strictly confined to the cervix (*extension to the corpus should be disregarded*). |
| IA | Invasive cancer identified only microscopically. All gross lesions, even with superficial invasion, are stage IB cancers. |
|  | Invasion is limited to measured stromal invasion with a maximum depth of 5 mm and no wider 7 mm. (*The depth of invasion should not be more than 5 mm taken from the base of the epithelium, either surface or glandular, from which it originates. Vascular space involvement, either venous or lymphatic, should not alter the staging.*) |
| IA1 | Measured invasion of the stroma is no greater than 3 mm in depth and 7 mm in width. |
| IA2 | Measured invasion of the stroma is greater than 3 mm but no greater than 5 mm in depth and no greater than 7 mm in width. |
| IB | Clinical lesions confined to the cervix or preclinical lesions greater than stage IA. |
| IB1 | Clinical lesions no greater than 4 cm in size. |
| IB2 | Clinical lesions are greater than 4 cm in size. |
| II | The carcinoma extends beyond the cervix but has not extended onto the pelvic wall; the carcinoma involves the vagina, but not as far as the lower third. |
| IIA | No obvious parametrial involvement. |
| IIB | Obvious parametrial involvement. |
| III | The carcinoma has extended on to the pelvic wall; on rectal examination, no cancer-free space separates the tumor and the pelvic wall; the tumor involves the lower third of the vagina; all cases with hydronephrosis or a nonfunctioning kidney should be included, unless they are known to have another cause. |
| IIIA | No extension onto the pelvic wall but involvement of the lower third of the vagina. |
| IIIB | Extension onto the pelvic wall, or hydronephrosis, or a nonfunctioning kidney. |
| IV | The carcinoma has extended beyond the true pelvis or has clinically involved the mucosa of the bladder or the rectum. |
| IVA | Spread to adjacent organs. |
| IVB | Spread to distant organs. |

and clinical behavior of adenocarcinomas are clearly associated.[28,29]

- *Anemia:* some investigators have reported an association between a low hemoglobin level before or during treatment for cervical carcinoma and a poor prognosis.[30,31]
- *Overall treatment time:* the survival rate and local-regional control rate becomes worse when the overall treatment time increases.[32]

## 4.4. Endometrium

- *Stage:* pathologic stage is prognostic for survival and local recurrence in cases of endometrial cancer.
- *Histopathologic grade:* one of the most sensitive indicators of prognosis in endometrial cancer. Grade is directly associated with the depth of myometrial invasion[5] and the frequency of lymph node involvement.[5,33]
- *Age:* younger patients with endometrial cancer, especially those younger than 60 years, have a better prognosis than older patients.[34,35]

- *Depth of myometrial invasion:* one of the most important predictors of lymph node involvement and prognosis in cases of endometrial cancer.[5,35]
- *Cervical invasion:* tumors that involve the endocervical stroma are associated with a poorer prognosis and have a higher likelihood of extrauterine involvement and disease recurrence than other types of cervical cancer.
- *Tumor size:* the predictive value of tumor size seems to be independent of the tumor's grade or depth of invasion.[36]
- *Lymph node involvement:* a strong association exists between lymph node involvement, particularly para-aortic node involvement, and a poorer prognosis in cases of endometrial cancer.[37]
- *Tumor cells in peritoneal washings:* the importance of tumor cells in peritoneal washings is controversial. However, in a multivariate analysis, Milosevic and colleagues concluded that although the presence of tumor cells in peritoneal washings was strongly associated with disease recurrence, this finding was largely due to the association

**TABLE 21-5. INTERNATIONAL FEDERATION OF GYNECOLOGY AND OBSTETRICS TNM CLASSIFICATION FOR CARCINOMA OF THE ENDOMETRIUM**

**Primary Tumor (T) (with FIGO Stage)**

| | |
|---|---|
| TX | Primary tumor cannot be assessed |
| T0 | No evidence of primary tumor |
| Tis | Carcinoma in situ |
| T1 (I) | Tumor confined to corpus uteri |
| T1a (IA) | Tumor limited to endometrium |
| T1b (IB) | Tumor invades as much as half of the myometrium |
| T1c (IC) | Tumor invades more than half of the myometrium |
| T2 (I) | Tumor invades cervix but does not extend beyond uterus |
| T2a (IIA) | Endocervical glandular involvement only |
| T2b (IIB) | Cervical stromal invasion |
| T3 (III) | Local and/or regional spread as specified in T3a/b and/or N1 and IIIA/B/C (see below) |
| T3a (IIIA) | Tumor involves the serosa and/or adnexa (direct extension or metastasis) or cancer cells are found in ascites or peritoneal washings |
| T3b (IIIB) | Vaginal involvement (direct extension or metastasis) |
| N1 (IIIC) | Metastasis to the pelvic and/or para-aortic lymph nodes |
| T4 (IVA) | Tumor invades the bladder mucosa and/or bowel mucosa (bullous edema is not sufficient to classify a tumor as T4) |
| M1 (IVB) | Distant metastasis, excluding metastasis to the vagina, pelvic serosa, or adnexa but including metastasis to intra-abdominal lymph nodes other than para-aortic or inguinal lymph nodes |

**Regional Lymph Nodes (N)**

| | |
|---|---|
| NX | Regional lymph node cannot be assessed (e.g., previously removed) |
| N0 | No regional lymph node metastasis |
| N1 | Regional lymph node metastasis |

**Distant Metastasis (M)**

| | |
|---|---|
| MX | Distant metastasis cannot be assessed |
| M0 | No distant metastasis |
| M1 | Distant metastasis |

**Stage Grouping**

| | | | |
|---|---|---|---|
| Stage 0 | Tis | N0 | M0 |
| Stage IA | T1a | N0 | M0 |
| Stage IB | T1b | N0 | M0 |
| Stage IC | T1c | N0 | M0 |
| Stage IIA | T2a | N0 | M0 |
| Stage IIB | T2b | N0 | M0 |
| Stage IIIA | T3a | N0 | M0 |
| Stage IIIB | T3b | N0 | M0 |
| Stage IIIC | T1 | N1 | M0 |
| | T2 | N1 | M0 |
| | T3a | N1 | M0 |
| | T3b | N1 | M0 |
| Stage IVA | T4 | Any N | M0 |
| Stage IVB | Any T | Any N | M1 |

FIGO, International Federation of Gynecology and Obstetrics.

**TABLE 21-6. INTERNATIONAL FEDERATION OF GYNECOLOGY AND OBSTETRICS TNM CLINICAL STAGING FOR CARCINOMA OF THE VULVA**

**Primary Tumor (T)**

| | |
|---|---|
| TX | Primary tumor cannot be assessed |
| T0 | No evidence of primary tumor |
| Tis | Carcinoma in situ (preinvasive carcinoma) |
| T1 | Tumor (≤2 cm in greatest dimension) confined to the vulva or vulva and perineum |
| T1a | Tumor (≤2 cm in greatest dimension) confined to the vulva or vulva and perineum with stromal invasion no greater than 1 mm |
| T1b | Tumor (≤2 cm in greatest dimension) confined to the vulva or vulva and perineum with stromal invasion greater than 1 mm |
| T2 | Tumor (>2 cm in greatest dimension) confined to the vulva or vulva and perineum |
| T3 | Tumor of any size with adjacent spread to the lower urethra and/or vagina or anus |
| T4 | Tumor invades the upper urethral mucosa, bladder mucosa, or rectal mucosa or is fixed to the pubic bone |

**Regional Lymph Nodes (N)**

| | |
|---|---|
| NX | Regional lymph node cannot be assessed |
| N0 | No regional lymph node metastasis |
| N1 | Unilateral lymph node metastasis |
| N2 | Bilateral lymph node metastasis |

**Distant Metastasis (M)**

| | |
|---|---|
| MX | Distant metastasis cannot be assessed |
| M0 | No distant metastasis |
| M1 | Distant metastasis (including pelvic lymph node metastasis) |

**Stage Grouping (American Joint Committee on Cancer and International Federation of Gynecology and Obstetrics)**

| | | | |
|---|---|---|---|
| Stage 0 | Tis | N0 | M0 |
| Stage IA | T1a | N0 | M0 |
| Stage IB | T1b | N0 | M0 |
| Stage II | T2 | N0 | M0 |
| Stage III | T1 | N1 | M0 |
| | T2 | N1 | M0 |
| | T3 | N0 | M0 |
| | T3 | N1 | M0 |
| Stage IVA | T1 | N2 | M0 |
| | T2 | N2 | M0 |
| | T3 | N2 | M0 |
| | T4 | Any N | M0 |
| Stage IVB | Any T | Any N | M1 |

**TABLE 21-7. INTERNATIONAL FEDERATION OF GYNECOLOGY AND OBSTETRICS CLINICAL STAGING SYSTEM FOR CARCINOMA OF THE VAGINA**

| Stage | Tumor Description |
|---|---|
| 0 | Carcinoma in situ, intraepithelial carcinoma |
| I | The carcinoma is limited to the vaginal wall |
| II | The carcinoma has involved the subvaginal tissues but has not extended onto the pelvic wall |
| III | The carcinoma has extended onto the pelvic wall |
| IV | The carcinoma has extended beyond the true pelvis or has clinically involved the mucosa of the bladder or rectum. The presence of bullous edema does not require a case to be classified as stage IV |
| IVA | Spread to adjacent organs and/or direct extension beyond the true pelvis |
| IVB | Spread to distant organs |

**TABLE 21-8. FREQUENCY OF NODAL INVOLVEMENT AND 5-YEAR SURVIVAL RATES BY INGUINAL NODE STATUS IN PATIENTS WITH VULVAR CANCER**

| Node Status | No. Patients (%) | % 5-Year Survival |
|---|---|---|
| Negative | 385 (65.5) | 90.9 |
| Positive | 203 (34.5) | 57.2 |
| 1–2 nodes | 124 (62.5) | 75.2 |
| 3–4 nodes | 40 (20.0) | 36.1 |
| 5–6 nodes | 19 (9.5) | 24.0 |
| ≥7 nodes | 16 (8.0) | 0 |
| Total | 588 (100) | |

Adapted from: Homesley HD, Bundy BN, Sedlis A, et al. Assessment of current International Federation of Gynecology and Obstetrics staging of vulvar carcinoma relative to prognostic factors for survival (a Gynecologic Oncology Group study). *Am J Obstet Gynecol* 1991;164:997–1004.

of malignant cytology with other adverse prognostic factors that dominate the clinical presentation.[38]

# 5. GENERAL MANAGEMENT

## 5.1. Vulvar Cancer

### 5.1.1. Surgical Management

- Minimally invasive vulvar tumors that infiltrate less than 1 mm beyond the most superficial basement membrane have a very low risk (<1%) of regional metastasis and can be treated with wide local excision alone. Any tumor that invades at a distance of more than 1 mm beyond the most superficial basement membrane requires treatment aimed at both the local tumor and the regional nodes.
- Traditional surgical management of vulvar cancer was en bloc resection and lymph node dissection, which were extremely morbid. Now, the surgeries are more individualized with the use of more tissue-sparing types of procedure.
- Most early-stage vulvar cancers are treated with wide local excision with inguinal node dissection. The excision should extend down to the inferior fascia of the urogenital diaphragm, and an effort should be made to obtain a tumor-free margin of at least 1 to 2 cm, unless doing so would compromise the function of a major organ.
- The standard treatment for the inguinal nodes is a radical lymphadenectomy that removes both the superficial and deep inguinofemoral nodes. The contralateral groin need not be dissected if the primary lesion is a well-lateralized T1 tumor. However, if the primary lesion approaches the midline or involves the anterior labia minora, bilateral nodal dissection should be performed.

- Pelvic nodal dissection is usually not performed because of the morbidity of the procedure. The current standard practice is to administer RT to the pelvis for patients with regional disease, thus reducing morbidity.
- Complications from radical inguinal lymphadenectomy are common, despite the use of separate inguinal incisions for the primary tumor resection and lymphadenectomy, and include wound complications, chronic lymphedema, and thrombotic complications. The perioperative mortality rate is 2% to 5%. Performing only a superficial inguinal node dissection can reduce perioperative mortality; however, a 5% to 7% groin recurrence rate with this procedure has been reported, even with tumor-free surgical margins.[39,40] Several investigators are also exploring the use of lymphatic mapping and sentinel lymph node biopsy of inguinal nodes as a way to reduce morbidity and recurrence.
- Five-year disease-specific survival rates of approximately 98% and 85% can be expected for patients treated with surgery alone for stage I (T1N0M0) and stage II (T2N0M0) disease, respectively.[9]

### 5.1.2. Postoperative Radiotherapy

- Postoperative RT is usually indicated for vulvar cancers with more than one positive inguinal node, one grossly positive inguinal node, extracapsular extension of the nodal disease, small tumors in patients with medical problems prohibiting radical inguinofemoral lymph node dissection, or a tumor-free vulvar resection margin of less than 8 to 10 mm.
- In 1986, investigators in the GOG published reports of a randomized trial that evaluated the role of postoperative RT in patients who had inguinal lymph node metas-

tases.[41] This trial was stopped early because of the significant relapse-free survival difference between the treatment arms at 2 years. The survival advantage for RT at 2 years (68% overall survival for RT vs 54% for pelvic node dissection) was statistically significant only for patients with metastases in two or more groin nodes (63% survival for RT vs 37% for pelvic node dissection).[41] Since this trial, elective pelvic lymphadenectomy is rarely performed, and regional adjuvant RT has become the standard adjuvant therapy for patients with metastasis to two or more groin nodes.

- In patients who had close or positive surgical margins, Faul and colleagues[42] reported a local recurrence rate of 16% in patients who received postoperative RT compared with 58% in patients who did not receive RT ($p = 0.04$).

- In patients receiving postoperative RT for groin node involvement, the RT fields should include at least both groin areas and the caudal external iliac nodes on the side of the involved groin nodes.

- If there is no clinical or radiographic evidence of involvement of the pelvic nodes, the top of the RT field should encompass the caudal external iliac nodes and should generally not extend more cephalad than the middle of the sacroiliac joints.

- A 2-cm margin lateral to the medial bony margin of the pelvis will assure adequate coverage of the lymph nodes that may lie lateral to the external iliac vessels.

- If there has been extensive nodal involvement, the caudal border of the treatment area should encompass the vertical chain of the inguinal lymph nodes in the upper medial thigh between the femoral vein and the saphenous vein.

- At The University of Texas M.D. Anderson Cancer Center (MDACC), the area of the primary tumor is also irradiated in most cases requiring irradiation of the inguinal nodes and pelvic nodes. A substantial risk for recurrence in tissues shielded by a midline block has been reported during postoperative RT directed at the groin and pelvic nodes.[41,43]

### 5.1.3. Preoperative Radiotherapy

- Patients should be considered for preoperative RT when their tumors encroach on normal tissues. Examples include tumors encroaching on the anal sphincter, abutting the pubic arch, involving more than the distal urethra, approaching the clitoris, invading the clitoral hood or frenulum, or extending more than minimally past the vaginal introitus.

- Moderate doses (36–54 Gy) of preoperative RT followed by excision of any residual tumor have resulted in surgical specimens with no evidence of residual primary cancer in 50% of cases.[44–46]

- Moore et al. described results of 71 patients with FIGO stages III or IV treated with preoperative RT and chemotherapy.[47] Residual unresectable disease persisted in only 2 patients, and bowel and bladder continence were preserved in all but 3 patients.

- Using the same preoperative RT approach, Montana et al. were able to convert approximately 90% of 46 cases of initially unresectable inguinal nodes to a resectable or potentially resectable status.[48]

### 5.1.4. Definitive Radiotherapy

- The superior results obtained by synchronous chemotherapy and RT in randomized comparison with RT alone for the treatment of cancer of the anal canal have prompted widespread extrapolation of this approach to the treatment of cancer of the vulva (Table 21-9).

**TABLE 21-9. REPORTED RESULTS OF CONCURRENT CHEMOTHERAPY IN PATIENTS WITH LOCALLY ADVANCED OR RECURRENT CARCINOMA OF THE VULVA**

| Author | No. Patients | Drugs | RT Dose (Gy) | CR (%) | Subsequent Failure | F/u (mo) |
|---|---|---|---|---|---|---|
| *Previously Untreated Patients* | | | | | | |
| Thomas et al.[119] | 24 | 5-FU±Mito | 40–64 | 6 (67%) | 3 (50%) | 5–43 |
| Berek et al.[120] | 12 | 5-Fu±CDDP | 44–54 | 8 (67%) | 0 | 7–60 |
| Russell et al.[121] | 18 | 5-Fu±CDDP | 47–72 | 16 (89%) | 2 (13%) | 2–52 |
| Koh et al.[122] | 14 | 5-FU±CDDP or Mito | 34–63.1 | 8 (57%) | 1 (17%) | 1–75 |
| Cunningham et al.[123] | 14 | 5-FU±CDDP | 50–65 | 9 (64%) | 1 (11%) | 7–81 |
| *Patients with Recurrent Disease* | | | | | | |
| Thomas et al.[119] | 15 | 5-FU±Mito | 40–64 | 8 (53%) | 0 | 5–43 |
| Russell et al.[121] | 7 | 5-FU±CDDP | 54–72 | 4 (57%) | 1 (25%) | 2–35 |

RT, radiation treatment; CR, complete response; F/u, follow-up; FU, fluorouracil; Mito, mitomycin; CDDP, cisplatin.

- Although results of this approach are encouraging, aggressive multimodality regimens should be used with particular caution in patients who have concurrent medical problems or diminished performance status.
- Because of potential enhancement of late normal-tissue effects and the possibility of exploiting the skin-sparing effects of megavoltage radiation when treating what is fundamentally a skin cancer, one should not exceed a dose of 54 Gy in 30 fractions, 59.5 Gy in 35 fractions, or 64 Gy in 40 fractions to the gross disease when chemoradiation is used.
- Treatment fields need to be individualized, taking into consideration any vulnerable normal tissues, including the femoral necks, small bowel, bladder, urethra, clitoris, and anus. A technique followed in this regard at MDACC is the simultaneous use of a large, wide, anterior low-energy photon field (4 or 6 MV) to encompass the entire target volume area; a narrower posterior high-energy photon field (10 to 20 MV) to encompass the perineum and pelvic nodes while excluding the femurs; and supplemental anterior electron fields to supplement the dose to the groin areas that overlie the femoral necks. After 40 to 45 Gy of radiation has been administered, the dose to the vulva and nodes is then boosted with appositional electrons, to reach the desired total dose.

## 5.2. Vagina

- RT is the treatment of choice for most patients with invasive vaginal cancers.
- Early tumors of the upper posterior vagina can sometimes be treated with radical hysterectomy and partial vaginectomy or, if the patient has no uterus, radical upper vaginectomy.[49]

### 5.2.1. Radiotherapy Alone

- Some small, very superficial tumors can be treated with brachytherapy alone. Chyle and colleagues[12] and Perez and colleagues[13] reported pelvic disease control rates of 87% and 88%, respectively, for small lesions treated with intracavitary RT alone. For apical lesions, surface doses of 90 to 100 Gy of RT are needed; for lesions in the middle or lower third of the vagina, the preferred treatment is a surface dose of 65 to 70 Gy with intracavitary brachytherapy and an added single-plane interstitial implant to increase the total dose to the tumor to 80 to 85 Gy.
- For palpable tumors, particularly those more than 2 to 3 mm thick, pelvic nodes need to be treated; therefore, external beam RT needs to be added to the regimen.
- External beam RT in patients with vaginal cancer is generally delivered by means of anteroposterior-posteroanterior fields. For tumors of the apical area, the fields should include the true pelvis, with at least a 4-cm distal margin. If the lesion involves the distal third of the vagina, then the medial inguinal nodes should be included in the radiation field.
- Brachytherapy should be tailored to the volume and distribution of the tumor. Apical tumors that are less than 3 to 4 mm thick may be treated with a vaginal cylinder. For more distal tumors, a combination of intracavitary and interstitial brachytherapy may be more appropriate.
- The dose of radiation depends on the patient's response to initial external beam RT, tumor size, extent of the disease, and ability to deliver brachytherapy. If brachytherapy can be delivered accurately, then an effort should be made to deliver a dose of 75 to 85 Gy to the tumor. When brachytherapy is not possible, one should try to deliver a dose of 60 to 66 Gy to the tumor using shrinking external beam fields.
- The 5-year disease-specific survival rates for patients with vaginal cancer treated with definitive RT range from 75% to 95% for stage I disease, 50% to 80% for stage II disease, 30% to 50% for stage III disease, and 15% to 30% for stage IVA disease.[12,13,15,50–52]
- Complication rates of definitive RT for vaginal cancers tend to be higher than those for cervical cancers. Chyle and colleagues reported a 19% incidence of major complications at 20 years for 301 patients treated with definitive RT.[12]

### 5.2.2. Chemotherapy

- Reports of using chemotherapy in patients with vaginal cancer are anecdotal. However, because vaginal cancer is similar to cervical cancer in its epidemiology and natural history, it may be reasonable to extrapolate from the randomized trials in cervical cancer that the use of concurrent cisplatin-based chemotherapy regimens with RT for selected patients with high-risk features is beneficial.
- Cisplatin-containing chemotherapy is used for patients with metastatic or recurrent vaginal cancer, but reported response rates are poor.[56,57]

## 5.3. Endometrium

- The mainstay of treatment for adenocarcinoma of the endometrium is surgical removal of the uterus.
- The role of adjuvant RT is still difficult to define. Such adjuvant treatment definitely improves local control, but its effects on survival are still unclear.

### 5.3.1. Surgical Management

- Total abdominal hysterectomy with bilateral salpingo-oophorectomy is widely regarded as the preferred treatment for most patients.
- Controversy currently exists in the gynecologic oncology community about the proper extent and the therapeutic

value of lymphadenectomy. Some investigators believe that complete lymphadenectomy improves survival,[58-60] whereas others have concluded that lymphadenectomy provides prognostic information only.[61-64]

### 5.3.2. Radiotherapy Alone

- Although hysterectomy is the primary treatment for early-stage endometrial cancer, patients at high risk for complications from surgery can be treated with RT alone. Disease-specific survival rates of 75% to 85% and local recurrence rates of 10% to 20% have been reported for patients with clinical stage I or II endometrial cancer who were treated with RT alone. Prognosis in these patients is associated with clinical stage and histologic grade.[65-71]

- Brachytherapy alone provides excellent local control in most patients with small uteri who have grade 1 tumors.

- Most patients with endometrial cancer, however, receive a combination of external beam RT and brachytherapy.

- External beam RT fields used for treating endometrial cancer are similar to those used in cervical cancer (described in the section below) encompassing the entire true pelvis, and RT is usually delivered by means of opposed anteroposterior-posteroanterior fields, to a total dose of 40 to 45 Gy.

- In endometrial cancer, it is very important to cover the uterine fundus adequately with brachytherapy. If the uterus is small, then a single small intrauterine tandem with increased activity at the tip should be used to broaden the radiation dose distribution in the fundus. However, in patients with large cavities, Heyman packing, Simon capsules, or two tandems in the right and left cornu of the uterus may be needed to provide adequate coverage to the fundus. With low-dose-rate brachytherapy, uterine applicators are commonly loaded with 45 to 50 mg RaEq and are left in place for two 48-hour treatments after 40 to 45 Gy of external beam radiation is delivered to the pelvis.

- Recently, high-dose-rate brachytherapy has been used. Kucera and colleagues reported a 5-year overall survival rate of 59.7% and a disease-specific survival rate of 85.4% in patients with clinical stage I disease who were treated with brachytherapy alone.[72]

- For patients with recurrent isolated pelvic recurrences whose initial treatment was hysterectomy alone, 5-year local control rates of 40% to 80% and 5-year overall survival rates of 30% to 80% can be achieved with definitive RT alone.[73,74]

### 5.3.3. Combined Surgery and Radiotherapy

- The role of adjuvant RT is controversial. Two studies showed that compared with surgery alone, surgery plus RT reduced local recurrences of endometrial cancer

significantly, but did not affect overall survival in patients with intermediate risk features after surgery compared to surgery alone.[75,76]

- In the study by Creutzberg and colleagues, the majority of patients after pathology review had grade 1 tumors rather than grade 2 tumors, putting them in a low-risk group rather than intermediate-risk group.[75]

- Patients with endometrial cancer who have low- to intermediate-risk factors, such as invasion of the inner or middle third of the myometrium and grade 1 to 2 disease, have a 3% risk for pelvic and para-aortic nodal involvement and may benefit from vaginal brachytherapy alone (Tables 21-2 and 21-3).

- If external beam radiation is not given, the usual recommended brachytherapy dose is either 60 to 70 Gy, administered at a low-dose rate over 72 hours, or 6 Gy, administered using high dose rate, prescribed to the vaginal surface or a depth of 0.5 cm for five fractions.

- Table 21-10 shows the result of patients treated with vaginal cuff radiation therapy alone who had favorable prognostic indictors.

- The optimal treatment for patients with clinical stage II endometrial cancer is controversial. Patients with clinically positive cervical stroma involvement have a substantial risk for occult paracervical and parametrial disease and for pelvic nodal disease.

- Although no prospective studies have been performed on patients with clinical stage II disease, we know that RT can sterilize occult parametrial and pelvic nodal disease and that surgery provides better control of central uterine disease. Thus, common treatment schemes use preoperative external beam RT with or without brachytherapy followed by hysterectomy. Overall survival rates range between 70% and 85% for therapies combining RT and surgery.

- Treatment recommendations for patients with pathologic stage III disease must be made on a patient-by-patient basis. Patients with pelvic nodes that are positive for cancer and para-aortic nodes that are negative can be treated with RT to the pelvis after surgery, and have an approximately 70% 5-year overall survival rate with combination therapy.

- Patients with positive para-aortic nodes can be treated postoperatively with extended-field RT, which results in reported 5-year survival rates of 30% to 50%.[37,77,78]

- Pelvic RT may be delivered using a four-field technique to spare small bowel. Doses of 40 to 50 Gy are used to control microscopic diseases. Serious complications are observed in 5% to 15% of patients who undergo postoperative pelvic RT; however, the risk for complications may be greater in patients who have had a staging lymphadenectomy.

- For extended-field RT, the fields should extend to the T11 or T12 vertebra to ensure coverage of perirenal nodes that are at risk for direct spread via the tubo-ovarian vessels. Four fields are usually used to spare both

**TABLE 21-10. INCIDENCE OF PELVIC RECURRENCE AFTER VAGINAL RADIOTHERAPY ALONE IN PATIENTS WITH FAVORABLE PROGNOSTIC INDICATORS**

| Study | No. Patients | Risk Factors* | Median F/u (Yr) | Recurrence Rate (%) |
|---|---|---|---|---|
| *No Lymphadenectomy* | | | | |
| Kucera et al.[124] | 376 | <2/3, G1 | Not stated | 0.8 |
| | | <1/3, G1–3 | Not stated | 0.8 |
| Eltabbakh et al.[125] | 303 | Stage IB, G1–2 | 8.1 | 0 |
| *Lymphadenectomy* | | | | |
| Morrow et al.[37] | 49 | <1/3, G1–3 | Not stated | 0 |
| Orr et al.[58] | 126 | Stage IB, G1–2 | 3.25 | 0 |
| | | Stage IC, G1 | | 0 |
| Mohan et al.[59] | 131 | Stage IB, G1 | 8 | 0 |

\* <2/3, middle third myometrial invasion; <1/3, inner third myometrial invasion; G, histologic grade.
From: Greven KM. Tailoring radiation to the extent of disease for uterine-confined endometrial cancer. *Semin Radiat Oncol* 2000;10:29–35.

the kidneys and small bowel. Doses of 45 Gy to 50 Gy are used to control microscopic disease.

## 5.4. Cervix

- For patients with cervical cancers that are less than or equal to FIGO stage IB1, radical hysterectomy is generally the preferred treatment. However, patients with stage IB1 tumors frequently require postoperative RT because of high-risk features. Patients receiving such treatment have more than a 90% 5-year overall survival rate.
- For patients with FIGO stage IB2 disease, surgery followed by RT is favored by some clinicians, whereas others treat with concurrent chemotherapy and RT. An ongoing trial from the GOG is randomizing patients with FIGO IB2 to either surgery followed by chemoradiation or definitive chemoradiation alone.
- Most patients with stage IIB or higher disease are treated with concurrent chemotherapy and RT.

### 5.4.1. Surgical Management

- Simple extrafascial hysterectomy is considered the standard definitive treatment for women with stage IA1 cervical cancers. This type of hysterectomy provides curative treatment for virtually all women with microscopic invasion.
- Radical hysterectomy with pelvic lymphadenectomy is considered standard treatment in the management of stage IA2, IB, and sometimes IIA cervical cancers. Radical hysterectomy involves the en bloc removal of the uterus, cervix, parametrial tissues, and upper vagina. Pelvic lymphadenectomy involves dissection of the nodal groups that primarily drain the cervix, namely the obturator and the external, internal, and common iliac nodes.

Some clinicians will also perform a para-aortic lymph node dissection.

- Type III radical hysterectomy is commonly used in patients with stage IB tumors. With type III radical hysterectomy, the lateral ligamentous uterine attachments are severed at or near the pelvic wall, the uterosacral ligaments are transected near their base, and the upper third of the vagina is removed.[79] Reported 5-year survival rates for women with stage IB1 cervical cancer treated with radical hysterectomy and pelvic lymphadenectomy are approximately 80% to 90%.[19,80,81]

### 5.4.2. Radiotherapy Alone

- Patients with stage IB1 and small IIA tumors have a similar outcome, whether they are treated with combined external beam RT and brachytherapy or radical hysterectomy and bilateral pelvic lymphadenectomy.
- The overall 5-year survival rate in patients with FIGO stage IB1 tumors is 80% to 90% with either surgery alone or RT alone (Table 21-11).
- Primary RT is effective in treating stage IB2 disease, with a 90% local control rate.[20,82,83] Eifel and colleagues reported central recurrence rates of only 1% for tumors smaller than 5 cm and 3% for exophytic tumors measuring 5 to 7.9 cm.[20]
- Even with the excellent local control rate with RT alone, several investigators have recommended initial surgery for patients with stage IB2 tumors. However, after initial surgery, most patients require postoperative RT.
- In a randomized trial comparing surgery to RT in patients with stage I disease, Landoni and colleagues reported that 84% of the patients who received initial surgery required postoperative RT and had more complications than patients who had RT alone.[80]

**TABLE 21-11. REPORTED 5-YEAR SURVIVAL RATES FOR PATIENTS WITH STAGE IB\* CARCINOMA OF THE CERVIX**

| Study | Year | Radiation Therapy | | Radical Hysterectomy | |
|---|---|---|---|---|---|
| | | No. Patients | 5-Yr Survival Rate | No. Patients | 5-Yr Survival Rate |
| Fuller et al.[109] | 1989 | | | 285 | 86% |
| Kenter et al.[126] | 1989 | | | 178 | 87% |
| Lee et al.[108] | 1989 | | | 237 | 86% |
| Alvarez et al.[127] | 1989 | | | 401 | 85% |
| Hopkins and Morley[128] | 1991 | | | 213 | 89% |
| Burghardt et al.[18] | 1992 | | | 443 | 83% |
| Coia et al.[129] | 1990 | 168 | 74% | | |
| Lowrey et al.[83] | 1992 | 130 | 81% | | |
| Perez et al.[82] | 1992 | 394 | 85% | | |
| Eifel[130] | 1994 | 1,494 | 81% | | |
| Barillot et al.[131] | 1997 | 478 | 83.5% | | |
| Landoni et al.[80] | 1997 | 167 | 74% | 170 | 74% |

\* International Federation of Gynecology and Obstetrics Staging.

- The GOG presently is conducting a trial that is randomizing patients with FIGO stage IB2 disease to either initial surgery with or without chemoradiation or definitive chemoradiation alone; it is hoped that this study will determine whether surgery is needed in patients with stage IB disease.

- Stage IIB through IVA disease is generally treated with RT alone. Five-year overall survival rates for this treatment are 62%, 62%, 50%, and 20% for stage IIB, IIIA, IIIB, and IVA cancer, respectively.

- In 1999, investigators reported five prospective trials demonstrating improved survival rates when patients with cervical cancer were treated with a combination of concurrent chemotherapy and RT.[53–55,84,85] All the chemotherapy was cisplatin based, and the patients in the trials had disease ranging from stage IB2 to IVA. Therefore, for these stages, the standard treatment now recommended is concurrent cisplatin-based chemotherapy and pelvic RT.

- The entire pelvis is usually treated with high-energy photons, using either a 4-field (anterior, posterior, right lateral, and left lateral) technique or a 2-field (anterior and posterior) technique. If using the 4-field technique, one needs to be careful not to shield potential sites of disease in the lateral field, particularly the presacral areas and the cardinal ligament.

- Brachytherapy plays a crucial role in the treatment of patients with an intact cervix. Brachytherapy allows high doses of radiation to reach the area of the tumor without exceeding normal tissue tolerance and is usually delivered via afterloading applicators, whether a low-dose rate or high-dose rate is used, that are placed in the uterine cavity and vagina. The most commonly used system is the Fletcher-Suit-Declos system. Vaginal packing is used to hold the tandem and colpostats in place and to maximize the distance between the sources and the bladder and rectum.

- The dose for external beam RT for cervical cancer ranges from 40 to 45 Gy delivered in 20 to 25 fractions. An effort should be made to deliver at least an additional 40 to 45 Gy using brachytherapy at a low-dose rate (or its equivalent at a high-dose rate) to point A in patients having bulky central disease. This can be accomplished without exceeding a dose of 75 Gy to the bladder reference point or 70 Gy to the rectal reference point, if the brachytherapy system is optimally placed.

- Patients with positive para-aortic nodes should be treated with extended-field RT. The abdominal portion of the field should be treated with either 4-field or conformal RT to reduce the dose to the small bowel and kidneys.

- An appropriate dose for microscopic disease is 45 to 50 Gy, and gross disease should be treated with higher doses such as 55 to 60 Gy, if possible.

- A study by Cunningham and colleagues reported a 48% 5-year survival rate in patients with para-aortic node involvement discovered at the time of hysterectomy who were treated with RT.[86]

- The addition of weekly cisplatin treatments may improve local control, but may also add to morbidity.

- Most late complications of RT involve the rectum, bladder, or small bowel. For patients with cervical cancer, overall estimates of the risk for major complications of RT usually range between 5% and 15%.[87–90] The risk for developing a major complication is greatest in the first 3 years. However, major complications, particularly bladder complications, have been reported as late as 30 years.

### 5.4.3. Combined Surgery and Radiotherapy

- The role of adjuvant RT still needs to be defined in cases of cervical cancer. As mentioned previously, most small tumors are treated with surgery; however, in the series conducted by Landoni and colleagues, 84% of their patients required adjuvant RT because of high-risk factors.[80]
- Most clinicians believe that patients who have more than one positive lymph node, parametrial involvement, or surgical margins positive for disease require postoperative RT. Results of a recently reported trial in which such patients were randomly assigned to receive postoperative RT alone or postoperative RT plus chemotherapy (concurrent cisplatin, with fluorouracil) showed a marked improvement in survival with chemotherapy plus RT.[54]
- In a prospective GOG trial, women whose hysterectomy specimens had various combinations of deep stromal invasion (i.e., invasion of one-third to two-thirds of the stroma), lymphovascular space invasion, or a large tumor diameter (≥5 cm) were randomly assigned to receive either postoperative RT or no further therapy.[91] The investigators reported a 44% reduction in the risk for recurrence when postoperative pelvic RT was given (19% vs 31%, $p = 0.009$). However, no difference in the overall survival rate was noted between the two arms of the study, which was attributed in part to the salvage of 8 pa-

tients in the group who underwent surgery with RT. Six percent of the patients in the RT group experienced grade 3 or 4 adverse events, compared with 2.1% in the surgery-only group. However, the 8 patients who were salvaged with RT were not included in the toxicity data.

- To eradicate microscopic residual disease, doses of 45 to 50 Gy (or 55 to 60 Gy if surgical margins are positive for disease or if extracapsular extension has occurred) may be delivered to the primary tumor bed and pelvis beginning 4 to 6 weeks after surgery.

## 5.5 Effect of Chemotherapy in the Pelvis

- In 1999 and 2000, the results of five prospective randomized trials demonstrated significant improvements in overall survival, disease-free survival, and local control rates when cisplatin-containing chemotherapy was administered concurrently with RT in patients with local-regionally advanced cervical cancer (Table 21-12).[53–55,84,85] These trials have resulted in the National Institutes of Health changing the standard treatment of locally advanced cervical cancer from RT alone to concurrent chemotherapy and RT.
- Three recent randomized trials have compared RT alone with RT plus non–cisplatin-containing regimens.[92–94]
- In one of those trials, Lorvidhaya and colleagues randomly assigned 926 patients to receive conventional RT, conventional RT followed by adjuvant chemotherapy, conventional RT plus concurrent chemotherapy, or conventional RT plus concurrent chemotherapy followed by adjuvant chemotherapy.[94] Concurrent chemotherapy consisted of intravenously administered mitomycin C

**TABLE 21-12. PROSPECTIVE RANDOMIZED TRIALS OF CONCURRENT RADIOTHERAPY AND CHEMOTHERAPY IN PATIENTS WITH LOCAL-REGIONALLY ADVANCED CERVICAL CANCER**

| Study | Stage | No. Patients | CT: Investigational | Control | Relative Risk for Death |
|---|---|---|---|---|---|
| Rose et al.[84] GOG 120 | FIGO IIB-IVA | 526 | Cisplatin 40 mg/m²/wk Cisplatin 50 mg/m² 5-FU 4 g/m²/96 HU 2 g/m² (2x/wk) | HU 3 g/m² (2x/wk) plus pelvic RT | 0.61 |
| Keys et al.[85] GOG 123 | IB2 | 369 | Cisplatin 40 mg/m²/wk | Pelvic RT | 0.54 |
| Whitney et al.[55] GOG 85 | IIB-IVA | 368 | Cisplatin 50 mg/m² 5-FU 4,000 mg/m² | HU 3 g/m² (2x/wk) plus pelvic RT | 0.72 |
| Morris et al.[53] RTOG 90-01 | IB2-IVA | 403 | Cisplatin 75 mg/m² or 5-FU 4 g/m²/96 hr for 3 cycles | Extended-field RT | 0.58 |
| Peters et al.[54] SWOG 8797/ GOG 109 | IB-IIA | 268 | Cisplatin 70 mg/m² or 5-FU 4 g/m²/ 96 hr for 2 cycles | Pelvic RT | 0.5 |

CT, chemotherapy; HU, hydroxyurea; RT, radiation treatment.

and orally administered 5-fluorouracil, and adjuvant chemotherapy consisted of only orally administered 5-fluorouracil. The investigators found that patients in either group receiving concurrent chemotherapy had a significantly better 5-year overall survival rate compared with patients who received conventional RT alone (82.7% vs 71.5%, $p = 0.001$).

- Although cisplatin-containing chemotherapy has produced some impressive responses in patients with cervical cancer, none of the randomized trials comparing RT with and without neoadjuvant chemotherapy has demonstrated improved survival rates with neoadjuvant chemotherapy.[95–97]

- More recently, investigators have tried to use neoadjuvant therapy in hopes of making patients with bulky lesions, who would otherwise be poor candidates for radical hysterectomy, better candidates for surgery.

- One of these trials randomized 205 patients with stage IB cervical cancer to receive either surgery alone or neoadjuvant chemotherapy followed by surgery.[98] All patients received postoperative RT. The authors reported that the survival rate was significantly higher in the group who received neoadjuvant chemotherapy than in the group who had surgery only (81% vs 66%, $p < 0.05$). The GOG recently completed a similar trial, but results are still pending. Ultimately, this approach may need to be compared with optimized chemoradiation to determine the most effective, least toxic treatment for these patients.

- Agents and methods that selectively enhance the effects of RT on the tumor, such as hypoxic cell sensitizers, chemical modifiers, hyperthermia, and high linear-energy-transfer RT, are under investigation.

## 6. INTENSITY-MODULATED RADIOTHERAPY IN THE FEMALE PELVIS

### 6.1. Target Volume Determination and Delineation

- In gynecologic cancers, the use of IMRT is most frequently seen in the postoperative setting to the pelvis. Multiple studies have shown that theoretically, IMRT reduces dose to the small bowel compared to standard 4-field pelvis treatment.[99–101]

- Figure 21-9 shows an example of isodose lines in a patient treated with 4-field pelvis compared to the same patient treated with IMRT, showing significant reduction in the dose to small bowel.

- The clinical target volume (CTV) of IMRT generally includes all areas of gross and potentially microscopic disease, namely the upper half of the vagina, parametrium, and regional lymph nodes.

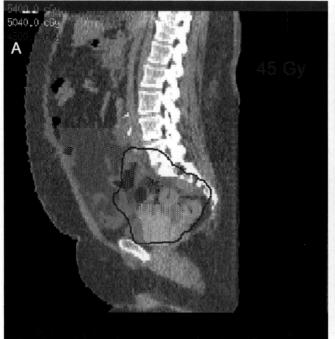
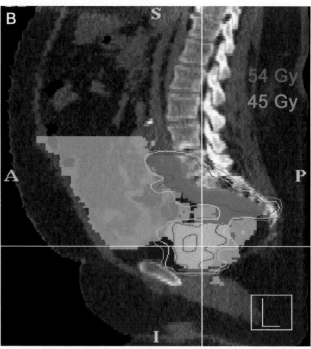

**FIGURE 21-9. A:** Typical isodose distribution of a standard 4-field pelvis used in postoperative patients. Contoured organs: bladder (*purple*), vagina and parametrial tissue (*yellow*), rectum (*green*), nodes (*orange*), small bowel (*blue*). **B:** Isodose lines in the same patient using an 8-field IMRT plan. There is a significant reduction in the dose to the small bowel using IMRT. Contoured organs: bladder (*dark blue*), vagina and parametrial tissue (*yellow*), rectum (*green*), nodes (*orange*), small bowel (*blue*).

- The upper half of the vagina is quite mobile and dependent on bladder and rectal filling (Fig. 21-10). At MDACC, RT simulation imaging is performed with a full and empty bladder, and images are fused. The upper vagina is contoured on the fused image so the CTV is actually an integrated target volume or ITV (Fig. 21-11).
- The regional lymph nodes targeted by IMRT include the common, internal, and external lymph nodes for both uterine and cervical carcinoma, as well as the sacral lymph nodes of the cervical carcinoma (Fig. 21-11).
- The presacral region, extending to level S3, is contoured in patients with cervical cancer to ensure coverage of the presacral lymph nodes and uterosacral ligament.
- The remaining lymph nodes include the normal lymphatic vessels or clips from surgery that were placed in the lymphatic beds with at least a 1-cm margin around them.
- All lymphocysts should be contoured, as well as a CTV.
- The CTV is usually enlarged by adding the 1-cm margin to create the planning target volume to account for organ motion and setup uncertainty.

## 6.2. Normal Tissue Delineation

- The normal tissues encompassed by IMRT of the pelvis include the bladder, rectum, small bowel, and (sometimes) bone marrow.
- The rectum is usually defined from the level of anus to the sigmoid flexure.

- The outermost extent of the small bowel loops within the peritoneal cavity are outlined. Individual loops of small bowel are not usually contoured separately.
- Figure 21-12 shows a typical 8-field plan used at MDACC for a patient who needed postoperative radiation therapy for endometrial carcinoma. The majority of patients are treated with 6 MV photon beams.

## 6.3. Other Uses for IMRT in Gynecologic Cancers

- IMRT may be used to provide a boost of radiation to nodes larger than 2 cm in patients with cervical cancer. At MDACC, we boost the dose of radiation to nodes with IMRT between the two bracytherapy implants in cervical cancer patients with such nodes.
- Figure 21-13 shows a patient receiving an IMRT boost to a large node in 1999; this patient still has no evidence of disease at last follow-up.
- IMRT may be used as a definitive treatment for metastatic disease to para-aortic and regional nodes and most likely delivers a reduced dose to the small bowel, kidneys, and spinal cord than is delivered by conventional RT.
- Figure 21-14 shows the plan for a patient treated with IMRT to the para-aortic region and pelvic nodes. One can treat the positive node at a slightly higher dose-per-fraction than disease with microscopic disease as occurred in this case.

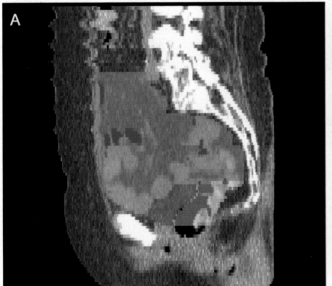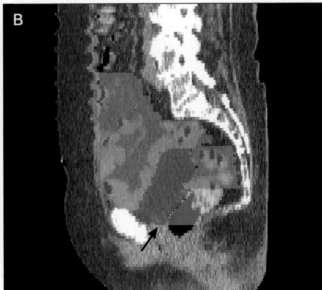

**FIGURE 21-10. A:** Sagittal view of a patient with an empty bladder with organs contoured. **B:** Sagittal view of the same patient with a full bladder shows the contour of the same patient. All three organs (vagina, small bowel, and rectum) move significantly with just bladder filling. Bladder (*purple*), vagina (*red*), rectum (*yellow*), small bowel (*green*).

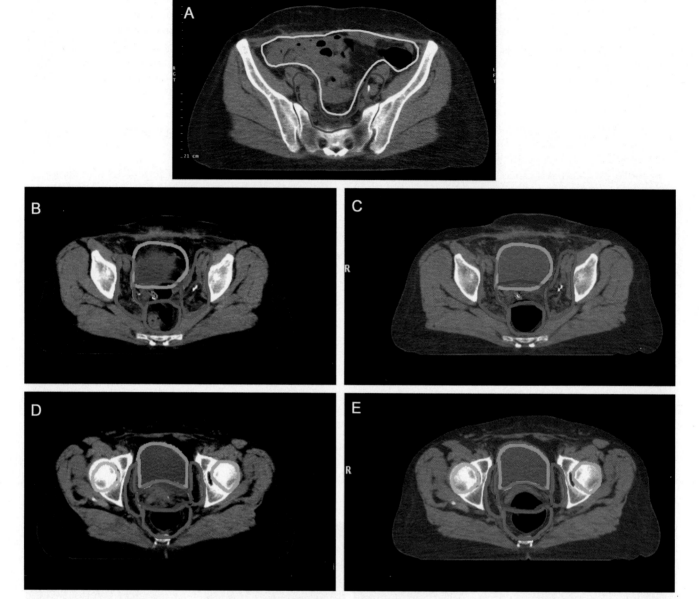

**FIGURE 21-11.** Axial views of the contours in a patient treated with postoperative IMRT. **B, D:** Contours of the vagina plus all other organs with an empty bladder. **C, E:** Contours with the bladder full. As can be seen from these images, we combine the position of the vagina with the bladder empty and full and use this as our integrated target volume (ITV) in *blue*. Axial view of the contours higher in the pelvis (**A**) is shown specifically to illustrate delineation of the nodes (outlined in *red*). Rectum (*purple*), ITV (*blue*), bladder (*green*), nodes (*red*).

- IMRT may also be useful in patients with vulvar carcinoma. At MDACC, we have treated several such patients, in whom we knew in advance that we could not boost the radiation dose to the vulva or the nodal disease using electrons, with definitive IMRT.
- As shown in Figure 21-15, we treated the gross nodal disease with a higher dose-per-fraction and a higher total dose, while the microscopic disease simultaneously received 50 Gy of radiation.

## 6.4. IMRT Results

- Using IMRT according to conventional guidelines, Roeske et al. found that the small bowel volume that received the prescribed dose was reduced by a factor of 2 compared with a traditional 4-field pelvic field approach. In addition, the volume of the rectum and bladder receiving the prescribed dose was reduced by 23%.[102]

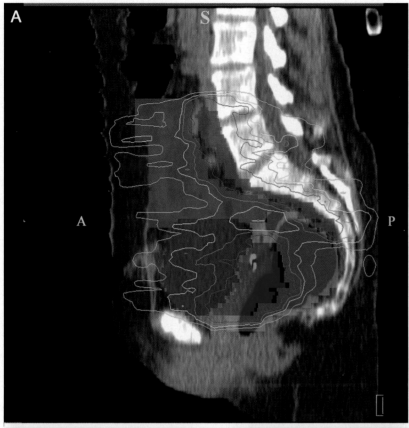

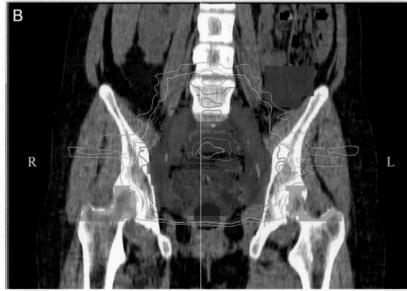

**FIGURE 21-12.** Sagittal and coronal views of a typical IMRT plan used in a patient who needed postoperative radiation therapy. Organ contours: nodal volume (*orange*), ITV (*red*) of the vagina and parametrial tissues (combination of contours from an empty and full bladder CT scan), small bowel (*blue*), rectum (*green*). Isodose lines: 50 Gy (*red*), 45 Gy (*orange*), 40 Gy (*yellow*), 30 Gy (*green*).

- After treating 40 patients with IMRT according to conventional guidelines, Mundt et al. reported a lower rate of acute grade 2 gastrointestinal toxicity in their patients compared with similar patients previously treated at their institution with conventional 4-field whole-pelvis RT. Also, the percentage of their IMRT patients requiring no or only infrequent antidiarrheal medications was 75%, compared with 34% in the patients who had received traditional four-field RT ($p = 0.001$).

- Mundt and colleagues also looked at chronic gastrointestinal toxicity in 36 patients treated with IMRT.[104] They found that IMRT caused a lower rate of chronic gastrointestinal toxicity than traditional 4-field pelvic RT had (11.1 vs 50%, $p = 0.001$). In a multivariate analysis

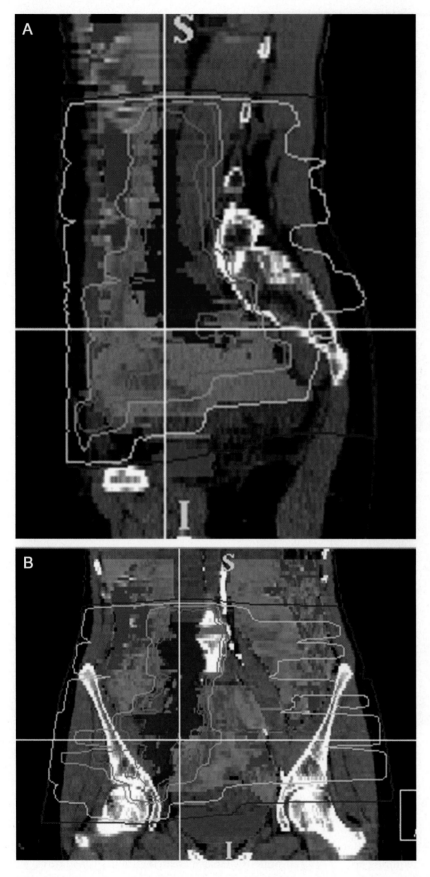

**FIGURE 21-13.** IMRT plan of a patient treated with IMRT boost to the gross nodal disease in between her two implants. This patient is still alive at last follow-up. Organ contours: small bowel (*mustard*), nodal area (*blue*), bladder (*pink*). Isodose lines: 20 Gy (*light purple*), 18 Gy (*red*), and 15 Gy (*green*).

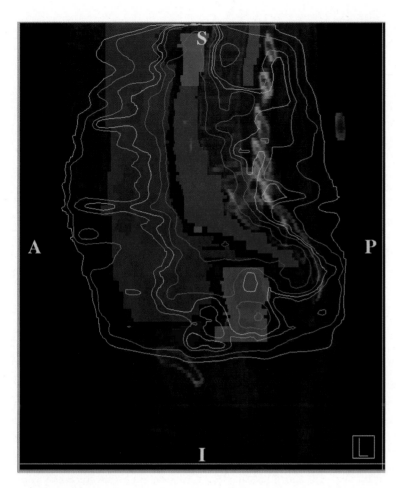

**FIGURE 21-14.** IMRT plan of a patient with grossly positive para-aortic nodes and pelvic nodes. Organ contours: small bowel (*blue*), rectum (*green*), bladder (*purple*), CTV—grossly positive nodes (*red*), microscopic positive nodes (*orange*). Isodose lines: 20 Gy (*light blue*), 30 Gy (*outer green*), 40 Gy (*inner green*), 45 Gy (*yellow*), 50 Gy (*purple*), 60 Gy (*red*). The plan was prescribed to 60 Gy at 200 cGy per fraction.

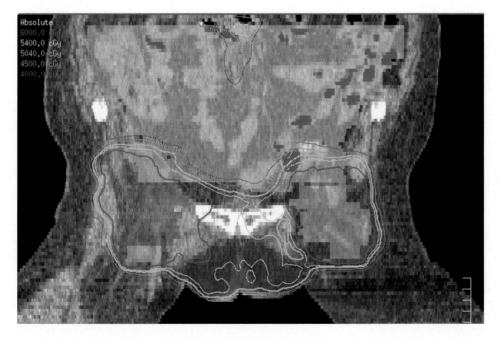

**FIGURE 21-15.** IMRT plan of a vulvar carcinoma patient with two positive inguinal nodes on the right side and three positive inguinal nodes on the left. Pelvic nodes by CT scan were negative. The patient had a history of multiple abdominal surgeries and therefore would be better treated with IMRT to spare the small bowel. Organ contours: vulva (*maroon/dark red*), small bowel (*mustard*), pelvic nodes (*yellow*), inguinal nodes (*light and dark blue*). Isodose lines: 40 Gy (*green*), 45 Gy (*orange*), 50.4 Gy (*blue*), 54 Gy (*yellow*), 60 Gy (*red*).

controlling for age and other clinical factors, IMRT retained a statistically significant effect on the incidence of chronic toxicity.[104]

- These investigators also found that IMRT can reduce the dose to the bone marrow, compared with traditional 4-field plans, which may be clinically significant in patients being treated with concurrent chemotherapy and RT.[105]
- Clinical data on the use of IMRT in other settings besides postoperatively for patients with gynecological cancers are not available. However, increasingly more studies are looking at IMRT as an adjuvant treatment for the intact cervix and vulva, as a way of providing a radiation boost to the lymph nodes, and as a primary treatment for regional lymph nodes. It is hoped that these studies will help identify areas for which IMRT is the treatment of choice.

# REFERENCES

1. Rutledge F, Smith JP, Franklin EW. Carcinoma of the vulva. *Am J Obstet Gynecol* 1970;106:1117–1130.
2. Morris JM. A formula for selective lymphadenectomy. Its application to cancer of the vulva. *Obstet Gynecol* 1977;50:152–158.
3. Al-Kurdi M, Monaghan JM. Thirty-two years experience in management of primary tumors of the vagina. *Br J Obstet Gynaecol* 1981;88:1145–1150.
4. Davis KP, Stanhope CR, Garton GR, et al. Invasive vaginal carcinoma: analysis of early-stage disease. *Gynecol Oncol* 1991;42:131–136.
5. Creasman W, Morrow C, Bundy B, et al. Surgical pathologic spread patterns of endometrial cancer. A Gynecologic Oncology Group Study. *Cancer* 1987;60:2035–2041.
6. Kim MJ, Chung JJ, Lee YH, et al. Comparison of the use of the transrectal surface coil and the pelvic phased-array coil in MR imaging for preoperative evaluation of uterine cervical carcinoma. *AJR Am J Roentgenol* 1997;168:1215–1221.
7. Yu KK, Hricak H, Subak LL, et al. Preoperative staging of cervical carcinoma: phased array coil fast spin-echo versus body coil spin-echo T2-weighted MR imaging. *AJR Am J Roentgenol* 1998;171:707–711.
8. Grigsby PW, Siegel BA, Dehdashti F. Lymph node staging by positron emission tomography in patients with carcinoma of the cervix. *J Clin Oncol* 2001;19:3745–3749.
9. Homesley HD, Bundy BN, Sedlis A, et al. Assessment of current International Federation of Gynecology and Obstetrics staging of vulvar carcinoma relative to prognostic factors for survival (a Gynecologic Oncology Group study). *Am J Obstet Gynecol* 1991;164:997–1004.
10. Sedlis A, Homesley H, Bundy BN, et al. Positive groin lymph nodes in superficial squamous cell vulvar cancer. A Gynecologic Oncology Group study. *Am J Obstet Gynecol* 1987;156:1159–1164.
11. Heaps JM, Fu YS, Montz FJ, et al. Surgical-pathologic variables predictive of local recurrence in squamous cell carcinoma of the vulva. *Gynecol Oncol* 1990;38:309–314.
12. Chyle V, Zagars GK, Wheeler JA, et al. Definitive radiotherapy for carcinoma of the vagina: outcome and prognostic factors. *Int J Radiat Oncol Biol Phys* 1996;35:891–905.
13. Perez CA, Grigsby PW, Garipagaoglu M, et al. Factors affecting long-term outcome of irradiation in carcinoma of the vagina. *Int J Radiat Oncol Biol Phys* 1999;44:37–45.
14. Eddy GL, Marks RD, Miller MC, et al. Primary invasive vaginal carcinoma. *Am J Obstet Gynecol* 1991;165:292–298.
15. Kucera H, Vavra N. Radiation management of primary carcinoma of the vagina: clinical and histopathological variables associated with survival. *Gynecol Oncol* 1991;40:12–16.
16. Urbanski K, Kojs Z, Reinfuss M, et al. Primary invasive vaginal carcinoma treated with radiotherapy: analysis of prognostic factors. *Gynecol Oncol* 1996;60:16–21.
17. Dixit S, Singhal S, Baboo HA. Squamous cell carcinoma of the vagina: a review of 70 cases. *Gynecol Oncol* 1993;48:80–87.
18. Burghardt E, Hofmann HMH, Ebner F, et al. Results of surgical treatment of 1028 cervical cancers studied with volumetry. *Cancer* 1992;70:648–655.
19. Alvarez RD, Potter ME, Soong SJ, et al. Rationale for using pathologic tumor dimensions and nodal status to subclassify surgically treated stage IB cervical cancer patients. *Gynecol Oncol* 1991;43:108–112.
20. Eifel PJ, Morris M, Wharton JT, et al. The influence of tumor size and morphology on the outcome of patients with FIGO stage IB squamous cell carcinoma of the uterine cervix. *Int J Radiat Oncol Biol Phys* 1994;29:9–16.
21. Fyles AW, Pintilie M, Kirkbride P, et al. Prognostic factors in patients with cervix cancer treated by radiation therapy: results of a multiple regression analysis. *Radiother Oncol* 1995;35:107–117.
22. Perez C, Kurman R, Stehman F, et al. Uterine cervix. In: Hoskins W, Perez C, Young R, eds. *Principles and practice of gynecologic oncology.* Philadelphia: Lippincott; 1992:591–662.
23. Dawtlaty R LO, Cross PA, et al. Prognostic factors in surgically-treated stage IB-IIB squamous cell carcinoma of the cervix with positive lymph nodes. *Int J Gynecol Cancer* 1998; 8:460–470.
24. Inoue T, Morita K. The prognostic significance of number of positive nodes in cervical carcinoma stages IB, IIA, and IIB. *Cancer* 1990;65:1923–1927.
25. Kim PY, Monk BJ, Chabra S, et al. Cervical cancer with paraaortic metastases: significance of residual paraaortic disease after surgical staging. *Gynecol Oncol* 1998;69:243–247.
26. Kamura T, Tsukamoto N, Tsuruchi N, et al. Multivariate analysis of the histopathologic prognostic factors of cervical cancer in patients undergoing radical hysterectomy. *Cancer* 1992;69:181–186.
27. Kristensen GB, Abeler VM, Risberg B, et al. Tumor size, depth of invasion, and grading of the invasive tumor front are the main prognostic factors in early squamous cell cervical carcinoma. *Gynecol Oncol* 1999;74:245–251.
28. Eifel PJ, Burke TW, Delclos L, et al. Early stage I adenocarcinoma of the uterine cervix: treatment results in patients with tumors greater, less than, or equal to 4 cm in diameter. *Gynecol Oncol* 1991;41:199–205.
29. Raju K, Kjorstad KE, Abeler V. Prognostic factors in the treatment of stage IB adenocarcinoma of the cervix. *Int J Gynaecol Obstet* 1991;1:69–74.
30. Logsdon MD, Eifel PJ. Figo IIIB squamous cell carcinoma of the cervix: an analysis of prognostic factors emphasizing the balance between external beam and intracavitary radiation therapy. *Int J Radiat Oncol Biol Phys* 1999;43:763–775.
31. Kapp DS, Fischer D, Gutierrez E, et al. Pretreatment prognostic factors in carcinoma of the uterine cervix: a multivariable analysis of the effect of age, stage, histology and blood counts on survival. *Int J Radiat Oncol Biol Phys* 1983;9:445–455.
32. Fyles A, Keane TJ, Barton M, et al. The effect of treatment duration in the local control of cervix cancer. *Radiother Oncol* 1992;25:273–279.
33. Wharton JT, Mikuta JJ, Mettlin C, et al. Risk factors and current management in carcinoma of the endometrium. *Surg Gynecol Obstet* 1986;162:515–520.

34. Greven KM, Corn BW. Endometrial cancer. *Curr Probl Cancer* 1997;21:65–127.

35. Grigsby PW, Perez CA, Kuten A, et al. Clinical stage I endometrial cancer: prognostic factors for local control and distant metastasis and implications of the new FIGO surgical staging system. *Int J Radiat Oncol Biol Phys* 1992;22:905–911.

36. Schink JC, Rademaker AW, Miller DS, et al. Tumor size in endometrial cancer. *Cancer* 1991;67:2791–2794.

37. Morrow C, Bundy B, Kurman R, et al. Relationship between surgical-pathological risk factors and outcome in clinical stage I and II carcinoma of the endometrium: a Gynecologic Oncology Group study. *Gynecol Oncol* 1991;40:55–65.

38. Milosevic MF, Dembo AJ, Thomas GM. The clinical significance of malignant peritoneal cytology in stage I endometrial carcinoma. *Int J Gynecol Cancer* 1992;2:225–235.

39. Burke TW, Levenback C, Coleman RL, et al. Surgical therapy of T1 and T2 vulvar carcinoma: further experience with radical wide excision and selective inguinal lymphadenectomy. *Gynecol Oncol* 1995;57:215–220.

40. Stehman FB, Bundy BN, Dvoretsky PM, et al. Early stage I carcinoma of the vulva treated with ipsilateral superficial inguinal lymphadenectomy and modified radical hemivulvectomy: a prospective study of the Gynecologic Oncology Group. *Obstet Gynecol* 1992;79:490–497.

41. Homesley HD, Bundy BN, Sedlis A, et al. Radiation therapy versus pelvic node resection for carcinoma of the vulva with positive groin nodes. *Obstet Gynecol* 1986;68:733–740.

42. Faul CM, Mirmow D, Huang Q, et al. Adjuvant radiation for vulvar carcinoma: improved local control. *Int J Radiat Oncol Biol Phys* 1997;38:381–389.

43. Dusenbery KE, Carlson JW, LaPorte RM, et al. Radical vulvectomy with postoperative irradiation for vulvar cancer: therapeutic implications of a central block. *Int J Radiat Oncol Biol Phys* 1994;29:989–998.

44. Hacker NF, Berek JS, Lagasse LD, et al. Individualization of treatment for stage I squamous cell vulvar carcinoma. *Obstet Gynecol* 1984;63:155–162.

45. Acosta AA, Given FT, Frazier AB, et al. Preoperative radiation therapy in the management of squamous cell carcinoma of the vulva: preliminary report. *Am J Obstet Gynecol* 1978;132:198–206.

46. Jafari K, Magalotti M. Radiation therapy in carcinoma of the vulva. *Cancer* 1981;47:686–691.

47. Moore DH, Thomas GM, Montana GS, et al. Preoperative chemoradiation for advanced vulvar cancer: a phase II study of the Gynecologic Oncology Group. *Int J Radiat Oncol Biol Phys* 1998;42:79–85.

48. Montana GS, Thomas GM, Moore DH, et al. Preoperative chemo-radiation for carcinoma of the vulva with N2/N3 nodes: a gynecologic oncology group study. *Int J Radiat Oncol Biol Phys* 2000;48:1007–1013.

49. Stock RG, Chen ASJ, Seski J. A 30-year experience in the management of primary carcinoma of the vagina: analysis of prognostic factors and treatment modalities. *Gynecol Oncol* 1995;56:45–52.

50. Kirkbride P, Fyles A, Rawlings GA, et al. Carcinoma of the vagina—experience at the Princess Margaret Hospital (1974–1989). *Gynecol Oncol* 1995;56:435–443.

51. Lee WR, Marcus RB, Sombeck MD, et al. Radiotherapy alone for carcinoma of the vagina: the importance of overall treatment time. *Int J Radiat Oncol Biol Phys* 1994;29:983–988.

52. Spiritos N, Doshi B, Kapp D, et al. Radiation therapy for primary squamous cell carcinoma of the vagina: Stanford University experience. *Gynecol Oncol* 1989;35:20–26.

53. Morris M, Eifel PJ, Lu J, et al. Pelvic radiation with concurrent chemotherapy compared with pelvic and paraaortic radiation for high-risk cervical cancer. *N Engl J Med* 1999;340:1137–1143.

54. Peters WAI, Liu PY, Barrett R, et al. Cisplatin, 5-fluorouracil plus radiation therapy are superior to radiation therapy as adjunctive therapy in high-risk, early-stage carcinoma of the cervix after radical hysterectomy and pelvic lymphadenectomy. Report of a Phase III Intergroup Study. *Gynecol Oncol* 1999;72:443.

55. Whitney CW, Sause W, Bundy BN, et al. A randomized comparison of fluorouracil plus cisplatin versus hydroxyurea as an adjunct to radiation therapy in stages IIB–IVA carcinoma of the cervix with negative para-aortic lymph nodes: a Gynecologic Oncology Group and Southwest Oncology Group study. *J Clin Oncol* 1999;17:1339–1348.

56. Slayton R, Blessing J, Beecham J, et al. Phase II trial of etoposide in the management of advanced or recurrent squamous cell carcinoma of the vulva and carcinoma of the vagina. *Cancer Treat Rep* 1987;71:869–870.

57. Thigpen T, Blessing J, Homesley HD, et al. Phase II trial of cisplatin in advanced or recurrent cancer of the vagina: a Gynecologic Oncology Group study. *Gynecol Oncol* 1986;23:101–104.

58. Orr JW, Jr., Holimon JL, Orr PF. Stage I corpus cancer: is teletherapy necessary? *Am J Obstet Gynecol* 1997;176:777–789.

59. Mohan DS, Samuels MA, Selim MA, et al. Long-term outcomes of therapeutic pelvic lymphadenectomy for stage I endometrial adenocarcinoma. *Gynecol Oncol* 1998;70:165–171.

60. Kilgore LC, Partridge EE, Alvarez RD, et al. Adenocarcinoma of the endometrium: survival comparisons of patients with and without pelvic node sampling. *Gynecol Oncol* 1995;56:29–33.

61. Carey MS, O'Connell GJ, Johanson CR, et al. Good outcome associated with a standardized treatment protocol using selective postoperative radiation in patients with clinical Stage I adenocarcinoma of the endometrium. *Gynecol Oncol* 1995;57: 138–144.

62. Chuang L, Burke TW, Tornos C, et al. Staging laparotomy for endometrial carcinoma: assessment of retroperitoneal lymph nodes. *Gynecol Oncol* 1995;58:189–193.

63. Piver MS, Hempling RE. A prospective trial of postoperative vaginal radium/cesium for grade 1–2 less than 50% myometrial invasion and pelvic radiation therapy for grade 3 or deep myometrial invasion in surgical stage I endometrial adenocarcinoma. *Cancer* 1990;66:1133–1138.

64. Kucera H, Vavra N, Weghaupt K. Benefit of external irradiation in pathologic stage I endometrial carcinoma: a prospective clinical trial of 605 patients who received postoperative vaginal irradiation and additional pelvic irradiation in the presence of unfavorable prognostic factors. *Gynecol Oncol* 1990;38:99–104.

65. Grigsby P, Kuske R, Perez C, et al. Medically inoperable stage I adenocarcinoma of the endometrium treated with radiotherapy alone. *Int J Radiat Oncol Biol Phys* 1987;13:483–488.

66. Jones D, Stout R. Results of intracavitary radium treatment for adenocarcinoma of the body of the uterus. *Clin Radiol* 1986;37:169–171.

67. Kupelian PA, Eifel PJ, Tornos C, et al. Treatment of endometrial carcinoma with radiation therapy alone. *Int J Radiat Oncol Biol Phys* 1993;27:817–824.

68. Landgren R, Fletcher G, Delclos L, et al. Irradiation of endometrial cancer in patients with medical contraindication to surgery or with unresectable lesions. *Am J Roentgenol Radium Ther Nucl Med* 1976;126:148–154.

69. Lehoczky O, Bosze P, Ungar L, et al. Stage I endometrial carcinoma: treatment of nonoperable patients with intracavitary radiation therapy alone. *Gynecol Oncol* 1991;43:211–216.

70. Rose PG, Baker S, Kern M, et al. Primary radiation therapy for endometrial carcinoma: a case controlled study. *Int J Radiat Oncol Biol Phys* 1993;27:585–590.

71. Rouanet P, Dubois JB, Gely S, et al. Exclusive radiation therapy in endometrial carcinoma. *Int J Radiat Oncol Biol Phys* 1993;26:223–228.

72. Kucera H, Knocke TH, Kucera E, et al. Treatment of endometrial carcinoma with high-dose-rate brachytherapy alone in medically inoperable stage I patients. *Acta Obstet Gynecol Scand* 1998;77:1008–1012.

73. Greven K, Olds W. Isolated vaginal recurrences of endometrial adenocarcinoma and their management. *Cancer* 1987;60:419–421.

74. Wylie J, Irwin C, Pintilie M, et al. Results of radical radiotherapy for recurrent endometrial cancer. *Gynecol Oncol* 2000;77:66–72.

75. Creutzberg CL, van Putten WL, Koper PC, et al. Surgery and postoperative radiotherapy versus surgery alone for patients with stage-1 endometrial carcinoma: multicentre randomised trial. PORTEC Study Group. *Lancet* 2000;355:1404–1411.

76. Roberts JA, Brunetto VI, Keys HM, et al. A phase III randomized study of surgery vs surgery plus adjunctive radiation therapy in intermediate-risk endometrial adenocarcinoma (GOG No. 99) (abstract). *Gynecol Oncol* 1998;68:135.

77. Corn B, Lanciano R, Greven K, et al. Endometrial cancer with para-aortic adenopathy: patterns of failure and opportunities for cure. *Int J Radiat Oncol Biol Phys* 1992;24:223–227.

78. Onda T, Yoshikawa H, Mizutani K, et al. Treatment of node-positive endometrial cancer with complete node dissection, chemotherapy and radiation therapy. *Br J Cancer* 1997;75:1836–1841.

79. Piver MS, Rutledge F, Smith JP. Five classes of extended hysterectomy for women with cervical cancer. *Obstet Gynecol* 1974;44:265–272.

80. Landoni F, Maneo A, Colombo A, et al. Randomised study of radical surgery versus radiotherapy for stage Ib–IIa cervical cancer. *Lancet* 1997;350:535–540.

81. Delgado G, Bundy B, Zaino R, et al. Prospective surgical-pathological study of disease-free interval in patients with stage IB squamous cell carcinoma of the cervix: a Gynecologic Oncology Group study. *Gynecol Oncol* 1990;38:352–357.

82. Perez CA, Grigsby PW, Nene SM, et al. Effect of tumor size on the prognosis of carcinoma of the uterine cervix treated with irradiation alone. *Cancer* 1992;69:2796–2806.

83. Lowrey GC, Mendenhall WM, Million RR. Stage IB or IIA-B carcinoma of the intact uterine cervix treated with irradiation: a multivariate analysis. *Int J Radiat Oncol Biol Phys* 1992;24:205–210.

84. Rose PG, Bundy BN, Watkins J, et al. Concurrent cisplatin-based chemotherapy and radiotherapy for locally advanced cervical cancer. *N Engl J Med* 1999;340:1144–1153.

85. Keys HM, Bundy BN, Stehman FB, et al. Cisplatin, radiation, and adjuvant hysterectomy for bulky stage IB cervical carcinoma. *N Engl J Med* 1999;340:1154–1161.

86. Cunningham MJ, Dunton CJ, Corn B, et al. Extended-field radiation therapy in early-stage cervical carcinoma: survival and complications. *Gynecol Oncol* 1991;43:51–54.

87. Eifel PJ, Levenback C, Wharton JT, et al. Time course and incidence of late complications in patients treated with radiation therapy for FIGO stage IB carcinoma of the uterine cervix. *Int J Radiat Oncol Biol Phys* 1995;32:1289–1300.

88. Lanciano RM, Won M, Hanks GE. A reappraisal of the International Federation of Gynecology and Obstetrics staging system for cervical cancer. *Cancer* 1992;69:482–487.

89. Montana GS, Fowler WC. Carcinoma of the cervix: analysis of bladder and rectal radiation dose and complications. *Int J Radiat Oncol Biol Phys* 1989;16:95–100.

90. Perez CA, Camel HM, Kuske RR, et al. Radiation therapy alone in the treatment of carcinoma of the uterine cervix: a 20-year experience. *Gynecol Oncol* 1986;23:127–140.

91. Rotman MZ, Sedlis A, Bundy B, et al. Postoperative irradiation of women with stage IB-IIA cervical cancers with poor prognostic features: a gynecologic oncology group study. [abstract]. *Int J Radiat Oncol Biol Phys* 2003;57:S189.

92. Thomas G, Dembo A, Ackerman I, et al. A randomized trial of standard versus partially hyperfractionated radiation with or without concurrent 5-fluorouracil in locally advanced cervical cancer. *Gynecol Oncol* 1998;69:137–145.

93. Wong LC, Ngan HY, Cheung AN, et al. Chemoradiation and adjuvant chemotherapy in cervical cancer. *J Clin Oncol* 1999;17:2055–2060.

94. Lorvidhaya V, Chitapanarux I, Sangruchi S, et al. Concurrent mitomycin C, 5-fluorouracil, and radiotherapy in the treatment of locally advanced carcinoma of the cervix: a randomized trial. *Int J Radiat Oncol Biol Phys* 2003;55:1226–1232.

95. Souhami L, Gil R, Allan S, et al. A randomized trial of chemotherapy followed by pelvic radiation therapy in Stage IIIB carcinoma of the cervix. *Int J Radiat Oncol Biol Phys* 1991;9:970–997.

96. Tattersall MHN, Larvidhaya V, Vootiprux V, et al. Randomized trial of epirubicin and cisplatin chemotherapy followed by pelvic radiation in locally advanced cervical cancer. *Am J Clin Oncol* 1995;13:444–451.

97. Leborgne F, Leborgne JH, Doldán R, et al. Induction chemotherapy and radiotherapy of advanced cancer of the cervix: a pilot study and phase III randomized trial. *Int J Radiat Oncol Biol Phys* 1997;37:343–350.

98. Sardi JE, Giaroli A, Sananes C, et al. Long-term follow-up of the first randomized trial using neoadjuvant chemotherapy in stage Ib squamous carcinoma of the cervix: the final results. *Gynecol Oncol* 1997;67:61–69.

99. Ahamad A, D'Souza W, Salehpour M, et al. Intensity modulated radiation therapy (IMRT) for post-hysterectomy pelvic radiation: selection of patients and planning target volume (PTV). *Int J Radiat Oncol Biol Phys* 2002;54(Suppl 1):42.

100. Mundt AJ, Roeske JC, Lujan AE, et al. Initial clinical experience with intensity-modulated whole-pelvis radiation therapy in women with gynecologic malignancies. *Gynecol Oncol* 2001;82:456–463.

101. Kavanagh BD, Schefter TE, Wu Q, et al. Clinical application of intensity-modulated radiotherapy for locally advanced cervical cancer. *Semin Radiat Oncol* 2002;12:260–271.

102. Roeske JC, Lujan A, Rotmensch J, et al. Intensity-modulated whole pelvic radiation therapy in patients with gynecologic malignancies. *Int J Radiat Oncol Biol Phys* 2000;48:1613–1621.

103. Mundt AJ, Lujan AE, Rotmensch J, et al. Intensity-modulated whole pelvic radiotherapy in women with gynecologic malignancies. *Int J Radiat Oncol Biol Phys* 2002;52:1330–1337.

104. Mundt AJ, Mell LK, Roeske JC. Preliminary analysis of chronic gastrointestinal toxicity in gynecology patients treated with intensity-modulated whole pelvic radiation therapy. *Int J Radiat Oncol Biol Phys* 2003;56:1354–1360.

105. Lujan AE, Mundt AJ, Yamada SD, et al. Intensity-modulated radiotherapy as a means of reducing dose to bone marrow in gynecologic patients receiving whole pelvic radiotherapy. *Int J Radiat Oncol Biol Phys* 2003;57:516–521.

106. Girardi F, Haas J. The importance of the histologic processing of pelvic lymph nodes in the treatment of cervical cancer. *Int J Gynecol Cancer* 1993;3:12–17.

107. Averette HE, Nguyen HN, Donato DM, et al. Radical hysterectomy for invasive cervical cancer. A 25-year prospective experience with the Miami technique. *Cancer* 1993;71:1422–1437.

108. Lee Y-N, Wang KL, Lin M-H, et al. Radical hysterectomy with pelvic lymph node dissection for treatment of cervical cancer: a clinical review of 954 cases. *Gynecol Oncol* 1989;32:135–142.

109. Fuller AF, Elliott N, Kosloff C, et al. Determinants of increased risk for recurrence in patients undergoing radical hysterectomy

for stage IB and IIA carcinoma of the cervix. *Gynecol Oncol* 1989;33:34–39.

110. Barber H. Cervical cancer: pelvic and para-aortic lymph node sampling and its consequences. *Baillieres Clin Obstet Gynaecol* 1988;2:769–777.

111. Creasman WT, Soper JT, Clarke-Pearson D. Radical hysterectomy as therapy for early carcinoma of the cervix. *Am J Obstet Gynecol* 1986;155:964–969.

112. Sudarsanam A, Charyulu K, Belinson J, et al. Influence of exploratory celiotomy on the management of carcinoma of the cervix. A preliminary report. *Cancer* 1978;41:1049–1053.

113. Stehman FB, Bundy BN, Disaia PJ, et al. Carcinoma of the cervix treated with radiation therapy. I. A multivariate analysis of prognostic variables in the Gynecologic Oncology Group. *Cancer* 1991;67:2776–2785.

114. LaPolla JP, Schlaerth JB, Gaddis O, et al. The influence of surgical staging on the evaluation and treatment of patients with cervical carcinoma. *Gynecol Oncol* 1986;24:194–206.

115. Berman ML, Keys H, Creasman W, et al. Survival and patterns of recurrence in cervical cancer metastatic to periaortic lymph nodes (a Gynecologic Oncology Group study). *Gynecol Oncol* 1984;19:8–16.

116. Ballon SC, Berman ML, Lagasse LD, et al. Survival after extraperitoneal pelvic and paraaortic lymphadenectomy and radiation therapy in cervical carcinoma. *Obstet Gynecol* 1981;57:90–95.

117. Lagasse LD, Creasman WT, Singleton HM, et al. Results and complications of operative staging in cervical cancer: experiences of the Gynecologic Oncology Group. *Gynecol Oncol* 1980;9:90–98.

118. Nelson AJ, Fletcher GH, Wharton JT. Indications for adjunctive conservative extrafascial hysterectomy in selected cases of carcinoma of the uterine cervix. *Am J Roentgenol* 1975;123:91–99.

119. Thomas G, Dembo A, DePetrillo A, et al. Concurrent radiation and chemotherapy in vulvar carcinoma. *Gynecol Oncol* 1989;34:263–267.

120. Berek JS, Heaps JM, Fu YS, et al. Concurrent cisplatin and 5-fluorouracil chemotherapy and radiation therapy for advanced-stage squamous carcinoma of the vulva. *Gynecol Oncol* 1991;42:197–201.

121. Russell AH, Mesic JB, Scudder SA, et al. Synchronous radiation and cytotoxic chemotherapy for locally advanced or recurrent squamous cancer of the vulva. *Gynecol Oncol* 1992;47:14–20.

122. Koh WJ, Wallace HJ, Greer BE, et al. Combined radiotherapy and chemotherapy in the management of local-regionally advanced vulvar cancer. *Int J Radiat Oncol Biol Phys* 1993;26:809–816.

123. Cunningham MJ, Goyer RP, Gibbons SK, et al. Primary radiation, cisplatin, and 5-fluorouracil for advanced squamous carcinoma of the vulva. *Gynecol Oncol* 1997;66:258–261.

124. Kucera P, Berman M, Treadwell P, et al. Whole-abdominal radiotherapy for patients with minimal residual epithelial ovarian cancer. *Gynecol Oncol* 1990;36:338–342.

125. Eltabbakh GH, Piver MS, Hempling RE, et al. Excellent long-term survival and absence of vaginal recurrences in 332 patients with low-risk stage I endometrial adenocarcinoma treated with hysterectomy and vaginal brachytherapy without formal staging lymph node sampling: report of a prospective trial. *Int J Radiat Oncol Biol Phys* 1997;38:373–380.

126. Kenter GG, Ansink AC, Heintz APM, et al. Carcinoma of the uterine cervix stage I and IIA: results of surgical treatment: complications, recurrence, and survival. *Eur J Surg Oncol* 1989;15:55–60.

127. Alvarez RD, Soong SJ, Kinney WK, et al. Identification of prognostic factors and risk groups in patients found to have nodal metastasis at the time of radical hysterectomy for early-stage squamous carcinoma of the cervix. *Gynecol Oncol* 1989;35:130–135.

128. Hopkins MP, Morley GW. Squamous cell cancer of the cervix: prognostic factors related to survival. *Int J Gynecol Cancer* 1991;1:173–177.

129. Coia L, Won M, Lanciano R, et al. The Patterns of Care Outcome Study for cancer of the uterine cervix. Results of the second national practice survey. *Cancer* 1990;66:2451–2456.

130. Eifel PJ. Problems with the clinical staging of carcinoma of the cervix. *Semin Radiat Oncol* 1994;4:1–8.

131. Barillot I, Horiot JC, Pigneux J, et al. Carcinoma of the intact uterine cervix treated with radiotherapy alone: A French cooperative study: update and multivariate analysis of prognostic factors. *Int J Radiat Oncol Biol Phys* 1997;38:969–978.

# SUBJECT INDEX

Page numbers followed by findicate figures; page numbers followed by tindicate tables.

superior mediastinal lymph
nodes/highest mediastinal
lymph nodes, 266
tracheobronchial lymph nodes, 266
upper lobar lymph nodes, 267
three dimensional-conformal radiation
therapy/intensity modulated
radiation therapy, 266–273
tracheobronchial lymph nodes, 274
Lymph nodes
axillary, breast cancer and, 238
esophageal cancer and, 289, 289*t*
head and neck cancer, magnetic resonance
imaging, computed
tomography, positron emission
tomography, compared, 65*t*
iliac, bipedal lag, delineating target
volumes with, 306*t*
inguinal, bipedal lag, delineating target
volumes with, 306*t*
location, relative to adjacent anatomic
structures, 306*t*
nasopharynx carcinoma, prognostic
factors, 143
of neck, 38–43
normal anatomy, 38–41, 40*f*–43*f*
pathology, 41–43, 43*f*
paranasal sinus carcinomas and, 126*t*
thyroid carcinoma and, 211–214, 214*f*

**M**
Magnetic resonance imaging, 30–32
anatomic delineation
cervix, 57–58
uterus, 57–58
of brain, 30–46
of cervix
protocol, 56–57
techniques, 56–57
sagittal T1-weighted images, 57
sagittal T2-weighted fast spin echo,
57, 57*f*
computed tomography compared
brain, 32–33, 33*f*
head and neck, 32–33, 33*f*
positron emission tomography
head and neck cancer, lymph node
metastasis, 65*t*
head and neck cancer recurrence, 66*t*
cross-sectional imaging, basics of, 30–34
head and neck imaging, 31–32, 33*f*
interpretation, fundamentals of, 33*f*,
33–34, 34*f*
neck cancers, 30–46
prostate, 47–52, 51*f*–56*f*
treatment planning, 56
registration with bony landmarks,
prostate, 52–56
registration with fiducial markers,
prostate, 56
skull base, 30–46
uterus
techniques/protocol, 56–57
axial T1-weighted images, 57

axial T2-weighted fast spin echo, 57,
57*f*
sagittal T1-weighted images, 57
sagittal T2-weighted fast spin echo,
57, 57*f*
for treatment planning, 59*f*, 59–60, 60*f*
Magnetic resonance spectroscopy imaging
of cervix, 59
of uterus, 59
Mammary chain, internal, breast cancer and,
238–240, 240*f. See also* Breast
cancer
Margins, delineation of, 22, 23*f*
Mastectomy. *See also* breast cancer
radiation in conjunction with, 244*t*
recurrence rates, 244*t*
Maxilla, alveolar ridge, anatomy, 154
Maxillary sinus tumors
clinical target volume determination
guidelines, 130*t*
management, 129
Mediastinal lymph nodes, in lung cancer,
274
computed tomography compared,
metastasis, positron emission
tomography, 64*t*
highest mediastinal lymph nodes, target
volume determination, 266
Mediastinum, lymph node involvement,
according to tumor location,
265*t*
Medical necessity of intensity-modulated
radiation therapy, 3
Medulloblastoma
Chang and Harisiadis (Langston
modification) classification, 91*t*
posterior fossa, skull, 87–88, 88*f*, 92–93
staging, 89
Meningioma
intracranial, Simpson's classification,
extent of resection, 90*t*
posterior fossa, skull, 85, 86*f*, 91
staging, 89
Mesothelioma, 275–285
18FDG-PET, 276
acute toxic effects of IMRT post-EPP, 284*t*
anatomy, 275
chemotherapy, 277–278
chest x-ray, 275
classification, 276*t*
computed tomography of chest, 275
conformal radiotherapy (after extrapleural
pneumonectomy), 278
diagnosis/staging, 275–276, 276*t*
physical examination, 275
signs/symptoms, 275
imaging, 275–276
intensity-modulated radiation therapy,
278–284
anterior-medial pleural reflection, 279
medial extent of crus of diaphragm,
279–281
normal tissue delineation, 281, 282*f*
normal tissue doses, 281–282, 282*t*
results of therapy, 284, 284*t*

target doses, 281–282, 282*t*
target volume
determination/delineation
(after extrapleural
pneumonectomy), 278–281,
279*f*, 280*f*, 281*f*
variable inferior extent of diaphragm,
279
verification process, 282–284, 283*f*,
284*f*
invasive staging, 276
laparoscopy, 276
mediastinoscopy, 276
magnetic resonance imaging, 276
management, 277–278
organs at risk, target doses, dose-volume
constraints of, 282*t*
palliation, 278
prognostic factors, 276–277
histology, 276
performance status, 276
treatment related factors, 277
prophylaxis, 278
radiation therapy, 278
surgery, 277, 277*t*
extrapleural pneumonectomy (EPP),
277
potential problems, 277
Meta-analysis data, cross-tabulation of site,
T stage, treatment modality,
128*t*
Metastatic carcinoma in neck node with
unknown primary, 232–237
diagnosis/staging, 232–233, 233*t*
imaging, 232
intensity-modulated radiation therapy,
234–236
normal tissue delineation, 234
normal tissue doses, 234
results, 234
target doses, 234
target volume delineation, 234, 235*f*,
236*f*
target volume determination, 234, 234*t*
management, 233–234
chemotherapy, 234
irradiation alone, 233
radiotherapy to ipsilateral neck, 233,
233*t*
surgery, with irradiation, 233
surgical, 233
Middle thoracic esophagus, 286
Mouth floor carcinoma
anatomy, 154
imaging, 155–156
management, 161–162, 162*t*
treatment results, 162*t*
Multimodality image fusion, defined, 5
Multiple simultaneous treatments, 3

**N**
Nasal cavity carcinoma, 123–135
actuarial locoregional control, survival
rates according to treatment
modality, 129*t*